Routledge Handbook of Philosophy and Nursing

Philosophy offers a means of unpacking and grappling with important questions and issues relevant to nursing practice, research, scholarship, and education. By engaging in these discussions, this *Handbook* provides a gateway to new understandings of nursing.

The *Handbook*, which is split loosely into seven sections, begins with a foundational chapter exploring philosophy's relationship to and with nursing and nursing theory. Subsequent sections thereafter examine a wide range of philosophic issues relevant to nursing knowledge and activity.

- Philosophy and nursing, philosophy and science, nursing theory.
- Nursing's ethical dimension is described.
- Philosophic questions concerning patient care are investigated.
- Socio-contextual and political concerns relevant to nursing are unpacked.
- Contributors tackle difficult questions confronting nursing.
- Difficulties around speech, courage, and race/otherness are discussed.
- Philosophic questions pertaining to scholarship, research, and technology are addressed.

International in scope, this volume provides a vital reference for all those interested in thinking about nursing, whether students, practitioners, researchers, or educators.

Martin Lipscomb is a Senior Lecturer at the University of Worcester's Three Counties School of Nursing and Midwifery (UK).

Routledge Handbook of Philosophy and Nursing

Edited by Martin Lipscomb

Routledge
Taylor & Francis Group

LONDON AND NEW YORK

Designed cover image: © Getty Images

First published 2024
by Routledge
4 Park Square, Milton Park, Abingdon, Oxon OX14 4RN

and by Routledge
605 Third Avenue, New York, NY 10158

Routledge is an imprint of the Taylor & Francis Group, an informa business

British Library Cataloguing-in-Publication Data
A catalogue record for this book is available from the British Library

Library of Congress Cataloging-in-Publication Data
Names: Lipscomb, Martin, editor.
Title: Routledge handbook of philosophy and nursing /
edited by Martin Lipscomb.
Description: Abingdon, Oxon; New York, NY: Routedge, 2024. |
Includes bibliographical references and index.
Identifiers: LCCN 2023010186 | ISBN 9781032114606 (hardback) |
ISBN 9781032547671 (paperback) | ISBN 9781003427407 (ebook)
Subjects: LCSH: Nursing—Philosophy. | Nursing ethics. | Nurse and patient.
Classification: LCC RT84.5 .R658 2024 | DDC 610.7301—dc23/eng/20230601
LC record available at https://lccn.loc.gov/2023010186

ISBN: 978-1-032-11460-6 (hbk)
ISBN: 978-1-032-54767-1 (pbk)
ISBN: 978-1-003-42740-7 (ebk)

DOI: 10.4324/9781003427407

Typeset in Sabon
by codeMantra

Contents

Contributors

Ghadah Abdullah Nurse Consultant and Director of Nursing, King Abdulaziz University Hospital, Jeddah (Saudi Arabia). Ghadah Abdullas' work is accessible via https://www.researchgate.net/profile/Ghadah-Abdullah

Hisham M Alfayyadh Assistant Professor, Translation Studies, King Saud University (Saudi Arabia). Hisham M Alfayyadh's work is accessible via https://www.researchgate.net/profile/Hisham-Alfayyadh

Peter Allmark Retired nurse, nurse teacher, and active part time researcher at the School of Nursing and Midwifery, University of Sheffield (UK). Peter Allmark's work is accessible via https://philpeople.org/profiles/peter-allmark

Mutlaq B Almutairi Senior Nurse Instructor, Quality Improvement and Nursing Education, King Fahad Medical City, Riyadh (Saudi Arabia). Mutlaq B Almutairi's work is accessible via https://www.linkedin.com/in/mutlaq-almutairi-717ab512b/

Fatma S Alsolamy Assistant Professor, Islamic Sciences and Literature, Jeddah University (Saudi Arabia). Fatma S Alsolamy's work is accessible via https://www.uj.edu.sa/DRS-0017048.aspx

Abdulaziz M Alsufyani Regional Director, Comprehensive Rehabilitation Center, Nursing and Infection Control Department, Ministry of Social Affairs (Saudi Arabia). Abdulaziz M Alsufyani's work is accessible via https://www.researchgate.net/profile/Abdualziz-Alsufyani

Mattia Andreoletti Postdoctoral Researcher at the Department of Health Sciences and Technology, ETH Zurich (Switzerland). Mattia Andreoletti's work is accessible via https://scholar.google.it/citations?user=Njvn2RwAAAAJ&hl=it

Miriam Bender Associate Professor at the Sue & Bill Gross School of Nursing at University of California Irvine (USA) and Founding Director of the school's Center for Nursing Philosophy. Miriam Bender's work is accessible via https://www.faculty.uci.edu/profile.cfm?faculty_id=6106

Patricia Benner Professor Emeritus at the University of California, San Francisco, School of Nursing (USA). Professor Benner's work is accessible via https://sociology.ucsf.edu/emeriti

Robyn Bluhm Professor in the Department of Philosophy and Lyman Briggs College at Michigan State University (USA). Professor Bluhm's work is accessible via https://philpeople.org/profiles/robyn-bluhm

Mustafa M Bodrick Consultant Advisor, Organizational Development and Excellence, Saudi Commission for Health Specialties, Adjunct Professor Nursing, MAHSA University (Malaysia), King Saud University, (Saudi Arabia), and Johns Hopkins University (USA). Professor Bodrick's work is accessible via https://www.linkedin.com/in/professor-mustafa-m-e-bodrick-74267148/

Annette J Browne Professor and Distinguished University Scholar at the University of British Columbia School of Nursing (Canada). Professor Browne's work is accessible via https://nursing.ubc.ca/our-people/annette-browne

Lawrence Burns Lecturer in the History of Medicine at King's University College at Western University (Canada). Lawrence Burns' work is accessible via https://www.researchgate.net/profile/Lawrence-Burns

Mary K Canales Professor at the University of Wisconsin-Eau Claire (USA). Professor Canale's work is accessible via https://www.researchgate.net/profile/Mary-Canales

Havi Carel Professor of Philosophy in the Department of Philosophy at the University of Bristol (UK). Professor Carel's work is accessible via https://www.bristol.ac.uk/people/person/Havi-Carel-8cf2a5a5-9182-419b-b1dc-a60fe075db51/

Franco A Carnevale Professor at the Ingram School of Nursing, McGill University, Montreal (Canada). Professor Carnevale's work is accessible via https://www.mcgill.ca/nursing/about/faculty/faculty-directory/franco-carnevale

Christine Ceci Associate Professor in the Faculty of Nursing at the University of Alberta (Canada) and a founder of the Care Practices Research Network. Christine Ceci's work is accessible via https://apps.ualberta.ca/directory/person/ceci and carepractices.org

Vico Chung Lim Chiang Former Associate Professor of Nursing, The Hong Kong Polytechnic University (Hong Kong SAR, China). Vico Chung Lim Chiang's work is accessible via https://orcid.org/0000-0002-6973-7241

Daniele Chiffi Assistant Professor of Philosophy, Politecnico di Milano (Italy). Daniele Chiffi's work is accessible via https://sites.google.com/site/chiffidaniele

M Murat Civaner Professor at Bursa Uludag University School of Medical School (Turkey). Professor Civaner's work is accessible via http://deontoloji.uludag.edu.tr/kadro/civaner/civaner_eng.htm

Chloe Crosschild PhD candidate the University of British Columbia School of Nursing (Canada), and Assistant Professor, Nursing Program, University of Lethbridge (Canada). Chloe Crossland's work is accessible via https://www.ulethbridge.ca/healthsciences/profile/chloe-crosschild

Jessica Dillard-Wright Assistant Professor in Elaine Marieb College of Nursing at University of Massachusetts Amherst (USA). Jessica Dillard-Wright's work is accessible via https://www.compostcollaborative.online/

Denise J Drevdahl Professor in the School of Nursing and Healthcare Leadership at the University of Washington Tacoma (USA). Professor Drevdahl's work is accessible via https://directory.tacoma.uw.edu/employee/drevdahl

Jacqueline Fawcett Professor, Department of Nursing, Robert and Donna Manning College of Nursing and Health Sciences, University of Massachusetts Boston and Professor Emerita, School of Nursing, University of Pennsylvania, Philadelphia, PA (USA). Professor Fawcett's work is accessible via https://www.umb.edu/academics/cnhs/faculty_staff/faculty/jacqueline_fawcett

Dawn Freshwater Vice-Chancellor of the University of Auckland (New Zealand). Adjunct clinical Professor in Mental Health at University of Western Australia, and the University of Leeds. Professor Dawn Freshwater's work is accessible via https://research-repository.uwa.edu.au/en/persons/dawn-freshwater/publications/

Thomas Foth RN and Associate Professor at the School of Nursing, Faculty of Health Sciences at University of Ottawa (Canada). Thomas Foth's work is accessible via https://www.uottawa.ca/faculty-health-sciences/nursing/our-professors/thomas-foth

Marsha D Fowler Adjunct Professor at Trinity Western University, British Columbia (Canada). Marsha D Fowler's work is accessible via https://www.twu.ca/profile/marsha-fowler

Freda DeKeyser Ganz Professor and Dean of the Faculty of Life and Health Sciences, Jerusalem College of Technology (Israel). Professor Ganz's work is accessible via https://www.jct.ac.il/facultyresearch/2017-2021/101/

Pamela J Grace Associate Professor Emerita, Boston College, Massachusetts (USA). Pamela J Grace's work is accessible via https://www.bc.edu/bc-web/offices/office-of-university-communications/for-the-media/boston-college-faculty-experts/pamela-grace.html

Sigríður Halldórsdóttir Professor at Faculty of Graduate Studies in Health Sciences, School of Heath, Business and Natural Sciences, University of Akureyri (Háskólinn á Akureyri) (Iceland). Professor Halldórsdóttir's work is accessible via https://www.unak.is/english/moya/ugla/staff/sigridur-halldorsdottir

Ingrid Hanssen Professor Emeritus at Lovisenberg Deaconal University College, Oslo (Norway). Professor Hanssen's work is accessible via https://ldh.box.com/s/58atqboi5 34ewoksrjw8fkf0qt1b45mc

Ken Hok Man Ho Assistant Professor of the Nethersole School of Nursing at The Chinese University (Hong Kong SAR, China). Ken Hok Man Ho's work is accessible via https://orcid.org/0000-0003-4934-2450

Michael Igoumenidis Assistant Professor at the Department of Nursing, School of Health Rehabilitation Sciences, University of Patras (Greece). Michael Igoumenidis' work is accessible via https://nurs.upatras.gr/index.php/en/anthropin-2/academi/67-faculty/academic/169-michael-igoumenidis.html

Favorite Iradukunda Assistant Professor in Elaine Marieb College of Nursing at University of Massachusetts Amherst (USA). Favorite Iradukunda's work is accessible via www.iradukunda.com

Debra Jackson Professor of Nursing at the Susan Wakil School of Nursing, University of Sydney (Australia). Professor Jackson is also editor-in-chief of the *Journal of Advanced Nursing*. Her work is accessible via https://www.sydney.edu.au/medicine-health/about/our-people/academic-staff/debra-jackson.html

Harkeert Judge PhD candidate in the Faculty of Nursing at the University of Alberta (Canada). Harkeert Judge's work is accessible via carepractices.org

Marit Kirkevold Professor and Head of Institute at Oslo Metropolitan University (Norway). Professor Kirkevold's work is accessible via https://www.oslomet.no/en/about/employee/maritkir/

Martin Lipscomb Senior Lecturer at the University of Worcester's Three Counties School of Nursing and Midwifery (UK). Martin Lipscomb's work is accessible via https://eprints.worc.ac.uk/view/author/Lipscomb=3AMartin=3A=3A.html

Graham McCaffrey Associate Professor in the Faculty of Nursing at the University of Calgary (Canada). Graham McCaffrey's work is accessible via https://nursing.ucalgary.ca/contacts/graham-mccaffrey

Martin McNamara Professor and Programme Director at University College Dublin (Ireland). Professor McNamara's work is accessible via https://people.ucd.ie/martin.mcnamara/publications

Maurice Nagington Lecturer and Researcher at the University of Manchester (UK). Maurice Nagington's work is accessible via https://research.manchester.ac.uk/en/persons/maurice.nagington/publications/

Roger Newham Associate Professor in the School of Nursing, University of Birmingham (UK), and Executive member of the International Philosophy of Nursing Society (https://ipons.online/about-ipons/). Roger Newham's work is accessible via https://research.birmingham.ac.uk/en/persons/roger-newham/publications/

Jing-Bao Nie Professor at the Bioethics Centre, Dunedin School of Medicine, The University of Otago (New Zealand). Professor Nie's work is accessible via https://www.otago.ac.nz/bioethics/people/academic/profile/?id=665

Inge van Nistelrooij Associate professor of Care Ethics at the University of Humanistic Studies, Utrecht, and Professor by special appointment 'Dialogical Self Theory' at Radboud University, Nijmegen, (Netherlands). Inge van Nistelrooij's work is accessible via www.ingevannistelrooij.com

John Paley Honorary Fellow at the University of Worcester's Three Counties School of Nursing and Midwifery (UK). John Paley's work is accessible via https://john-paley.com/

Evridiki Papastavrou Associate Professor (now Adjunct) at the School of Health Sciences, Cyprus University of Technology (Cyprus). Evridiki Papastavrou's work is accessible via https://www.cut.ac.cy/faculties/hsc/nur/staff/teaching-and-research/e.papastavrou/

Amélie Perron Professor at the School of Nursing at the University of Ottawa and Co-President of the Nursing Observatory (Canada). Professor Perron also edits the journal *Aporia*. Her work is accessible via https://www.uottawa.ca/faculty-health-sciences/nursing/our-professors/amelie-perron

Barbara Pesut Professor and Principal Research Chair in Palliative and End-of-Life Care at the University of British Columbia, Okanagan (Canada). Professor Pesut's work is accessible via https://nursing.ok.ubc.ca/about/contact/barbara-pesut/

Olga Petrovskaya Assistant Professor in the University of Victoria School of Nursing (Canada). Olga Petrovskaya's work is accessible via https://www.uvic.ca/hsd/nursing/people/home/faculty/profiles/petrovskaya-olga.php

Louise Racine Professor in the College of Nursing at the University of Saskatchewan (Canada). Professor Racine's work is accessible via https://nursing.usask.ca/people/louise-racine.php

Mark Risjord Professor of Philosophy, Emory University (USA). Professor Risjord's work is accessible via http://ila.emory.edu/people/faculty/risjord-mark.html

Paul Snelling Principal Lecturer in Adult Nursing at the University of Worcester's Three Counties School of Nursing and Midwifery (UK). Paul Snelling's work is accessible via https://eprints.worc.ac.uk/view/author/Snelling=3APaul=3A=3A.html

Ismalia De Sousa PhD candidate at the University of British Columbia School of Nursing (Canada). Ismalia De Sousa's work is accessible via https://ismaliadesousa.com/

Ruth De Souza VC Fellow at RMIT University, Melbourne (Australia). Ruth De Souza's work is accessible via www.ruthdesouza.com

Fredrik Svenaeus Professor of Philosophy at the Centre for Studies in Practical Knowledge, Södertörn University (Sweden). Professor Svenaeus' work is accessible via https://www.sh.se/english/sodertorn-university/contact/researchers/fredrik-svenaeus?tab=svid10_40cb2fd2166620ee92947b01

Holly Symonds-Brown Assistant Professor in the Faculty of Nursing at the University of Alberta (Canada). Holly Symonds-Brown's work is accessible via https://apps.ualberta.ca/directory/person/hsymonds and carepractices.org

Wayne Thompson Assistant Professor and Programme Director at University College Dublin (Ireland). Wayne Thompson's work is accessible via https://people.ucd.ie/wayne.thompson/publications

Sally Thorne Professor at the University of British Columbia (Canada). Sally Thorne is also the editor-in-chief of the journal *Nursing Inquiry*. Sally Thorne's work is accessible via https://nursing.ubc.ca/our-people/sally-thorne

Michael Traynor Professor of Nursing at Middlesex University (UK). Professor Traynor's work is accessible via https://www.mdx.ac.uk/about-us/our-people/staff-directory/profile/traynor-michael

Claire Valderama-Wallace Associate Professor in the Department of Nursing, California State University East Bay (USA). Claire Valderama-Wallace's work is accessible via https://www.researchgate.net/profile/Claire-Valderama-Wallace

Helen Vandenberg Associate Professor in the College of Nursing at the University of Saskatchewan (Canada). Helen Vandenberg's work is accessible via https://nursing.usask.ca/people/helen-vandenberg.php#Biography

Colleen Varcoe Professor Emeritus at the University of British Columbia School of Nursing (Canada). Professor Varcoe's work is accessible via https://nursing.ubc.ca/our-people/colleen-varcoe

Roger Watson Academic Dean, Southwest Medical University (China), and Editor-in-Chief of *Nurse Education in Practice*. Roger Watson's work is accessible via https://orcid.org/0000-0001-8040-7625

Simon van der Weele Assistant Professor at the Department of Citizenship and Humanisation of the Public Sector, University of Humanistic Studies, Utrecht (Netherlands). Simon van der Weele's work is accessible via https://orcid.org/0000-0001-9931-2394

Jason A Wolf President and CEO of *The Beryl Institute*, Founder and President of the *Patient Experience Institute* (USA) and Founding Editor of the *Patient Experience Journal*. Jason A Wolf's work is accessible via https://www.theberylinstitute.org/page/SpeakerWolf

Martin Woods Honorary Research Associate/Teaching Fellow at Victoria University Wellington (New Zealand). Martin Woods' work is accessible via https://www.research-gate.net/profile/Martin-Woods-3

Lydia Wytenbroek Assistant Professor and Co-Lead of the Consortium for Nursing History Inquiry at the University of British Columbia School of Nursing (Canada). Lydia Wytenbroek's work is accessible via https://nursing.ubc.ca/our-people/lydia-wytenbroek

Dan Zahavi Professor of Philosophy and Director of Center for Subjectivity Research at University of Copenhagen (Denmark). Professor Zahavi's work is accessible via https://cfs.ku.dk/staff/?pure=en/persons/34520

1 Introduction

Martin Lipscomb

Despite the bold and pithily plausible declamatory pronouncements that litter introductory texts, there is no substantive consensus on what "philosophy" is, means, includes/excludes, looks like, or is supposed (if anything) to achieve. Thorny problems also surround the important question of who philosophy benefits, as well as what benefit entails. "Nursing" similarly defies a simplistic description, and the word "handbook" can be interpreted in more than one way. Yet complication aside, you have before you the first edition of the *Routledge Handbook of Philosophy and Nursing*. We hope you enjoy it.

Enjoyment and agreement need not however cohere, and readers probably will not (and nor should they) accept everything argued herein. Indeed, given the hot button nature of several topics covered, readers will almost certainly disagree with at least some of what they encounter; and this is "okay". It is of course satisfying when the perspectives of readers and authors find themselves convivially attuned. Yet whatever the value of philosophic thought/writing, value does not come only or simply from engaging with others who articulate our thoughts and beliefs, others we agree with. Instead, value is as likely – it may be more likely – to derive from confronting ideas previously unconsidered. We might reject these new ideas or we might find ourselves troubled when fresh thinking lends credence to viewpoints we thought we knew but had rejected. Nonetheless, in contemplating what is new, where we decline what is proposed, and when we find ourselves compelled to modify or reposition existing beliefs, we may more fully come to grasp or realise our own views.

Dispute can therefore have merit, and in addition to disagreement about what is said, aforementioned contrasting opinions regarding the scope, remit, purpose, and limit of philosophy are also worth considering. For example, many but by no means all nurses with an interest in philosophy intend enquiry to play, ultimately, some part in nursing actions broadly defined. That is, they want philosophic discourse or engagement to produce and have "use value" (practical or beneficial outcomes) in clinical care, education, research, scholarship, *etc*. This perfectly reasonable albeit somewhat instrumental way of thinking about the value of thinking makes sense so long as the ties between thought and action are not too tightly drawn, and philosophic rumination/analysis may play this role. It can and no doubt does inform thought and thereby (tangentially) action. Perhaps it often should.

Yet, this is not the only way of considering value, and while aligning our understanding of what nursing is/could be with instrumentally orientated ideas about use value mirrors key facets of the technological, scientific, economic, and ideological structures that make up modern society, thinking for thinking's sake also has its adherents. Personally, I am drawn to the issues and questions that philosophers worry over because these

DOI: 10.4324/9781003427407-1

issues/questions possess, for me, inherent interest. The objects of concern may be (they generally are) unanswerable in any definitive or final sense, and this self-evidently complicates naïve assumptions concerning philosophy's judgement informing and/or action guiding potential. Further, whatever it is that is learnt from philosophic discourse, insofar as this learning resists straightforward summary or synopsis, it frequently defies simple elucidation. Thus, for me, it is entanglement with the intricacies and possibilities of argument rather than concluding a "result" or "answer" that maintains interest, and while attempting to understand philosophic ideas might later inform my thinking about practical nursing matters, this is neither guaranteed nor necessary. Some issues/questions are simply worth pondering, and I do not feel compelled to justify this assertion. Unsurprisingly, and quite properly, this anthology links ideas to or with nursing at varying degrees of abstraction. Yet, complementing my own no doubt idiosyncratic "take" on the value of philosophy, within this work, readers might be struck by the way issues and questions burst or run out beyond the confines of nursing practice. Thinking thus defies or mocks disciplinary restrictions, and the borders of "nursing philosophy" as well as "philosophy of/for nursing" – along with questions about thought's beneficiary (does/should philosophy aid only the thinker and/or others) – remain gloriously open.

Given that meaningful definitional agreement is absent regarding almost every aspect of philosophy, in this book, a spectrum of styles and positions are embraced. Readers will thus find chapters that talk to the works of named philosophers, chapters engaging specific philosophic ideas, chapters discussing ideas and practices which, in their handling, can be considered philosophic and – for want of a better phrase – experimental writing/discourse. This variety will antagonise some people. However, offering a range of approaches may – it is intended – to stimulate thought, and a strict *"this and only this is philosophy"* stance was shunned when securing contributions. Contributors, all of whom are experts in their respective fields, take up philosophy in their own distinctive ways. Further, although the text's title includes the word "handbook", contributors were encouraged to present a case or argue a point. Forms of argumentation were left to contributors. However, "handbook" does not here signify a work providing instructions or guidance in what might be thought of (at least in nursing) as the usual directive sense of that word. This is not an instruction manual. Contributors were thus told they could but need not provide balanced arguments where balance implies painful fence sitting, and in this way, it is anticipated or hoped that "imbalance" or a polemical timbre gives contributions that take this approach greater zest. Whether readers concur with or reject what is proposed, we seek to encourage or prompt reflection and reaction.

Moreover, chapter writers come from a range of disciplines, standpoints, and physical locations/geographies (variations in sentence construction/grammar hint at these differences). The overwhelming majority of contributors are, as might be expected, nurse scholars, and pleasingly, many of today's most thought-provoking and inspiring nurse writers agreed to participate in the work. These contributions provide a philosophically orientated snapshot of current interests and perceived problems confronting nursing, and perhaps predictably, where explored chapter themes and questions overlap, argumentative conflict as well as consensus is, as noted, discernible. In addition, the work includes non-nurse philosophers/scholars interested in nursing-healthcare, and non-nurse philosophers/scholars whose work matches nursing concerns but is not specifically or always about nursing-healthcare. This breadth of input is important. Including non-nurses alongside nurse scholars helps mitigate against insularity and parochialism, and in my view this practice enriches the offering presented. That said, naturally, despite enrichment, even a large text such as this barely grazes the surface of the subjects engaged, and to state the obvious, more is left out than is included. Thus, not only are contrasting views possible on every one of the subjects covered, but many pertinent and relevant issues are not mentioned at all. More positively, a great deal is achieved, and while shortly before the work was scheduled for submission we unfortunately lost some African, Latin American, and other voices to sickness and workload pressure (to the detriment of diversity), a varied set of question-problems are pursued. Indeed, despite its limitations, optimistically, if the ideas and arguments presented here appeal to readers, and if engagement encourages or spurs on thinking, further reading, and conversation, the book will be deemed a success.

To facilitate comprehension, chapters are divided into seven sections (see the chapter list). However, the subject matter of submissions often overlap and interleave, and parcelling contributions in this way forces a coherence onto sections that, inevitably, cannot but misidentify and misalign some of what is said. Placing contributions proved to be exceptionally difficult. I remain dissatisfied with the result, and no doubt better ways than the schema employed here are available. It should also be recognised that because contributors come from a variety of countries/locations, and because English is not always the first language of contributors, syntactic and stylistic differences between chapters will, as hinted at above, be apparent. When editing work, a deliberately minimalist approach to corrections was taken. Robust rewriting risks distorting what is argued, and an overly interventionist tack might (quite reasonably) be thought presumptuous. Nonetheless, in conclusion, caveats aside, we are pleased with our collective achievement. While anthologies can be accused of lacking scholarly kudos, they may also be of great value and hopefully this is one such offering. Lastly, I want to say a personal thanks to everyone involved in the project. Thus, thank you to contributors (your patience was greatly appreciated), and thank you to Routledge (Grace McInnes) for commissioning the book. We hope readers find much to attract, intrigue, and interest them within these 47 chapters, the work of 67 scholars. The work was a pleasure to assemble.

Part 1

Philosophy and nursing

2 Nursing, philosophy, and nursing philosophy

Mark Risjord

Introduction

What is the relationship between nursing and philosophy such that the philosophy *of* nursing, or a nursing *philosophy*, could emerge as a field of inquiry? Or to put the question another way, what is the value of philosophy to nursing clinicians, scholars, leaders, and educators? And what is the value of nursing to academic philosophers? One common answer to these questions is that nursing philosophy is foundational to nursing. Fawcett endorsed this role for philosophy and made it part of nursing's disciplinary structure when she wrote:

> [T]he metaparadigm of a discipline identifies the phenomena about which ontological, epistemic, and ethical claims are made. The unique focus and content of each conceptual model then reflect certain philosophical claims. The philosophies therefore are the foundation for other formulations, including conceptual models, grand theories, and middle-range theories.
>
> (Fawcett, 2005, p. 22)

The broad idea is that nursing philosophy asks "second-order" questions inquiring into the presuppositions or assumptions of nursing. Nursing practice and scholarship depend on answers to philosophical questions, but it cannot ask or answer those questions by itself. Nursing philosophy provides answers by drawing on an established body of knowledge in the discipline of philosophy. Pure[1] philosophy thus provides resources that nursing philosophers apply to critique, problematize, analyze, and revise presuppositions at the foundation of nursing, thereby improving the "first-order" practice. Let us call this the "foundational picture" of nursing philosophy.

While the idea that nursing philosophy is foundational to nursing practice and scholarship is attractive, I will argue that it is deeply flawed. I will recommend that the foundational picture be replaced by a picture wherein the philosophy of nursing is an interdisciplinary inquiry, distinct from, but related to, both pure philosophy and nursing. On the interdisciplinary picture, nursing philosophy does not ask second-order questions; it asks conceptual questions arising as part of nursing practice and scholarship. Its contribution is not to derive answers from pure philosophy, but to communicate a kind of translation that enables nurse philosophers to directly engage the conceptual challenges of nursing.

While the foundational picture is common and there is broad consensus on the picture's elements, Steven Edwards has done the most to articulate its details in a complete

DOI: 10.4324/9781003427407-3

and coherent account (Edwards, 2001, 1997). In "What is Philosophy of Nursing?" he argues that philosophical inquiry has three features (Edwards, 1997, p. 1091): (1) Philosophical inquiry employs distinctive methods, roughly, conceptual analysis and the assessment of argument. (2) Philosophical inquiry is concerned with a body of specific problems, broadly identifiable as questions of metaphysics, epistemology, and ethics. (3) Philosophical questions have a distinctive character or level, inquiring into the presuppositions of nursing. This chapter will begin by elucidating Edwards' analysis and it will demonstrate how these features generate the foundational picture. After a critique of the foundational picture, the final section will sketch the alternative picture of nursing philosophy as an interdisciplinary field.

Philosophy, conceptual analysis, and argumentation

Edwards' first feature uses methodology to distinguish philosophy from the empirical sciences, on the one hand, and from other kinds of humanistic inquiry on the other, as many have done when circumscribing nursing philosophy (Grace and Perry, 2013; Kikuchi, 1999, 1992; Pesut and Johnson, 2008; Sarvimäki, 1999; Schröck, 1981, Silva, 1977). Scientific inquiry is *empirical* in the sense that the knowledge produced is ultimately grounded (in large part) by experience. Scientific claims are tested against observation; they are falsifiable. By contrast, philosophical claims are conceptual, and in this way, they are remote from experience. The question of whether humans have free will, for example, is not answerable by any experiment or survey, at least not directly. Answering it requires trying to understand what it would mean to have a free will, to understand how human action fits into a world of causes. What Edwards meant by "conceptual analysis," I suggest, is the broad idea that philosophical inquiry depends on methods that interpret concepts and relate them to each other. To be sure, in its more theoretical reaches, scientific inquiry can also be concerned with the articulation and refinement of concepts. And in their most abstract and highly general form, conceptual critique and modification in science can take on a philosophical dimension, having consequences for both philosophy and the sciences.

The humanistic disciplines are, like philosophy, not directly responsive to empirical observation. Their raw material is some form of cultural production: a text, painting, musical performance, sculpture, or dance. Philosophy distinguishes itself from the other humanities in two related ways. First, it is more self-consciously *normative* in the sense that it is concerned with persuading the reader to think about something in a particular way.[2] A critical analysis of Melville's *Moby-Dick* may provide insight into the human condition, but its goal is to provide an interesting interpretation of the text, not to persuade the reader to adopt Melville's perspective on mortality and divinity. A philosophical analysis of Descartes' *Meditations on First Philosophy*, by contrast, will provide a way of interpreting Descartes' arguments that make them both intelligible and persuasive to the reader. While, in the end, one might not be convinced that the mind is distinct from the body, interpreting Descartes' argument requires expressing its logical force.

Philosophy's concern with argumentation is the second way in which it is distinct from the other humanities. Philosophical writing styles vary, and not all philosophers appeal to formal logic or put their arguments right on the surface of the prose.[3] But all philosophical writing provides reasons in support of a conclusion, and one cannot understand a philosopher's point of view without critically understanding the reasons supporting it. The critical understanding so distinctive of philosophy is enshrined in the structure of Plato's dialogues, where Socrates' interlocutors probe his arguments. Socrates' views are deepened and developed by responding to his companions' objections. Again, not all philosophical writing styles make the underlying dialectic apparent. And often, the dialectical movement is not in the text at all, but between the author and the reader. It follows that understanding a philosophical text requires looking for flaws in the author's reasoning and considering how they would respond to potential objections.

While these methodological characteristics of philosophy capture much that is central to philosophical practice, we would not want to identify either pure philosophy or nursing philosophy with these methods. As Edwards argues, it would truncate the relation between philosophy and nursing. If philosophy were identified with method, it would portray philosophy as merely provided conceptual engineering consults for nursing, shoring up arguments here, realigning concepts there. It isn't clear why nurses themselves couldn't do this for themselves, or why philosophers would be particularly helpful. So, while the distinctive methodology of philosophy must be a part of the contribution it makes to nursing, methodology cannot be the whole story.

Second-order questions and the foundational picture

Edwards argues that because the methodological criterion alone is insufficient, a philosophy of nursing requires a "more substantial conception of philosophy" (Edwards, 1997, p. 1091). His second and third characteristics flesh out the substance: philosophy is concerned with a body of specific problems, and it poses questions "of a distinctive character or level" (Edwards, 1997, p. 1091). In his writing on the philosophy of nursing, Edwards described philosophical questions in two ways: as "second-order" (Edwards, 2001, p. 7) and as "external" (Edwards, 1997, p. 1091). As we will see, these descriptions are closely related, and they generate the foundational picture.

Writing on nursing philosophy has often used a distinction between "first-order" and "second-order" questions to identify philosophical inquiry (Edwards, 2001; Sarvimäki, 1999; Schröck, 1981). Edwards draws on the philosopher Anthony Quinton, who described the second-order character of philosophy as "thinking about thinking" (Quinton, 1995, p. 666). Edwards illustrates the difference between first- and second-order questions in this way:

> Suppose it is said 'Smith is better now'. What is meant by 'better'? Or 'Smith is healthy'. What is meant by 'healthy'? Or, 'Smith is a good nurse'. What is meant by 'is a good nurse'? These are all second-order questions. Answers to them are presupposed at the first-order level. Answers to first-order questions will be inadequate if the answers to the second-order queries they provoke are inadequate.
>
> (Edwards, 2001, p. 8)

While the image of "thinking about thinking" is suggestive, the difference between the first- and the second-order needs elucidation. In particular, why do second-order questions ask about *presuppositions* of the first-order level? And why would the accuracy of first-order inquiries be inadequate, unless second-order questions could be adequately answered? Edwards fills in these important details in his 1997 essay by appealing to Carnap's conception of a linguistic framework and his distinction between "internal" and "external" questions (Carnap, 1950).

Carnap's distinction between "internal" and "external" questions arises from ambiguity in questions about existence. The question "Does a greatest prime number exist?" is a mathematical question, to be answered by finding a mathematical proof. By contrast, the question "Do numbers exist?" could not be answered by finding a mathematical proof. The question of whether there is a greatest prime number is "internal" to the practice of mathematics. Carnap conceptualized mathematical practice as a "linguistic framework" that included a network of concepts, presuppositions, assumptions, and methods of answering questions. Given the framework of mathematics, Euclid could prove that there is no greatest prime. However, the question of whether numbers exist is a question *about* the framework itself. It cannot be raised or answered within the framework of mathematics, since that framework presupposes the existence of numbers. In this sense, the question of whether numbers exist is "external" to the framework. On this kind of view, both ordinary language and academic disciplines provide linguistic frameworks, and any linguistic framework depends on presuppositions about the meaning of its fundamental concepts. First-order questions are internal and thus depend on these presuppositions. Second-order questions are external to the first-order framework, asking about its conceptual presuppositions.

Edwards deviates from Carnap's conception of an external question in one very significant way: Carnap thought that external questions had no substantive answers. For Carnap, a second-order question like "Do numbers exist?" *cannot* be answered by philosophical debate. Rather, in Carnap's view, it is a purely practical matter of choosing a framework that will suit one's needs. Clearly, Edwards could not accept Carnap's pragmatism about external questions since it would make nursing philosophy impossible. Unlike Carnap, then, Edwards must assume that the discipline of philosophy contains a body of knowledge that can be used to answer (or try to answer) second-order questions about the presuppositions of linguistic frameworks. This is the sense in which nursing philosophy must be *substantive*.

The picture of nursing philosophy as a foundational enterprise thus flows directly from conceptualizing philosophical questions as second-order (or external) and from treating second-order questions as substantive. The presuppositions of a linguistic framework are analogous to the axioms of a mathematical system. They must be implicitly assumed if any use is to be made of the system. And these presuppositions can be adequate or inadequate in substantive ways; we can be wrong in our fundamental assumptions about, say, knowledge or justice. Should the presuppositions be flawed, the whole framework is flawed. Second-order inquiry into the basis of the framework is thus necessary to ensure that the framework is sound. Philosophy as a field of study has developed a vast library of work exploring such fundamental concepts. An applied philosophy, like the philosophy of nursing, draws on these resources to identify—and perhaps to address—flaws in the presuppositions of a particular framework.

Against the foundational picture

The foundational picture has both conceptual and practical flaws that make it inappropriate as a way of understanding the philosophy of nursing. Conceptually, it rests on a problematic notion of meaning and conceptual content. And practically, while critiquing foundations is advertised as making nursing thought and practice better (Ellis, 1983; Fawcett, 2005; Kikuchi, 1992; Pesut and Johnson, 2008; Sarvimäki, 1999; Schröck, 1981; Silva, 1977), the asymmetry of the foundations picture undermines its practical capacity to do so.

The foundational picture assumes that conceptual inconsistency or unclarity is always problematic and needs to be addressed by second-order inquiry. Consider Edwards' example of health. The conception of a linguistic framework leads him to suggest that "Smith is healthy" depends on an assumption about the meaning of "health." Insofar as the meaning is unclear or the usage inconsistent, agreeing that Smith is a paragon of health is somehow suspect. But, as Wittgenstein pointed out, it is quite absurd to require precise definitions as a condition of using a language: "When I give the description: 'The ground was quite covered with plants'—do you want to say I don't know what I am talking about until I can give a definition of a plant?" (Wittgenstein, 1953, Section 70). The context of use determines whether a conceptual inconsistency or unclarity is a problem to be addressed by a more precise definition. And the particular kind of clarification required depends on the purposes of our use and the specific errors or misinterpretations that might arise. There is no standing demand for second-order inquiry just because we mobilize a concept like health.

Of course, communication obviously requires a shared language, and this requires shared meanings. The levels picture mistakenly moves from this platitude to the notion that in asserting "Smith is healthy," we must assume a particular definition of health. In both ordinary life and scholarly inquiry, "health" is ambiguous. Indeed, it is a good example of an "essentially contested concept" (Gallie, 1955), where the dimensions of meaning conflict in such a way as to make agreement on a single, precise definition impossible. Far from undermining our ability to conduct health research or engage in health care, the inconsistencies and conflicts among our varied usages of "health" are productive. The different, but interrelated, usages facilitate a rich variety of ways of thinking about health. Settling on a single, precise notion—even if grounded in beautiful philosophical argumentation—would arguably truncate health care and research. The idea that we need adequate answers to second-order questions so as to have adequate answers to first-order questions is thus mistaken.

The foundational picture also problematically entails that philosophy and nursing are asymmetrically related. As the foundation, philosophy does not depend on nursing in the way that nursing depends on philosophy. Philosophical reflection on ontology, epistemology, and ethics proceeds without reference to nursing. On the foundational picture, philosophers of nursing take the concepts of, e.g., knowledge or health as clarified in pure philosophy and use them to clarify the concepts of nursing knowledge or nursing client health. With the conceptual foundation secured, the foundational picture proposes, nurses and nurse scholars can go about their first-order business in better ways. This asymmetry is problematic for two closely related reasons. First, the agenda for nursing philosophy seems to be set by pure philosophy rather than by nursing. To be sure, the concepts to be clarified are fundamental to the nursing framework, but the second-order inquiry (philosophy) determines whether and how the concepts need clarification. The specific conundrums and conceptual difficulties faced by nurses appear to play little role in shaping nursing philosophy, much less the pronouncements of pure philosophy. At the very least, this seems inconsistent with the practice of most nursing philosophers working today. Second, as suggested above, both whether a concept needs clarification and the kind of clarification required depend intimately on the context of use. This means that the first- and second-order questions cannot be as independent as the levels picture would have it.

If we accept that we can communicate even if meanings are inevitably unclear and sometimes even incoherent, then the foundational picture undermines nursing philosophy's possible contributions to nursing. On the foundational picture, the pressing business of nursing is, and must be, entirely first-order. Unless the conceptual confusions bring the first-order business to a halt, the second-order questions will be superfluous. Seeking foundations puts philosophers of nursing in a predicament similar to that of the philosopher Ted Cohen. Cohen demonstrated that the rules of baseball were logically inconsistent and brought the inconsistency to the Rules Committee of the National Baseball League. They refrained from changing the rules on the grounds that the contradiction had no practical consequences (Cohen, 2018). Since ambiguity—or even logical inconsistency!—is tolerable, one can see why both clinicians and nurse scholars would regard a second-order inquiry as a rather pointless exercise. The foundational picture, then, practically undermines the very activity it is intended to support.

Philosophy of nursing as an interdisciplinary field

Wilfred Sellars once wrote that "The aim of philosophy, abstractly formulated, is to understand how things in the broadest sense of the term hang together in the broadest sense of the term" (Sellars, 1963, p. 1). Sellars pictured philosophy as a matter of making sense, not securing foundations. In a Sellarsian spirit, I would like to sketch an *interdisciplinary* picture of nursing philosophy as an alternative to the foundational picture. On the interdisciplinary picture, nursing philosophy is a field wherein we try to understand how nursing, in the broadest sense of the term, hangs together, and doing so requires blending philosophical and nursing concerns. I will argue that this picture preserves the insights on which the levels picture is based. But it eschews the conception of a linguistic framework and the corresponding distinction between first- and second-order questions. By doing so, the picture of nursing philosophy as an interdisciplinary field avoids the pitfalls of foundationalism.

On the foundational picture, since the philosopher of nursing is asking second-order questions, their inquiry cannot be part of the nursing discipline and must be part of philosophy. By contrast, to treat nursing philosophy as an interdisciplinary inquiry is to say that it is *neither* part of the discipline of philosophy *nor* part of the discipline of nursing. While disciplinary boundaries are historically contingent and socially maintained, disciplines have distinctive areas of interest, typical kinds of question, and typical methods for answering them. Interdisciplinary inquiries ask questions that fall between disciplinary concerns. And to answer their questions, interdisciplinary scholars must draw on the conceptual, theoretical, and methodological resources of more than one discipline. Nursing philosophy is an interdisciplinary field of inquiry because it must draw on both philosophy and nursing, though it draws on these disciplines in different ways.

Nursing provides nursing philosophy with its questions. These are, contrary to the foundational picture, questions that arise within the nursing discipline as part of its normal inquiry and practice. For example, "What is nursing?" and "What is a nurse?" are often mentioned as a question of nursing philosophy (Edwards, 1997, p. 1092, 2001, p. 15; Ellis, 1983, p. 212; Schröck, 1981, p. 13). Far from being a question that could not be asked with the framework, the question "What is a nurse?" arose within nursing in response to specifically nursing concerns. One of the earliest explicit calls for philosophy was Dorothy Johnson's "A Philosophy of Nursing," which began with the lines:

> What is nursing? A philosophical question of a few years ago has become an urgent cry as professional nurses seek to find and establish anew their identity in a rapidly expanding group of health workers.
>
> (Johnson, 1959, p. 198)

Answering the "what is nursing?" question was (and remains) pressing for political reasons. This philosophical question is a means by which nursing can demonstrate its unique contribution to health care. Questions about nursing knowledge and expertise also arose from a broadly political concern to position nursing within health care. These conceptual questions arise from intellectual needs specific to nursing, and nurse scholars *qua* nurse scholars need to answer them; they are not external to nursing. Nursing philosophy must thus draw on nursing expertise to formulate the questions it will address.

Because the questions of nursing philosophy arise from intellectual and practical issues within nursing, the answers must satisfy the intellectual demands of those who asked. This means that nursing philosophy must contribute to nursing. The questions are conceptual and normative—which is what makes them require philosophical methods—but the concepts get their life from nursing practice and discourse. It follows that the substance of nursing philosophy needs to be conceptually embedded into nursing, related to other concepts mobilized by nurses in their practice and scholarship. Only by keeping the concepts connected to nursing discourse can the answers help understand how nursing, in the broadest sense of the term, hangs together.

Turning to nursing philosophy's relation to pure philosophy, questions like "What is nursing?" or "What is nursing knowledge?" are *philosophical* because they are conceptual, normative, and not answerable empirically. They are conceptual in the sense that their answers require conceptual articulation. They are normative and not empirical in the sense that we cannot answer the "What is nursing?" question by determining what most nurses think nursing is (though this might be interesting and useful to know). Answering these questions requires a normative argument that, e.g., nursing ought to be thought about in one way rather than another. It follows that the interdisciplinary field of nursing philosophy must draw on the methods of philosophy: argument, critique, and conceptual analysis.

If philosophy of nursing is an interdisciplinary field, what is the relationship between the substance of philosophy—the topics of metaphysics, epistemology, and value theory—to the questions of nursing philosophy? It must differ in at least two ways from the foundational picture. On the foundational picture, philosophy secured the foundations of nursing. Since the presuppositions must be sound, the philosophical theses and concepts on which they rest have to be properly understood. The philosopher of nursing has to "get it right" and produce answers that are, to put it bluntly, true. On the interdisciplinary picture, the philosopher of nursing is not charged with being sure that the presuppositions of nursing are sound. Criteria for whether and how a philosopher of nursing "gets it right" are not beholden to pure philosophy. A second way in which the two pictures differ is that, on the foundational picture, specifics of nursing are added to the generalities of philosophy. Pure philosophy generates a conception of knowledge that applies to all human activities. Nursing knowledge is then pictured as a species of the genus, and the job of the nursing philosopher is to discover its specific differences. If nursing philosophy is interdisciplinary, by contrast, there is no need for the concept of, e.g., nursing knowledge to be related to the concept of human knowledge as species to genus. It is entirely possible that the answer to nursing questions about knowledge bears on concerns quite different from those that have traditionally occupied philosophers.

Rejecting the idea of a second-order inquiry distances nursing philosophy from pure philosophy, and it thereby runs the risk of re-instantiating the problematic idea that different inquiries require their own frameworks or paradigms. If nursing philosophy is not responsible in some way to pure philosophy, one might object, then nursing philosophers seem free to invent their own set of conceptual tools, independent of any other field of inquiry. The resulting picture would then have each discipline standing on its own, and I have explored the pernicious consequences of this idea elsewhere (Risjord, 2011). The solution to the conundrum is to refuse the temptation of thinking that disciplinary lines of inquiry could be independent. There is no bright line separating nursing from any other discipline, nor any line separating philosophy from the sciences. This means that our concepts draw their content from a variety of uses, and we cannot simply ignore the use of, e.g., "knowledge" in another domain, simply because it conflicts with one's imme- diate concern. To understand how things in the broadest sense of the term hang together in the broadest sense of the term, our conceptual articulations and normative arguments to be responsible to the broadest senses of the terms in question.

To understand how the substance of nursing philosophy might be "responsible to" the discipline of philosophy, I suggest that nursing philosophy's use of traditional philo- sophical literature should be understood as analogous to *translation*.[4] Translation is always a communicative act. The translator begins with a text that is incomprehensible to an audience. From it, they derive a message to be communicated in terms that are both relevant to, and understandable by, the audience. Thus, while translation does not depend on "getting it right," the translator needs to know the language well enough to be able to extract a message appropriate for the audience. This means that the philoso- pher of nursing needs to know the source material of traditional philosophy well enough to identify relevant ideas and arguments. Indeed, nursing philosophers need expertise in philosophy, and the deeper the expertise, the better they will be able to respond to the conceptual questions that arise from nursing. The task of a nursing philosopher is to find relevant ideas (where relevance is established by nursing) from philosophy and develop them in the context of nursing thought and practice. The goal is to show how thinking about a phenomenon in a new way will help nurses answer the conceptual question they posed.

Thinking of the philosophy of nursing—indeed, all "applied philosophy"—as a kind of translation not only preserves the independence of nursing philosophy as an interdis- ciplinary field, but also lets nursing philosophy talk back to pure philosophy. Nursing philosophy can talk back to pure philosophy precisely because answers to the questions of nursing philosophy will take on a life of their own in nursing discourse. Nurses will take up views about what it means to have a nursing identity, or what it means to have nursing expertise, and use them in their scholarship and to guide their practice. The ways that "identity" and "knowledge" play out in nursing are further uses, and as such ought to be relevant to our broader, philosophical understanding of these concepts. By standing between philosophy and nursing, the interdisciplinary field of the philosophy of nursing is positioned to contribute to both.

Conclusion: the value and limits of pictures

I have deliberately characterized foundationalism as a "picture," and not as a "(meta) philosophical theory," because I doubt that anyone—including Stephen Edwards—would fully endorse it. Rather, the picture grows out of natural and common ways of describing what we are up to when doing nursing philosophy and how it orients our practice. It is a lens through which we can view what we do in nursing philosophy in order to see its significance. But our thought and action always outrun the boundaries of any picture.

Thus, in offering interdisciplinarity as an alternative picture, I am not recommending that our practice changes dramatically. Rather, I suggest that by viewing the activities of nursing philosophers through the lens of interdisciplinarity, we get a less distorted image of what we are doing and why it matters. Viewed in this way, we can see that the practice of nursing philosophy has always been interdisciplinary, and this in-between status has always been the source of both our successes and frustrations.[5]

Notes

1 I doubt that there is a pure philosophy in any sense that one might attach to the word "pure." I use it here to distinguish philosophy which is independent of nursing concerns from the philosophy of nursing.
2 While developing the point is outside of the scope of this chapter, I submit that this normative character distinguishes the discipline of philosophy from personal philosophies ("my philosophy of nursing") on the one hand and from ideology on the other. The focus on normativity is consonant with, but distinct from Edwards' (1997), Kikuchi's (1999), and Pesut and Johnson's (2008) similar distinctions.
3 Sarvimäki (1999) has a useful overview of different approaches to philosophy, ranging from logical analysis to "philosophical poems."
4 See Risjord, 2022 for further development of this idea.
5 I would like to thank my colleagues and students in Emory's Institute for the Liberal Arts for helping me think about my work in interdisciplinary terms.

References

Carnap, R., 1950. Empiricism, Semantics, and Ontology. *Revue Internationale de Philosophie* 4(11), 20–40.

Cohen, T., 2018. There Are No Ties at First Base, in: Herwitz, D. (Ed.), *Serious Larks*. Chicago: University of Chicago Press, pp. 93–104.

Edwards, S.D., 1997. What is Philosophy of Nursing? *Journal of Advanced Nursing* 25, 1089–1093.

Edwards, S.D., 2001. *Philosophy of Nursing: An Introduction*. New York: Palgrave.

Ellis, R., 1983. Philosophic Inquiry. *Annual Review of Nursing Research* 1(1), 211–228.

Fawcett, J., 2005. *Contemporary Nursing Knowledge: Analysis and Evaluation of Nursing Models and Theories*, 2nd ed. Philadelphia: F. A. Davis.

Gallie, W.B., 1955. Essentially Contested Concepts. *Proceedings of the Aristotelian Society* 56, 167–198.

Grace, P.J., Perry, D. J., 2013. Philosophical Inquiry and the Goals of Nursing. *Advances in Nursing Science* 36(2), 64–79.

Johnson, D.E., 1959. A Philosophy of Nursing. *Nursing Outlook* 7, 198–200.

Kikuchi, J. F., 1992. Nursing Questions That Science Cannot Answer, in: Kikuchi, J. F. and Simmons, H. (Eds.), *Philosophic Inquiry in Nursing*. Newbury Park, CA: Sage, pp. 26–37.

Kikuchi, J.F., 1999. Clarifying the Nature of Conceptualizations about Nursing. *Canadian Journal of Nursing Research* 30(4), 115–128. .

Pesut, B., Johnson, J., 2008. Reinstating the 'Queen': Understanding Philosophical Inquiry in Nursing. *Journal of Advanced Nursing* 61, 115–121.

Quinton A., 1995. Philosophy, in: Honderich, T. (Ed.) *The Oxford Companion to Philosophy*. Oxford: Oxford University Press, pp. 666–70.

Risjord, M., 2011. *Nursing Knowledge: Science, Practice, and Philosophy*. Oxford: Wiley-Blackwell.

Risjord, M., 2022. The Nurse Philosopher as Translator, in: Lipscomb, M. (Ed.), *Complexity and Values in Nurse Education: Dialogues on Professional Education*. London: Routledge, pp. 205–206.

Sarvimäki, A., 1999. Answering Philosophical Questions Facing Contemporary Nursing Practice. *Western Journal of Nursing Research* 21, 9–15.

Schröck, R., 1981. Philosophical Issues, in: Hockey, L. (Ed.) *Current Issues in Nursing*. Edinburgh: Churchill Livingstone, pp. 3–18.

Sellars, W., 1963. *Science, Perception and Reality*. London: Routledge and Kegan Paul, pp. 1–40.

Silva, M., 1977. Philosophy, Science, Theory: Interrelationships and Implications for Nursing Research. *Image: Journal of Nursing Scholarship* 9(3), 59–63.

Wittgenstein, L. 1953. *Philosophical Investigations*. London: Basil Blackwell.

3 On the contribution of the nursing theorists

Sally Thorne

A new graduate student wonders what the nursing theory movement was really all about and why it matters. Does anyone actually read or use those conceptual models for nursing these days? And why should nurses care how each of the model builders conceptualized patient or any of the other "metaparadigm concepts" of nursing?

Why nursing theory?

Although nursing has, from the time of Florence Nightingale and Mary Seacole, possessed a fairly strong sense of itself as a discipline distinct from, but intersecting with, the practice of medicine, articulating and explaining the scope and boundaries of that distinctive disciplinary domain have never been straightforward. From nursing's perspective, there has always been something it would consider a "medical model" – generally a curative approach to diseases and abnormalities organized by an understanding of the distinct organ systems that make a human body function. And while nurses have always been taught to understand and work with how physicians think about their patients, they have been quite steadfast in their conviction that what nursing brought to the table was something distinct from and complementary to that particular disciplinary world view.

A century after Nightingale's *Notes on Nursing* (1959/1946), as health care, science and technology were rapidly evolving, professional nursing began to appreciate the urgency of articulating exactly how the role of the nurse differed from that of other health care providers (Chinn & Kramer 2019; Engebretson 1997). To do so, it sought to establish a scientific basis for practice (Field 1987), and to advance the education of practitioners in possession of the competencies to enact practice that was grounded in that science (Cull-Wilby & Peppin 1987; Jones 1997). In this context, it became clear that teaching nursing students using the conventional medical model as an organizing framework was ineffective (Dean 1995; Orem & Parker 1964). In response, by the 1960s and 1970s, our thought leaders began to experiment with alternative ways to conceptually structure the central ideas of the discipline in a manner that would more strongly socialize new practitioners in fixing a distinctly nursing lens upon the phenomena of interest, and allow for the development of a nursing science informed by theories that were specific to the requirements of nursing disciplinary knowledge (Fawcett 1980; Meleis 2018).

Who were the nursing theorists?

Hildegard Peplau (1952) is generally considered the first of these modern "nurse theorists." A psychiatric nurse, she articulated a theory of interpersonal relations between

DOI: 10.4324/9781003427407-4

nurse and client that she believed would revolutionize the treatment of persons with behaviour and personality disorders in a humane direction. She envisioned shared experiences between nurse and client facilitated by observation, description, formulation, interpretation, validation and intervention, rather than the more passive assumption that nurses simply carried out physician orders in doing things to passive patients. Ida Jean Orlando (1961) expanded on Peplau's thinking to articulate nursing as a deliberative process based on interpretation of the behaviours that represent a patient's need for help. The five steps embedded in her approach to producing favourable outcomes or patient improvement became standardized in the discipline as the *nursing process* – the iterative sequence of assessment, diagnosis, planning, implementation and evaluation. Virginia Henderson, who had first published a conceptualization of nursing as a profession oriented towards supporting people to meet their basic human needs, following the tradition of Maslow's hierarchy of needs in 1955, expanded this idea into a theory of nursing in her 1966 text *The Nature of Nursing* (Henderson 1955, 1966).

By the 1970s, a number of nursing theorists were explicitly taking up the idea of theorizing the discipline, and we can begin to see in their works various ways of conceptualizing how nursing understands the patient, as well as its aspirations for that patient and its interpretation of its role in facilitating those aspirations. Martha Rogers (1970) began to conceptualize the patient as a unitary entity, irreducible into parts and inseparable from its environment. Dorothea Orem (1971) understood the need for nursing as addressing a deficit in the ability to provide one's self with the self-care that sustains health and life. Joyce Travelbee (1971) focused her thinking on human suffering and the person-to-person relationship that helps people find meaning within it and maintain hope. Dorothy Johnson (1959, 1974) pioneered the consideration of a patient as a behavioural system seeking equilibrium. Sr. Callista Roy (1976), in addition to the systems approach, viewed the person as continuously adapting in physiology, self-concept, role function and independence, with the nurse's role during illness and health being to promote that adaptation. Among the many other well-known nurse theorists who entered the field over subsequent years with their own brand of conceptualizing the discipline was Rosemarie Parse (Parse 1981), whose human becoming theory guided nurses to focus on quality of life from each person's own perspective.

Depending on how you count, the list of formal conceptual models for nursing grew to include several (i.e. three or four) dozen over these years. The vast majority of the authors that we think of as *nursing theorists* (and whose contributions we find listed in the many nursing theory texts and websites devoted to recording the nursing theory tradition) were based in the USA. Although each of their theories had a formal title (e.g., *Theory of Transpersonal Nursing*, *The Conservation Model*, *Health as Expanding Consciousness*, *Theory of Culture Care Diversity and Universality*, *Conceptual System and Theory of Goal Attainment*), most were best known in the nursing world by the name of their author and champion (respectively, Jean Watson, Myra Levine, Margaret Newman, Madeleine Leininger, Imogene King), and so on (Alligood 2021). A handful of nursing models were published outside of the USA, by theorists such as Scandinavians Kari Martinsen (*Philosophy of Caring*) and Katie Eriksson (*Theory of Carative Caring*), Canadians Evelyn Adam (*Conceptual Model of Nursing*) and Moyra Allen (*The McGill Model of Nursing*). And in some instances, models were co-authored by teams, including Margaret Campbell, Mary Cruise and Rose Murakami (*University of British Columbia Model for Nursing*) in Canada and Nancy Roper, Winifred Logan and Alison Tierney

(*The Roper-Logan-Tierney Model for Nursing*) in the United Kingdom. However, despite these few exceptions, the syntax of the nursing theory movement continues to be navigated primarily in terms of the theorists' names.

What were they theorizing?

In critically reflecting on the diversities within the evolving conceptualizations, Yura and Torres (1975) made the early observation that four key concepts were common to them all – "man," "society," "health" and "nursing." Fawcett (1978) responded by reframing "man" as "person" and "society" as "environment" to remove sexism and to more fully express the idea of the wider context in which health and illness unfold. Looking back to the work of those early theorists, revisionists redefined that work as aligning with these concepts, therefore constituting distinct conceptual frameworks for nursing (Flaskerud & Halloran 1980; Kim 1983). On that basis, drawing upon the idea that a "metaparadigm" of any discipline constituted "a statement or group of statements identifying its relevant phenomena," Fawcett (1984) reviewed the available theoretical literature, providing numerous examples of what she interpreted as evidence of agreement on the existence of these central concepts as representative of a metaparadigm of nursing, and claimed to have found no "contradictory statements" (p. 84). She further observed that these same recurring themes could also be found in the works of nurse scholars since Nightingale. In declaring these recurring themes as "nursing's metaparadigm concepts," Fawcett established a common language that, from the mid-1980s onwards, would continue to distinguish the theorizing associated with nursing conceptual models from all other forms of what we might call more "substantive" theorizing within the discipline (Donnelly 2001). According to Deets (1990), however, this declaration of an established paradigm was arguably an attempt at legitimization that seemed to ignore conventional understandings of how a scientific paradigm actually comes into being – something identifiable after the fact on the basis of the activity of a scientific community. In Deets' view, in its hurry to establish itself as a mature discipline, nursing had "short circuit[ed] the process of developing a tradition" (p. 150). Nevertheless, as the nursing models era evolved, with dozens of theorists offering their own distinctive versions, these metaparadigm concepts formed the core and became the framework against which the various theories were assessed, evaluated and critiqued (Meleis 2018).

Although all of the theorists included ideas about the metaparadigm concepts in their conceptual models as they proposed and developed them over time, the vast majority of their effort was placed on how the nurse was to understand the patient as *client* of nursing. Indeed, the term client became popularized in many of the models as a device to distinguish the passive recipient of medical care (*patient*) from the active agent with whom nursing engaged in the process of preventing illness or returning to health. Assessment, as the entry point into the nurse-client relationship and the foundation for the entire nursing process, required that the nurse be able to conceptualize that which was most relevant about the person for the purpose of making decisions with respect to nursing interventions and goals of care. In this manner, the "hallmark" of the nursing models became their "depiction of a framework for organizing data about the individual person as the basic focus of nursing's attention" (Thorne et al. 1998, p. 1258).

In that the various conceptual models had been constructed on the basis of understandings of human experience borrowed from (and therefore legitimized by) various prominent theorists in the social sciences, the specific gaze each called for in its assessment framework was often shaped by ideas derived from those other disciplines and applied to the nursing context.

Many of these distinctions in the writings of the various nurse theorists are most evident in their choice of terminology within these frameworks, including the (often) idiosyncratic language each chose to characterize the fundamental elements associated with the person that the practising nurse was expected to assess. To illustrate, *Roy's Adaptation Theory*, which was derived from the systems theory of Austrian biologist Ludwig Von Bertalanffy and the adaptation theory of American psychologist Harry Helson (Roy 1988), contains philosophical assumptions characterized by humanism, veritivity and cosmic unity and scientific assumptions such as the ideas that "[s]ystems of matter and energy progress to higher levels of complex self-organization" and "[s]ystem relationships include acceptance, protection, and fostering interdependence" (Roy 2009, p. 31). Within this framework, the individual is conceptualized as an adaptive system, defined as a whole with parts that function as a unity for a purpose. Nursing assessment therefore orients the focus of attention on the various parts of that human system in interaction with one another. In contrast, Parse's *Human Becoming Theory* (formerly "Man-Living-Health") developed the idea of nursing as a human science based on the work of German philosopher Wilhelm Dilthey, among others (Parse 2002). It asks nurses to consider that

> ...humans live at multidimensional realms of the universe all-at-once as they prereflectively and reflectively choose from options incarnating imaged value priorities. Through languaging, humans disclose and hide all-at-once the who that they are, while living the opportunities and limitations of being close to and apart from others. Humans change moment-to-moment as they actualize dreams and hopes through inventing new ways to propel beyond what is to what is not-yet.
>
> (Parse 1999, p. 8)

Because "humans co-author their becoming in mutual process with the universe, cocreating distinguishable patterns which specify the uniqueness of both humans and the universe" (p. 5), the objective of nurses is to discern and support those patterns so that the human person under their care was fully supported in "transcending multidimensionality with the possibles" (p. 6).

During the nursing theory heyday, it became an imperative for nursing education programmes to build curriculum according to the guidance of a specified nursing model in order to signify progressive development of nursing knowledge and skills towards application of that model across any nursing practice setting. Failure to explicitly adopt a nursing conceptual framework as a framework for curriculum implied a programme that was stuck in medical model thinking, and mechanisms for assessing best practices in nursing education, such as approval and accreditation systems, included the idea of nursing frameworks as an expected organizing principle. Likewise, numerous hospitals and health authorities (at least across North America) explicitly adopted one specific conceptual framework for nursing, ensured that all of their nursing staff were well versed in at least its basic ideas and implemented documentation systems (such as admission guides, nursing assessment frameworks and nursing charting requirements) according to the ideas and emphases that their particular model addressed. There was significant dialogue between institutions using the same model to share ideas and resources. Educators and administrators working within specific models came together to develop shared knowledge as to how best to prepare new nurses and deliver care that was model-based.

What went wrong?

Before I describe some of what I believe to be the most impressive and valuable contributions made by the nursing model movement to our current understanding of the nature of nursing, it seems important to reflect on what, at least from my perspective, derailed this intensive theorizing and philosophizing movement into what became a contentious and ultimately dysfunctional period of scholarly discourse.

One key factor had to do with the alignment between the nursing theory movement and the concurrent focus on the advancement of nursing science. Although some philosophical terminology had found its way into the model literature in its very early days, and certainly all or most model builders articulated philosophical principles as part of the values underpinnings of their work, it seems fair to argue that the theorists primarily saw themselves as contributors to nursing science rather than philosophy, and therefore envisioned their models as the theoretical basis for nursing research and practice into the future. It is important to remember how influential the ideas of Thomas Kuhn had become across many disciplines during the 1970s and 1980s. His *Structure of Scientific Revolutions* (1962) had described the manner in which competing scientific paradigms eventually led to scientific progress within a specific field or discipline, such that major advancements in science were revolutionary in nature rather than evolutionary. In this light, the various approaches to working out nursing's metaparadigm concepts became conflated with the idea of disciplinary maturity, including the assumption that ultimately one of the theoretical models would come to serve as the agreed-upon foundation for all of nursing's mature disciplinary science.

Jaqueline Fawcett, in her 1980 paper, had tried valiantly to untangle the confusion within nursing between conceptual models and theories. She had pointed out quite early on in the model movement that a conceptual model for nursing is not a theory in the true sense, in that it does not contain detailed explanations of postulated relationships among variables. Rather, conceptual models were intended to serve as abstractions, mental maps, organizers for the ideas of concern to the discipline, and were therefore capable of providing only general guidelines for scientific endeavours and practice decisions (Ellis 1968; McKay 1969). Regardless, the language of "nursing theory" stuck to the model building enterprise, and with it came the persistent conviction that the role of nurse theorists was to compete for their theory's pre-eminence within the discipline. Towards this end, nurse theorists and the communities of scholars working to promote the various theories attempted to demonstrate with some precision how practice based on their distinctive conceptual framework, including their detailed conceptualization of the person as focus for nursing action, would be preferable to practice based on competing models. They also pressed forward the idea of nursing research explicitly scaffolded upon their theoretical model rather than research into the more substantive questions nurses were often asking (Alghase & Whall 1993). While some of the model-based research may well have yielded interesting insights about the clinical phenomena in question, much of it tended to reflect exemplars of the model's application rather than adding specific value to knowledge for the wider field. And since the language and conceptual structure of each model was so intricately embedded in its application, the findings from nursing research based on one conceptual model were often unintelligible to nurses working within a different nursing framework. The high level of particularity associated with each model meant that nurses were communicating with one another within the distinctive theoretical camps rather than as a more cohesive professional community.

As the competition for primacy heated up, some nurse theorists sought to discredit others by positioning groups of models into what they termed paradigms or mutually incommensurate "world views" in the Kuhnian sense of the term. The language of *simultaneity paradigm*, first articulated by Parse in 1987, referred to a particular style of nursing conceptual model that was explicitly unitary, seeing the whole of a person as something that could not be understood by knowledge of the parts, and inseparable from the entirety of the universe (Barrett 2002). The terminology used by the simultaneity proponents to refer to all other conceptual models was *totality paradigm*, implying the assumption that one can know the whole through study of the parts (Barrett 2002). As these terms found their way into the nursing theory lexicon, the simultaneity-totality division became a device through which proponents worked to extend the credibility of the simultaneity models by positioning them as inherently more holistic and philosophically superior to other models (Cody 1995; Nagle & Mitchell 1991; Newman 1992). In this context, the models branded as totality paradigm were understood by simultaneity theorists as committed to an occult reductionism and discounted as remnants of a logical positivist form of science (Cody 1996; Cody & Mitchell 2002). And at this point, some of the discourse, both at nursing conferences and in the literature, became somewhat nasty, with some scholars attempting to alert the profession to the implications of the kinds of divisions that this extreme form of paradigm thinking can entail (Kikuchi & Simmons 1999; Thorne 2001; Thorne et al. 1998, 1999) and others rejecting the credibility of any critique from those whose scholarly work was external to their paradigmatic perspective (Cody 2000; Parse 1998).

For most nursing scholars, particularly those who had not been following the plot of the paradigm wars saga, this debate was sufficiently unseemly to justify abandoning the idea of prioritizing nursing theory development as a relevant and meaningful enterprise for the profession. The idea that there were fundamentally disparate species of nurses whose world views could not co-exist was highly problematic to educators, regulators and policy makers alike. They were also aware that the ideosynchratic language associated with many of the nursing theories was a liability within the world of interprofessional health education and practice. Ultimately, the discipline for the most part distanced itself from the model movement, abandoning the explicit reliance on conceptual models for education and practice, and took up alternative theoretical structures (drawn from ideas inside and outside of the discipline) to undergird its research (Engebretso 1997; Holden 1990). The model communities continued to exist (and still do today), but as a smaller fringe interest group, rather than the robust kind of discipline-wide conversation that they had once represented. The outcome is that most nurse scholars now pay very little attention to models as a legacy of nursing thinking. In educational programmes, where nursing theory courses involving in-depth study of multiple models were once a requisite component of all graduate education in nursing, today's newer scholars are more likely to be exposed to a different menu of ideas underpinning the discipline. The models as a whole still take up a chapter in introductory nursing textbooks and some (especially Rogers and Parse) continue to have communities of dedicated followers. But for the most part, they reside as an uncomfortable part of nursing's history, best forgotten and not particularly relevant to the ideas that are shaping the discipline today.

Why bother with nursing theories today?

While it is tempting to discredit the messy history of the nursing theory movement as an embarrassing intellectual departure with no particular relevance for the discipline today, I take a more charitable view and find considerable material within the works of many of the nursing theorists for helping us reflect on the profoundly interesting philosophical questions that continue to shape disciplinary thinking. From my perspective, these early theorists could not have fully appreciated the explicitly philosophical nature of their work, caught up as they were within the scientific advancement of the discipline that seemed so necessary to support the profession. In finding their way out from under the heavy dominance of medical science within health care, they sought legitimacy in alternative forms of science, particularly drawing upon the social sciences. And they worked hard to try to model out what it is that constituted the nature and structure of the discipline they loved within those terms. Some of the peculiar language they advocated within the application of their various conceptual models was explicitly chosen for the purpose of being so different from the typical languages of other disciplines within health care, helping nurses to understand that their profession held a distinctive social mandate and role within health care. They succeeded, within a time of rapid change and progress in health care education and administration, to take ownership of how nursing was taught, managed and enacted. Their aspirations were enormous, and their sincere commitment to the cause unquestionable. And although the body of scholarly work they developed in the interest of these aspirations and commitments may not have grown into the foundation of the profession that they imagined it to become, they did change our sense of the nature of this discipline.

Essentially, the problem they were confronting, and we still confront today, is the incredible complexity of this entity we call nursing. Of course, the nursing theorists lacked the benefit of understanding complexity in the manner we do today, as much of their work predated the 1987 advent of Gleick's *chaos theory* and the resultant development of *complexity science* in moving science beyond simple cause and effect relationships and towards ways of thinking about dynamic and interactive phenomena (Coppa 1993; Ray 1998). Nursing is at once both so straightforward that any child in the playground can explain with a reasonable degree of accuracy what a nurse is and does, and also so inherently complex that it defies operational definition in any form that satisfies the remarkable diversity of thought and action that go on in the name of the profession across roles, settings and contexts. The problem of defining nursing's unique mandate and function within health care continues to vex the profession and creates a pressing problem in the context of ongoing challenges with respect to national and global nursing workforce planning (as the COVID-19 pandemic has so graphically demonstrated). Our professional associations and policy bodies continue to have to keep a close eye on who is making decisions that affect nursing, and on what assumptive bases they are making those decisions. And despite our ongoing best efforts to explain nursing in that wider domain, to communicate the contributions nursing can, does and ought to be making to the health of our nations, we continue to face this central problem of capturing the essence of the discipline and its distinctive knowledge and skills.

The conceptual model builders we refer to as nurse theorists were not trained philosophers but were attempting to engage in essentially philosophical work within a world in which science was the prevailing paradigm. And if we think of their work in this manner, and sidestep the parts that reflect the consequent derailment, I believe that we can find much of current value to our ongoing efforts to wrestle with the deeper ontological and epistemological questions with which nursing is faced. What is the essential nature of nursing? What aspects transcend all cases and contexts in which nursing is so differently practised? How might we articulate the distinctive angle of vision that nursing brings to health care and patient care? And what is that delicate balance between respect for persons and the desire to intervene?

One of the most important contributions that I believe nurse theorists gave us was the sense of certainty that a distinctive angle of vision on "the person" was central to our discipline. Although it may well be that this angle of vision is better represented in variations suited to our different practice contexts than to being conceptualized within a singular conceptual framework emphasizing basic human needs, or adaptation, or system equilibrium for example, the idea that we "see" the person or persons under our care differently than do our colleagues in other disciplines is of fundamental importance to our continuing future (Taylor, Lynn & Bartlett 2018). Nursing's function is typically incredibly interdisciplinary (we take on functions of other disciplines during the hours they are not on duty, for example), and it requires that we know something of how all of the other disciplines are viewing the person so that we can mediate and navigate through the health care system on behalf of that person. But that aspect in which we are the disciplinary expert is and always has been rather invisible (beyond the task functions) to our interdisciplinary colleagues. Because of this, we are far too often still seen as the "housekeepers" of health care, necessary but not that exciting or expert, operating at the invisible margins of the truly important work. In this deeply and systemically embedded culture of health care, the need to be able to advocate for what we know persons need and deserve, and to create systems of nursing care in which they can attain their best possible outcomes, we need language and context and structure to try to embed nursing solidly and strongly into the way operations function. In order to keep that policy voice of the profession alive and functional, we will need to maintain a strong focus on the concept of person.

Person-centred care has become a watchword in health care across the spectrum – an objective of the patient advocacy movement and something that has now been recognized as essential by governments, health administrations and many disciplines. This is the modern linguistic framing of what the nursing theorists were attempting to articulate – that idea of how we can keep a strong focus of attention on the individual as he or she engages with our discipline and the wider health world in the business of seeking health. In order that we do not fall prey to the more simplistic interpretations of what person-centred care might entail (patient representatives on health boards, patient satisfaction surveys, use of patient-reported outcome measures in our clinical trials), we need thoughtful philosophizing about how nursing can and should be conceptualizing personhood, and ensuring that whatever else we do is also preserving it. Further, we need to retain a sense of that personhood as both patterned and diversified, such that as we build general knowledge about people, we can also be increasingly skilled at being attuned to the diversities of persons that justify individualized approaches (Thorne & Sawatzky 2014).

Since the time of the model builders, the idea of social determinants of health has gained purchase across our health care systems and communities. We now fully appreciate that the "causes" of disease and ill health are not limited to the biological kinds of insults that were the central focus of health professions and health care systems of an earlier era. The work done by nurse theorists to try to conceptualize the idea of "environment" as a metaparadigm concept of central concern to nursing has, I believe, directly contributed to the deeply established tradition of nursing's social mandate and comfort with engaging with the social realities that shape health. Nursing has a strong presence in community care and advocacy, in shining a spotlight on the vast array of injustices and inequities that continue to systematically and differentially disadvantage some persons and groups. The early work of our model builders seems to me to have legitimized that massive shift from the idea of nurses as physical care givers to the idea that they are also and always social advocates. The study of how model builders conceptualized that central function therefore seems informative to our current understanding of how we have come to legitimize social engagement as fundamental to responsible care of the person, and how truly individualized care cannot be realized without a critically reflective understanding of the complex social world the person inhabits.

Finally, I reflect on how the work of the model builders has taught us to be intrigued with the idea of health, far beyond the absence of disease and intricately connected with ideas of social context and existential well-being. The philosophical challenge of articulating what it is that drives us, both on behalf of an individual case and also more metaphorically on behalf of the aspirations of all peoples, remains a beacon of light towards which we all strive. Amidst the complexities of ethical reasoning, political strategizing and social engineering, nursing shares a sense of right action that has stood it in good stead across time and space. Ideas such as harm reduction or cultural safety that have revolutionized our practices across multiple contexts depend highly on that capacity for a collective professional understanding of how to work within multiple and competing agendas for a path towards the greater good for individuals as well as communities.

In conclusion, I believe that what the nurse theorists were struggling with remains philosophically interesting as the central challenge of nursing's identity and self-definition. Their collective explorations through ideas such as complexity, personhood, social determinants of health and quality of life (although those precise concepts were not yet available to them) have played an important role in securing the widespread confidence we now recognize within our discipline that nursing represents a distinctive angle of vision and has a powerful role to play in the evolution of health care worldwide. On this basis, I think that the works of this cadre of scholars are well worth ongoing explicitly philosophical consideration as a treasure trove of historical insights into how marvellously complicated and fascinating these fundamentally ontological and epistemological questions can be. Whether the scholars that constitute the next generation of thinkers within our discipline consider their own work as substantive or philosophical in nature, they all stand to benefit from recognizing that the current maturity of conviction nursing displays with respect to very real complexities inherent in our disciplinary mandate rests on a profound intellectual project that absorbed some of the finest minds of its time.

References

Alghase, DL & Whall, AF 1993. Rosemary Ellis' views on the substantive structure of nursing. *Image: Journal of Nursing Scholarship*, vol. 25, no. 1, pp. 79–72.

Alligood, MR 2021. *Nursing theorists and their work* (10th ed.), Mosby, St. Louis, MO.

Barrett, EAM 2002. What is nursing science? *Nursing Science Quarterly*, vol. 15, no. 1, pp. 51–60.

Chinn, PL & Kramer, MK 2019. *Integrated knowledge development in nursing* (10th ed.), Mosby, St. Louis, MO.

Cody, WK 1995. About all those paradigms: Many in the universe, two in nursing. *Nursing Science Quarterly*, vol. 8, pp. 144–147.

Cody, WK 1996. Occult reductionism in the discourse of nursing theory. *Nursing Science Quarterly*, vol. 9, pp. 140–142.

Cody, WK 2000. Paradigm shift or paradigm drift? A meditation on commitment and transcendence. *Nursing Science Quarterly*, vol. 13, no. 2, pp. 93–102.

Cody, WK & Mitchell, GJ 2002. Nursing knowledge and human science revisited: Practical and political considerations. *Nursing Science Quarterly*, vol. 15, no. 1, pp. 4–13. https://doi.org/10.1177/08943180222108705

Coppa, DF 1993. Chaos theory suggests a new paradigm for nursing science. *Journal of Advanced Nursing*, vol. 18, no. 6, pp. 985–991.

Cull-Wilby, BL & Peppin, JI 1987. Towards a coexistence of paradigms in nursing knowledge development. *Journal of Advanced Nursing*, vol. 12, no. 4, pp. 515–521.

Dean, H 1995. Science and practice: The nature of knowledge, in A Omery, CE Kasper & GG Page (eds.), *In search of nursing science*, Sage, Thousand Oaks, CA, pp. 275–290.

Deets, C 1990. Nursing's paradigm and a search for its methodology, in N Chaska (ed.), *The nursing profession: Turning points*, Mosby, St. Louis, MO, pp. 149–154.

Donnelly, E 2001. An assessment of nursing theories as guides to scientific inquiry, in N Chaska (ed.), *The nursing profession: Tomorrow and beyond*, Sage, Thousand Oaks, CA, pp. 331–346.

Ellis, R 1968. Characteristics of significant theories. *Nursing Research*, vol. 17, no. 3, pp. 217–222

Engebretson, J 1997. A multiparadigm approach to nursing. *Advances in Nursing Science*, vol. 20, no. 1, pp. 21–33.

Fawcett, J 1978. The what of theory development, in *Theory development: What, why, and how*, National League for Nursing, New York, pp. 17–33. [Proceedings, Third Nursing Theory Conference, NLN (15–1708)].

Fawcett, J 1980. A framework for analysis and evaluation of conceptual models of nursing. *Nurse Educator*, vol. 5, no. 6, pp. 10–14.

Fawcett, J 1984. The metaparadigm of nursing: Present status and future refinements. *Image: Journal of Nursing Scholarship*, vol. 16, no. 3, pp. 84–87.

Field, PA 1987. The impact of nursing theory on the clinical decision-making process. *Journal of Advanced Nursing*, vol. 12, no. 5, pp. 563–571.

Flaskerud, JH & Halloran, EJ 1980. Areas of agreement in nursing theory development. *Advances in Nursing Science*, vol. 3, no.1, pp. 1–7.

Gleick, J 1987. *Chaos: Making a new science*, Penguin, New York.

Henderson, V 1955. *Harmer and Henderson's textbook of the principles and practice of nursing*, Macmillan, New York.

Henderson, V 1966. *The nature of nursing*, Macmillan, New York

Holden, RJ 1990. Models, muddles and medicine. *International Journal of Nursing Studies*, vol. 27, no. 3, pp. 223–234.

Johnson, DE 1959. A philosophy of nursing. *Nursing Outlook*, vol. 7, no. 4, pp. 198–200.

Johnson, DE 1974. Development of theory: A requisite for nursing as a primary health profession. *Nursing Research*, vol. 23, no. 5, pp. 372–377.

Jones, M 1997. Thinking nursing, in SE Thorne & VE Hayes (eds.), *Nursing praxis: Knowledge and action*, Sage, Thousand Oaks, CA, pp. 125–139.

Kikuchi, J & Simmons, H 1999. Practical nursing judgment: A moderate realist conception. *Scholarly Inquiry for Nursing Practice*, vol. 13, no. 1, pp. 43–55.

Kim, SH 1983. *The nature of theoretical thinking in nursing*, Appleton-Century-Crofts, Norwalk, CT.

Kuhn, TS 1962. *The structure of scientific revolutions*, University of Chicago Press, Chicago.

McKay, R 1969. Theories, models, and systems for nursing. *Nursing Research*, vol. 18, no. 5, pp. 393–400.

Meleis, AI. 2018. *Theoretical nursing: Development and progress* (6th ed.), Wolters Kluwer, Philadelphia, PA.

Nagle, LM & Mitchell, GJ 1991. Theoretic diversity: Evolving paradigmatic issues in research and practice. *Advances in Nursing Science*, vol. 14, no. 1, pp. 17–25.

Newman, MA 1992. Prevailing paradigms in nursing. *Nursing Outlook*, vol. 40, no.1, pp. 10–13, 32.

Nightingale, F 1859/1946. *Notes on nursing: What it is, and what it is not*, Harrison, London. [Reprinted by Lippincott, 1946].

Orem, DE 1971. *Nursing: Concepts of practice*, McGraw Hill, New York.

Orem, DE & Parker, KS 1964. *Nursing content in preservice nursing curriculums*, Catholic University of America Press, Washington, DC.

Orlando, IJ 1961. *The dynamic nurse–patient relationship: Function, process, and principles*, P. Putnam's Sons, New York.

Parse, RR 1981. *Man–living–health: A theory of nursing*, Wiley, New York.

Parse, RR 1987. *Nursing science: Major paradigms, theories, and critiques*, W. B. Saunders, Philadelphia, PA.

Parse, RR 1998. The art of criticism. *Nursing Science Quarterly*, vol. 11, p. 43.

Parse, RR 1999. Theoretical conceptualizations, in RR Parse (ed.), *Illuminations: The human becoming theory in practice and research*, Jones and Bartlett, New York, pp. 5–8.

Parse, RR 2002. Editorial: 15th anniversary celebration. *Nursing Science Quarterly*, vol. 15, no. 1, p. 3.

Peplau, HE 1952. *Interpersonal relations in nursing*, G. P. Putnam's Sons, New York.

Ray, MA 1998. Complexity and nursing science. *Nursing Science Quarterly*, vol. 11, no. 3, pp. 91–93.

Rogers, ME 1970. *An introduction to the theoretical basis of nursing*, F. A. Davis, Philadelphia, PA.

Roy, C 1976. *Introduction to nursing: An adaptation model*, Prentice Hall, Englewood Cliffs, NJ.

Roy, C 1988. An explication of the philosophical assumptions of the Roy Adaptation Model. *Nursing Science Quarterly*, vol. 1, no. 1, pp. 26–34.

Roy, C 2009. *The Roy adaptation model* (3rd ed.), Prentice Hall Health, Upper Saddle River, NJ.

Taylor, C, Lynn, P & Bartlett, JL 2018. *Fundamentals of nursing: The art and science of person-centered care* (9th ed.), Wolters Kluwer, Philadelphia, PA.

Thorne, S 2001. People and their parts: Deconstructing the debates in theorizing nursing's clients. *Nursing Philosophy*, vol. 2, pp. 259–262.

Thorne, S, Canam, C, Dahinten, S, Hall, W, Henderson, A & Kirkham, SR 1998. Nursing's metaparadigm concepts: Disimpacting the debates. *Journal of Advanced Nursing*, vol. 27, no. 6, pp. 1257–1268.

Thorne, S, Reimer Kirkham, S & Henderson, A 1999. Ideological implications of paradigm discourse in nursing research, education and practice theory. *Nursing Inquiry*, vol. 6, pp. 123–131.

Thorne, S & Sawatzky, R 2014. Particularizing the general: Sustaining theoretical integrity in the context of an evidence-based practice agenda. *Advances in Nursing Science*, vol. 37, no. 1, pp. 5–18.

Travelbee, J 1971. *Interpersonal aspects of nursing*, F. A. Davis, Philadelphia, PA.

Yura, H & Torres, G 1975. Today's conceptual frameworks within baccalaureate nursing programs. *National League for Nursing Publications*, vol. 15–1558, pp. 17–25.

4 Philosophy of science and nursing research

Robyn Bluhm

In the foreword to a recent edited volume on nursing theory, Michael Traynor notes:

> I do wonder whether whole generations of nurse researchers, educators and prac-
> titioners have been put off theory by the way in which the profession approaches
> theory-building from the 1960s to, approximately, the 1980s. Instead of teams
> driven by curiosity about puzzling events working to develop explanations, it seems
> that a handful of nurses in prominent, mainly U.S., university positions looked
> at established academic disciplines and noticed they that they had theories. They
> started to put it about that if we too had theories, people would have to take us
> seriously. Cue decades of obscure elaboration of facile ideas alongside the frankly
> bizarre. Cue a million headaches as credulous nurses worldwide are encouraged to
> 'use' these theories to help organize patient care.
>
> (2017, p. xii)

As a philosopher of science, I can't comment on how accurate Traynor's description is of
the impact of "theory" on nursing education and practice. I do, however, think that to
the extent to which it is accurate, it is the result not just of nursing theorists' "elaboration of ideas", but also of the understanding of theories that they adopted (and adapted)
from then-contemporary philosophy of science. Moreover, if the goal is to use theories
(or at least the results of research) in patient care, nurse researchers may find more recent
trends in philosophy of science more useful. Specifically, in the past couple of decades,
philosophers of science have emphasized the importance of scientific models, as well as
or instead of theories, and have paid increasing attention to scientific practice. In this
chapter, I provide an overview of the logical empiricist approach to science and its influence on nursing theory. In doing so, I draw on work by a number of philosophers and
nurses, including Silva and Rothbart (1984), Suppe and colleagues (Lenz et al. 1995,
1997; Suppe and Jacox 1985), and Risjord (2010), to show how logical empiricism has
influenced – not always for the good – nursing scholars' conceptualization of theories. I
then discuss recent work by Risjord (2010, 2019) and Bender (2018) that argues for the
importance of models for nursing research. In the final section of this chapter, I further
develop this work on models to emphasize the importance of attending to the practice
of modelling.

Current nursing theory has its roots in mid-20th-century attempts to establish nursing
as an academic discipline with a specialized knowledge base. The goal of establishing a
unique knowledge base for nursing was driven by several related issues: delineating the
scope of nursing's professional activities; developing nursing education; and legitimating

DOI: 10.4324/9781003427407-5

nursing as a profession. Early books and journal articles addressed all three of these issues. Risjord (2010) distinguishes among three kinds of nursing research publications during the 1950s and early 1960s. First were studies examining the role and responsibilities of nurses and the nature of nursing education. These studies were effectively sociological studies of nurses, rather than research on the practice or the science of nursing. Second, over time, more studies were published that "either examined the effectiveness of nursing interventions or proposed a useful way of approaching nursing problems" (p. 11). These theories can be understood as what Dickoff and James (1968) call "situation-producing theories" – they are theories designed to help to achieve a (nursing) goal, rather than simply to make predictions or to explain a phenomenon. Third were systematic works that had several aims, the analysis of nurse-patient interactions, the explication of the role of nurses and the process of nursing, and the articulation of the nature of nursing itself: "what was special, important, or essential to, nursing" (Risjord 2010, p. 11). This last category of nursing scholarship provided a number of different conceptual frameworks for nursing as a practice that are still influential. As nursing scholars were increasingly influenced by philosophy of science, in part because of their need to characterize the nursing role and academic nursing education, their understanding of the latter two kinds of research changed.

Logical empiricism and nursing theory

Philosophy of science during the mid-20th century was characterized by a consensus regarding a number of issues, including the structure of scientific theories, the relationship between different areas of scientific research, and the centrality of laws to scientific explanation. As the name of this consensus – logical empiricism – indicates, philosophers of this era were interested in the logical structure of theories, rather than in the practical details of how they were developed and tested. The actual process of doing science was viewed as a matter for historians and sociologists, rather than for philosophers. Putting this point somewhat differently, philosophy was concerned with the justification of theories, not with how they were discovered. A philosophical approach to some area of science therefor involved developing a "rational reconstruction" of an area of science, "a logical substitute rather than real processes" (Reichenbach 1938, p. 5).

Viewed from this logical perspective, theories are sets of sentences, and they are justified when appropriate logical relationships exist among the set of sentences that comprise the theory. Because this view of theories focuses on logical relations among the sentences of the theory, it is known as the syntactic view. Philosophers also often refer to it as the "received view". In addition, within a scientific domain, theories were held to exist at different levels of abstraction. "Higher" level theories are more abstract and make more general claims about a phenomenon, while "lower" level theories are derived in part from these higher level theories, and also contain more specific information about the domain the theories cover that shows how the theory applies in particular circumstances. How this works can more easily be seen in the context of the logical empiricist account of explanation, which has the same logical structure as the account of theories. On this "covering law" or "deductive-nomological" view, explanations are deductive arguments that consist of an explanandum, which describes the event or phenomenon to be explained, and an explanans, which consists of sentences that deductively entail the explanandum and that includes at least one scientific law, plus sentences with additional contextual information related to the phenomenon or event, such as descriptions of antecedent conditions. Scientific laws were explained the same way, with more abstract, general laws featuring in the explanans and explaining lower-level laws.

At the lowest level, theories were understood to make testable empirical claims, which means that the sentences that made up a theory needed language that "linked" the theory to the world. This was accomplished by including observation terms in the theory that were defined by how they related to observable, sensory properties of objects (e.g., "hot", "red", or "large"). Claims about theoretical concepts used in the sentences of the theory must, in order to be meaningful, be logically translatable to claims about observable sensory properties. Leaving aside some important criticisms of this idea (see Risjord 2010, pp. 110–112 for an overview of these), stipulating that the *meaning* of theoretical terms must be given in terms of their observational consequences, raised problems in accounting for changes in theories over time, including extending the theory to cover new concepts and laws. The inability of the received view of theories to account for theory development and change is perhaps unsurprising, given the logical empiricists' initial focus on theory justification; however, as interest grew in scientific discovery and in the historical development of science, alternatives to the received view were developed. I will return to this point below.

The influence of logical empiricism can be seen in nursing scholarship from about the mid-1960s to the mid-1970s. Mark Risjord (2010) shows that a number of nursing papers and textbooks from this time either explicitly cited philosophers who accepted the logical empiricist view of theories or used ideas and terminology that echoed the received view[1] (see also Silva and Rothbart 1986). Of particular note are two papers published in 1974, by Jacox and by Hardy, that articulate similar approaches to the development of theory in nursing. Hardy echoes the logical empiricists' grounding of theories in observable phenomena, when she describes concepts as "labels, categories, or selected properties of objects to be studied" and says that they are "the bricks from which theories are constructed" (1974, p. 100). Jacox emphasizes the hierarchical building of theories on these observable foundations, with more abstract theories being connected to observables through logical relationships among concepts (p. 3). Note, though, that Jacox and Hardy both emphasize the *construction* of theories, not just their logical analysis. That is, they draw on the logical empiricist' understanding of how scientific theories are justified, but apply it in the process of theory development, which (as I noted earlier) the logical empiricists themselves viewed as outside of the concerns of philosophy.

Over time, discussions of the hierarchical nature of nursing theories settled on a description of three broad kinds of theories: grand theories (a term taken from sociology) were abstract descriptions of the basic concepts of nursing; practice theories were intended to provide guidance in specific nursing situations; and middle-range theories (also a sociological term) were to bridge the gap between the two other levels. Although different scholars use different terminologies, use the same terms slightly differently, or add additional levels to the hierarchy, this basic structure was broadly accepted. Moreover, acceptance of this understanding of theories, and the relationships among them, meant that logical empiricism continued to shape nursing research during the remainder of the 1970s and the 1980s. In the next section, I draw on work by Risjord (2010) and by Silva and Rothbart (1984) to outline two ways in which adherence to the tenets of logical empiricism shaped, and even distorted, continuing discussions in the nursing literature, by leading nurses to reinterpret earlier work in nursing theory. Recall that early nursing research included, in addition to discussion of nursing theory, the development of conceptual frameworks and studies designed to inform nursing practice. As nursing knowledge increasingly came to be understood as involving a hierarchy of theories, the way in which these two kinds of work were understood changed to fit this hierarchy.

Reinterpreting conceptual frameworks and research on nursing practice

One way in which logical empiricism distorted the nursing literature was in shaping the continuing development of conceptual frameworks for nursing. This was one of the earliest areas of nursing scholarship and represented efforts to delineate the scope of nursing practice and to clarify the values and goals that shaped this practice, an understanding of this work that Risjord (2010) describes as the *orientation* picture of conceptual frameworks.[2] By expressing the fundamental goals and values that guide nursing research and practice, conceptual frameworks orient nurses to the discipline. This use is reflected in the fact that the developers of early conceptual frameworks were explicitly motivated by their experiences as educators and the need to teach students how to think like nurses. These early works were not conceived of as theories. For example, in an interview on her work, Hildegard Peplau described it as providing a set of concepts or a framework that could be applied in different nursing situations, but denied that it was a nursing theory (Peplau 1983, cited in Suppe and Jacox, pp. 243–4).

As the ideas of logical empiricism became more influential, however, conceptual frameworks were increasingly understood as being grand theories of nursing and therefore sources from which middle-range, testable, theories could be deduced. Risjord calls this the *abstraction* view of conceptual frameworks, on which conceptual frameworks express "the fundamental concepts of a theory" (Risjord, p. 174). Nurses who accepted this abstraction view interpreted the work of early nursing theorists such as Peplau and Orlando, not as articulating models of nursing's goals and values, but as providing abstract theories that could be used to derive lower-level, testable theories. Similarly, Silva and Rothbart note that even as late as the early 1970s, the conceptual framework literature continued to develop separately from the literature on the nature of nursing theories. But by the later 1970s, some authors were revising work they had published earlier in the decade and altering their terminology so that it was more congruent with logical empiricist metatheory, using terms such as "concept" and "proposition" in developing their frameworks.

Despite the fact that the orientation and the abstraction pictures of conceptual models are incompatible, Risjord notes that they are often conflated. Not all nursing theorists distinguished between theories and conceptual frameworks, using the terms "grand theory", "conceptual model", and "conceptual framework" interchangeably (p. 173). He further shows that regardless of terminology, they are often described in terms that reflect both the orientation and the abstraction picture. This conflation is important because conceptual frameworks (understood on the orientation view) and theories are intended to serve different purposes and should therefore be evaluated differently. Suppe and Jacox (1985) emphasize that conceptual frameworks are not empirically testable, but rather "provide a perspective from which specific theories or hypotheses are developed and evaluated" (p. 249). While theories are evaluated based on their empirical adequacy, conceptual models are evaluated only in part on the basis of the adequacy of the theories they give rise to.

A second way in which the continuing influence of logical empiricism has shaped nursing research is in the literature on middle-range theories. Reflecting the logical empiricists' hierarchy of theories, middle-range theories are understood as being derived from grand theories. Risjord notes that during the 1990s, appeal to middle-range theories became extremely popular as a way of developing theories that would be useful for nursing practice, and that discussion of these theories has continued to view them as a way of connecting grand theory with nursing practice. However, he argues, this framing of the role of middle-range theories misinterprets a major contribution of the paper that "is routinely cited as the origin of the middle-range theory movement" (p. 142). The paper, "Collaborative development of a middle-range theories: toward a theory of unpleasant symptoms" (Lenz et al. 1995) actually proposed middle-range theories as a *replacement for*, rather than a *supplement to*, grand theory. The authors "recast the definition of middle range theories" (Lenz et al., p. 3), "divorcing" it from its positivist origins, by saying that the defining feature of a middle-range theory is that the entities of the theory (and the relationships among them) can be defined and measured. Risjord notes that this understanding of middle-range theories aligns them with the semantic view of theories, a philosophical successor to the syntactic view of theories that focuses on the content, rather just on than the form (or syntax) of a theory (Risjord 2010, p. 142; see also Risjord 2019). I will say more about this in the following section.

In summary, nursing scholarship has been, and continues to be, influenced by logical empiricism. When a nursing literature emerged that addressed questions about the scope of nursing and the nature of nursing knowledge, it included conceptual frameworks that specified the nature and goals of nursing, as well as research that was directly relevant to nursing practice. However, as the literature became increasingly shaped by discussions of the nature of nursing theory, it was assumed that both conceptual frameworks and theories relevant to practice would fit into a hierarchy of theories that resembled logical empiricism's received view.

Theories – and models – after logical empiricism

A number of authors have remarked on the irony of the fact that, just as nurses were beginning to look to logical empiricism for guidance on developing nursing theories, philosophers were coming to reject this approach to philosophy of science. To some extent, more recent developments in philosophy of science have been taken up by nursing theorists, but there is no single approach that has a similarly strong influence. In this section, I discuss work in philosophy of science that replaced the logical empiricists' syntactic view of theories, including the semantic view briefly mentioned above, and the increasingly vibrant and diverse work on the use of models in science. I then show how this work has been taken up by Risjord (2010, 2019) and Bender (2018) in the context of philosophy of nursing.

As problems with the received view of theories became increasingly apparent, philosophers of science began to develop alternative accounts of scientific knowledge. The concept of a model is central to many of these accounts. Scientific models, as we shall see, are notoriously diverse in form and function. Daniela Bailer-Jones suggests that, despite this diversity, the core feature of a model is that it "is an interpretive description of a phenomenon that facilitates access to that phenomenon" (1999, p. 108). Similarly, Risjord suggests that, "[t]o understand something as a model is to emphasize the way it represents different elements of a system working together to produce a larger phenomenon" (2019, p. 3).

One way that philosophers have developed the idea of a model has been to retain the formal or mathematical structure of theories (as understood on the received view), but to supplement syntactic theories with a semantic interpretation – a model – that connects the logical structure of the theory with the world. This approach reflects the relationship between theories and models found in logic: a theory is "a set of sentences in a formal language", while a model "is a structure…that makes all sentences of a theory true when its symbols are interpreted as referring to objects, relations, or functions of a structure" (Frigg and Hartmann 2020). This "semantic view" of theories was often adopted by philosophers who focus on highly mathematical sciences (especially physics), but has also been developed in Suppe and colleagues' work on middle-range theories in nursing, described above.

More promising for nursing research is a second way of developing the idea of a model, which takes formal logical or mathematical models to be just one kind of model – one way of providing an interpretive description of a phenomenon of interest. On this account, models can take the form of physical objects (such as scale models or model organisms), diagrams or graphs, computer simulations, or analogies, in addition to mathematical models. Although this broader range of kinds of model can be paired with the traditional view of theories as formal structures (Craver 2002; Winther 2021), increasingly philosophers of science interested in the use of scientific models accept what Rasmus Winther calls the "pragmatic view" of theories, which, among other things, takes theories to be (at least in part) non-formal, to be continuous with scientific practice, and to (like models) take a plurality of forms.

This brief overview of models, and their role in contemporary philosophy of science, provides useful context for recent discussions of the role of models in nursing research. Both Mark Risjord (2010, 2019) and Miriam Bender (2018) have argued that nursing philosophy should focus on models, rather than on theories. Risjord builds on work by Frederic Suppe and colleagues to show that middle-range theories, on their account, are best understood as models, while Bender draws on recent work in philosophy of science (including by Craver and his colleagues) that views models as mechanisms.

Risjord (2019) has argued that middle-range theories should be understood as models – not because they are derived from higher level theories to mediate between the theory and the phenomenon to be explained, but because they meet the characteristic he sees as definitive of a model; they "are representations of how and why a phenomenon arises" (p. 3). This understanding is achieved by addressing three questions: (1) "What is the phenomenon modelled?" (2) "What are the elements of the model?" and (3) "What are the relations among the elements?" (p. 7). Bender also emphasizes that models aim to describe and explain the dynamic nature of the phenomenon being modelled, as opposed to theories which consist of static descriptions of concepts and the relationships among them.

Another important characteristic of models is that they require selection of which features of a phenomenon to model. Scientists will not generally try to incorporate all aspects of the phenomenon of interest in a model, as that would make it too unwieldy to work with. Instead, they simplify the phenomenon by incorporating only the elements and characteristics that are of particular interest. Because of this, Risjord argues, models have both epistemic and pragmatic components. Like a map, which portrays only some features of the terrain it represents, models can be evaluated separately on the question of whether they are accurate (do they adequately represent the terrain or phenomenon?) and the question of whether they are useful (do they do what the user needs them to do?). The London Tube map, for example, achieves its pragmatic ends despite very low accuracy. (It needs only to be accurate about the relative order of the stations on a line and the location of transfer points between lines.)

For models developed in health care research, both the epistemic and the pragmatic dimensions of a model are judged in large part by how well they guide the development of interventions. The nursing "terrain" has to be modelled accurately enough to facilitate the pragmatic aim of helping patients. Both Bender and Risjord argue that models are more closely connected to practice than are theories, so they can provide guidance as to how to intervene in the kind of situation being modelled. Bender also cites Risjord's (2010) discussion of the theory of unpleasant symptoms, and points out that the developers of that work claim that including multiple factors in their theory/model makes it "particularly valuable for individualizing interventions to fit the patient's characteristics and unique patterns of symptoms" (Lenz et al. 1997, p. 23; cited in Bender 2018, p. 7). In the final section of this chapter, I expand on this idea by connecting the work of Lenz et al. (1995, 1997) with another important development in philosophy of science – an increasing focus on scientific practice.

From models to modelling – the importance of practice

Philosophers of science have only quite recently considered the epistemic importance of understanding scientific practice. Recall that the logical empiricists viewed scientific practice as the province of historians and sociologists: they focused on the context of justification, not the context of discovery. Beginning with Kuhn, philosophers began to pay attention to the history of science, and for the past couple of decades, they have increasingly studied the actual work of *doing* science – the experimental techniques and methodological choices made by scientists. The models and mechanisms emphasized by Risjord and Bender are the results (or, more accurately, are works-in-progress) of these practices.

In their discussion of the usefulness of middle-range theories for nursing research and practice, Lenz et al. (1995) do not just provide a description of the theory. Because their paper aims not just to introduce the theory of unpleasant symptoms, but also to show how it can serve as a model for the development of middle-range theories, they describe their scientific process in some detail. Because of this, we have some insight into the building of their theory/model, including the motivation for various choices they made.

Overall, they suggest that developing middle-range theories requires, first, "descriptors" of relevant phenomena that are precise enough to make them "measurable or objectively codable" (p. 4). Next, regularities between the descriptions are identified and must be precise enough to enable the regularities to be used to guide nursing practice. With regard to the development of descriptors, Lenz et al. show how early works contributing to the theory involved developing a description of dyspnea. An initial understanding of the phenomenon was developed through reviewing the existing literature, which suggested that dyspnea has various dimensions (including, similar to pain, psychological, and physiological aspects) and that it is not correlated with pulmonary function. These studies, however, were intended to elucidate the physiological mechanisms of dyspnea and so used induced dyspnea – which did not accurately reflect actual patients' experiences. The investigators therefore conducted a study designed to compare individual patients' experiences during periods of dyspnea to their experiences when not dyspneic, and finally returned to the literature to contextualize and interpret their empirical results. The outcome of this part of the research was a multi-faceted concept of dyspnea, formulated in such a way as to facilitate intervention on each of the components. A similar process was undertaken in (initially separate) work done to understand fatigue during childbearing, with initial reviews of the literature being combined with qualitative interviews, clinical observation, and a quantitative questionnaire.

Once these descriptions were developed, the investigators noticed similarities in the ways in which dyspnea and fatigue had been conceptualized, as well as in factors that could precipitate or exacerbate these symptoms, and the symptoms' effect on patients' lives and activities. Comparison also led to further refinement of both concepts and, ultimately, the development of an initial theory (model) to guide further research. A second paper published two years later provided an update on the theory: for example, the relationships among precipitating factors, symptoms, and the effects of symptoms had been further refined to model feedback among the three kinds of variables.

The paper also describes a study in which the theory, the nurse-researchers' clinical experience, and prior research were used to develop an intervention to help new mothers who were having difficulty breastfeeding their infants. Because both pain and fatigue are common during this period, the theory was used to identify an array of factors (e.g., lack of rest, depression, and lack of support) that might contribute to the symptoms. The intervention developed based on the theory was also multi-faceted, enabling nurses to address situational or psychological factors influencing the symptoms, as well as the symptoms themselves, as required to help a particular patient. In other words, the model was complex enough to incorporate the wide variety of potentially relevant factors, but also depicted the relationships among these factors in ways that allowed isolation of the factors that were most relevant in a particular case. In Risjord's terms, above, the model had both epistemic and pragmatic values: it both tells us about the nature of the phenomenon being modelled and provides guidance for alleviating unpleasant symptoms.

Attending to the practice of modelling draws our attention to a number of important features of the scientific process: the need for a variety of research methods; the crucial contribution of clinical experience; the way previous literature informs, but does not determine, the research; and the importance of collaboration. It therefore leads to a better understanding of science, one that is more useful for both philosophers and nursing researchers than could be obtained by thinking about science knowledge as a monolith of theories.

Notes

1 He also argues that these influences can still be seen in contemporary nursing texts.
2 Risjord mainly uses the term "conceptual models", but because of the extensive discussion of models later in this chapter, I will use the synonym "conceptual frameworks".

References

Bailer-Jones, D.M. (1999) Tracing the development of models in the philosophy of science. In *Model-Based Reasoning in Scientific Discovery*, Ed. Lorenzo Magnani, Nancy J. Nersessian, and Paul Thagard. New York: Springer, pp. 23–40.

Bender, M. (2018) Models versus theories as a primary carrier of nursing knowledge: A philosophical argument. *Nursing Philosophy* 19(1): e12198.

Craver, C.F. (2002) Structures of scientific theories. In *The Blackwell Guide to the Philosophy of Science*, Ed. P. Machamer, M. Silberstein. New York: Wiley and Sons, pp. 55–79.

Dickoff, J., James, P. (1968) A theory of theories: A position paper. *Nursing Research* 17(3): 197–203.

Frigg, R., Hartmann, S. (2020) Models in science. In *The Stanford Encyclopedia of Philosophy*, Ed. Edward N. Zalta. URL = <https://plato.stanford.edu/archives/spr2020/entries/models-science/>.

Hardy, M.E. (1974) Theories: components, development, evaluation. *Nursing Research* 23(2): 100–107.

Jacox, A. (1974) Theory construction in nursing: An overview. *Nursing Research* 23(1): 4–13.

Lenz, E.R., Suppe, F., Pugh, L.C., Milligan, R.A. (1995) Collaborative development of middle-range theories: Toward a theory of unpleasant symptoms. *Advances in Nursing Science* 17(3): 1–13.

Lenz, E.R., Pugh, L.C., Milligan, R.A., Gift, A., Suppe, Frederick. (1997) The middle-range theory of unpleasant symptoms: An update. *Advances in Nursing Science* 19(3): 14–27.

Reichenbach, H. (1938) *Experience and Prediction: An Analysis of the Foundations and Structure of Knowledge.* Chicago: University of Chicago Press.

Risjord, M. (2010) *Nursing Knowledge: Science, Practice, and Philosophy.* West Sussex: Wiley-Blackwell.

Risjord, M. (2019) Middle-range theories as models: New criteria for analysis and evaluation. *Nursing Philosophy* 20(1): e12225.

Silva, M.C., Rothbart, D. (1984) An analysis of changing trends in philosophies of science on nursing theory development. *Advances in Nursing Science* January: 1–13.

Suppe F., Jacox, A.K. (1985) Philosophy of science and the development of nursing theory. *Annual Review of Nursing Research* 3(1): DOI: 10.1891/0739–6686.3.1.241.

Traynor, M. (2017) Foreword. In *Social Theory and Nursing Theory*, Ed. M. Lipscomb. Abingdon: Routledge, pp. x–xii.

Winther, R.G. (2021) The structure of scientific theories. In *The Stanford Encyclopedia of Philosophy*, Ed. Edward N. Zalta, <https://plato.stanford.edu/archives/spr2021/entries/structure-scientific-theories/>.

5 What is the art in the art and science of nursing?

Graham McCaffrey

Good nursing practice demands scientific knowledge and technical skills, and a capacity to respond with attention to the outlook and concerns of each individual person in need of care. This combination is often bundled up into the catch-all "art and science of nursing," but that capacity to be open to others and respond to them in deliberate, therapeutic ways does not just happen. Hidden in the so-called "art" of nursing, there is a world of skills and knowledge that can be articulated and put to use in nursing practice, education, and research. Doing so demands careful, intentional sounding out of how arts and humanities constitute a vital dimension of nursing. This chapter is an introduction to dimensions of how arts and humanities are necessary to fully understand and value the recognition of human experience that is so crucial to humane nursing practice.

The "art and science of nursing" is a conventional term, both over-used and under-used; over-used as a shortcut to get to a sense of different kinds of knowledge and experience at play in nursing practice, and under-used as a gateway to thinking through the possibilities of the "art" side of the equation. The coupled term reflects a genuine challenge to capture the epistemological basis of nursing. There is an epistemological plurality that is intrinsic to nursing knowledge (McCaffrey, 2021). Scientific knowledge by itself is not sufficient to conduct good nursing practice; yet, good nursing practice is impossible without it; likewise, responsive awareness to other people's circumstances and interests is vital to good nursing practice, but by itself could be nice but useless to its recipient. Against this background of epistemological plurality, in this chapter, I will look more closely at the art side of the equation.

In this chapter, I focus on art as forms of human creativity and reconnect it with humanities, to encompass a related set of fields of knowledge and practices, mediums of expression, and disciplines that we can decide may or may not have useful applications for nursing knowledge. I look again at the common idea in nursing of art-as-practice-in-motion and suggest how enactivist thinking can help to put flesh on the ephemeral. Finally, I come back to the coupling of art and science.

Arts and humanities

Art in its endless variety is a constant of human cultures. It contains a multitude of ways in which people strive to make sense of their world to themselves, to each other, and to their societies. Art is one of humanity's best ways of reflecting upon itself, seeking, claiming, affirming, disputing meaning. Meaning for human beings is in practice a profusion of

DOI: 10.4324/9781003427407-6

multiple meanings, constantly in play with each other, changing through time, and bound up with human passions and purposes.

Arts and humanities are commonly bracketed together as overlapping realms of attention. Approximately, the arts are primary forms of expression, whereas the humanities are scholarly disciplines, some of which are concerned with arts directly, like literary studies. Other humanities disciplines, such as philosophy or history, have their own modes of expression and creativity through language, as well as codes of factual reference and logical analysis. Unlike the tense pairing of arts and sciences, arts and humanities are associated as a connected range of fields of meaning mapping and making.

With regard to nursing, arts and humanities fit under the broad interdisciplinary field of health humanities (Crawford et al., 2015). Health humanities has evolved out of medical humanities, itself a subset of medical education sustained by doctors who recognize the place of arts and humanities in connecting medical knowledge with human experience, diagnosis with illness, or treatment with healing. Medical and now health humanities, however, have largely bypassed nursing in its disciplinary singularity. Meanwhile, nursing for its part has elided the full potential of the arts and humanities in its embrace first of nursing grand theory, then of the amorphous "art and science" of nursing.

Art and nursing: examples from literature

Art forms can bring us into other people's worlds in an immediate sense, even across vast spaces of time, geography, and culture. Art bridges spaces between people. It is communicative and relational. By itself, that does not necessarily mean that experiences of art lead directly to compassionate attitudes, let alone actions, as is sometimes claimed. Art itself can evoke an empathetic response that need not translate into empathy towards others in real life. However, what art can do is expose us to otherness as an ineluctable quality of social life. Otherness can be received as identification or as awareness of difference, or both at once. It is an exposure to the relational open-endedness that is constantly mobilized in nursing practice. To that extent, art has a useful and important role to play in self-understanding and transmission of what it is to do nursing.

Here is one example of exposure to otherness from literature. I have used poetry, partly because literary work is easier to discuss in a written chapter and because among all art forms, I am most drawn to and most familiar with poetry. Other art forms, including visual arts, music, or theatre, all evoke connection and response according to their own range of expressive means.

Walt Whitman in a series of poems about his time as an orderly during the American Civil War used lyrical concentration to describe his own tactile experience with wounded soldiers as they presented themselves to him. In his poems, he captures the exposure of nurses to others' pain and trauma, purposefulness amidst pain, unique personal responses within a society-level crisis, and for all that, the fleetingness of compassionate connection as the wound dresser moves from wounded soldier to wounded soldier.

From the stump of the arm, the amputated hand,
I undo the clotted lint, remove the slough, wash off the matter and blood,
Back on his pillow the soldier bends with curv'd neck and side falling head,
His eyes are closed, his face is pale, he dares not look on the bloody stump,
And has not yet look'd on it.

(Whitman, 2005, p. 263)

If there is a theory practice gap, then Whitman sutures together its edges in a way that has its place in nursing thought at least as much as theoretical papers or studies.

There is some affinity between poetry that evokes moments of intense experience and attempts by phenomenological researchers to get at experience. These are not phenomenological accounts although they do convey experience vividly and immediately, cutting across time and space. Arguably, poetry exceeds the limits of phenomenology with its obligations towards academic coolness. Tu Fu (2020) says something about what it is like to be a refugee that lends insight into a nurse in Manchester, Toronto, or Warsaw caring for a patient from Syria, Somalia, or Ukraine. Whitman economically presents a compacted moment of practice that includes observation, action, and assessment as well as vivid presentness.

Examples of contemporary literary works represent nursing by nurses in the form of memoirs. Christie Watson (2018) and Molly Case (2019) from the UK and Tilda Shalof (2005) from Canada have written vivid accounts of their nursing practice which convey how expert skills and knowledge are folded into each human situation, evoking ethical decision making, team relationships, and affective life. Stretching literary genres to include comics, MK Czerwiec (2017) wrote and drew a book-length account of working on an HIV/AIDS unit through the most difficult period of the AIDS epidemic.

Art bridges inner human experience and shared worlds. It can render us recognizable to each other and introduce us to experiences in their otherness. But if we see something new and understand the world differently, then we may have a greater repertoire of response. None of this is inevitable, nor does it determine which responses are going to be good responses, without other criteria such as ethics and evidence of clinical effectiveness. Art lends itself to seeing the complicatedness of things, which can, in turn, lead to humility in the face of complexity.

The art of nursing: aesthetics

The "art of nursing" has been complicated by the related term "aesthetics" famously introduced as one of Carper's (1978) four ways of knowing. Aesthetics for her is the personal. This is confusing since the conventional meaning has to do with beauty, with harmonious balance, in appearances or sounds, especially in relation to works of art. Etymologically, in Greek, it meant the science of sensory perceptions.

Gadamer (2004) retrieved aesthetics from its limited sense of refined taste to convey something closer to its original meaning, as a felt change in one's sense of the world in response to a work of art. He used artworks and our response to them as a starting point for his account of hermeneutics, or interpretation as a fundamental mode of human life. He argued that art is not a rarefied part of life that we may visit once in a while, but is more like a prism through which aspects of life are refracted in ways that give us a connection to life with a sense of immediacy, such that we can be changed by encounters with art; our horizon of how we see the world can be altered.

At best, there may be beauty in nursing in some limited sense, such as a gracefully achieved dressing change or a well-composed moment of connection, but it feels like this is straining to find the aesthetic in any strict sense. Gadamer's argument is helpful insofar as it is one of the building blocks of his phenomenology of understanding, of interpretation as an integral part of human engagement in the world. Not only artworks, but encounters with others as patients, family members, or colleagues have their effects on us just as we contribute our own effects in a constant dialectic of call and response. New knowledge and ideas too are not merely acquired but subtly affect our horizons (to borrow a Gadamerian metaphor) on the world, changing how we see as well as what we know.

Aesthetics in its original meaning points to the work of the senses, of perception. The senses are of great interest for nursing, since so much of a nurse's consciousness *qua* nurse is taken up with and guided by making sense of – among other things – sensory perceptions. Even in high-tech healthcare, where "basic" tasks of toileting and washing are delegated to nursing aides, nurses remain close to the physical reality of human bodies, full of blood, viscera, bones, muscles, mucus, urine, faeces, any of which might make an irregular appearance outside the envelope of the body. Nurses see, touch, smell, hear, and less often taste sensations that in most areas of life we do our best to avoid or at least keep under careful control.

Ways to think with sense: enactivism

The word "sense" has a number of senses, as Richard Kearney (2015) has pointed out. It can mean the bodily senses, or clear thinking, or intuition, or meaning itself. Sense-making in these multiple meanings is one way of thinking about how "art and science" may both be present in practice, in the way nurses draw naturally and (mostly) unreflectively on different kinds of knowledge, including aspects of their own experiences, in making decisions about what to do.

Sense-making itself invokes a need for a way of understanding how this comes about.

Enactivism is a version of embodied cognition theory that takes human cognition as an embodied process, in interaction with the environment. It is itself hybrid, drawing on neurological science and phenomenological ideas (Thompson, 2007) to propose a model of embodied cognition that rejects the back-projected computer metaphor of the brain as a processing unit and sees cognition as a distributed process. Cognition is embodied, embedded, extended, and enactive (Gallagher, 2017). Cognition is therefore contextualized and social, where kinesthetic action and thought are parts of one process. It provides, in my view, a far more meticulously articulated understanding of what happens in an event of nursing practice than a vague appeal to the "art of nursing." Enactivist models rely heavily on the previous work of Merleau-Ponty and his phenomenology of embodied being-in-the-world, combined with scientific knowledge of brain functioning. Knowing about the neural pathways implicated in addiction, for example, helps to understand something about addiction as an organic feedback loop, but as soon as a pathway is referred to as the "reward" system, meaning is implicated in terms of what constitutes a reward in the eyes of a particular person and how that has come about. The pathway leads out of the brain and into the world.

Enactivism gives us a way of thinking about the person that is detailed and dynamic. It recognizes that physiological, social, and cultural processes are in play in human health or illness behaviours, while insisting on their inherent complexity without a leap to an imagined "whole person." It supports the importance of discernment and judgement in nursing practice, deciding which connections matter for any given event of nursing action, rather than claiming a comprehensive vision that is more rhetorical than practical.

Encultured practice

Thompson (2007) argues that cognition is not only embodied but also produced through dynamic interaction with environments and others. "One of the most important reasons that human mentality cannot be reduced simply to what goes on inside the brain of an individual is that human mental activity fundamentally social and cultural" (Thompson, 2007, p. 403). It is intersubjective and, because human beings are also cultural beings, it is enculturated. Art-as-culture suffuses nursing practice as it does any sphere of human activity. By culture here, I am not thinking only of cultural artefacts, rituals, or activities but of the mesh of meanings in which those things are alive in human interactions. Cultural competence for nurses is not a question of memorizing lists of aggregated characteristics and preferences of cultural groups – though knowledge is not a bad thing – but about discernment and attunement to the condition of finding oneself in interaction with another person who lives within a different mesh of meanings.

Culture cuts through time and each of us carries traces of histories of our origins – not always consciously and not always comfortably, but we live with, through, and sometimes against our cultural inheritances. It is a way of understanding that requires perspectives, resources, and skills from the humanities to be able to articulate and bring into practice just as nurses bring scientific knowledge into practice. Naming the arts and humanities is the one way of giving nurses leverage to work with the cultural engagements that are entailed in nursing work.

History is layered in healthcare, from the medical history in which professionals, primarily doctors, define what counts as important, through personal history, where a person defines for themselves what matters, to capital H history that can crash into people's lives with often long-lasting health effects from traumas of wars, civil wars, or environmental disasters. The concept of intergenerational trauma gives a language for trying to understand how it is that trauma at community or societal levels can have repercussions across extended periods of time. I once carried out a mental health assessment of an elderly Chinese man who answered my questions, through an interpreter, levelly and politely. Then as I asked about his life story, he talked about losing his small business in Saigon when the North Vietnamese took over in 1975, about 30 years earlier. Suddenly, he showed a visceral anger as if it had happened a week ago. The past is part of our emotional life, and mental health, in the present and sometimes knowledge of history is needed to help make connections with patients to make sense of the present.

Trauma-informed care draws attention to narrative, to a person's sense of self in the world, that is in a network of acculturated meanings. The defining slogan for trauma-informed care is to ask not "what's wrong with you?" but "what happened to you?" One question asks for symptoms and leaves diagnosis up to the professional; the other asks for access to a world of meaning into which the professional must try to find a place to stand where, with their professional knowledge and skills, they can collaborate to reorient the ongoing narrative.

The art of nursing: research

Having explored how arts and humanities make available resources for thinking about nursing as a culturally engaged practice, here I offer some observations of how they appear in research and education, though not always explicitly recognized as such. Nursing researchers use a lot of qualitative research (notoriously for some). The underlying reason for that is the orientation of nursing towards wanting to know about the experiences of people receiving and/or providing nursing care. Arguments about the method are important, but do not obviate the underlying impulse to want to know about what it is like to experience x, on the assumption that it will help us to do nursing better if we are better informed about what the people we work with are going through. This impulse, which seems obvious enough, and justified as a basis for research (doctors and healthcare organizations are increasingly interested in "patient stories") brings in its academic train a host of arguments about methodological rigour and value.

It is outside the scope of this chapter to address those debates but since it would appear qualitative research is not going away, I will point to some of the ways in which qualitative research draws on knowledge from the humanities, often unacknowledged. Among qualitative methods, some strive more than others for at least a patina of scientific prestige by claiming versions of objectivity. (Grounded Theory, for example, which comes from social science, operates on its own reductionist formula of stepped textual analysis). Others, notably phenomenology and its close relation hermeneutics, claim a specific philosophical heritage which roots them in the humanities. Both are based on accounts of experience, with hermeneutics being more accommodating of the creative role of the researcher in interpreting accounts of experience (Moules et al., 2015). Narrative enquiry, as the name suggests, takes narrative as a route of access into allowing people to bring a structured, dense account of experience into being (Clandinin, 2013). Arts-based research, where drama, literature, or film-making, for example, is the medium of the research itself, is most explicitly and obviously in the realm of art and humanities knowledge (Knowles and Cole, 2008).

When seen as branches of humanities, it makes it easier to see what (some) qualitative research methods are trying to do. Their value needs to be registered in terms of humanities knowledge, not scientific knowledge. Greater precision about domains of knowledge, their limits and affordances, would take some heat out of debates in nursing literature about what constitutes "proper" nursing knowledge.

The art of nursing: education

Materials from the arts have long been used in nursing education as a means to getting under the skin of how people experience illness and healthcare encounters, exercising the imagination to widen nursing students' peripheral vision for patient perspectives. Here, I offer an example of how narrativity and character, which can be features of literary, visual, or performance art forms, are employed in a simulation to create a sense of genuine contact with another.

In simulation, educators talk about "fidelity" to mean the degree to which students are fooled into taking a simulated scenario seriously, to respond as if it is real, which means as if there is something at stake in the scenario itself, not only as a means to completing an assignment. This "as if" that bridges the simulacrum and the reality operates in the world of the humanities. When anyone reads a novel, or watches a TV drama, its success depends on the "as if" taking hold, at least enough to feel that there is something at stake for these people made of words and light, on the page or acted out on screen.

A colleague of mine, Michelle Cullen, created a simulation she has called "Turk Talks" (suggested by her collaborator, Dr. David Topps, in reference to a chess-playing automaton presented to a Turkish Sultan, which was operated by a person hidden inside the figure). Turk Talks are designed to help students learn communication skills in mental health and addictions nursing, by conducting interviews within a scenario, with a facilitator – usually students play the nurse, and facilitators the patients, though the roles can easily be reversed. I have taken part in the simulations many times and I have noticed that, although "conversation" is conducted remotely, by typing into chat boxes, often with unnaturally long pauses, a genuine affective experience happens. As I play the part of a patient, interacting with several students at once, I can find myself responding in distinctly individuated ways. With one, I might find the initial introduction pleasant and agreeable, and as "the patient," I feel inclined to work with that "nurse" and answer questions; another, who starts off with assertions about my situation, can get my back up and I immediately feel annoyed, defensive, and therefore become uncooperative. I am not claiming any special acting ability; quite the opposite, I am noting a normal human inclination to read into others' intentions and to have a spontaneous organic response that is affective before it is rational, felt before it is turned into words. All this takes place without any facial expression, body language, and in made-up scenarios that I will step out of and forget about once the class is over. In the moment, however, I cared about these people who did not exist, who were made only of words. It mattered to me what happened to them and I was invested in trying to work out how best to help them in my imagined role as their nurse.

Art and science: together again

"Physics, literary criticism, political theory, geology and ethics should all notice that they share a world" (Midgley, 2006, p. 193). Mary Midgley in her work *Science and Poetry* uses the metaphor of an atlas to show how we readily understand that different kinds of knowledge co-exist for us. She suggests that to anyone schooled in how to read an atlas, it presents no challenge that there will be several maps of the same territory. One might show political boundaries and cities, another climate patterns, and another locations of raw materials. We understand that these are all different aspects of the same place, separated out to provide particular types of information but nonetheless simultaneous and meaningful depictions of the territory. "We are not looking for the relations between places on the same map. We are trying to understand the relation between two maps of different kinds…" (p. 112). She is not talking about nursing, but it strikes me as having a particular application for nurses, where the simultaneous mobilization of the objective and the subjective, science and art, is constantly in play. And not only that, but enacted through speech, thought, and action. In the atlas of nursing, the map showing science is well delineated, and much annotated in the margins, while the map for art is poorly sketched, lacking outline or well-delineated features.

Michel Serres, sometime ship's engineer and mathematician before becoming a philosopher, felt quite at home in the sciences and humanities, since for him the question was only ever about how they speak to each other. Across a large body of work, he tried various metaphorical and explanatory strategies to get across his ideas about the interpenetration of art and science. He observed that for science, time is a flat present, forever the culmination of accumulated knowledge, whereas culture always stretches away into the past and the past continues to live through culture. What he called the "third-instructed" is a consciousness that is irretrievably inside of the scientific worldview and at the same time part of nature and culture. One is bright, rational, and objective, while the other gives us reasons for being and acting, "not only from what we think, but from what we suffer. This latter reason cannot be learned without cultures, myths, arts, religions, tales, and contracts" (Serres, 1997, p. 71). "Science meets culture when science is incarnated and encounters or produces pain, evil, and poverty. That moment never ends, because it bears the world and history" (Serres, 1997, p. 70). Nursing is in attendance at this crossroads, responsive to suffering and pain, cognizant of science, cognizant of human meanings.

Serres here is talking about human consciousness in the modern world, unavoidably using and subject to technology, while experiencing the same embodied life in relation to cultural meanings that human beings have always done. But for nurses, there is a special appositeness, working with people in situations of overt suffering, using not abstract science but technologic scientific means to attempt to relieve suffering felt by its subject from the inside out. "The state of things seems to me to be an intersecting multiplicity of veils, the interlacing of which bodies forth a three-dimensional figure. The state of things is creased, crumpled, folded, with flounces and panels, fringes, stitches and lacing" (Serres, 2016, p. 82). Serres is a philosopher of empiricism for whom that means palpable, sensory experience of the material world, where sciences, arts, and humanities all have a part. "Empiricism plunges one into a many-splendoured reality that requires great patience and intense powers of abstraction" (Serres, 2016, p. 26). This is a mode of empiricism for nursing which all depends, as Serres also says, "on time, place and circumstance" demanding "patience…and infinite exploration" (p. 27). Practice in other words is unending, the right response to the needs of another is never wholly clear, or available and abstract knowledge, cultural knowledge, and the work of the senses are mingled.

Art and science, as in Midgley's atlas analogy, co-exist, folding over and into each other imperceptibly in moment-to-moment practice. One limitation of Gadamer's analysis of aesthetic knowledge is that in trying to rehabilitate the humanities, he maintains the separation between art and science (even if only tactically) in a way that is inadequate for a full account of what nursing is like. Michel Serres (2016) used the metaphor of the threads on the back of an embroidery to see how different tracks of knowledge are criss-crossed and knotted together to make what, on the front, is a complete image. It takes input from the humanities, the art side of nursing, to contemplate how the picture is made, of the art and science of nursing.

Conclusion

The art and science of nursing can be more than a slogan that gestures towards plurality in nursing knowledge. We can do better in understanding what we mean by art for nursing, and in bringing the resources of the arts and humanities into the fold of nursing thought in a much more intentional way. One aspect of using arts and humanities knowledge more effectively is to find better ways of articulating what happens in nursing practice, rather than falling back into academic shadow boxing over the so-called paradigms. We would do well to learn to think with hybridity. Enactivism, itself hybrid, part science, part philosophy, part concrete, part conceptual lends itself to understanding what happens in nursing practice, working back from nursing practice. Philosophy of science already relies on humanities traditions and in nursing we should also turn to philosophers of hybridity like Serres and Midgely, and of dialogue like Gadamer and Kearney.

Art presents the human predicament in a way that science simply cannot. Great artworks persist in their power and fascination because they go on drawing new generations into their inexhaustible fields of meaning. This matters to nursing because nursing is a practice that is centrally about interactions between human beings – embodied, emotive, culturally loaded, stuffed with meanings – and more than that, interactions that often occur at moments of crisis in human lives, brought about by illness, trauma, loss, and pain. Arts and humanities work to comprehend and communicate truths about exactly those pressure points where nursing lives and does its work.

References

Carper, B.A. (1978). Fundamental patterns of knowing in nursing. *Advances in Nursing Science*, 1 (1), pp. 13–24. doi:10.1097/00012272–197810000-00004

Case, M. (2019). *How to treat people: A nurse at work*. London: Viking.

Clandinin, D.J. (2013). *Engaging in narrative inquiry*. Walnut Creek, CA: Left Coast Press.

Crawford, P., Brown, B., Baker, C., Tischler, V., and Abrams, B. (2015). *Health humanities*. Basingstoke: Palgrave Macmillan.

Czerwiec, M.K. (2017). *Taking turns: Stories from HIV/AIDS Care Unit 371*. University Park, PA: The Pennsylvania State University Press.

Gadamer, H.G. (2004). *Truth and method*. Translated from German by Joel Weinsheimer and Donald G. Marshall. New York: Continuum.

Gallagher, S. (2017). *Enactivist interventions: Rethinking the mind*. Oxford: Oxford University Press.

Kearney, R. (2015). The wager of carnal hermeneutics. In Kearney, R. and Treanor, B., eds. *Carnal hermeneutics*. New York: Fordham University Press, pp. 15–56.

Knowles, J.G. and Cole, A.L., eds. (2008). *Handbook of the arts in qualitative research*. Thousand Oaks, CA: Sage.

McCaffrey, G. (2021). Kasulis' intimacy/integrity heuristic and epistemological pluralism in nursing. *Nursing Philosophy*, 22(2), p.e12333-n/a. https://doi.org/10.1111/nup.123333

Midgley, M. (2006). *Science and poetry*. London: Routledge.

Moules, N.J., McCaffrey, G., Field, J., and Laing, C. (2015). *Conducting hermeneutic research: From philosophy to practice*. New York: Peter Lang.

Serres, M. (1997). *The troubadour of knowledge*. Translated from French by Sheila Faria Glaser and William Paulson. Ann Arbor, MI: The University of Michigan Press.

Serres, M. (2016). *The five senses: A philosophy of mingled bodies*. Translated from French by Margaret Sankey and Peter Cowley. London: Bloomsbury.

Shalof, T. (2005). *A nurse's story: Life, death and in-between in an intensive care unit*. Toronto: McClelland & Stewart.

Thompson, E. (2007). *Mind in life: Biology, phenomenology, and the science of mind*. Cambridge, MA: Belknap Harvard.

Tu Fu. (2020). *The selected poems of Tu Fu*. Translated from Chinese by David Hinton. New York: New Directions Publishing.

Watson, C. (2018). *The language of kindness: A nurse's story*. London: Chatto & Windus.

Whitman, W. (2005). *Leaves of grass*. New York: Signet.

6   The knowledge of nursology

Jacqueline Fawcett

Nursologists are visiting several people in their homes. They wonder what they are to think about when they go into each person's home. Specifically, they wonder what is the knowledge of nursology needed for practice and for any scholarly projects they may want to conduct.

The purpose of this chapter is to present my personal perspective of the knowledge of the discipline of nursology, which I conceptualize as a holarchy. This perspective "embraces epistemological plurality. In [nursology], there is a commitment to recognizing different ways of knowing to support [the discipline's] mandate to consider the individual holistically and in context" (Ou et al., 2017, p. 7). That mandate has recently extended to populations and to the entire planet as nursology takes planetary conditions and planetary health into account (Kuehnert et al., 2022).

Discussion in this chapter encompasses my beliefs about what constitutes nursology knowledge, an explanation about the components of the holarchy of nursology knowledge, and thoughts about how nursology knowledge is found to be or not to be empirically adequate. The chapter content reflects an admitted post-positivist theory-laden philosophy that is consistent with Popper's (1965) "horizon of expectations" (p. 47) and his philosophy of refutation of knowledge that undergirds theory development. Although it is possible that the holarchy of nursology knowledge is the same as the structure for knowledge in other disciplines, my area of expertise is limited to nursology. The chapter ends with a brief discussion of the need to decolonize nursology knowledge.

Nursology

I believe that nursology is the proper name for the discipline that has been called nursing. Nursology is defined as "knowledge of the phenomena of interest to nursologists, which are [why, when, where, and how] nursologists collaborate with other human beings as they experience wellness, illness, and disease, within the context of their environments" (Fawcett, 2019, p. 919). This definition provides the lens for a discussion of discipline-specific knowledge. I also believe that all members of the discipline of nursology are appropriately called nursologists (rather than nurses). Referring to the discipline as nursology and to its members as nursologists has substantial practical and political implications for the place of the discipline within the academy, such that the members of our discipline are true partners with members of all other disciplines in the development, dissemination, and utilization of knowledge.

DOI: 10.4324/9781003427407-7

Table 6.1 Definitions for Components of the Holarchy of Nursology Knowledge

Components of the Holarchy of Nursology Knowledge	Definitions
Metaparadigm	"the global concepts that identify the phenomena of central interest to a discipline, the global propositions that describe the concepts, and the global propositions that state the relations between the concepts" (Fawcett & DeSanto-Madeya, 2013, p. 6).
Philosophy	"a statement encompassing ontological claims about the phenomena of central interest to a discipline, epistemic claims about how those phenomena come to be known, and ethical claims about what the members of a discipline value" (Fawcett & DeSanto-Madeya, 2013, p. 8).
Conceptual Model	"a set of relatively abstract and general concepts that address the phenomena of central interest to a discipline, the propositions that broadly describe those concepts, and the propositions that state relatively abstract and general relations between two or more of the concepts" (Fawcett & DeSanto-Madeya, 2013, p. 13).
Theory	"one or more relatively concrete and specific concepts that are derived from a conceptual model, the propositions that narrowly describe those concepts, and the propositions that state relatively concrete and specific relations between two or more of the concepts" (Fawcett & DeSanto-Madeya, 2013, p. 15).
Methods of scholarly inquiry	Ways in which data are collected, including design of scholarly projects, people who participate in the projects, interview guides or questionnaires, data collection procedures, protection of study participants, and data analysis techniques (Fawcett & Garity, 2009).

The holarchy of nursology knowledge

Furthermore, I believe that the knowledge of nursology is a holarchy, which means that each component of knowledge is whole within itself and is also a part of the larger whole (Wilbur, 1998). In nursology, the larger whole is contemporary knowledge of the discipline of nursology. Thus, each component of contemporary knowledge of nursology is a complete whole and is also a part of the larger whole (Fawcett & DeStanto-Madeya, 2013).

My perspective of the holarchy of nursology knowledge is that it comprises five components: a single metaparadigm and multiple philosophies, conceptual models, theories, and methods of scholarly inquiry (Fawcett & DeSanto-Madeya, 2013). Although I recognize and acknowledge others' definitions for each of these components, the definitions I use are given in Table 6.1. The metaparadigm is the most abstract component of nursology knowledge and guides the development of all other components – philosophies, conceptual models, theories, and methods of scholarly inquiry, which are the least abstract components.

The metaparadigm

The idea for a component of knowledge called the metaparadigm arose in discussion of the multiple meanings Kuhn (1962) had given to the term, paradigm. Masterman (1970) pointed out that one meaning reflected a metaphysical rather than scientific notion or entity and labeled that meaning as the metaparadigm. Hardy (1978) explained that the

Table 6.2 Metaparadigm Concepts and Definitions

Metaparadigm Concepts	Definitions
Human Beings	"the individuals, if individuals are recognized in a culture, as well as... the families, communities, and other groups or aggregates who are participants in [nursology]" (Fawcett & DeSanto-Madeya, 2013, p. 6).
Environment	"human beings' significant others and physical surroundings, as well as... the settings in which [nursology practice and research] occur, which range from private homes to health care facilities to communities to society as a whole... [as well as] all local, regional, national, and worldwide cultural, social, political, and economic conditions that are associated with human beings' health" (Fawcett & DeSanto-Madeya, 2013, p. 6). Environment extends to the planet and planetary conditions, including climate and climate change (Kuehnert et al., 2022). Planetary health is "an attitude towards life and a philosophy for living, It emphasizes people not disease, and equity, not the creation of unjust societies" (Horton, 2014, as cited by Kalogirou et al., 2020, p 6).
Health	"human processes of living and dying" (Fawcett & DeSanto-Madeya, 2013, p. 6).
Nursologists' Activities	"the definition of [nursology, such as caring], the actions taken by [nursologists] on behalf of or in conjunction with human beings, and the goals or outcomes of [nursologists'] actions... [which] are viewed as a mutual process between the participants in [nursology] and [nursologists]. The process encompasses activities that are frequently referred to as assessment; labeling, or what some [nursologists] refer to as diagnosis; planning; intervention; and evaluation" (Fawcett & DeSanto-Madeya, 2013, p. 6).

metaparadigm "is the broadest consensus within a discipline. It provides the general parameters of the field and gives scientists a broad orientation from which to work" (p. 38). The specific function of the metaparadigm is to identify the concepts and propositions that represent the very abstract and general subject matter of the discipline.

My version of the metaparadigm of nursology encompasses four concepts, their definitions, and propositions stating linkages between the concepts. The concepts and their definitions are given in Table 6.2.

The four propositions that link the metaparadigm concepts are as follows:

1. The discipline of [nursology] is concerned with the principles and laws that govern human processes of living and dying.
2. The discipline of [nursology] is concerned with the patterning of human health experiences within the context of the environment.
3. The discipline of [nursology] is concerned with [nursologists'] actions or processes that are beneficial to human beings.
4. The discipline of [nursology] is concerned with the human processes of living and dying, recognizing that human beings are in a continuous relationship with their environments

(Fawcett & DeSanto-Madeya, 2013, p. 6)

Philosophies

"Philosophy in its broadest sense is wondering and being curious about the 'big' or fundamental questions that humans have grappled with throughout history" (Kessler, 1998, as cited in Bruce et al., 2014, p. 567). The function of a philosophy is to articulate disciplinary beliefs and values for ontological, epistemic, and ethical claims (Bruce et al., 2014). Nursology philosophies articulate these claims for each of the metaparadigm concepts.

Each nursology philosophy reflects one of three worldviews, and each worldview provides a different perspective of the metaparadigm concepts, the relations between the concepts, and ways to develop knowledge about the concepts and their relations.

1 The features of the **Reaction World View** are as follows:

- *Humans are biopsychosocialspiritual beings.*
- *Human beings react to external environmental stimuli in a linear, causal manner.*
- *Change occurs only for survival and as a consequence of predictable and controllable antecedent conditions.*
- *Only objective phenomena that can be isolated, observed, defined, and measured are studied.*

(Fawcett & DeSanto-Madeya, 2013, p. 9)

2 The features of the **Reciprocal Interaction World View** are as follows:

- *Human beings are holistic; parts are viewed only in the context of the whole.*
- *Human beings are active, and interactions between human beings and their environments are reciprocal.*
- *Change is a function of multiple antecedent factors, is probabilistic, and may be continuous or may be only for survival.*
- *Reality is multidimensional, contextdependent, and relative.*

(Fawcett & DeSanto-Madeya, 2013, p. 9)

3 The features of the **Simultaneous Action World View** are as follows:

- *Unitary human beings are identified by pattern.*
- *Human beings are in mutual rhythmical interchange with their environments.*
- *Human beings change continuously, unpredictably, and in the direction of more complex selforganization.*
- *The phenomena of interest are personal knowledge and pattern recognition.*

(Fawcett & DeSanto-Madeya, 2013, p. 10)

Conceptual models

Conceptual models arise from empirical observations, intuition, and innovative deductions. The function of each conceptual model is to provide a distinctive frame of reference for nursologists' activities. The content of each conceptual model addresses the metaparadigm concepts (see Table 6.2), and each conceptual model is based on features from one or more of the three philosophical worldviews.

Fawcett (2017) described nine widely recognized nursology conceptual models and discussed their uses as guides for nursology quality improvement projects; literature reviews, instrument development; descriptive, correlational, experimental, and mixed methods research; and practice. These conceptual models, many of which are summarized on the nursology.net website, are as follows:

Johnson's Behavioral System Model
King's Conceptual System
Levine's Conservation Model
Neuman's Systems Model
Orem's Self-Care Framework
Rogers' Science of Unitary Human Beings
Roy's Adaptation Model
    The AACN Synergy Model for Patient Care
    Meleis' Transitions Framework

Four other nursology conceptual models that focus specifically on health policy and/or population health are as follows:

- The Conceptual Model of Nursing and Health Policy (Fawcett & Russell, 2001; Russell & Fawcett, 2005).
- The Conceptual Model of Nursing and Population Health (Fawcett & Ellenbecker, 2015).
- The Conceptual Model of Nursology for Enhancing Equity and Quality: Population Health and Health Policy (Fawcett, 2021a).
- The Consensus Paper Conceptual Framework (Kuehnert et al., 2022).

Theories

Popper (1968) explained, "Theories are nets cast to catch what we call 'the world': to rationalize, to explain, and to master it. We endeavour to make the mesh ever finer and finer" (p. 59). Accordingly, I believe that the function of nursology theories, which are implicitly or explicitly derived from conceptual models, is to provide relativity direct guidance for nursologists' activities. This belief about theories is at least somewhat consistent with Lauden's (1996) claim that theories are the answers to the problems of science (or more broadly, to the problems of nursology research, practice, education, and administration). Lauden (1996) wrote:

> [T]he aim of science is to secure theories with a high problem-solving effectiveness and that scientific progress is possible when empirical data [are] diminished. Indeed… it is possible that a change from an empirically well-supported theory to a less well-supported one could be progressive, provided that the latter resolved significant conceptual difficulties confronting the former. Finally, the better theory solves more conceptual problems while minimizing empirical anomalies.
>
> (pp. 77–87)

Nursology theories encompass three levels of abstraction – grand theories, middle-range theories, and situation-specific theories. Grand theories are the most abstract and are applicable to the entire population that is the focus of scholarly inquiry. Middle-range theories are generalizable to the entire population that is the focus of scholarly inquiry. Situation-specific theories are about a particular group of persons who are experiencing a particular health condition and are not generalizable or transferable beyond these people and this health condition.

Eight ways of knowing in nursology, which I consider as types of theories that can be middle-range or situation-specific, are listed here with their focus:

- **Empirical knowing** encompasses all that is involved in operationalizing nursology science (Carper, 1978).
- **Aesthetic knowing** encompasses all that is involved in realizing the art of nursology (Carper, 1978).
- **Ethical knowing** encompasses all that is involved in articulating nursology beliefs and values (Carper, 1978).
- **Personal knowing** encompasses all that is involved in expressing each nursologist's authentic self in relation to others (Carper, 1978).
- **Sociopolitical knowing** encompasses all that is involved in nursologists' understanding health care cultures and politics (White, 1995).
- **Emancipatory knowing** encompasses all that is involved in nursologists' creation of change toward ever higher quality of their activities (Chinn & Kramer, 2008).
- **Spiritual knowing** encompasses all that is involved in each nursologist's understanding of existence in a spiritual sense (Willis & Leone-Sheehan, 2019).
- **Unknowing** encompasses all that is involved in nursologists' not explicitly knowing of nursology, yet knowing how to be authentically present (Munhall, 1993).

My own and others' theory-development research has led me to realize that a series of related situation-specific theories can be combined or integrated to form a middle-range theory (Fawcett, 2021b). For example, a situation-specific theory of functional status during low-risk childbearing could be combined with a situation-specific theory of functional status during high-risk childbearing to develop a middle-range theory of functional status during childbearing.

Methods of scholarly inquiry

Methods of scholarly inquiry encompass how theories are generated and tested via research and how theories are used in nursology practice. The functions of methods of inquiry are the actual procedures used to conduct research or engage in practice. My perspective of the methods is that research findings are conditional and can be false. Indeed, conceptual and theoretical reflections and thinking and new methods can uncover new knowledge that replaces what had been thought to be empirically adequate. This perspective acknowledges that knowledge evolves slowly through successive programs of scholarly inquiry, or evolves rapidly though revolutions when reflection and scholarly inquiry uncovers innovations in thinking, such as unpacking black boxes of knowledge.

Empirical adequacy is determined by comparing research findings or results of practice with the theory that guided the research or practice. New theories are generated by means of qualitative methodologies, which usually are ways to obtain subjective data in the form of people's words and stories of their experiences of some phenomenon. In contrast, existing theories are tested by means of quantitative methodologies, which usually are ways to obtain objective data in the form of people's responses to questionnaires made up of numerical items. If the theory and the research findings or practice results are consistent, the theory is regarded as empirically adequate, at least until a new theory is developed. Although many researchers regard lack of empirical adequacy as a problem of method (e.g., too small a sample and lack of reliable and valid questionnaires), Popper (1965) declared that rejection – of refutation – of a theory leads to development of a better theory.

Methods for obtaining both objective and subjective knowledge are needed for "multidimensional understanding of the client within the context of situation, family and environment" (Ou et al., 2017, p. 7). I believe that multidimensional understanding is best determined by conducting scholarly inquiry for the purpose of development of situation-specific theories.

A challenge is to uncover implicit or tacit knowledge, that is, "the knowledge gained from experience, interactions, and the acquisition and combination of skills" (Zander, 2007, p. 8). Another especially important challenge is to avoid the primacy of a particular method, such as a qualitative approach or a quantitative approach. Still, another important challenge is to avoid primacy of method over theory. Accordingly, I believe that a balance of theory and method, with method only for the development of theory, is needed.

Decolonizing nursology knowledge

Given the dominant Euro-centric while privilege perspective of most, if not all, nursology knowledge (Chinn, 2021), there is a crucial need for decolonizing our disciplinary knowledge. This means that the components of nursology knowledge (existing metaparadigm, philosophies, conceptual models, theories, and methods of scholarly inquiry) have to be revised or discarded in favor of perspectives of knowledge that clearly include the ethnic and cultural diversities of all nursologists, with special attention to nursologists of color.

Decolonizing nursology knowledge involves developing knowledge that

is an interchange between [culturally and contextually relevant] theory and practice and [is] guided by [culturally and contextually relevant] philosophy [that] is like a kind of pendulum where all three elements [that is, culturally and contextually relevant philosophy, theory, practice] are treated as equals.
(Hoeck & Delmar, 2018, p. 1)

Chinn (2021) pointed out that much of the work of decolonizing can be achieved through an emphasis on development of situation-specific theories by inviting people to tell their stories of their health experiences. Continuing, she explained that the "situation-specific theories are grounded in the actual realm of human experience and the social and political context in which experience is embedded" (Chinn, 2021, p. 34). The stories can be analyzed within the context of a particular situation and the people's culture. It is important, though, to avoid stereotyping of the story-tellers on the basis of their culture.

Therefore, one possible starting point for decolonizing nursology knowledge is to select an existing conceptual model to identify – at an abstract level – a phenomenon of interest to the discipline. The phenomenon of interest is the topic for a situation-specific theory, which can be used to support or revise the conceptual model or develop a new conceptual model. For example, Roy's adaptation model (RAM) can be used to guide a study with a group of women and their partners to tell their stories of their experiences of high-risk childbearing. The findings from analysis of the stories is a situation-specific theory, which then can be used to determine whether RAM needs to be revised or a new model of adaptation or other phenomenon needs to be developed. Decolonizing might take RAM cultural assumptions into account. These assumptions are as follows:

- Experiences within a specific culture will influence how each element of the RAM is expressed (Roy, 2009, p. 31).
- Cultural expressions of the elements of the RAM may lead to changes in practice activities such as nursing assessment (Roy, 2009, p. 31).

Conclusion

My perspective of nursology knowledge is admittedly a Euro-centric view arising from my white privilege. Thus, in keeping with efforts of decolonize nursology knowledge, I welcome the critique and outright rejection of the holarchy of nursology knowledge in part or in whole by readers of this chapter, with the expectation of a better way of thinking about one or all of the components of nursology knowledge or even if there are components of nursology knowledge.

Nursologists who are visiting several people in their homes now know a lot about the knowledge of nursology and understand that they may select one of many nursology conceptual models to guide their practice and may apply an integration of the eight types of theories for each person they visit. They also understand that the conceptual model and theories they are using will serve as guides for their scholarly projects. Furthermore, they now understand how important it is to listen to each person's story of health conditions within the context of that person's culture, so that all that they do is not based on an Euro-central white privilege perspective of nursology knowledge.

References

Bruce, A., Rietze, L., & Lim, A. (2014). Understanding philosophy in a nurse's world: What, where and why? *Nursing and Health* 2(3): 65–71, http://www.hrpub.org DOI: 10.13189/nh.2014.020302.

Carper, B. A. (1978). Fundamental patterns of knowing in nursing. *Advances in Nursing Science* 1(1): 13–23.

Chinn, P. L. (2021). Equity and social justice in developing theories. In E-O Im & A. I. Meleis (Eds.), *Situation specific theories: Development, utilization, and evaluation in nursing* (pp. 29–37). Springer Nature Switzerland.

Chinn, P. L., & Kramer, M. K. (2008). *Integrated theory and knowledge development in nursing* (7th ed.). Mosby Elsevier.

Fawcett, J. (2017). *Applying conceptual models of nursing: Quality improvement, research, and practice.* Springer.

Fawcett, J. (2019). Nursology revisited and revived [Editorial]. *Journal of Advanced Nursing 75*: 919–920. DOI: 10.1111/jan.13925.

Fawcett, J. (2021a). The conceptual model of nursology for enhancing equity and quality: Population health and health policy. In M. Moss & J. Phillips (Eds.), *Health equity and nursing: Achieving equity through policy, population health and interprofessional collaboration* (pp. 101–117). Springer.

Fawcett, J. (2021b). Middle range theories and situation specific theories: Similarities and differences. In E-O. Im & A. Meleis (Eds.), *Situation specific theories: Development, utilization, and evaluation in nursing* (pp. 39–47). Springer, Nature Switzerland.

Fawcett, J., & DeSanto-Madeya, S. (2013). *Contemporary nursing knowledge: Analysis and evaluation of nursing models and theories* (3rd ed.). F. A. Davis.

Fawcett, J., & Ellenbecker, C. H. (2015). A proposed conceptual model of nursing and population health. *Nursing Outlook 63*(3): 288–298. DOI: 10.1016/j.outlook.2015.01.009.

Fawcett, J., & Garity, J. (2009). *Evaluating research for evidence-based nursing practice.* F. A. Davis.

Fawcett, J., & Russell, G. (2001). A conceptual model of nursing and health policy. *Policy, Politics, and Nursing Practice 2*(2): 108–116. DOI: 10.1177/152715440100200205.

Hardy, M. E. (1978). Perspectives on nursing theory. *Advances in Nursing Science 1*(1): 37–48.

Hoeck, B., & Delmar, C. (2018). Theoretical development in the context of nursing—The hidden epistemology of nursing theory. *Nursing Philosophy 19*(1): 10 pages. DOI: 10.1111/nup.12196.

Kuehnert, P., Fawcett, J., DePriest, K. Chinn, P. Cousin, L., Ervin, N., Flanagan, J., Fry-Bowers, E., Killion, C., Maliski, S. Maughan. E. D., Meade, C., Murray, T., Schenk, B., & Waite, R. (2022). Defining the social determinants of health for nursing action to achieve health equity. A consensus paper from the American Academy of Nursing. Nursing Outlook, 70(1), 10–27. DOI: 10.1016/j.outlook.2021.08.003

Kuhn, T. S. (1962). *The structure of scientific revolutions.* University of Chicago Press.

Lauden, L. (1996). *Beyond positivism and relativism.* Westview Press. Quotation retrieved from Wikipedia. https://en.wikipedia.org/wiki/Larry_Laudan).

Masterman, M. (1970). The nature of paradigm. In I. Lakatos & A. Musgrave (Eds.), *Criticism and the growth of knowledge* (pp. 59–89). Cambridge University Press.

Munhall, P. L. (1993). "Unknowing." Toward another pattern of knowing in nursing. *Nursing Outlook* (3): 126–129.

Ou, C. H. K., Hall, W. A., & Thorne, S. E. (2017). Can nursing epistemology embrace p-values? *Nursing Philosophy 18*(4): 9 pages. DOI: 10.1111/nup.12173.

Popper, K. R. (1965). *Conjectures and refutations: The growth of scientific knowledge.* Harper and Row.

Popper, K. R. (1968). *The logic of scientific discovery.* Harper Torchbooks.

Roy, C. (2009). *The Roy adaptation model* (3rd ed.). Pearson.

Russell, G. E., & Fawcett, J. (2005). The conceptual model for nursing and health policy revisited. *Policy, Politics, and Nursing Practice 6*(4): 319–326. DOI: 10.1177/1527154405283304.

White, J. (1995). Patterns of knowing: Review, critique, and update. *Advances in Nursing Science 17*(4): 73–86. DOI: 10.1891/RTNP-D-20–00095.

Wilbur, K. (1998). *The marriage of sense and soul: Integrating science and religion.* Random House.

Willis, D. G., & Leone-Sheehan, D. M. (2019). Spiritual knowing; Another pattern of knowing in the discipline. *Advances in Nursing Science 42*(1): 58–68. DOI: 10.1177/0894318414558606.

Zander, P. E. (2007). Ways of knowing in nursing. The historical evolution of a concept. *Journal of Theory Construction and Testing 11*(1): 7–11.

Part 2

An ethical profession

7 (Normative) moral theory and nursing practice

Paul Snelling

Introduction

It's quite a task to write succinctly on moral theory and nursing practice not least because of the problem of almost infinite regress. The challenge is to say something of interest to and, importantly, of everyday use to nurses in their practice, whilst avoiding both trite oversimplification and disappearing down the rabbit hole of abstract and detailed philosophising. John Rawls' definition of moral theory is a case in point:

> Moral theory is the study of substantive moral conceptions, that is, the study of how the basic notions of the right, the good, and moral worth may be arranged to form different moral structures. Moral theory tries to identify the chief similarities and differences between these structures and to characterise the way in which they are related to our moral sensibilities and natural attitudes, and to determine the conditions they must satisfy if they are to play their expected role in human life.
>
> (Rawls 1974, p. 5)

If this isn't necessarily a definition I would recommend to an undergraduate class of nurses, it nevertheless captures the point that understanding the nature and function of moral theory (as academic study as well as intended action guide) also requires some understanding of prior moral concepts. Later in the same paper, Rawls refers to 'a correct theory of right and wrong, that is, a systematic account of what we regard as *objective* moral truths' (1974, p. 7, emphasis added), introducing a metaethical question that many nurses will regard as unnecessary as they navigate their moral environment. Moral theory can be understood to have two functions. A theoretical (metaethical) purpose concerned with the features of moral properties and words, what makes things good or bad, right or wrong (Timmons 2021), and a practical (normative) purpose, to articulate a decision procedure which anyone can use to justify right action in a given situation. This chapter considers normative moral theories.[1]

Must nurses know about moral theories? Should they?

A starting point in considering the place of moral theory in nursing practice might be the questions of how much moral theory should (all) nurses know – and how much they must know. The answer to this lies, at least for the latter question and for UK nurses, in the Nursing and Midwifery Council[2] document '*Future nurse: Standards of proficiency for registered nurses*', the nearest there is to a national curriculum for nursing.

DOI: 10.4324/9781003427407-9

The document '…provides clarity to the public and the professions about the core knowledge and skills that they can expect every registered nurse to demonstrate' (NMC 2018a, p. 6). This document doesn't mention the word 'moral' but uses the word 'ethics'[3] twice. Once in relation to research ethics and once to require that at the point of registration the registered nurse will be able to 'understand and apply relevant legal, regulatory and governance requirements, policies, and ethical frameworks' (NMC 2018a, p. 8). That's all there is – there's no more detail about what this entails or includes, or whether a moral theory can be regarded as a framework. The details are for individual universities to decide within curricula, provided they meet the standards.

By contrast, the Institute for Medical Ethics (IME)[4] collaborates with the General Medical Council, the UK medical regulator, to produce a core curriculum for undergraduate medical ethics and law, detailing that students should be able to 'Recognise different approaches to ethical theory, values, and reasoning that inform decisions in medical practice, policy and law' (Institute of Medical Ethics 2019, p. 6).[5] There's clearly a difference here which may have an impact on discussions and ethical decision making within multidisciplinary teams. It is argued (Tschudin & Marks-Maran, 1993) that nursing ethics can be regarded as distinct from medical and other healthcare ethics, but the application of moral theory to which all parties in a discussion can refer to provides a common moral framework upon which to approach moral dilemmas. This is only possible when contributors, or at least those in professional roles, can all draw upon a working knowledge.

But this is not to suggest that ethical dilemmas can be resolved solely by reference to moral theories. In the environment of professional healthcare, these decisions are influenced by many other factors, most importantly the law. Some decisions, for example whether to accede to a request for Medical Aid in Dying (MAiD), are governed by statute, varying between jurisdictions. A nurse or doctor who argues that MAiD in a specific circumstance is morally allowable or obligatory, risks a very great deal by *acting* upon their moral conviction where it is prohibited by law, even where it is well argued, supported by this or that moral theory. In addition, regulated healthcare professionals follow a code of ethics[6] which guides and directs practice, and if many of these documents are more akin to legal than ethical prescriptions (Snelling 2016), transgressions, even if they are not unlawful, can be career ending. These consequences for individuals can be built into calculations in some moral theories, but moral theories and moral thinking more generally are better understood in the context of professional healthcare as judgement-informing rather than action-guiding.

Case studies and dilemmas

Though there is a moral dimension to everything that moral agents do, or choose not to do, in teaching, research and discussion of moral matters, it is common to focus on dilemmas, which can be thought of as instances where moral reasoning identifies two or more defensible courses of action which are mutually exclusive. Nurses do not need a code of ethics or a moral theory to tell them not to steal from their patients, but ask any class of students to discuss anything from their practice that has troubled them morally and there will likely be a range of experiences offered. This is from my experience as a ward manager many years ago: A patient with sickle cell crisis was experiencing severe pain. At that time, the analgesic of choice was Pethidine, an opiate drug supplied in vials of 100 mg/2 ml. The prescription was for 150 mg, taken to the patient as an injection of 3 ml of clear fluid in a syringe. There were some concerns about dependency, and it was also considered that the patient was exaggerating their pain[7] and so the prescription was reduced to 100 mg. However, fearing a difficult discussion and likely confrontation with the patient during the night shift, nurses added 1 ml of saline to the (now) 2 ml of Pethidine in the reduced dose so that when they went to the patient with the Pethidine, the syringe still contained 3 ml fluid. Looking at the syringe, the patient asked 'is that my Pethidine?' Stephanie, the registered nurse, replied that it was.[8]

What moral theories are we talking about?

There are many moral theories, all with many varieties. Books on moral theories commonly include sections on egoism, hedonism, existentialism, contractarianism and rights theories (Graham 2004; LaFollette and Persson 2013; Timmons 2021). Books on nursing ethics also come in many varieties. Many, perhaps the majority (Avery 2013; Buka 2020; Tingle and Cribb 2014; Wheeler 2012), cover both law and ethics and as we have seen, this combination is probably more useful for practising nurses as action guide. These books tend to cover three main ethical theories briefly: First, consequentialist moral theories commonly referred to for simplicity as utilitarianism and associated with Mill and Bentham. Second, non-consequentialist theories with various versions of Kantian deontology most commonly referred to and finally, agent-centred moral theories, commonly virtue ethics associated with Aristotle. Some texts (Wheeler 2012) include versions of feminist and care ethics as similar in some respects to virtue ethics though focussing on relationships with others rather than solely the character of the moral agent.[9]

Each of these three theories had been proposed, rejected, discussed, amended and generally picked over at great length and in great detail for centuries, millennia in the case of the virtues, and explanations of a few paragraphs leave the merest transient scratch upon the surface. They can be regarded more as developing projects rather than quasi-religious texts fixed in the time and cultural context of initial writing. Aristotle owned slaves and believed that women were naturally inferior to men. Kant also believed in the subordination of wives to their husbands and was unambiguous in his racism. Mill, though for his time a champion of women's rights,[10] also accepted and defended the racism and colonialism of his age (Sterba 2005). None could have anticipated anything of modern nursing practice, but the principles which have guided discussion and development of their theories remain of great importance.

Consequentialism

Consequentialism is a group of moral theories of which the utilitarianism (Mill 1998) of John Stuart Mill (1806–1873) is the best known, which holds that the morally correct action is the one that produces the best or least bad outcomes. This seems plausible; much of what we do is done with the future in mind. When Stephanie deceived her patient into believing that the dose of Pethidine had not been reduced, she was likely thinking of everyone in the ward. The patient would have a more peaceful night without the confrontation and the arguments; she herself would be able to spend more time with other patients who would be able to sleep better in a quieter environment. The consequences for everyone would be better if she just added a little saline to the syringe. Who amongst us hasn't told a lie to prevent a greater harm?

Though intuitively attractive, in its more abstract formulations, utilitarianism poses some very difficult questions. What is the thing that we must maximise? How can we make the calculations? Do we have to make the calculations for every moral action? The latter question produced two distinct versions. In act utilitarianism, a calculation is made (for all acts) which compares likely outcomes of available options. The moral choice is the option which produces the best outcomes, as far as we are able to predict. Apart from the matters of what to maximise and how, act consequentialism requires very many calculations as well as, on occasion, requiring some acts which seem counterintuitive to moral life, exemplified in several famous thought experiments.[11]

In rule consequentialism, rules that tend to maximise outcomes are developed. Generally speaking, the world goes better if people tell the truth, and so to prevent people from having to stop to calculate consequences before every act, it would be better simply for everyone to follow a rule of not lying. Again, an appealing development but it wouldn't take too long to encounter an issue where it would be significantly better to tell the lie, if it prevented a death, or two, or ten, or a hundred. At some point, it would be (much) better to tell the lie, and so the question is asked: When can the rules be discarded? One way to address this is not to discard the rule but to amend it. In this way, rules are reformulated and repeatedly specified, and rule consequentialism collapses back into act consequentialism. Two-level theory theories have been proposed as one way to recognise the value of following rules and on occasion, casting them aside (see, for example, the English utilitarian R.M Hare [1981]).

Reconciling rules and acts in this way may seem rather complex but healthcare professionals do this as part of their everyday practice. For example, in the matter of disclosure of information, a rule explicit in Codes of Ethics is that confidential information should not be disclosed. Sound consequentialist reasoning requires this; if healthcare professionals gossiped about their patients, this would likely result in a reduction of trust and fewer people seeking medical help, causing poorer health. However, there are some instances where keeping a confidence could lead to very poor consequences, if serious communicable disease or an intention to harm others was disclosed. In deciding right action, healthcare professionals must consider consequences for the individual act of disclosure but also consider the risk of undermining the general rule of confidentiality. The below quotation is from guidance applying to all health professionals released by the UK government.[12]

>…Exceptional circumstances that justify overruling the right of an individual to confidentiality in order to serve a broader societal interest. Decisions about the public interest are complex and must take account of both the potential harm that disclosure may cause and the interest of society in the continued provision of confidential health services.
>
> (Department of Health 2010)

Utilitarian reasoning is frequently seen in issues of population health, for example, in rationing decisions, where the process of allocating resources using the Quality Adjusted Life Year (QALY) is an attempt to calculate benefit between conditions so that outcomes within financial constraints can be maximised (Spencer et al. 2022). During the COVID-19 pandemic, calculations of maximising benefit were seen in population health measures like lockdowns and the possibility of allocation of ventilators (Savulescu, Persson and Wilkinson 2020). Rule utilitarianism would require Stephanie to tell the truth, and this could be overruled by an act calculation if the consequences were severe.

Deontology

Deontological moral theories focus on duty. Deon is the Greek word for duty. In a sense, the word 'duty' is commonplace in professional language, without implying a Kantian approach. The NMC Code mentions a duty of confidentiality (NMC 2018b, p. 8) and the professional duty of candour. Deontological theories, largely associated with the work of the German philosopher Immanuel Kant (1724–1804), require that we do our duties for their own sake – only then has any act moral worth (Walker 2023). But there is no list of duties. Instead, Kant provided a maxim or guiding principle which requires that moral agents 'act according to a maxim which can at the same time be valid as a universal law'[13] (Kant 1994, p. 24). This means that you should act only in a way that everybody should act, that universality is the essence of morality, arrived at through reason rather than any subjective consideration favouring either the moral agent or anyone else. There is no emotion, no special account of relationships. Your duty must be undertaken just because it is your duty. Kant has a reputation for promoting rigid exceptionless manifestations of the principle which cannot be set aside by appeal to unfavourable consequences. He is unambiguous with respect to lying in an essay entitled 'On a Supposed Right to Lie Because of Philanthropic Concerns' published towards the end of his life in 1798: 'To be truthful (honest) in all declarations is, therefore, a sacred and unconditional commanding law of reason that admits of no expediency whatever' (Kant 1994, p. 164).

Some of the reasoning in his short paper will be familiar to critics of various forms of utilitarianism, that it is impossible to know what consequences are. Walker (2023), amongst others, considers that Kant is not very good at setting out his case and refers to 'that unfortunate paper' (Walker 2023, p. 122). It is simple to think of examples where it would be extremely challenging to accept that lying is wrong. What if truth-telling resulted in the death, or two, or ten, or a hundred? If a terrorist asked you if you knew where a battery needed to complete an explosive device was located? In the matter of lying, Kant was clear but without this awkward pronouncement – or in other moral circumstances where he was less prescriptive – the rule of universality could be specified in a similar fashion to the move from rules back to acts in utilitarianism. Even with the clarity provided in the case of lying, 'most deontologists reveal themselves to be of the threshold variety' (Alexander 2008, p. 86). The moral law is followed to a certain point after which consequentialist considerations overrule what the deontologists regard (below the threshold) as something *intrinsically* right. Even if the location of the threshold is impossible to identify, threshold deontology does at least ameliorate intuitive misgivings about rules followed to the extreme. This should not bother Stephanie were she to take a deontological approach. She should not lie.

Virtue ethics (and care ethics)

Virtue ethics has its roots in ancient times, most famously in the writings of the Greek philosopher Aristotle (384BCE–322BCE). Virtue ethics focusses not on deciding right action, but instead on considering the features of a good life and how to be a good person, on character rather than action, with the assumption and expectation that good people do good things. To do this, moral agents cultivate virtues, which can be described as traits of character resulting in a disposition to think, feel and act in certain ways. These dispositions are not innate but can be cultivated through habituation. Acquiring the virtues involves some circularity as Aristotle demonstrated with regard to the virtue of temperance: 'It is by refraining from pleasures that we become temperate, and it is when we become temperate that we are most able to abstain from pleasures' (Aristotle 1953, pp. 34–35).

Aristotle (1953) discusses a number of virtues in *Nicomachean Ethics*, each of which is to be cultivated in the mean between excess and deficiency. For example in the sphere of self-expression, the mean of truthfulness lies between the excess of boastfulness and the deficiency of understatement. The list of Aristotelian virtues is not fixed and can be amended or enlarged. Begley (2005), for example, gives a list, including compassion, honesty, kindness, tolerance and courage; some of these virtues will be familiar to UK nurses as they form part of the nursing strategy '*Compassion in Practice*' (Department of Health 2012).[14]

Virtue ethics has been subject to a number of criticisms (Ferkany and Newham 2019), but perhaps the most significant for Stephanie is that it fails to deliver action guidance and is therefore of little practical use. Begley's (2005) refutation of this charge, borrowing from Hursthouse (1999), relies in large part on comparisons with competing theories; it's not so much that the virtues fail to give action guidance, more that the other competing theories are poor in this regard as well. The virtues can be regarded as implying rules (Hodkinson 2008); the virtue of truthfulness reformulated as a rule to tell the truth. If this lacks application, so do utilitarian and deontological rules, which is why they need detailed specification. Aristotle acknowledges that only general rules can be given, that questions of conduct and expedience are not fixed and that general rules are not precise:

> [...] but the agents are compelled to think out for themselves what the circumstances demand, just as happens in the arts of medicine and navigation.
> (Aristotle 1953, p. 33)

It's not clear that this helps Stephanie very much either. Thinking about the best course of action may help Stephanie to become a virtuous practitioner, guided by professional phronesis (wisdom), but until complete, the journey to phronesis itself provides scant guidance. Virtue theory can't tell Stephanie what to do, but there is clear presumption on telling the truth (Hodkinson 2008).

Nursing has provided fertile ground for agent-centred moral theories,[15] likely due to the account within utilitarianism and deontology of an ethic which is both impersonal and, in different ways, calculating – requiring the moral agent to step away from a situation and have a good think about what is the best thing to do. This is not to say that agent-centred theories don't require careful consideration, but they also allow or require some connectedness with the situation and with other people. Though rarely attained, abstract moral thinking involving universalisable principles was characterised as the highest level of moral development in Lawrence Kohlberg's work on moral development (McLeod-Sordjan 2014). However, as his erstwhile research assistant pointed out, Kohlberg's research sample consisted only of boys. In her seminal work *In a Different Voice*, Carol Gilligan (1982) argued that women's values centred on caring relationships rather than impersonal justice. The book is widely considered a starting point for feminist ethics of care developed by others, including Nel Noddings (1984), Joan Tronto (1994) and specifically related to nurses, Helga Kuhse (1997), finding a natural home within nursing's purpose rooted in care[16] and an overwhelmingly female workforce.

As a normative moral theory, care ethics possibly has little to offer Stephanie other than she should care for her patients. Appealing though it may be to those who see the nurse-patient relationship as based on emotional attachment, care ethics has been criticised for being vague. Perhaps a more serious charge is that the empirical findings which provided the initial impetus (that is, women don't think like men) are unreliable (Paley 2006).

Moral theories in use – frameworks and empirical research

Perhaps the most commonly used framework in bioethics is the four principles approach by Tom Beauchamp and James Childress first published in 1977 and now in its eighth edition (Beauchamp and Childress 2019).[17] This book changed the field of bioethics when it first appeared in 1977, only five years after the end of the infamous Tuskegee experiment (Washington 2008) at a time when medicine was finally addressing the malaise of deeply paternalistic practice which disempowered patients and marginalised other professionals. This text, sometimes referred to as a theory it its own right proposed that the eponymous principles (respect for autonomy, non-maleficence, beneficence, justice) could be derived from all the moral theories. In decision-making processes then, detailed referral and discussion to Mill, Kant or Aristotle was unnecessary. Once accepted, the principles are explanation enough of what should guide action. Later editions emphasised the importance of common morality rather than moral theory, that is constructing the principles from below rather than deriving them from above (Baker 2022). This change in emphasis is perhaps of greater interest to philosophers than to practitioners, but there is at least one common theme: Practitioners don't need to know a great deal of moral theory to make moral decisions. There is some evidence, however, that they do find moral theories useful (Monteverde 2014).

If the question of how much detail about moral theory that nurses need will be hotly debated, not least because of competing priorities in increasingly crowded pre-registration curricula,[18] there are other ways of assessing the use of moral theory in nursing practice. There are, for example, many examples of ethical decision-making frameworks, some of which make explicit reference to theories. Park (2012) identified and integrated 20 models, producing a rather complex model which includes consideration of ethical rules, principles, theories, professional ethics, legal aspects, personal conscience and institute or society's values. The review of existing models suggested that most applied a version of 'ethical pluralism applying diverse ethical theories' (Park 2012, p. 141). Consequentialism and deontology were predominantly used; care and virtue ethics were uncommon. Decision-making frameworks can be helpful in directing thinking but it's not clear how they can be of use, except in retrospect and upon reflection, to Stephanie, whose moral decision was made in the moment.

Rules (which can be internalised) are helpful for these situations. In a study which used a version of Stephanie as a case study (Kristjansson et al. 2017), over 80% of participants responded that they would refuse to follow the practice of deception. Having indicated the decision, participants were then asked to identify, from a list, their reasons for their decision. The list gave six reasons, two of which represented virtue-based reasoning, two represented consequentialist reasoning and two represented duty-based reasoning. The headline message from a range of results specified by scenario and sub-sample is that the commonest justification was duty-based reasoning for all groups. This propensity for experienced nurses to rely on rules was described as 'a disconcerting picture' in a further publication from the study (Varghese and Kristjansson 2018, p. 151).

A challenge for research like this is to make the reasons sufficiently specific so that the link between the reason and the moral theory is clear. One of the responses to the scenario designated as a deontological reason is that 'You are professionally obligated not to deceive your patients' (Kristjansson et al. 2017, p. 25). However, this reason could equally refer to professional rather than ethical reasons, following a rule in a code of ethics. Surveys are rather blunt instruments because it is difficult to distinguish between reasons for rule following. A rule (or clause in the code) can be adhered to because it's your duty, or because it's derived from virtue or because it tends to maximise outcomes, or complied with (just) to avoid sanction (Spielthenner 2015). Qualitative research enquiring about how nurses understand their moral environment tends to focus on experiences rather than a detailed discussion whether or how this or that moral theory is utilised in shared decision making or dilemmas addressed (for example, see Karlsson et al. 2015).

Conclusion

There has also not been enough space to consider other perhaps stronger influences on our individual moral outlook – culture, religion and education, and the professional and legal context has been considered only in passing. That noted, would any of this chapter be of any assistance to Stephanie and her specific decision or any of the others that she would need to consider during her work? The moral theories I have introduced all argue in various ways and supported by survey evidence, that she was wrong, but I suggest that act utilitarianism provides the most plausible defence. For my own part, though I admit to utilitarian tendencies, my objection was mainly deontological. Would Stephanie admit to being a utilitarian for all decisions? Kristjansson et al.'s (2017) study does not report data on whether participants were consistent in their approach across the six scenarios presented. Many nurses, I suspect, will follow Gallagher (2018, p. 105) in describing themselves as 'pragmatic pluralists' as far as normative moral theory is concerned even if this is not so much concerned with identifying right action as its justification and the way the decision is undertaken.

It seems to matter whether care is delivered because of its consequences, or for the sake of duty, or because the nurse is genuinely caring, a trait which leads them to want to care, and/or has an emotional connection with the patient. As well as often arriving at the same normative conclusion, there can be common ground in the approaches such that a virtuous person can favour utilitarian arguments, for example. I would hope that Stephanie would benefit from understanding the broad approaches to normative moral theory, and I suggest that she would agree that there's no single *correct* moral theory for nursing practice.

Notes

1 Possibly unwisely. Prior to any discussion of morally right action, we should ask ourselves what is the purpose of nursing? What is it for? How can you recognise a good nurse or assess your own nursing care? What outcomes are we trying to maximise? Health, objectively measured, or patients' individual preferences? (Snelling 2018). Answers to these questions underpin any normative enquiry.

2 The Nursing and Midwifery Council is the statutory regulator of nurses and midwives in the UK. It sets educational standards and maintains a register.

3 In this context, I regard these words as virtually synonymous – that is, a moral theory is an ethical theory.

4 The Institute of Medical Ethics is 'Dedicated to improving education and debate in medical ethics. As a charitable organisation we promote and support the impartial study and understanding of medical ethics and its integration into clinical practice through education, research, and publication' (IME n.d.).

5 To be fair, this is not an exact comparison. There is no mention of moral theories in the General Medical Council's 'Generic Professional Capabilities Framework' (GMC 2017), but the point is that there is detailed curricula guidance produced for doctors but not for nurses, certainly in the UK. Reviews of ethical competence and detailed suggestions of what should be taught are available but these haven't made their way into a process that informs and guides curricula in the same way as the IME (Lechasseur et al. 2018; Gallagher 2006).

6 Codes come in varying titles, forms and function, including Codes of Ethics, Codes of Conduct, Codes of Practice and various combinations (Snelling 2016). In this chapter, I lump them together as Codes of Ethics.

7 See Lipscomb (2022) and responses on this point.

8 Was Stephanie lying? A lie is told when an agent says something that she knows to be false with the intention that others accept that it is true. Stephanie could say that she didn't lie, but hers is certainly an act of deception (Carson 2010). To those who say I should have picked a clearer example of lying, I reply that moral life is complex and nuanced. However, much law and morality turn on wafer-thin distinctions; discussion about whether something is a lie or not can miss the point about the morality of the particular act. This could be the subject of a chapter in itself.

9 The question of whether care ethics can be considered as a completely different theory, or set of theories, than virtue ethics will be of great interest to many and of no interest to others. Space in both curricula and texts is always limited. Choices are made.

10 According to Reeves (2007, p. 414) no less a scholar than Martha Nussbaum referred to Mill as 'the first great radical feminist in the western philosophical tradition'.

11 For example, Philippa Foot's trolly problem (Foot 1967) which has been much enlarged and adapted (for example by Edmonds 2014). A trolley hurtles down a track heading for five men. But there is a side spur where a single man is standing. Can we deflect the train so that only one man is killed? Or can we push a man in front of the train to stop it but killing him in the process in order to spare the five? Both the deflection and the push save five lives at the cost of one. Are they morally equivalent? Thought experiments like this are very useful to test intuitive objections to moral theories.

12 Guidance on these matters is much more developed for the medical profession than others, and for nurses is largely non-existent though the same considerations apply (Snelling and Quick 2022).

13 The precise wording depends on translation.

14 This strategy was introduced in the wake of the Francis Report into a scandal of very poor care in the NHS, and articulated six values for nursing: Care, Compassion, Competence, Communication, Courage and Commitment. At least one evaluation – O'Driscoll et al. (2018) – showed professional resistance and anger amongst nurses that the strategy is a top-down initiative which fails to recognise structural constraints.

15 A CINAHL search (1999–2023) for the keywords Nurs* and Ethic* combined with Deontolog* scored 89 hits, combined with Utilitarian* OR Consequentialis* scored 63 hits and combined with virtue* scored 205 hits. A search in the journal *Nursing Ethics* 1994–2022 using the words utilitarian*, deontology and virtue* scored 228, 136 and 632 hits, respectively. There are book-length applications of virtue ethics in nursing (Armstrong 2007; Sellman 2011) but none that I am aware of for utilitarianism or deontology. Hardly a bibliographic analysis but perhaps indicative of the field.

16 And, as a reminder, Care is the first of the 6Cs.

17 A nursing 'version' of this classic text was produced by Edwards in 1996 with a second edition in 2009.

18 In my own university and in addition to a research-based literature review dissertation, there is space for a module on evidence-based practice but not for one on ethics.

References

Alexander, L. (2008). Scalar properties, binary judgments. *Journal of Applied Philosophy*, 25(2), 85–104.

Aristotle (1953). *The Nicomachean Ethics*. Translated by J.A.K. Thomson. London: Penguin.

Armstrong, A. (2007). *Nursing Ethics: A Virtue-Based Approach*. London: Palgrave Macmillan.

Avery, G. (2013). *Law and Ethics in Nursing and Healthcare: An Introduction, Second Edition*. London: Sage.

Baker, R. (2022). Principles and duties: A critique of common morality theory. *Cambridge Quarterly of Healthcare Ethics*, 31(2), 199–211.

Beauchamp, T.L. & Childress, J.F. (2019). *Principles of Biomedical Ethics, Eighth Edition*. New York: Oxford University Press.

Begley, A.M. (2005). Practising virtue: a challenge to the view that a virtue centred approach to ethics lacks practical content. *Nursing Ethics*, 12(6), 622–637.

Buka, P. (2020). *Essential Law and Ethics in Nursing*. London: Routledge.

Carson, T.L. (2010). *Lying and Deception: Theory and Practice*. Oxford: Oxford University Press.

Department of Health (2010). *Confidentiality: NHS Code of Practice – Supplementary Guidance: Public Interest Disclosures*. [online] https://assets.publishing.service.gov.uk/government/uploads/system/uploads/attachment_data/file/200147/Confidentiality_-_NHS_Code_of_Practice_Supplementary_Guidance_on_Public_Interest_Disclosures.pdf (last accessed 26th January 2023).

Department of Health (2012). *Compassion in Practice. Nursing, Midwifery ad Care Staff: Our Vision and Strategy*. [on line] https://www.england.nhs.uk/wp-content/uploads/2012/12/compassion-in-practice.pdf (last accessed 26th January 2023).

Edmonds, D. (2014). *Would You Kill the Fat Man?* Princeton: Princeton University Press.

Edwards, S.D. (2009). *Nursing Ethics, A Principle Based Approach*. London: Palgrave MacMillan.

Edwards, S.D. (2016). *Nursing Ethics, A Principle Based Approach, Second Edition*. London: Palgrave MacMillan.

Ferkany, M. & Newham, R. (2019). A comparison of approaches to virtue for nursing ethics. *Ethical Perspectives*, 26(3), 427–457.

Foot, P. (1967). The problem of abortion and the doctrine of the double effect. *Oxford Review*, 5.

Gallagher, A. (2006). The teaching of nursing ethics: Content and methods. Promoting ethical competence. In Davis, A.J., Tschudin, V., & de Reave, L. (Eds.) *Essentials of Teaching and Learning in Nursing Ethics*. Edinburgh: Churchill Livingstone Elsevier. Chapter 20 pp. 223–239.

Gallagher, A. (2018). Progress in nursing ethics: Something old, something new… In Carr, D (Ed.) *Cultivating Moral Character and Virtue in Professional Practice*. London: Routledge, Chapter 7, pp. 96–107.

General Medical Council (2017). Generic professional capabilities framework. [online] https://www.gmc-uk.org/-/media/documents/generic-professional-capabilities-framework--2109_pdf-70417127.pdf#page=8 (last accessed 26th January 2023).

Graham, G. (2004). *Eight Theories of Ethics*. London: Routledge.

Gilligan, C. (1982). *In a Different Voice*. Cambridge: Harvard University Press.

Hare, R.M. (1981). *Moral Thinking. Its Levels, Method and Point*. Oxford: Oxford University Press.

Hodkinson, K. (2008). How should a nurse approach truth-telling? A virtue ethics perspective. *Nursing Philosophy*, 9(4), 248–256.

Hursthouse, R (1999). *On Virtue Ethics*. Oxford: Oxford University Press.

Institute of Medical Ethics (n.d.). https://ime-uk.org/ (last accessed 26th January 2023).

Institute of Medical Ethics (2019). Core Curriculum for Undergraduate Medical Ethics and Law. [online] https://ime-uk.org/wp-content/uploads/2020/10/IME_revised_ethics_and_law__curriculum_Learning_outcomes_2019.pdf (last accessed 26th January 2023).

Kant, I. (1994). *Ethical Philosophy (Second Edition)*. Translated by J.W. Ellington. Indianapolis: Hackett Publishing.

Karlsson, M., Berggren, I., Kasén, A., Wärnå-Furu, C., & Söderlund, M. (2015). A qualitative metasynthesis from nurses' perspective when dealing with ethical dilemmas and ethical problems in end-of-life care. *International Journal for Human Caring*, 19(1), 40–48.

Kristjansson, K., Varghese, J., Arthus, J., & Moller, F (2017). Virtuous practice in nursing: Research Report. University of Birmingham, Jubilee Centre. [online] https://www.jubileecentre.ac.uk/1588/projects/virtues-in-the-professions/virtuous-practice-in-nursing (last accessed 26th January 2023).

Kuhse, H. (1997). *Caring: Nurses, Women and Ethics*. Oxford: Blackwell.

LaFollette, H., & Persson, I. (Eds.) (2013). *The Blackwell Guide to Ethical Theory, Second Edition*. Oxford: Wiley Blackwell.

Lechasseur, K., Caux, C., Dollé, S., & Legault, A. (2018). Ethical competence: An integrative review. *Nursing Ethics*, 25(6), 694–706.

Lipscomb, M. (2022). Pain is (or may not be) what the patient says it is – professional commitments: objects of study or sacrosanct givens? In Lipscomb, M. (Ed.) *Complexity and Values in Nurse Education*. Oxford: Routledge.

McLeod-Sordjan, R. (2014). Evaluating moral reasoning in nursing education. *Nursing Ethics*, 21(4), 473–483.

Mill, J.S. (1998). *Utilitarianism*. Oxford: Oxford University Press.

Monteverde, S. (2014). Undergraduate healthcare ethics education, moral resilience, and the role of ethical theories. *Nursing Ethics*, 21(4), 385–401.

Noddings, N. (1984). *Caring: A Feminist Approach to Ethics and Moral Education*. Berkley: University of California Press.

Nursing and Midwifery Council (2018a). Future nurse: Standards of proficiency for registered nurses. [on line] https://www.nmc.org.uk/globalassets/sitedocuments/standards-of-proficiency/nurses/future-nurse-proficiencies.pdf (last accessed 26th January 2023).

Nursing and Midwifery Council (2018b). The Code: Professional standards of practice and behaviour for nurses, midwives and nursing associates. [online] https://www.nmc.org.uk/globalassets/sitedocuments/nmc-publications/nmc-code.pdf (last accessed 26th January 2023).

O'Driscoll, M., Allan, H., Liu, L., Corbett, K., & Serrant, L. (2018). Compassion in practice—Evaluating the awareness, involvement and perceived impact of a national nursing and midwifery strategy amongst healthcare professionals in NHS Trusts in England. *Journal of Clinical Nursing*, 27(5–6), e1097–e1109.

Paley, J. (2006). Past caring. The limitations of one-to-one ethics. In Davis, A.J., Tschudin, V., & de Reave, L. (Eds.) *Essentials of Teaching and Learning in Nursing Ethics*. Edinburgh: Churchill Livingstone Elsevier. Chapter 14 pp. 149–164.

Park, E.J. (2012). An integrated ethical decision-making model for nurses. *Nursing Ethics*, 19(1), 139–159.

Rawls, J. (1974). The independence of moral theory. *Proceedings and Addresses of the American Philosophical Association*, 48, 5–22.

Reeves, R. (2007). *John Stuart Mill: Victorian Firebrand*. London: Atlantic Books.

Savulescu, J., Persson, I., & Wilkinson, D. (2020). Utilitarianism and the pandemic. *Bioethics*, 34(6), 620–632.

Sellman, D. (2011). *What Makes a Good Nurse*. London: Jessica Kingsley.

Snelling, P.C. (2016). The metaethics of nursing codes of ethics and conduct. *Nursing Philosophy*, 17(4), 229–249.

Snelling, P.C. (2018). The subversion of Mill and the ultimate aim of nursing. *Nursing Philosophy*, 19(1), e12201.

Snelling, P. & Quick, O. (2022). Confidentiality and public interest disclosure: A framework to evaluate UK healthcare professional regulatory guidance. *Medical Law International*, 22(1), 3–32.

Spencer, A., Rivero-Arias, O., Wong, R., Tsuchiya, A., Bleichrodt, H., Edwards, R.T., ... Clarke, P. (2022). The QALY at 50: One story many voices. *Social Science & Medicine*, 296, 114653.

Spielthenner, G. (2015). Why comply with a code of ethics? *Medicine, Health Care and Philosophy*, 18(2), 195–202.

Sterba, J.P. (2005). *The Triumph of Practice over Theory in Ethics*. Oxford: Oxford University Press.

Timmons, M. (2021). *Moral Theory: An Introduction*. New Delhi: Dev Publishing.

Tingle, J. & Cribb, A. (Eds.) (2014). *Nursing Law and Ethics*. Oxford: Wiley Blackwell.

Tronto, J.C. (1994). *Moral Boundaries: A Political argument for an Ethic of Care*. New York: Routledge.

Tschudin, V. & Marks-Maran, D. (1993) *Ethics: A Primer for Nurses. Workbook*. London, Balliere Tindall.

Varghese, J. & Kristjansson, K. (2018). Experienced UK Nurses and the missing U-curve of virtue based reasoning. In Carr, D. (Ed.) *Cultivating Moral Character and Virtue in Professional Practice*. London: Routledge, Chapter 11, pp. 151–165.

Walker, R. (2023). Kant. In Angier, T. (Ed.) *Ethics: The Key Thinkers (Second Edition)*. London: Bloomsbury Academic.

Washington, H.A. (2008). *Medical Apartheid: The Dark History of Medical Experimentation on Black Americans from Colonial Times to the Present*. New York: Anchor Books.

Wheeler, H. (2012). *Law, Ethics and Professional Issues for Nursing: A Reflective and Portfolio-Building Approach*. London: Routledge.

8 Nursing

A moral profession?

Roger Newham

Could there be an immoral profession? Perhaps 'the oldest profession' could be. Even this question raises a host of others about the nature of morality and thus immorality. It is doubtful as to whether prostitution is a profession. Even though definitions of a profession are contested, prostitution does not fit with the various sociological descriptions of a profession though perhaps other occupations now do. This chapter leaves it open as to the moral status of prostitution. There does seem to be a historical thread based on the act of 'profession' or professing to serve others that has been and still is used to distinguish professions from other occupations (Pellegrino, 2001a). Perhaps prostitution could fit such an account. Although the association with professing is based on serving the public as a form of altruism, yet nurses in most institutions, perhaps all, are paid for their service. However, the altruistic service is again an 'ideal type' and need not reflect any actual practice of nursing. For the sake of this chapter, the assumption is that nursing is a profession or at least a semi-profession (Etzioni, 1969). It might not meet the usual sociological accounts of a profession that includes a strong autonomous stance especially concerning organisation of its work, though, today, this is not confined to the nursing profession. Nevertheless, it does seem to have a particularly strong claim to being a profession as an 'ideal type' as altruistic service providing an essential good or more likely goods (for human beings?). What nursing's distinctive good is, if anything, will be picked up later but it is of note that dustbin collectors also serve human goods as do ballet dancers and farmers and more contentiously health service managers and prostitution and some ballet dancers are professional ballet dancers. Perhaps goods of health and justice served by the professions of medicine (nursing) and law are more fundamental or at least more important than other goods. There needs be some account of how and why this might be. One way to do so is to connect the goods to morality. Morality matters, but how much and how does it connect with the idea of goods or value?

If nursing has recently become a profession, then being a profession is not an essential part of being a nurse; it cannot be the essence of nursing that it is a profession. Nursing may directly connect to morality when it was not a profession. Depending on one's account (or the true account?) of morality, nurses in religious orders might be such an example, but also nurses more generally. But if, as is very plausible, morality encompasses all professions and occupations, this would not distinguish nursing from many other occupations. This raises the point that professions connection to morality is meant to be something more than morality been applied to them as it is applied everywhere else.

DOI: 10.4324/9781003427407-10

Rather, the claim seems to be that professions have a divergent or even different morality (Williams, 1983; Rhodes, 2022).

> What gives interest to the idea of a professional morality is the possibility that such a morality may diverge from 'ordinary' or 'everyday' morality. Indeed, it is this possibility that gives content to the idea of a professional morality at all, as opposed merely to a set of conventions or styles of etiquette associated with certain professions.
>
> (Williams, 1983, 192)

But understanding in what sense professional morality can diverge from or differ from ordinary morality is hard to grasp. Ordinary morality allows that certain acts can only be done in special, specified circumstances if they are not to be immoral, that the same act can be (morally) acceptable in some circumstances and not in others (Williams, 1983, p. 194). It is of note that Williams holds divergence and possible conflict can occur because of professional dispositions or sentiments. He was writing a chapter for an American book about good lawyers, and lawyers having (some) professional dispositions most might find ethically poor. But in relation to nursing, this may have resonance from a different angle about how nurses should be. Where the weight expected of nurse's dispositions and sentiments for providing altruistic service results in mystification of the idea of the nursing profession.

> What will be needed in concrete social terms will be a respect for the profession that takes the form of appropriate sentiments and is expressed in certain practices. If too much is asked of those sentiments, they will break down or will have to fall back on mystification.
>
> (Ibid, 198)

There seem to be two broad attempts in the literature at connecting morality to professions that are the theories approach and the practice approach. In fact, the practice approach divides, with one approach being much more radical in its understanding of morality than the other. These, in turn, are based on what account is given of the nature of morality, being meta-ethical, epistemological, and normative. Briefly and crudely, morality as theory is 'applied' to practice. Morality as theory holds that norms discovered as a part of reality, or as constitutive of agency or constructions of reason, do not depend upon any social roles or practices for their nature and authority. Principles derived from the theory are applied to practice or, perhaps better, are enacted albeit with the necessity of judgement. Morality as practice begins by claiming norms, including moral norms arise from social practice, such as the context or standpoint of nursing practice. Often, the standpoint relates to moral theory that prioritises the Good via a specific type of Good or ends the practice taken as essential or at least focal. However, this cannot be all there is to the point of claiming nursing as a moral profession. It is perhaps more to do with the notion of context of nursing practice and in some sense the morality being dependent on the context, including the role or profession of being a nurse. It seems to be implying that the norms arising in the relationship between nurses and others depend for their justification and thus authority, perhaps even their existence, on the role and context, which are partial rather than impartial and that these norms are moral norms as opposed to non-moral norms, for example, professional norms or sociological norms.

Morality as practice also requires judgement. The emphasis given here on the need for judgement will become important later. The point for now is the claim that morality as theory cannot account for professional morality's special (moral) obligations or relationships, or importance. It needs a morality of practice in order to do so, to recognise nursing as a moral profession and to account for what acts nurses should and should not do as well as virtues they must have. Both accounts, however, have problems.

Moral theory approach

It is hard to state something general about moral theory that is not contested. Moral theory is, generally, an attempt to give an account of morality which is part of normativity and thus practical, aiming to change the world if the world does not fit with the moral norms. Its norms or its reasons have some special weight or authority grounded in either the right or the good (value) with its principles being universal, general, and impartial. But what is contested is how much authority moral norms or reasons have (Dorsey, 2016).

Nursing as a moral profession would be understood as the application or enactment of moral principles to their situations and potential actions. It is thought that *ultimately* morality makes roles irrelevant to the moral assessment of acts or potential acts. If moral theory entails moral norms as universal, general, and impartial, then it seems that there can be nothing morally distinctive of professions such as nursing. Either nursing is justified by morality or it is not. Either professions are justified by morality or they are not. Therefore, standpoints such as a nursing standpoint require conformity to moral norms. Failure to conform to one's moral norms entails a normative failure, and one acts wrongly. We blame people who fail to act morally. We blame a nurse, dustbin collector, or prostitute. Perhaps a lot more of nursing work is closely related to morality than say a dustbin collector and thus we may be praising and blaming nurses more frequently but that does not make for a divergent or distinct morality.

However, it seems what is expected of a moral theory approach is algorithmic action guidance. That is guidance known in advance of actual action as what particular acts (not the broader type of acts) should and should not be done *by nurses*. However, as Onora O'Neil (1990) as well as moral theorists such as Kant and Mill claim, this cannot be done. Judgement is always required. The expectation that moral theory should provide an algorithmic decision-making approach to nursing practice or anything else is mistaken.

Moral principles are connected to types of cases not tokens, and being normative are meant to change the world, not fit it. Rather than application, principles are enacted in contexts or situations. Thus, the idea of a moral profession as a specification of general moral principles will not take one all the way to knowledge of what to do in a particular case. In part because moral reasoning as, practical reasoning is about actions yet to be done moral principles as normative principles are 'ineliminably indeterminate' (O'Neil, 1990, 186). Practical judgement is always needed. Principles are defeasible but not dispensable (Ibid., 188). Additionally, there are usually many competing principles to be taken into consideration and this is perhaps especially so in nursing practice. Importantly, moral principles and other normative requirements need to jointly enact (O'Neil, 1990). So, on the moral theory approach, it seems as though a moral profession understood as providing clear principles for action in nursing contexts is somewhat redundant because as norms and in this case as moral norms, it cannot do so. Instead, the enactment of professional norms and ethical norms and probably other norms needs considering and at the end of the day, judgement will still be needed as to what one actually does. Taking advice from O'Neil:

> We need to move from discussions of principles relevant to specifiable situations and contexts to discussions of policies and institutions that support processes of practical judgement by making it easier to achieve adequate enactments of those principles in a wide variety of demanding situations.
>
> (192)

Thus, moral theory can account for moral norms and leave room for professional norms and other practical norms that matter. The point of claiming nursing as a moral profession becomes redundant but there can be professional norms as norms that are required as a nurse and for consistency in actions as nurses. It may or may not be that strong moral rationalism is true and that moral norms would override all other practical norms, but even if it were true, the point still holds though the consequences may be different.

Morality as a practice approach

The work of Edmund Pellegrino (for example, 2001a and 2001b) often in conjunction with David Thomasma (for example, 1981) is extremely instructive in recognising the problems of professions and the connection to morality and trying to provide a third way between a moral theory approach and MacIntyre's (1981) notion of a practice approach. It is particularly instructive because he wants to rely on the MacIntyrean account of a practice and internal goods; yet, he also sees the problem in doing so as did MacIntyre himself in works published after *After Virtue*. Both MacIntyre and Pellegrino ultimately saw that their accounts of a secular, socially constructed, practice-based approach required underpinning by very abstract (and a certain type of religious) moral theory via natural law which was then to be applied to professional morality or what it was to be a moral profession. They both end up with a moral theory approach with universal, general, impartial principles that is also strongly rationalistic.

But morality as a practice approach is meant to eschew moral theory especially its generality and impartiality and rely instead on either the special context and relationships of, for example, nursing practice or particular action judgements by people with practical wisdom (*phronesis*). Sellman (2011) claims that a worry of such a (virtue) practice approach is that it is conservative. This need not be the case as thoughtful nurses within the practice and those outside of the practice can change it. Rather, the worry has to do with what morality is taken to be. A practice approach to morality that is in any sense reliant on norms of groups will not be authoritative for those not a part of the group and even perhaps not for some within the group (O'Neil, 1990).

Perhaps morality matters more than etiquette or convention, but some account is needed as to the nature of such a morality. Practice-based accounts of morality are on most accounts a partial or ethnocentric approach to moral norms. The socially constructed ends are not all there is to the practice approach; additionally, there is the idea of nurses' dispositions or sentiments and the broader claim about a unity of an individual life and how such dispositions contribute to the good life. So, a moral profession and a professional morality does not on a practice approach create goods based on whatever norms are socially constructed at a particular time for a particular community; rather, the goods themselves must be part of the wider good, the moral good. Hence, it seems to slide towards a moral theory approach. Often, the practice approach is linked to virtue ethics and for nursing as a moral profession, the unifying factor would be its sense of purpose related to ends of nursing and the idea of commitment and identity. Foot's (2001) account of 'natural goodness' might seem to fit quite well with healthcare professions being about functioning of human beings but tying such goods of human function to both a distinct end for humans in reason and morality is problematic (and Foot denies her approach is to be labelled virtue ethics). Though nurses have or must have certain dispositions and also character traits as virtues, it is dispositions or sentiments that seem to be the point of Williams' (1983) account of how professional morality can diverge though not be distinct from 'ordinary' morality. And it is a virtue account of nursing practice that seems to (but ultimately does not) allow for a distinct or divergent morality for nurses giving sense to the idea of a moral profession. But a virtue account of nursing practice needs an account of the end or ends of nursing practice.

A particularly acute problem for understanding nursing as a moral profession with a professional morality is providing an account, or better, the account of what nursing is (Edwards, 1997). It should not be *a* philosophy of nursing as though there could be many such philosophies. Philosophy of nursing must be able to provide the end(s) of nursing that are distinct from other healthcare professionals based on what nursing (essentially?) is. There are already some signs of this problem in Pellegrino's (2001a and 2001b) accounts where, dependent on the level of generality, it slides towards a healthcare worker's profession to all professions having a common internal morality to morality more generally and then to religion or spiritual and transcendent (Adams, 2002) good which is taken to be ultimate and overriding. At some point, the internal will become external. It is plausible to claim that nursing sees its distinctiveness in understanding the whole person who is a patient promoting their well-being as a whole. Yet, a focus on promoting the well-being of the whole person is an essential part of clinical medicine in Pellegrino's philosophy of medicine, where the end of medicine includes not only curing but helping to die well, though, of course, for Pellegrino and many others, never intentionally acting to end a life (Pellegrino, 2005). Pellegrino, like MacIntyre, ends up ultimately with morality as having overriding force. One immediate concern with morality being understood to be overriding in its force, such that, for example, prostitution is always morally wrong or always bad (for human beings or human agency), regardless of time and place and particular situation, is that nurses will in many cases be breaching their terms of employment and also the law and probably be at odds with what the patient thinks good and right.

Nursing as a moral profession has been articulated by nurses as something more than an ability to carry out evidence-based skills or tasks using measurable, pre-determined outcomes (Newham et al., 2013). Nursing has been called a *praxis*, rather than a *techne* or *poesis* whereby *praxis* is morally laden and/as intrinsically good. Nursing's professional morality has been articulated using Aristotle and the idea of virtuous character, so rather than just a focus on how something is done, focus is also given to the way it is done (Armstrong, 2010; Sellman, 2011). *Phronesis* has been used to explicate the idea that nursing, or at least expert nursing, is a type of practical wisdom that is essentially moralised and unlike *poesis* it cannot be separated from the moral character of the person. But without some account of what nursing is, its ontology, we cannot understand how such practical wisdom can be nursing practical wisdom. In any case, *phronesis* entails much more than nursing, being about how to live generally. Additionally, the moral epistemology of such an approach is hard to understand; how does one know about or how does reason provide access to such objective, usually non-natural goods?

So, the idea of nursing as a moral profession has highlighted the importance of what nursing is. We need a philosophy of nursing. Then perhaps we can start making the claim that because this is what nursing is, this is what nurses should and should not do and make the connection with morality. The use of morality is perhaps there to emphasise the importance of the claim. Morality matters and much of what nurses do matters and matters morally. The notion of right and good nursing practice is meant to provide a moral stance against other types of relationships a nurse might enter into, whether voluntarily or not, that would not be congruent with nursing's (essential) nature or ends. These could be broad political and economic activities such as perhaps 'managerialism' (Wong, 2004) or specific types of acts such as euthanasia (Pellegrino, 2005) and even theological stances about good acts (Welie, 2002). But it is not the nature of nursing or nursing as a profession that does this; it is morality. Nursing would be best to use its authority and respect it holds to argue for improvements to institutions so that professional norms, moral norms, and many other norms can best be accommodated within nursing practice, rather than focusing on knowing in advance what acts should and should not be done from a nursing and thus moral perspective and criticising others who emphasise different norms.

References

Adams, R. (2002) *Finite and Infinite Goods: A Framework for Ethics*, Oxford, Oxford University Press.

Armstrong, A. (2010) *Nursing Ethics: A Virtue Based Approach*, London, Palgrave Macmillan.

Dorsey, D. (2016) *The Limits of Moral Authority*, Oxford, Oxford University Press.

Edwards, S. (1997) What is philosophy of nursing? *Journal of Advanced Nursing*, 25, 1089–1093.

Etzioni, A. (1969) *The Semi Professions and their Organisation: Teachers, Nurses Social Workers*, New York, Free Press.

Foot, P. (2001) *Natural Goodness*, Oxford, Clarendon Press.

MacIntyre, A. (1981) *After Virtue: A Study in Moral Theory*, Notre Dame, University of Notre Dame Press.

Newham, R., Curzio, J., Carr, G., et al. (2013) Contemporary nursing wisdom in the UK and ethical knowing: problem explicating the ethics of nursing. *Nursing Philosophy*, 15, 50–56.

O'Neil, O. (1990) *Constructions of Reason: Explorations of Kant's Practical Philosophy*, Cambridge, Cambridge University Press.

Pellegrino, E. (2001) The internal morality of clinical medicine: paradigm for the ethics of the helping and healing professions. *Journal of Medicine and Philosophy*, 6, 559–579.

Pellegrino, E. (2005) Some things ought never be done: moral absolutes in clinical ethics. *Theoretical Medicine and Bioethics*, 26, 469–486.

Pellegrino, E., Thomasma, D. (1981) *A Philosophical Basis of Medical Practice*, New York, Oxford University Press

Rhodes, R. (2022) The uncommon ethics of the medical profession: a response to my critics. *Cambridge Quarterly of Healthcare Ethics*, 31(2), 212–219.

Sellman, D. (2011) *What Makes A Good Nurse: Why the Virtues Are Important for Nursing*. London, Jessica Kingsley Publishers.

Welie, J. (2002) The relationship between medicine's internal morality and religion. *Christian Bioethics*, 8(2), 175–198.

Williams, B. (1983) Professional morality and its dispositions in David Leuban (ed.), *The Good Lawyers: Lawyers' Role and Lawyers' Ethics*, New Jersey, Rowman and Allanheld, Ch 16.

Wong, W. (2004) Caring holistically within new managerialism. *Nursing Inquiry*, 11(1), 2–13.

9 Remembering the future
Nursing's social ethics

Marsha D. Fowler

Introduction

Bioethics, in itself and as imported into nursing, has a narrow compass. It is largely focused on medical clinical problems and conflicts such as end-of-life decisions, futile interventions, genetic advances, suicide and euthanasia, and patient refusal of treatment. Where *bioethics* takes a societal approach, usually deploying the concept of (distributive) justice, its focus is on access to care, cost of care, allocation of resources, and rationing. In recent years, this has enlarged to include concerns such as health inequalities, "greening" of hospitals, and triage in natural or human-made disasters. However, *nursing ethics*, that is the ethics generated by the nursing profession, prior to its importation of bioethics, more specifically from 1880s to 1965, has not been so pallid.

The development of modern nursing walks hand-in-hand with the development of nursing ethics, giving rise to an extraordinary body of literature, largely written by nurses for nurses. This includes approximately 100 textbooks and editions, and hundreds of journal articles. As the profession and its ethics take shape, it is profoundly affected by the social location of women, the first-wave feminism of early nursing leaders, the social concerns or the Progressive Era, and the related aspirations for the creation of a profession for women. These factors converge to shape the ethics of the profession *ab initio* as a distinctly social ethics. Yet 125 years later, nursing's movement into the university, its embrace of bioethics, and its loss of nursing humanities have caused its social ethics to languish and its ethics to become stunted. The way forward is for nursing to embrace its own capacious ethics, while using the more constricted bioethics as adjunctive. Reclaiming the plucky tradition of *nursing ethics* would create for nursing a clearer and brighter future with a stronger vision of the good society, the good nurse, and good patient care, by addressing issues of the social construction of health/illness, and even how an individual person became your patient in the first place.

Gendered barriers to the development of modern nursing

Nightingale had privileged access to men of power ready to further her ends, but those leaders who followed were hindered both by laws and by social norms that left women and the emerging modern nursing without formal power or authority. More specifically, it left them unable to create the structural framework for nursing. This would require the enfranchisement of women and overturning other legal disabilities that constrained women, such as a married woman's right to own property; to control her own money; to have child custody in a divorce; to engage a lawyer; to being a person under the law

DOI: 10.4324/9781003427407-11

(i.e., the abolition of coverture laws); rights of access to education, employment; and more (with national differences).[1] Social limitations ratcheted the legal manacles tighter. The political clout to form a profession required the power to vote and to pressure legislators formally in order to create legal structures such as licensure, registration, standardisation of education, and title protection. However, an educated, scientific, paid profession for women working outside the home flew in the face of the "cult of true womanhood" which "held that white women were rightfully and naturally located in the private sphere of the household and not fit for public, political participation or labor in the waged economy."[2,3] Kang notes that "the white middle-class leadership of the first wave [feminist] movement shaped the priorities of the movement, often excluding the concerns and participation of working-class women and women of color."[4] Issues of race, class, and gender played a part in early modern nursing. Most of the early nursing leaders were white, Christian, middle-class, educated (not necessarily schooled at this point), single women.[5] To prepare legal structures to undergird nursing was one thing – to prepare society for women to be formally educated professionals was yet another, implicitly constituting an assault upon True Womanhood. The barriers to professionalising nursing necessitated battling on two different fronts, with women in both camps. Then, as now, not all women believed in "equality for women."

The emergence of modern nursing is also set within the context of the wide-ranging social reforms of the Progressive Era. While progressivism in the US and the UK was different, they both sought to rectify social problems. These included problems of urbanisation, industrialisation, immigration, political corruption, and alcoholism. This was largely a middle-class movement that addressed myriad ills in domains of government policies, civil rights, politics, and society. Societal reforms included the education of children and women, the scientisation and professionalisation of academic disciplines, including medicine, social sciences, history, economics, education, political science, and the humanities. Early nursing leaders were engaged in an astonishing range of civic and social reforms.[6] Women's suffrage; women's, worker's, children's and animal rights, and broad social reforms – a plateful of activism even before adding lashings of nursing.

Nursing's social engagement

The early nursing leaders sought to imbue a commitment to social engagement in nursing students through curricular requirements and moral formation. The 1916 California Bureau of Registration of Nurses curriculum requirements for ethics mandated lectures and readings on "Democracy and Social Ethics," "Modern Industry," "Housing Reform," "The Spirit of Youth and the City Streets,"and other social-ethical concerns.[7,8] In 1917, the National League for Nursing Education published its "Standard Curriculum for Schools of Nursing." It mandated ethics lectures, including sequential sections on:

• Introduction: Customary Morality
• Personal or Reflective Morality
• Ethical Ideals and Standards
• Moral Judgement; Conduct and Character
• Place of "Self" in the Moral Life
• Social Virtues
• Ethical Principles as Applied to Community Life

- Principles of Ethics Applied to One's Work or Profession
- Principles of Ethics Applied to One's Personal Life[9,10]

Additional ethics content was expected to be taught. This ethics curriculum bears little resemblance to the narrower contemporary bioethics content. The content is overwhelmingly oriented towards social concerns, and there is little in the way of the dilemmatic content of today's curriculum. Instead, the emphasis is on the moral character of the nurse, the moral aspects of nursing relationships, including the moral obligations of the nurse to herself – which receive little attention in bioethics.

Nursing ethics was structured around classes of relationships. Harriet Camp wrote a six-part series on ethics in *Nurse and Hospital Review* (1889). She writes:

> For convenience sake I will divide the duties of a nurse into seven classes: 1st. Those she owes to the family. 2nd. Those she owes to the doctor. 3rd. Those owing the family, friends, and servants of the patient. 4th To herself. 5th. To her own friends. 6th To her own hospital or school. 7th. To other nurses.[11]

This configuration reflects the fact that nursing predominantly took place in the patient's home. Nursing ethics would continue to be structured around specific relationships, though the classes would be recombined and reconfigured over the years, most often into five relationships: (a) nurse to patient/family, (b) nurse to physician and other health professionals, (c) nurse to self, (d) nurse to profession and nurse colleagues, and (e) nurse to society. The nursing ethics textbooks dealt with each of these relationships, though some focused exclusively on the nurse-to-patient relationship. The ethics of nursing articulated through these relationships suffused the theoretical and practical curricula and the clinical apprenticeship. The ANA *Code of Ethics for Nurses* (2015), even today, retains a relational structure and is a vestigial remnant of nursing ethics in an era now dominated by bioethics.

In the nurse-to-society relationship, graduate nurses were formed into civic engagement through lectures, conference papers, association meetings, and more. The most basic level of the duties within this relationship became (after suffrage was passed) the duty to vote, or more precisely to be an informed voter. Even before suffrage, nursing leaders sought the rectification of social ills *as nurses*. However, the duty to vote, *as nurses*, met with very specific obstacles.

The Lynchpin: women's suffrage

Suffrage was a messy affair. It could be granted and then taken away, have restrictions such as voting in municipal but not national elections, and have lower voting criteria for men. The conditions for individual women to be enfranchised presented a problem for nurses. The condition for Local Government Franchise, upon which Parliamentary Franchise was based, was age 30, no legal incapacity, and six months tenancy with sole access. For nurses,

> Any woman…who inhabits any dwelling house by virtue of any office, service, or employment (namely, matron of a hospital, headmistress living in a school house, etc.), and the employer under whom she serves in such employment does not reside in the house, will be a tenant.[12]

Under the criteria, the matron qualified for the vote, but nurses did not as they did not have exclusive access to their rooms. "The control of nurse's rooms in English hospitals rests...in the matron and not in the nurse."[13] One British nurse proposed that

> if hospitals in this country would adopt the plan which has been introduced...in the United States, the difficulty...would be overcome...At those American hospitals the management of the nurses' homes or nurses' quarters is entirely in the hands of the nurses themselves...the matrons have nothing to do with them.[14]

Ultimately, both British[15] and American nurses were enfranchised.

Evil social conditions and the uprising of women

Lavinia Dock (1859–1956), an American nursing leader in the US, the UK, and the International Council of Nurses (ICN), expresses concern that younger nurses had forgotten the struggles that went before them, and what it meant for enabling nurses to engage in social change.

> I have felt greatly concerned about the nurses' attitude, because it shows that they had forgotten—or that the younger ones had never learned—the we owed our existence as an educated and respectable profession to the woman movement...The fact of this enormous debt, and that we would simply not exist, except as miserable Gamps and slaves, had it not been for the uprising of women (and I contend that the claim for the ballot cannot be separated from the general advance of women) makes the whole question...take on a very different aspect. For I feel that our younger members need to be told what has gone before...Oh, how much there is to be done that will never get done until women have power!...Child labor... the question of venereal disease... prostitution, will never really be solved until that day, when women...enact laws that will assist and encourage educational propaganda which must, of course go hand in hand with prevention... the glorious thing about education as to diseases is that it brings you straight and unerringly, and with no delay, down to the social causes which are contributory, and which need legislation for their removal. This strong light thrown on evil social conditions will show more urgent reasons for removing them than could be done by a century of argument.[16]

Notions of the social construction of the conditions of illness and disease and health disparities were pervasive among the early nursing leaders. The amelioration of "evil social conditions" was seen to be within the purview, expertise, and moral duty of nurses. Their nursing literature emphasises nurses' moral obligation to vote, to stand for office if so skilled, and to advocate for the social changes that would provide for the health and well-being of all the nations. To aide in this, the *Nursing Record* (later the *British Journal of Nursing*) regularly reported on and reprinted excepted minutes of the actions of Parliament.

The editor of the *Nursing Times* asks, "How shall I vote," and indicates that the answer to this question requires nurses to ask "the kind of government we think desirable" to address the countless social problems.

> With regard to domestic affairs...there are many questions of housing (we shall want a healthy home for everyone, at a cost within the means of the wage earners); questions

of equal pay for equal work; of divorce (is it fair that there should be inequality between men and women?); of infant life protection; of the motherhood of the nation; of the supply of pure milk; and so on.[17]

Not only were these thought to be questions women should tackle, but that nurses were particularly equipped to do so.

> ...such questions as education, housing, infant mortality and welfare come within the scope of women, and more especially of nurses, and all these are questions for Parliament...[18]

The whole of society, and the world, was nursing's walnut to crack, a vision for nursing that subsequently waned after the 1960s, as nursing left the hospital schools, entered the universities, gave up their hospital libraries, ceded ethics to philosophers, and embraced bioethics. The social concern of bioethics does not have nursing's wider compass. This is a thin overview of nursing's social engagement, one that a specific social issue, venereal diseases, will help to illustrate. The work of nurses, Albinia Broderick (1861–1955), Lavinia Dock, and Mary Burr, is noteworthy for our purposes here.

Venereal disease: it's not about sex

Pre-antibiotic venereal diseases were a global scourge, always worsening during wartime, or around military bases. Sir William Osler (1849–1919) called syphilis "the fourth killing disease, the other three being heart complaints, cancer, and tuberculosis."[19]

Concerns included the transmission of the venereal diseases between prostitutes and military men, prostitutes and civilian men, men and their wives, wives to an unborn child, and patients to nurses. As venereal disease ravaged society, it engaged various factions – including the military, nurses, physicians, church leaders, suffragists, and others. There were two different approaches: social morality and social hygiene. (*Social* is a pristinated term for *sexual*.) This is a Gordian knot that cannot be untied here, involving multiple intertwined movements, including feminism, suffrage, workers' rights, eugenics, birth control, sex education, prostitution, "white slavery," censorship and pornography, illegitimacy, temperance, drug abuse, rape, domestic violence, and much more. There are also issues of class, gender, and race that are likewise entailed. The social morality and hygiene movements are important to an understanding of the social-ethical engagement of early nursing with these issues.

The Social Morality Movement (or Abolitionist or Purity Movement) was an Anglo-American, middle-class, movement from the 1860s to about 1910 with some persistence today. The movement is rooted in the work in England of the remarkable Josephine Butler (1828–1906). Butler, a middle-class woman, campaigned for women's suffrage, for the right of women to better education; for the end of coverture in British (and American) law; for the abolition of female child prostitution; and for an end to "white slavery," that is, the trafficking of girls and British young women into Continental prostitution; and for an end to the prevailing sexual double standard. The movement's emphasis was on ending prostitution and attendant venereal disease, and on ending the sexual double standard. A concern for justice for women generally, and prostitutes specifically, and a good bit of anger, propelled this movement, to which working-class men were recruited.

An unexpected tsunami of women and feminist efforts was precipitated by the surreptitious passage of the UK Contagious Disease Acts of 1864, 1866, and 1869. The initial act sought to reduce the incidence of venereal disease among military men by controlling prostitution that was prevalent around military bases. The Acts required the forcible gynaecological examination of any woman thought to be, or reported to be, a prostitute. If she were found to be infected, she would be forcibly detained, for up to nine months, in a "lock hospital," until disease free.[20] There were plainclothes police, so-called "morality police" who trolled for these women, who had considerable independent discretion to bring charges.

In response to the Acts, Butler founded the Ladies National Association (LNA, 1869–1915), a brilliantly organised, effective, grass-roots movement that brought in women who had never before been politically active. The ladies of the LNA published "Women's Manifesto," which was signed by 2,000 women, including Florence Nightingale.[21,22] Victorian society in the UK and the US was unprepared for the force of this women's movement against the Acts and, more scandalously, for women to bring sex, sexual behaviour, sexually transmitted diseases, reproductive anatomy, and the sexual double standard into open discussion in polite society. The LNA held that these Acts were unconstitutional and morally wrong as they simultaneously established the business of prostitution, *de jure*; perpetuated both a sexual double standard and notions of male "sexual necessity"; and violated the constitutional rights of women. Butler maintained that her movement was an "abolitionist movement," not a "purity movement."

The Social Hygiene Movement was furthered by the military and the medical profession. Eventually, medicine realised that the regulation of prostitution was ineffective in disease control and called for its abolition. The military had a hardened general position that men could not be stopped from availing themselves of commercialised sex (prostitution) so that prostitution must be regulated.

In the end, the abolitionist movement transitions into a Social Hygiene Movement; the Acts are overturned; it is recognised that regulating prostitution is ineffective as a public health measure, that holding only women as the source and transmitter of venereal disease is absurd, and that the Acts did in fact violate the rights of women. This is an embarrassingly reductionistic version of these complex movements, but it is hoped sufficient to establish the context for the work of Broderick, Dock, and Burr, who present successive, coordinated, papers at the 1909 ICN Congress. Their papers were backed up by their clinical, political, and social action. These papers are demonstrative of the scope and depth of social ethics in nursing in the early part of the 1900s.

Albinia, Lavinia, and Mary

Albinia Broderick was a radical, Irish Republican, nurse. In 1909, she presented "Morality in Relation to Health," the first paper at the International Congress of Nurses.[23] Her paper detailed a vivid, dark, clinical picture of the three venereal diseases, the discovery of the causative microorganisms, a bit of the global history of the diseases, and the wreckage wrought by the transmission to prostitutes and servicemen, to husbands, to wives, to neonates, and to nurses in patient care. She notes that physicians hid the diagnosis from wives infected by their husbands and from nurses caring for infected patients: "it was common practice to hide from the woman the nature of her disease. She only knew that 'she had never been well since her marriage'."[24] While Broderick had first-hand nursing experience of patients with venereal disease, she was knowledgeable beyond clinical practice and ably addressed the history, scientific knowledge, clinical treatment, and global reach of the disease. Her central concern, however, was for the abolition of the Acts regulating prostitution and the sexual double standard. Her speech notes that such regulation had previously failed in every European country; it only captured the older, regular prostitutes and not the younger freelancing prostitutes; and that (she quotes a military report), "The isolation of a particular section of infected persons, namely of diseased prostitutes, cannot be considered an ideal method of arresting the disease, while large numbers of infected persons *of both sexes* remain free to spread the contagion"[25].

Broderick has specific recommendations: (a) forthright sex education for children, (b) teach children discipline and self-control, (c) make venereal disease reportable like other contagious diseases, (d) "open recognition. Bold acknowledgement of these diseases in our midst, and that they had to be met and treated," (e) "free and easily accessible treatment to which no moral stigma is attached," (f) punishment of infected persons who knowingly transmit the disease, and (g) the reduction of alcoholism. Much of her discussion is reminiscent of the early days of HIV/AIDS. She calls for nurses to be active in prevention, and that "scientific research should pursue its aims firmly and clearly, uninfluenced by the tyranny of custom and independent of prejudices."[26] Her paper is greeted with silence and "then the intense feeling it aroused found expression in a storm of applause which subsided only to be renewed again and again."[27]

Lavinia Dock's paper, "The Need of Education on Matters of Social Morality," followed. Dock applauds growth in the "candid teaching of physiology and hygiene of sex and the newest developments of preventive medicine." But she has harsh words for society that

> by reason of the deeply ingrained false shame, mock modesty, vulgar hypocrisy, and generally intensely pharisaic mental attitude that had been deeply ingrained in human society as the result of a double standard of morals, one for men and one for women.[28]

This double standard meant that women were not taught about reproductive physiology. She was particularly concerned that nurses knew and witnessed the clinical aspects and tragedies of venereal diseases, but they were

> lamentably ignorant of the real extent of this so-called 'social' or venereal disease... no moral or historical, humanly truthful teaching was heard as to the *reason why* of these horrible diseases...though nurses might talk amongst themselves of tragedies witnessed, they usually seemed to regard them vaguely as fixed conditions of a mysterious universe.[29]

Dock discusses the need to improve nursing education on venereal diseases that took into account the social context of the diseases, the "*reason why*" they existed beyond the causative microorganism. Dock then discusses prostitution,

> a subject so appalling and hideous that if one concentrated all one's thoughts upon it, especially on that branch called the white slave traffic, one could easily become deranged; yet in the efforts at the prevention of social diseases it could not be put aside.[30]

White slavery refers to the sex trafficking of British girls over the age of consent (13 years). Trafficking was essential to replacing the prostitutes who died of venereal diseases, and to satisfy the appetite for younger prostitutes. Dock notes that in the US, there were approximately 600,000 prostitutes whose "average life was 10 years, many dying after three to five years. Thus to keep up the supply about 60,000 fresh and once pure and healthy women were annually drafted into this death-dealing business."[31] She also notes that male prostitutes "were too often left out of consideration." Dock quotes Morrow, founder of the Society of Sanitary and Moral Prophylaxis (US): "Efforts should be directed not to making prostitution safe, but to prevent the making of prostitutes." She held that this was possible, but only if all women attained "the power such as could only be obtained through the possession of the franchise."[32]

Dock links nursing and women's power to eradicate social ills to women's authority based on enfranchisement. She, and all the leaders of early nursing, evidences an acute awareness of the social conditions that give rise to disease, and the necessity for their amelioration. In the case of prostitution and venereal disease, it was middle-class women advocating on behalf of outcast, lower-class women. Their position was not without flaws: they assume that all women in prostitution were forced or sold into the life. Some feminists today argue that the movement was patronising and classist. It may well have been. However, the close interaction nurses had with patients suffering from the devastating effects of venereal diseases engendered a measure of compassion as an impetus. Dock advocates for a fulsome agenda of teaching sex physiology and hygiene to the public, the abolition of the sexual double standard, and the educational preparation of nurses so that they might avoid becoming infected in the course of clinical practice. She also advocates for the improvement of women's education and wages, the ablation of social structures that reduce women to prostitution; for raising the age of consent from 13 to 16, and for the criminal punishment of white slave traffickers.

The third paper was presented by nurse Mary Burr (Director of the National Council of Trained Nurses of Great Britain and Ireland) on "Some Statistics of Criminal Assault Upon Young Girls." She acknowledges the extraordinary difficulty in obtaining adequate statistics and that some organisations "flatly refused to furnish information."[33] Burr investigates the number of cases of rape and sexual violence against girls, the number of subsequent prosecutions, the results of the prosecutions, and the ages of the victims. Because there were no comprehensive statistics to be had, she resorted to criminal statistics scrounged from various jurisdictions. In one jurisdiction, in 15 years there were reported 2,302 "cases of defilement [rape] of girls under 13 and 2442 cases of girls under 16 reported to the police."[34] Prosecutions were few, and convictions fewer still – 145 in total.[35] "On inquiry why prosecutions in cases of assault were so few, the reply received from all quarters was that the culprit was so often the father, step-father, or brother of the victim." Often, the children, as young as 10, were silenced, and if the girl were pregnant, she was "restrained by threats," and parents would not allow rescue workers to intervene. Burr was told that, in another jurisdiction, "convictions were very few, as relations were so often the culprits."[36]

As is the case today, some of the defendants blamed "...foreigners. But only one offender in all the reported cases for 1907 was an alien. These men who defiled women and violated their own offspring were British."[37] She continues, in conclusion,

> These men...had the power of helping to make the laws which women must obey, and of making them as easy as possible for the indulgence of their own lusts...Yet we are

told that men could well be trusted to look after women's interests and welfare. If such a state of things were the result of their care, the sooner women took matters in hand the better it would be for the nation's moral and physical condition.[38]

The discussants following the paper were from Germany, New Zealand, and Finland. Their words corroborated similar conditions, from all three papers, in their own counties.

In 1910, Dock published a nursing textbook, *Hygiene and Morality*.[39] It is a blistering, critique of British society. None of the socio-political structures escape unscathed. The jailers who abuse prostitutes, the disgruntled men who falsely accuse innocent women, the military that wants to assure safe illicit sex for its men, the judges who will not prosecute rapists and child molesters, the legislators and military who seek to contain venereal disease by cooping up and treating women alone, the Parliament that establishes laws that severely punish prostitutes but strenuously avoids abolishing prostitution, the MPs who make it a misdemeanour to kidnap a girl under 16 for sexual purposes – Dock gores all these and more. As a book written for nurses, it models both a vision for society and nursing activism.

What can be seen here is a concern for the individual person (prostitute), and a concern for the individual within a subclass of disadvantaged persons (lower-class, prostitute, outcast), and the subclass within a larger class (women in society). Broderick, Dock, and Burr undertake the critique of the entire ladder of social structures, from the physicians and hospitals, to the constabulary, to judges, to legislators, to the laws and how they are enacted, to Parliament/Congress. They critique legal, economic, political, military, medical, educational, and other social structures. They are equipped with facts, statistics, prowess in social critique, a commitment to social change, and an activist and reformist commitment fuelled by passion, values, and clinical experience. They cross national borders in their critique, making common cause for a shared nursing vision of global health. The health of society is at stake: its remedies cannot and may not come at the expense of vulnerable persons. Broderick, Dock, and Burr's nursing would not stand for this.

Social ethics: social criticism and social change

Social ethics is that division of applied ethics that engages in the critique of social structures with an emphasis on the socio-political conditions that foster social harms, including rigid social stratification, poverty, illness, exploitation, oppression, and injustice. It is the broader framework under which concerns for social justice are explored, but also embraces concerns for human dignity, well-being, and welfare; respect, community, freedom, and equality; the common good, social virtue, and more. Social justice is but one among many concepts within social ethics: it does not stand on its own. Social ethics is intrinsically political in nature and directed towards social policy. As Winter notes, social ethics is concerned with "issues of social order—the good, right, and ought in the organisation of human communities and the shaping of social policies. Hence the subject matter of social ethics is moral rightness and goodness in the shaping of human society."[40]

Dock, Broderick, and Burr had in-the-trenches first-hand experience of caring for persons suffering from conditions that were preventable, diseases that were the consequence of "evil social conditions." Their vision for nursing was not limited to the medical situation of the individual patient. Their vision extended to the context of the patient's illness and the social structures that affected health, illness, and treatment.

Conclusion

Contemporary nursing, by limiting its social concerns to those identified by bioethics, betrays our brilliant, expansive heritage. The justice literature in bioethics has broadened in recent years, and re-termed *social justice*; yet, it largely remains focused on access to care, the cost of care, and rationing. In addition, in recent years, nursing education has developed a blinkered focus on evidence-based practice, with diminished attention to philosophical, ethical, and social-ethical thinking. Today's nursing articles on sex trafficking (in CINAHL and PubMed databases) are limited to the clinical recognition of persons who have been trafficked, particularly in the emergency department, and do not address larger social or justice issues. It stands in stark contrast to the vision and social compass of Broderick, Dock, Burr, Fenwick, Nightingale, and others. Today, the *social critique* of trafficking is not found (CINAHL/PubMed) in the bioethics or nursing bioethics literature.

Social structures wound large segments of society, further harming those already disadvantaged. A sticking plaster on the patient does not ameliorate the social forces that damage individuals, families, and communities; forces that nursing is equipped to address. As Hurlston notes in 1911:

> To all thoughtful people who work among the poor in any of our large towns the questions must often present themselves: What is the cause all the disease we meet with among the children? Why, in the 20th century, in this so-called civilised country, is it allowed to exist? What are we all doing to improve this deplorable state of affairs?[41]

Indeed. Why are these conditions allowed to exist? What is nursing doing to improve this deplorable state of affairs? Perhaps remembering our foundational social ethics will provide nursing a vision for its future and even more cognisant clinical care.

Notes

1 Elizabeth Cady Stanton, "Declaration of Sentiments," *Report of the Woman's Rights Convention, Held at Seneca Falls, New York, July 19 and 20, 1848. Printed by John Dick.* (Rochester, NY: The North Star office of Frederick Douglass, 1848). Elizabeth Cady Stanton Papers, Manuscript Division, Library of Congress (007.00.00). https://www.loc.gov/exhibitions/women-fight-for-the-vote/about-this-exhibition/seneca-falls-and-building-a-movement-1776–1890/seneca-falls-and-the-start-of-annual-conventions/declaration-of-sentiments/

2 Barbara Welter, "The Cult of True Womanhood: 1820–1860," *American Quarterly*, 18, no. 2, Part 1 (Summer):151–174.

3 Milian Kang, Donovan Lessard, Lura Heston, and Sonny Nordmarken, *Introduction to Women, Gender, Sexuality Studies* (Amherst, MA: University of Massachusetts Amherst Libraries, 2917), https://openbooks.library.umass.edu/introwgss/front-matter/287-2/

4 Kang et al., *Women*, 117

5 Vern Bullough, Lilli Sentz, and Alice Stein, *American Nursing: A Biographical Dictionary*, vol. 2 (New York: Garland Publishing, 1992), xiv.

6 Marsha Fowler, Unpublished research (San Marino, CA: Huntington Library), rare documents archives, 1982.

7 Bureau of Registration of Nurses, California State Board of Health, *Schools of Nursing Requirements and Curriculum* (Sacramento: State Printing Office, 1916).

8 Marsha Fowler, "The Influence of the Social Location of Nurses-as-Women on the Development of Nursing Ethics," in *Nursing Ethics: Feminist Perspectives,* ed. Helen Kohlen and Joan McCarthy (London: Springer, 2020): 3–22.

9   National League for Nursing Education, *Standard Curriculum for Schools of Nursing* (New York: NLNE, 1917).

10 Fowler, *Influence*, 12.

11 HCC [Harriet C. Camp], "The Ethics of Nursing: Talks of a Superintendent with Her Graduating Class," *Trained Nurse* 12, no. 5 (May, 1889): 179.

12 Editor, "Votes for British Nurses," *The Nursing Times* XIV, no. 664 (January 19, 1918): 61–62.

13 Anon., "Nurses and the Vote," *The Nursing Times* XIV, no.781 (April 17, 1920): 475.

14 Anon., "Nurses and the Vote," 475.

15 Anon., "Nurses and the Vote," *The Nursing Times* XV, no. 749 (September 6, 1919): 893.

16 Lavinia Dock, "The Nursing Profession and the Vote," *The British Journal of Nursing* XLII, no. 1089 (February 13, 1909): 135.

17 Editor, "How Shall I Vote?," *The Nursing Times* XIV, no. 708 (November 23, 1918): 1171.

18 Editor, "Vote," 1171.

19 Anon. "Book review, *Address to Women on the Prevention of Venereal Disease*," *The Nursing Times* XIX, no. 955 (August 18, 1923): 782.

20 Judith Walkowitz, *Prostitution and Victorian Society: Women, Class, and the State* (Cambridge: Cambridge University Press, 1980), 1–9.

21 Walkowitz, *Prostitution*, 75–78, 281.

22 Women's Manifesto, https://archiveshub.jisc.ac.uk/search/archives/c1797273-1af3–349d-b16e-0ce3dacdce93

23 British Journal of Nursing, "International Congress of Nurses, Friday Morning July 23, 10 a.m. to 12:30PM," *British Journal of Nursing* XLIII, no. 1,117 (28 August, 1909): 171–173.

24 Albinia Broderick, "Morality in Relation to Health, ICN Congress," *British Journal of Nursing* XL111, no. 1,117 (28 August, 1909): 171.

25 Broderick, "Morality," 172.

26 Broderick, "Morality," 173.

27 Broderick, "Morality," 173.

28 Lavinia Dock, "The Need of Education on Matters of Social Morality," *British Journal of Nursing* XL111, no. 1,117 (28 August, 1909): 173.

29 Dock, "Need," 173.

30 Dock, "Need," 174.

31 Dock, "Need," 174.

32 Dock, "Need," 174.

33 Mary Burr, "Some Statistics of Criminal Assault Upon Young Girls," *British Journal of Nursing* XL111, no. 1,117 (28 August, 1909): 175.

34 Burr, "Statistics," 176.

35 Burr, "Statistics," 176.

36 Burr, "Statistics," 176.

37 Burr, "Statistics," 176.

38 Burr, "Statistics," 176.

39 Lavinia L. Dock, *Hygiene and Morality: A Manual for Nurse and Others Giving and Outline of the Medical, Social and Legal Aspects of Venereal Diseases* (New York: GP Putnam, 1910).

40 Gibson Winter, *Social Ethics: Issues in Ethics and Society* (London: SCM Press1968): 6.

41 Julia Hurlston, "Stray Thoughts for Nurses," *British Journal of Nursing* 1, no. 188 (Jan 7, 1911): 6–7.

10 Nursing and morality in China

The necessity and possibility of a Confucian ethics of care

Jing-Bao Nie

Introduction

Is there a Confucian ethics of nursing? And is there a Confucian ethics of care? The immediate answer to either of these two questions is negative. Human interpersonal and social life depends on care, caregiving, and care-receiving. Without them, no individual, family, community, or society could survive, let alone thrive. In many aspects, nursing embodies and exemplifies care and caregiving. But the nursing profession in the modern sense never existed in traditional Chinese society. Confucianism, like other major Chinese moral traditions such as Daoism (Taoism) and Buddhism, never produced explicitly and systematically any ethics of care. Only in recent years and as a response to the international development of the philosophy of care, particularly feminist ethics of care, have pioneering studies started to elaborate on Confucian outlooks and ideas on care.

In this chapter, I aim to argue for the necessity and possibility of developing a Confucian ethics of nursing and care.

Unfortunately, Confucianism has been severely ill-fated in modern and contemporary times. Confucianism constitutes the moral, political, and spiritual system of beliefs and practices that define Chinese civilization and, to a great extent, East-Asian cultural characteristics. But the sweeping intellectual and social movements of "radical anti-traditionalism" in 20th-century China treated Confucianism as the chief root of Chinese socio-political problems. Official communist attitudes have ranged from totally condemning it as being anti-revolutionary in Mao's regime to hijacking it to reinforce authoritarianism in recent years. Internationally, Confucianism has often been dismissed as having only historical interest and, at its best, Chinese and East-Asian relevance. Or it is supposed to be despotic in essence, and thus its stands as the "radical other" to Western morality, particularly the ethical and political principles of liberalism.

Despite the world-altering reach of globalization, transcultural and global bioethics, and cross-cultural understanding and scholarly comparative studies in general, suffer from many persistent but intellectually problematic and politically harmful ways of characterizing what cultural differences are and how we should respond to them. Problems include marginalizing bioethical issues concerning large populations in the developing world, and overlooking the relevance of ethical traditions of non-Western cultures that might profitably address today's bioethical challenges. In the past two decades, I have pursued an interdisciplinary methodology, integrating ethical enquiry with historical and sociological studies. Most of my research projects focus on bioethical issues in China and East Asia within a global context. Through this research, to overcome some of the malaises in transcultural and global bioethics, I have put forward and am still developing

DOI: 10.4324/9781003427407-12

a theoretical and methodological approach of "ethical transculturalism." Rooted in Chinese reality and nourished by Chinese moral traditions, particularly Confucianism, ethical transculturalism highlights five key elements: taking internal plurality seriously within every culture; overcoming the pervasive mindset that reinforces contrasting and dichotomizing cultures as "radical others" that are destined to clash; focusing not only on cultural differences but also on transcultural similarities and a common humanity; searching for the ways to stimulate genuine and more profound transcultural ethical dialogues; and upholding the primacy of morality over the tyranny of socio-political practices (Nie 2011, 2021; Nie and Fitzegerald 2016, 2021).

Operating from within the approach termed "ethical transculturalism," in this chapter, I will examine nursing and morality in the Chinese socio-cultural and -political contexts. First, the crisis of the nursing profession in China and the major Chinese ethical approaches to nursing are discussed. This discussion includes a critical description of official socialist medical ethics. Then, the possibilities of developing a Confucian ethics of nursing and care are explored. Overall, drawing upon the fundamental moral concepts of *ren* (benevolence, humaneness, or humanity; previously alphabetized as *jen*) and *yin nai renshu* (medicine as the art of humanity) in Confucian ethics and medical ethics, I elaborate a Chinese ethical vision of nursing and care, whose catchword is "nursing as *renshu*, the art of humanity."

The crisis of nursing and morality in China

The necessity of a Confucian ethics of nursing and care arises from the persistent crisis of nursing as a profession in China, and how official socialist medical ethics and healthcare organization impact on nursing and nursing ethical practice.

Defying the long-rooted and still popular stereotypes of Chinese society and cultures as being largely static and conservative, China has been in constant social and political change, including revolutionary change, since the 19th century. Within this context, the establishment and impressive development of nursing as a profession in China have co-existed with what can be called "the chronic crisis of nursing." Just as the crisis of values accompanies modernity in the West and globally, modern and contemporary China has been in a constant crisis of morality, with symptoms being graver at specific periods than others. So the continual crisis of nursing and care should be regarded as a manifestation of the relentless crisis of morality and values in modern and contemporary China. Inadequacies in implementing reforms instantiating the leading ethical approaches to nursing and care in China, including the Nightingale model, socialist medical ethics, and the bioethical framework, reflect this crisis.

Chinese nurses face a series of enduring challenges, including an acute labour shortage, low economic and social status, heavy workloads, multiple responsibilities, and moral distress. Nursing shortages trouble many countries. However, in China, despite tremendous progress, the shortage of nurses, especially well-trained nurses, has long been a serious and widespread problem. The number of nurses per thousand people in China rose from 1.52 in 2010 to 2.54 in 2016, and has continued to increase since 2016. But this number is still much lower than the international average of 4–5 nurses per thousand people. The shortage of *male* nurses has been even more severe ever since the start of nursing as a profession in the late 19th century. As in 2016, only 2.1% of registered nurses in China are male (Yang and Hao 2018). Due to substantial disparities and inequalities across different regions, and the existence of significant structural divisions between urban and rural areas, the number of available nurses is even lower in disadvantaged areas and populations.

As in other parts of the world, a large number of complicated and often interconnected factors have contributed to the shortage of nurses in China. They include not only low wages, heavy workloads, and poor working conditions but also the institutional problems of the healthcare system, nursing education infrastructures, and the social image of the nursing profession (Hu, She and Jian 2010). A loss of motivation to choose nursing as a career path among young people exacerbates the persistent shortage of nurses. One study indicates that subjective social status (internalized social image) exerted a significant indirect effect through job satisfaction on nurse turnover intention in China (Feng et al. 2017).

Twenty years ago, in her pioneering and still only book-length study on nursing and ethics in China in the English language, practising nurse and philosopher Samantha Mei-che Pang in Hong Kong explored how nurses in China, as elsewhere, faced conflicting moral values and competing professional duties (Pang 2003). She categorized 11 facets of Chinese nurses' multiple role responsibilities into four groups according to their relation to what and whom they are responsible for and to. Responsibilities in relation to society include the doctrine of socialist humanism (discussed below) and the issue of healthcare access. Responsibilities in relation to the patient and the patient's family include protective care and benevolence, quality of care, and holistic inclusion of family members in patient care. Responsibilities in relation to practice and the nurse's personal and professional qualities include attitudes to work, and respect for nursing and the nurse's dignity. Responsibilities in relation to health institutions include compliance with institutional rules and regulations (Pang 2003, Chapter 5).

Demanding multiple role responsibilities of nurses and the low economic and social status of the nursing profession have resulted in mental stress and moral distress. One study has documented that the nursing profession and work issues constitute the "strongest" mental stress factor affecting nurses in China and that shift work yielded the "highest" stress score (Qin et al. 2016). In recent decades, moral distress has emerged as a subject extensively discussed in healthcare bioethics including nursing ethics across Western countries (Gallagher 2010). Moral distress often occurs when practitioners experience conflict between competing duties and values. Nurses are, it is claimed, particularly vulnerable to moral distress. Interestingly, according to one empirical study, the level of moral distress among Chinese nurses is reportedly low, with the frequency and intensity of moral distress being low-to-moderate (Zhang et al. 2018). Yet, this result must be treated with caution. These findings do not necessarily mean that the actual level of moral distress among Chinese nurses is low. Instead, there may simply be a low *awareness* or *consciousness* of moral distress. It might be that this problem is so far unrecognized and/or is not yet addressed among nurses and other health professionals in China.

Corresponding to three distinctive periods of Chinese development since the second half of the 19th century, Chinese ethical approaches to nursing underwent radical transformations. Specifically, three models or frameworks of practice have been developed. Initially, Western medical missionaries played a leading role in establishing hospitals, setting up or formalizing medical education, and inaugurating the nursing profession in China in the modern sense. As a part of this process, missionary nurses introduced the Nightingale model of nursing along with its ethical precepts to China.

Thereafter, Mao's regime (1949–1976) heralded "socialist humanism," "socialist humanitarianism," or "revolutionary humanitarianism" (*gemin de rendao zhuyi*). This represented a new and dominant ethical approach to nursing and healthcare in general.

Proclaimed by Mao Zedong himself, its slogan is: "Heal the wonded, rescure the dying, and practice revolutionary humanitarianism." Fulfilling the requirements of the communist ideology and official political agenda became the primary and ultimate moral end of the nursing profession and nurses.

Since the 1980s, thanks to the world-changing social policies of "Economic Development" and "Reform and Openness," China has been experiencing an evolution from medical morality centred on socialist humanitarianism to a paradigm of medical ethics incorporating some international bioethical norms, including autonomy and rights. Yet, the official doctrine of socialist humanitarianism and socialist ethics remains, especially when Maoism is rapidly reemerging in recent years. Nevertheless, by and large, its impact is now less overpowering in healthcare practices and the academic fields of medical and nursing ethics. For example, most officially endorsed national medical and nursing school textbooks on medical ethics and nursing ethics often highlight respect, non-maleficence, beneficence, and justice as the basic ethical principles for medicine and nursing in China (Wang and Yi 2016; Wang and Yang 2020; Liu and Fan 2022), and this is, clearly, a modified version of the influential "four principles" of biomedical ethics that originated in American bioethics.

All three major ethical approaches to nursing were initially imported from the West. While they have been significantly sinonized in the Chinese socio-cultural and -political contexts, they are far from sufficient in China. One of the main inadequacies lies in their lack of deep Chinese cultural roots. Therefore, it is necessary to revive the traditional Chinese moral systems and values, such as those of Confucianism and Daoism, to develop an ethics of nursing and care in China. This ethics will facilitate individual nurses, the nursing profession, and society to cultivate a better moral sense of nursing in China and even globally.

Can there be a Confucian ethics of care?

Is the mission of developing a Confucian ethics of care possible? The answer is affirmative. This section will offer a highly selected brief review of the academic debate on whether there is, or can be, a Confucian ethics of care, and it will point out a potential Confucian moral framework. In the next section, based on the fundamental ethical concept of *ren*, I will sketch one promising Confucian ethical vision of nursing and care: "nursing as *renshu*, the art of humanity."

Since the 1990s, in response to international developments in the philosophy of care, particularly feminist care ethics, some pioneering studies occurred to elaborate on Confucian ethical outlooks and ideas on care. Mostly taking an approach of Chinese-Western comparative philosophy, these academic discussions acknowledge some basic historical and socio-political facts. They recognize that Confucianism has no explicit existing theories on the importance of care and caregiving. Despite many possible synonyms, hardly any direct counterparts of the words like nursing and care exist in the traditional Chinese language and, hence, Confucianism.

Moreover, structural gender discrimination and suppression against women have manifested in such practices and institutions as foot-binding, polygyny, and the systemic limitation of women's participation in economic and socio-cultural activities. The patriarchal social arrangements and cultural perceptions of women have contributed to the persistent low economic and social status of nursing as a profession and nurses as health professionals in modern and contemporary China. Confucianism has been widely believed to be the main cultural cause of systematic Chinese sexism. However, innovative feminist studies through creatively reinterpreting such foundational Chinese philosophies as *yin-yang* demonstrates that Confucianism does not inherently discriminate and oppose women (Rosenlee 2006).

In general, two central questions dominate the current academic debate on Confucian ethics of care. They are: Can there be a Confucian ethics of care? And if yes, is it compatible with the contemporary Western ethics of care? (Li 2000). Encouragingly, scholars have begun to identify more nuanced similarities and differences between Confucian care ethics and the ethics of care in the West. For example, according to one fascinating article, these two ethical outlooks highlight relations-based moral reasoning and decision-making, in contrast to the influential liberal ethical theories that overemphasize individual autonomy. But realizing this common ground should not overlook their actual and potential differences. Western care ethicists prioritize, for example, questions pertaining to inequality and equality, while Confucian ethics focus more on reciprocity. The other critical difference is that Confucian ethics treats care as a virtue in cultivating one's moral character and agency. By contrast, Western care ethics emphasize care as both a disposition and practice and "the caring relationship to be a primary means of moral evaluation." Furthermore, "For the care ethicists, the practice of care embraces communicative morality, within fluid, dynamic interpersonal relationships - in sharp contrast to Confucian care practices, which are constructed within formal standards and fixed, role-based relationships" (Wada 2014, 361).

Another groundbreaking work on comparative Confucian ethics and feminist ethics proposes that the Confucian ideal of reciprocity can empower women (and hence nurses) to achieve gender equality. Early Confucian texts and the belief in the unity of *Ren* with *Dao* reveal a Confucian socio-ethical version of egalitarianism. This extends the emphasis of both Confucian ethics and feminist care ethics by stressing humanity and interdependence – that is, interdependence between social individuals and groups within and beyond their communities and countries to address social justice and care on a global scale. Therefore, cultural traditions like Confucianism "can be undeniable sources for strengthening contemporary social ideas of humanity, democracy, equality, and freedom for all" (Yuan 2019, 9).

The potent Confucian notion of *ren* has come to occupy a central role in modern Chinese-Western comparative philosophical studies. This role is grounded in how it is used to compare Confucian and contemporary care ethics (Li 2000; Yuan 2019). As one scholar eloquently summarizes:

> Confucian ethics in the historical past may not have focused on women's rights and choices sufficiently. An appropriation of *ren* in the present is nonetheless a powerful tool for reforming the tradition in the present and future. Given the good track record of *ren*'s transformative power in moral agents and its radiating effect on the society for the betterment of the needy, one has good reason to be hopeful for future contributions of Confucian *ren* ethics to feminist philosophy and practice.
>
> (Pang-White 2011, 383)

Nursing as Renshu, the art of humanity: a Confucian socio-ethical vision of care

Constructing a Confucian social ethics of care and nursing is not only necessary but possible. In addition to the reason that care-receiving and caregiving constitute an elemental dimension of human existence, Confucianism has rich intellectual resources for such an undertaking. Its history over three millennia shows that it has always been open to new moral horizons. As existing research shows, one productive way to undertake this task is to not only compare but contrast Confucian ethics of care with alternative non-Confucian (here Western) care ethics.

Conceptually, Confucianism defines human life as constant moral cultivation which aims to manifest one's character, love, renovate other fellow humans, and ultimately, abide in the highest good. From this perspective, human existence should begin with the individual person but must extend to family, community, country, and thereafter the world. Its highest aspiration is for humans to reach genuine goodness and harmoniously unite with Earth and Heaven. Therefore, Confucianism treats care and nursing as fundamentally a moral undertaking. Being moral, including caring for others, constitutes the deepest source of joy and happiness humans can attain in this world. Through care and only through care can humans realize, individually and collectively, their true moral, social, and spiritual nature – as well as the joy of learning to be human through our journeys of life (professional life included) (Yuan 2009; Huang 2014; Nie 2021).

With many different schools of thought and practices, Confucianism has significant internal plurality and diversity. It thus has a great pool of potent ethical outlooks, concepts, principles, and ideals that should and can be mined to develop different versions of its ethics of care and nursing. In the healthcare setting, one of these possibilities is to extend the Confucian principle and ideal of *yi nai renshu*. This positions medicine as the art of humaneness or humanity. It defines medicine as a moral practice based on and promoting the essential Confucian virtue and social norm of *ren*, and this idea should and can be extended to the profession of nursing. In other words, Confucian ethics advocates "nursing as *renshu*, the art of humaneness or humanity."

As a core and potent concept in Confucianism, *ren* has been translated into English variously as "humaneness," "benevolence," "beneficence," "perfect virtue," "goodness," "human-heartedness," "love," "altruism," or "humanity." The idea of "medicine as the art of humanity" has been widely regarded as *the* fundamental principle of traditional Chinese medical ethics by contemporary Chinese and Western scholars (Unschuld 1979; Nie 2009, 2011; Wang and Yi 2016). And defining medicine as the art of humaneness and humanity underscores the ultimate moral ends and significance of the professional work of health professionals.

At the same time, along with reimaging nursing ethics along Confucian ethical lines and ideals, the economic, social, and medical status of nursing must be improved in China and elsewhere if "good" care is to be given. On the one hand, in traditional China, the social status of medicine as an occupation or profession was as low as other technical skills, certainly much lower than *rushu* (civil service and Confucian learning). Medical practitioners belonged to the lower social category of artisan or technician. Even Confucianism used to treat medicine as just a type of *ji* (technique or craftsmanship) or *shu* (craftsmanship or art). The Confucian tradition usually looked down on forms of craftsmanship, i.e., working with one's hands, and many Confucians were ashamed to learn or to practise medicine for this reason. On the other hand, medical works such as *The Yellow Emperor's Class of Medicine* (Neijing), a foundational text of traditional Chinese medicine as practised historically and today, call medicine "the Dao (way) of excellence and the business of great sages," "the ultimate virtue," and acupuncture "the superb craftsmanship" (Chen 1991a). Moreover, historically, the notion of "medicine as the art of humanity" was initially proposed and established to improve the social status of medical practitioners and medicine as an occupation in imperial China (Chen 1991b; Nie 2009, 2011).

The Confucian vision of nursing as the art of humanity enriches the moral sense of nursing. S. Mei-che Pang (2003) insightfully argued against the tendency of treating the work of nurses as merely a technical task (however important these tasks are). There is thus an absolute need to cultivate a moral sense of nursing in the clinical setting. The current view is that technical tasks are not important. This is erroneous. Moreover, cultivating a moral sense of nursing recasts and enhances the ethical meaningfulness of these technical tasks and it will enhance and develop professional role responsibilities.

One common understanding of Confucian ethics is that its focus on the moral cultivation of individual characters makes it merely a species or version of virtue ethics. This is not a mistaken view. However, it is a limited view. This characterization tends to ignore or at least downplay the sophisticated social dimensions of Confucian ethics. Cross-cultural empirical studies indicate that Chinese nurses are more virtue-based in their perceptions of ethical responsibilities. In contrast, American nurses are more principle-based, and Japanese nurses are more care-based (Pang et al. 2003). That said, these findings may reinforce the perception or stereotype of Confucian moral philosophy as largely virtue ethics.

Confucian ethics of care, however, prescribe or set out, for adherents, a much higher moral ladder to climb. Confucian ethics start with caring for oneself, especially one's moral character, but – as noted – this quickly extends to helping develop a caring relationship with and to the family, community, nation, and humankind as a moral commonwealth (Yuan 2009).

The practical and academic relevance of building Confucian care nursing ethics for China is straightforward. However, one should not then overlook the possibility and significance of developing a Confucian ethics of care in global settings. Among other options, Confucian care ethics can potentially help identify strengths, weaknesses, and blind spots among the leading and less influential schools of nursing philosophy and care ethics that originated and have been nourished in the Western socio-cultural context. Partly because of its inherent universalistic ethical spirit and outlook, Confucianism can be a constructive partner in transcultural and transglobal dialogues on existing and emerging challenges that face the nursing profession, nursing philosophy, and care ethics.

Conclusion

Developing a Confucian ethics of nursing and care is both necessary and possible. The necessity arises from the continual crisis of nursing as a profession in China. It is also needed – it can play a part – as a counterbalance to other prominent Chinese ethical approaches to nursing, including official socialist medical ethics. Confucianism has rich intellectual resources for the ethics of care and nursing. Among other possibilities, being centred on the fundamental ethical concept of *ren* (benevolence, humaneness, or humanity), Confucian ethics advocates for and positions nursing as moral practice or *renshu*, the art of humanity. Despite being ill-fated in the past century and a half, Confucianism can significantly contribute to better cultivating the morality of nursing and care in China and even globally.

References

Chen, M. (1991a) [First published in 1723] *Gujin Tushu Jicheng Yibu Quanlu* (Collection of Ancient and Modern Books, The Part of Medicine), Book 1: Huangdi Suwen and Lingyu Jing (Volumes 1–46 in original), Beijing: People's Health Press.

Chen, M. (1991b) [First published in 1723] *Gujin Tushu Jicheng Yibu Quanlu* (Collection of Ancient and Modern Books, The Part of Medicine), Book 12: General Discussions (Volumes 501–520 in original), Beijing: People's Health Press.

Feng, D., Su, S., Yang, Y., Xia, J., and Su, Y. (2017) Job Satisfaction Mediates Subjective Social Status and Turnover Intention among Chinese Nurses. *Nursing and Health Sciences* 19: 388–392.

Gallagher, A., (2010) Moral Distress and Moral Courage in Everyday Nursing Practice. *OJIN: The Online Journal of Issues in Nursing* Vol. 16 No. 2

Hu, Y., She, J., and Jian, A. (2010) Nursing Shortage in China: State, Causes and Strategy. *Nursing Outlook* 58: 122–128.

Huang, Y. (2014) *Why Be Moral?: Learning from the Neo-Confucian Cheng Brothers*, Albany, NY: State University of New York Press.

Li, C. (ed.) (2000) *The Sage and the Second Sex: Confucianism, Ethics and Gender*. Chicago and La Salle: Open Court.

Liu, J. and Fan, Y. (2022) *Huli Lunlixue* (Nursing Ethics) (3rd Ed.). Beijing: People's Health Press.

Nie, J.-B. (2009) "The Discourses of Practitioners in China," In: R. Baker and L. McCullough (eds.) *The Cambridge World History of Medical Ethics*, Cambridge and New York: Cambridge University Press. pp. 335-344.

Nie, J.-B. (2011) *Medical Ethics in China: A Transcultural Interpretation*. London and New York: Routledge.

Nie, J.-B. (2021) The Summit of a Moral Pilgrimage: Confucianism on Healthy Ageing and Social Eldercare. *Nursing Ethics* 28(3): 316–326.

Nie, J.B. and Fitzgerald, R. (Eds.) (2016) Special issue on "Transcultural and Transglobal Bioethics: A Search for New Methodologies." *Kennedy Institute of Ethics Journal* 26(3).

Nie, J.-B. and Fitzgerald, R. (2021) "Global Health and Ethical Transculturalism: A New Methodology," in: S. Benatar and G. Brock (eds.) *Global Health and Global Health Ethics*, 2nd edition, Cambridge: Cambridge University Press, pp. 326–338.

Pang, S.M. (2003) *Nursing Ethics in Modern China*. Amsterdam: Rodopi.

Pang, S.M., Sawada, A., Konishi, E., Olsen, D.P. Yu, P.L.H., Chan, M., and Mayumi, N. (2003) A Comparative Study of Chinese, American and Japanese Nurses' Perceptions of Ethical Role Responsibilities. *Nursing Ethics* 10(3): 295–311.

Pang-White, A.A. (2011) Caring in Confucian Philosophy. *Philosophy Compass* 18(1): 69–82.

Qin, Z., Zhong, X., Ma, J., and Lin, H. (2016) Stressors Affecting Nurses in China. *Contemporary Nurse* 52(4): 447–453.

Rosenlee, L.L. (2006) *Confucianism and Women: A Philosophical Interpretation*, Albany, NY: State University of New York Press.

Unschuld, P.U. (1979) *Medical Ethics in Imperial China*. Berkeley, CA: University of California Press.

Wada, Y. (2014) Relational Care Ethics from a Comparative Perspective: The Ethics of Care and Confucian Ethics. *Ethics and Social Welfare* 8(4): 350–363.

Wang, M. and Yi, M. (2016) *Yixue Lunlixue* (Medical Ethics) (2nd Ed.). Beijing: People's Health Press.

Wang, W. and Yang, M. (2020) *Huli Lunlixue* (Nursing Ethics) (3rd Ed.). Beijing: Tsinghua University Press.

Yang, J.S. and Hao, D.J. (2018) Dilemmas for Nurses in China [Correspondence]. *The Lancet* 392: 30.

Yuan, Y. (2009) [1812]. *Shisan Jing Zhushu* (The Thirteen Confucian Classics with Commentaries and Sub-commentaries). 5 Vols. Beijing, China Bookstore.

Yuan, L. (2019) *Confucian Ren and Feminist Ethics of Care: Integrating Relational Self, Power, and Democracy*. Lanham and Oxford: Lexington Books.

Zhang, W., Wu, X., Zhan, Y., Ci, L., and Sun, C. (2018) Moral Distress and Its Influencing Factors: A Cross-Sectional Study in China. *Nursing Ethics* 25(4): 470–480.

11 Islamic Humanism

Toward understanding nursing care for Muslim patients

Mustafa M. Bodrick, Jason A. Wolf, Ghadah Abdullah, Mutlaq B. Almutairi, Abdulaziz M. Alsufyani, Fatma S. Alsolamy, and Hisham M. Alfayyadh

Introduction

Caring is a fundamental aspect of nursing. As nursing practice continues to advance toward person-centricity, culturally sensitive care delivery that caters for individual philosophies and beliefs has become paramount. Consequently, different definitions of caring have emerged to address these differences in delivery, particularly in regard to whether it is administered from a personal or materialistic viewpoint. That said, there is limited information about the Islamic conception of care. Muslim patients frequent most clinics and practitioners worldwide. Numbered at 1.8 billion, Muslims account for 24% of the world's population and, presumably, of healthcare clinical visitors. Islam is also the second-largest-growing religion worldwide, and it, like most other social systems, should be acknowledged and accommodated by public services (Kolmar & Kamal, 2018). Yet, misunderstanding and neglect of Islam-specific care prevail within the nursing sector. Healthcare systems have failed to develop a landscape of care that responds to the unique needs and expectations of Muslim patients. Holistic nursing should integrate beliefs, philosophies, and cultures into the care plan, and, accordingly, practitioners must inquire into Islam and Islamic beliefs to effectively tend to Muslim patients. The Quran demonstrates four ways in which Islam portrays care: Almighty God's care for humankind, humans' care for one another, an individual's care for themselves, and the universe's care for humankind and vice versa. These four forms of Islamic care follow humanistic and holistic ideals, in that, an individual's experiences and their environment are essential aspects that should be accounted for in formulating the caring framework. While Islamic scriptures base care on divine commands and human nature, taking note of these fundamentals will help practitioners make informed decisions that will enhance holistic care. Such an outcome is only attainable with a person-centered care model. Popularized by Brendan McCormack, the person-centered model establishes and fosters a holistic therapeutic relationship that links care providers to patients and other persons who are significant in their lives (McCance et al., 2011; McCormack, 2003; McCormack & McCance, 2006; McCormack, Dewing & Mccance, 2011). Mutual respect, self-determination, and respect are the model's values (Ibid., 2011). This study highlights the humanistic perspective of Islamic care and its contribution as an Abrahamic religion to the healthcare scene. It will also explain the difference between Islamic humanism and humanistic Islam and appraise related concepts of patient care models. We find that, guided by the person-centered framework, it is possible to develop a standardized nursing care framework that, regardless of nationality, socioeconomic status, or gender, is responsive to Muslim patients' unique needs and expectations.

DOI: 10.4324/9781003427407-13

Overview of Islam and related considerations connecting to Islamic humanism

Nursing literature is dominated by Eurocentric nursing practices, and most existing studies lack adequate coverage on the concept of Islamic care. In criticizing this bias, Rassool (2000) states that "throughout the Western literature, the concept of caring is extensively examined in the context of the Judeo-Christian tradition" (p. 1477). However, the growing global Muslim population mandates extensive study of the topic. Practitioners should know about Islamic culture and its beliefs to deliver high-quality care to Muslim patients since most of them integrate religion into every facet of their lives and conduct (Rassool, 2000). For instance, the opening words of the Qu'ran, "In the Name of Allah (Almighty God), Most Gracious, Most Merciful" [Bismi Llah ir Rahman ir-Bahim]" – essential invocations that are to be mandatorily recited at the beginning of any action or word – demonstrate the religious relevance and influence of Almighty God in the lives of Muslim persons (Rassool, 2000, p. 1476). Moreover, the Islamic faith emphasizes the importance and connections between health, the environment, holism, and knowledge and elaborates on the "Oneness of Allah" and the unity of God, meeting the psychological, spiritual, physical, and environmental attributes of a holistic healthcare model (Rassool, 2000). In addition to the Western bias in nursing literature, the theoretical frameworks of care models portray profound inclination toward the secular perspective of nursing and healthcare. This state, in turn, begs the question of whether the secular nursing approach is as accommodative to Muslim as non-Muslim patients (Rassool, 2000). Ultimately, it is essential for healthcare stakeholders to explore the notion of Islamic care and examine its potential contribution to establishing effective holistic care.

The bias toward secular care in healthcare systems worldwide implies a disregard of the fundamental spiritual dimension of care and an overall lack of awareness about spiritual development's important role in healing. Therefore, one could justifiably surmise that the current care framework does not adequately embrace holism. From the description of Wong et al. (2022), holistic care incorporates physical, social, and cultural factors into a comprehensive care model. It also emphasizes the connectedness of the body, mind, and spirit. Therefore, because spirituality is a crucial component of holistic care, the patient's spiritual needs should be prioritized in care delivery. An essential philosophical dimension that underpins the religious considerations for Muslim patients are the concepts of diversity, equity, inclusion, and belonging (DEIB) (Chao et al., 2022; Jones & Jones, 2022). Further, if DEIB are to be authentic concepts in nursing care, then the religious components of patients' lives, that is, Muslims and other religious sectors, should be meaningfully recognized and validated insofar as religious inclusion is taken as an essential observance (Chao et al., 2022; Hasan, 2022; Jones & Jones, 2022). Mindful of this consideration, Islam is practiced globally by a variety of ethnicities and nationalities, and therefore adds impetus to having this focus on Islamic humanism.

A range of universally practiced Islamic tenets inform the actions and perspectives of Muslim patients regardless of location. Notably, the five pillars of Islam, *Shahada, Salat, Zakat, Sawm,* and *Hajj,* are defined in the Hadith. *Shahada* is the acknowledgment that Allah is the one and only true God, and Muhammad is his messenger (Edgar, 2002). *Salat* is the requirement for Muslims to pray at fixed times, and five prayers are upheld in this regard: Fajr (sunrise prayer), Zuhr (noon prayer), Asr (prayer before sunset), Maghrib (sunset prayer), and Isha (prayer before midnight) (Hussain, 2012). *Zakat* is the requirement for Muslims to engage in charity, while *Sawm* is the fasting observed during the month of Ramadhan (Hussain, 2012). Lastly, *Hajj* is the pilgrimage to Mecca

(Hussain, 2012). These pillars guide Muslim patients' lives, attitudes, and beliefs. As such, an awareness of the pillars and what they mean to Muslim patients' ways of living could be vital to implementing patient-centered care.

Alongside the five pillars of Islam, the six principles of Islamic doctrine could advise nursing practitioners' implementation of patient-centered care. The six principles are (1) belief in fate, (2) belief in the Judgment Day, (3) belief in the Books, (4) belief in angels, (5) belief in the Prophet and the guidance that rests on his wisdom, and (6) belief that Allah is the one and only true God (Al-Bar & Chamsi-Pasha, 2015). The Muslim patient's core beliefs and spiritual practices are embodied by the five pillars of Islam and the six principles of the faith. When observed in tandem, a nursing practitioner could tailor care to accommodate any unique set of values, beliefs, and expectations that an individual Muslim patient upholds. Thus, by paying attention to the fundamentals outlined in Islamic scriptures, the person-centered care framework would not only be culturally responsive, but it would also embrace the tenets that guide religious practice and shape the lives of Muslim patients.

Islamic humanism's contributions as an Abrahamic religion

Islamic humanism proposes a culturally responsive approach to nursing care for Muslim patients. It is widely accepted that the three Abrahamic religions of Judaism, Christianity, and Islam have significantly contributed to humanism. For instance, for believers, religious strictures about care and ethical behavior emanate from Almighty God, and given their historical-cultural impact, the Abrahamic religions have shaped the ethical landscape and orientation that, today, is reproduced in modern versions of secular and religious humanism (Rassool, 2000). Almighty God is considered the supreme being that provides a foundation for morality, and Islamic humanism is premised on principles derived from this morality (Rassool, 2000). Non-theistic perspectives are based on human experiences and aspects that are unique to this population. For example, there is a strong emphasis on compassion and empathy as critical parts of ethical behavior among individuals (Leirvik, 2020). This ethical orientation is apparent in Islamic humanism's desire for an Islam that exists harmoniously with fundamental values like socio-political justice, respect for the right to self-determination, and respect for people's innate dignity. Toward this end, Islamic humanism holds that the core values of care, compassion, kindness, and mercy are vital to developing a person-centered philosophy that cuts across all levels of patient care, including the primary, secondary, tertiary, and quaternary levels. It is a philosophy of nursing care that acknowledges and addresses the spiritual, emotional, physiological, mental, and physical dimensions of human suffering.

Integrating Islamic humanism into person-centered care avails a universal framework that all nurses, irrespective of their religious affiliation, can apply when caring for Muslim patients. This approach would recognize and differentiate human suffering from spiritual, emotional, mental, physiological, and physical perspectives. It would be a holistic combination of all these aspects that connect and affect a person's well-being.

The concept of the "person" forms the core of the person-centered approach and, accordingly, the care that should be administered to a Muslim patient (Santana et al., 2018). This conceptualization of care views a patient as an individual with unique needs that must be met for positive patient outcomes. A person has goals, problems, experiences, and other aspects of life that only apply to them and must be considered during care. In this regard, nurses must explore the concept of person-centric care by assessing the beliefs that distinguish Muslims from non-Muslim patients, the expectations and needs unique to the humanistic characteristics of Muslims, and the strategies for engaging with Muslim patients (McCormack et al., 2011). At the basic level, the concept of "person" consists of patients' humanness (Olsson et al., 2013). These values guide patients' construction of their lives (McCormack et al., 2011). Islamic humanism upholds kindness, mercy, compassion, affection, selflessness, and care as its underpinning values (Mohd, 2019). Ultimately, these ideals are encapsulated in the mantra of "loving your brother and neighbor as yourself", which is integral to the faith of the Muslim patient.

Appraising Islamic humanism and related concepts

Islam has often been portrayed by the media as a religion of violence, owing to the theocracies that implement the Sharia Law inhumanely, and deviate from the religion's core value of compassion. However, these adherents are not representative of Islam practice or Muslims and portraying the religion as violent undermines the efforts of the majority of believers who continue to vehemently challenge extremist oppression.

The Noble Quran and Prophet Muhammad's traditions reinforce tolerance and respect for all humankind regardless of gender, religion, race, and color (Mohd, 2019). Therefore, the majority of Muslims uphold that Islam centers on human welfare. However, political manipulation and an obsolete, outdated exegesis of the religion have relegated Islamic humanism. Arab scholar Mohammad Arkoun (2011) explains that Islamic humanism is strongly associated with classical Greek philosophy and ethics. He posits that European philosophers' extensive discussions about humanism caused the advancement of the humanist position in Western communities. Hence, non-European communities grew critical of humanism, viewing it as an atheistic or Christian ideology. He, however, holds that societies that are not likely to enter such debates "are cast disdainfully into the corner of a worthless heritage: a heritage of conservatism and primitive antiquity" (p. 156). Admittedly, there has been a significant shift from classical to modern versions of Islamic humanism. Leirvik (2020) states that while classical forms of humanism were associated with human virtues and personal formation, modern humanism in Islam is sharply criticized and perceived to be characterized by extremist and threatening religious acts. Islamic humanism is clearly constantly evolving following the need for human-rights-oriented "humanization" in Islam. Islamic scholar Nasr Hamid Abu Zayd developed the "humanistic" viewpoint to re-energize conjecture on humanism. Humanistic Islam pursues "the value of personhood that they find in their religion, and they balance its asperities with a lambent commitment to intellectual freedom and personal creativity" (Goodman, 2013, p. 1023). This school of thought allows individuals to leverage their spiritual heritage and interpret the Quran's teachings in ways that are affirmative of humanity. According to Abu Zayd and other humanistic intellectuals, Prophet Muhammad and many other Muslims in the medieval era pursued rational, scientific, and humanistic discourses in their interpretation of knowledge. Further, as per the American Humanist Association (2018), a vast range of Islamic literature reveals the view that classical Islam tolerated humanistic ideas of secularism, liberalism, individualism, and skepticism. Humanists advocate for a society where people can openly express themselves without fear (Khan, 2015). Additionally, a humanistic Islam entails no use of violence or acts of terror to drive ideals (American Humanist Association, 2014).

While the two concepts seem indistinguishable, there is an apparent difference. Humanism signals a religious obligation to human rights norms. Such values include equal treatment of people regardless of political, religious, or personal convictions. However, humanistic Islam calls for a critical perspective of religion and humanity. The humanistic viewpoint here implicitly urges individuals adhering to the religion to practice self-criticism and extensively examine systemic and religious practices through a humanistic perspective.

Islamic humanism manifested in nursing practice

Embracing the philosophy of Islamic humanism in nursing practice is best illustrated by the rediscovery of the legacy and contributions of Rufaidah Al-Aslamia from 620 AD, the first Muslim nurse and a pioneer of Islamic nursing since the beginning of Islam and Prophet Mohammed's (Peace and Blessings Upon Him – PBUH) era (Bodrick et al., 2022). Historical qualitative research conducted during 2021–2022 confirmed and elevated Rufaidah Al-Aslamia as a chief influencer, pioneer, and advocate for Islamic humanism in nursing.

Legacy of Islamic humanism in nursing by first Muslim nurse Rufaidah Al-Aslamia

The root of Islamic nursing dates back over 1,400 years when Rufaidah Al-Aslamia became the first Muslim practicing nursing in Madinah, the city of Prophet Mohammed (PBUH) (Bodrick et al., 2022). Few written accounts of Rufaidah as an Islamic nursing pioneer existed up until the publications by Hussain (1981) and Jan (1996) that triggered qualitative historical inquiry about her work, most of which were published between 2021 and 2022 (Bodrick et al., 2022).

Rufaidah was born in 597 AD in Madina and is known as the first Muslim nurse. Her father was a physician-surgeon who mentored her in medical practices and influenced her desire to help the Muslim community (Basha, 2020; Bodrick et al., 2022). Prophet Muhammad (PBUH) respected Al-Aslamia and gave her the resources to advance her knowledge and teach others new approaches for caring for wounded Muslim soldiers, a move that revolutionized public health and social work at the time (Hibbert & Al-Dossari, 2015). Rufaidah had witnessed the repercussions of war on the Muslim soldiers, compelling her to advocate for more female nurses. In this pursuit, she started a clinical teaching program for volunteering Ansar women to teach provision of care to the sick, which evolved into an established nursing school – the first of its kind – and enabled her to practice and propagate her system-focused approach (Bodrick et al., 2022). Rufaidah practiced nursing that catered to individual patient needs and, consequently, revolutionized nursing practice among Islamic nurses (Hibbert & Al-Dossari, 2015). Rufaidah's framework of considering patients' holistic needs was especially necessary in the battlefields, where nurses were untrained and did not understand patient needs (Abu Rabia et al., 2021). This revolution was notably impactful. Before her involvement, physicians worked with various resources at their disposal; yet, they had little consideration for the patient. She introduced hydration as an essential aspect of care delivery, emphasized hygiene when caring for wounded soldiers in battle, and recommended stabilizing patients before serious procedures like amputation (Abu Rabia et al., 2021) In doing so, Rufaidah showed that the simple details in care provision could positively impact the patients' well-being (Abu Rabia et al., 2021). For example, hygiene in the patient's environment would reduce the risk of infection and promote faster recovery. Rufaidah also advanced Islamic nursing by training nurses about appropriate healthcare procedures and actions that would ensure quality care for the patient (Bodrick et al., 2022). She worked with companions and traveled to battle-fields to care for soldiers, where Prophet Mohammed (PBUH) trusted her and allowed her to train other nurses in essential care during wars (Bodrick et al., 2022; Kadioğlu, 2021). This decision would prove influential for women in nursing. For example, many women wanted to contribute to the battles and accepted the training Rufaidah offered. She also changed the public's perceptions of female nurses by gaining the Prophet's respect from treating high-ranking soldiers in the Muslim army. Lastly, her focus on hygiene and patient care for severely injured solders was ground-breaking, and it stimulated the spread of her approaches, which presently form the fundamentals of Islamic nursing (Bodrick et al., 2022).

Rufaidah followed an open system technique that included input, output, throughput, and feedback elements (Bodrick et al., 2022). Her nursing model entailed multifaceted activities and portrayed effective management skills. Rufaidah oversaw the setup of the "Khaimah Rufaidah", a field tent remote clinic where she administered care to wounded soldiers (Bodrick et al., 2022). She also helped organize a tent in Madinah next to the grand mosque, where she tended to children and adults. In tandem with her leadership skills, Rufaidah also portrayed the importance of critical decision-making and practical problem-solving in holistic nursing as part of Islamic humanism (Bodrick et al., 2022). Rufaidah applied a positive nurse-patient relationship system to enhance quality of care. It would involve nursing individuals in the shade, ensuring sufficient ventilation and hygiene standards, and providing clean water. Rufaidah also ensured that the sites where patients lay were clean and comfortable (Bodrick et al., 2022). The Prophet (PBUH) appraised the nursing pioneer's organizational efficiency and found her devotion to providing care impressive, and rightly so. As a result, Rufaidah's nursing practice contained and inspired the modern crucial facets of holistic care. However, compared to other prominent nursing personalities like Florence Nightingale, Rufaidah's contributions are relatively under-explored.

In light of the core components of the "person" concept, there is a need to determine the considerations or strategies that would be ideal for Muslim patients. The values and practices that would be integral to the Muslim patient include acknowledging and respecting the presence of Prophet Muhammad (PBUH), reinforcing the person-centeredness of nursing care, highlighting the essence of fasting, creating opportunities for worship in the course of healing, respecting the charitable value of visiting people who are unwell, and respecting the privacy and modesty of Muslim patients. Furthermore, traditions unique to Muslims, such as fasting, must be considered during care, and practitioners need to make accommodations for them in their care delivery frameworks (Gustafson & Lazenby, 2019). Alongside these interventions, nurses could administer Islamic-specific end-of-life care that underpins Islamic humanism. This includes observing Muslim traditions and beliefs about transiting to the after-life, such as performing Shahada in the right ear of a baby or dying patient (Tackett et al., 2018). Islam-specific care should also extend to mentally disabled patients, parents, and senior citizens, all the while focusing on the spiritual aspects of the care delivery process, such as regarding illness as a test from Allah (Tackett et al., 2018). Within a clinical environment, the nurse can avail prayer carpets and handle the Holy Qur'an, with respect, given the significance it holds in Islamic religion as a sacred text that comes directly from God. Also, passing in front of a praying patient must be avoided, and holy Zam-Zam water, sometimes provided by the family, should be labeled as such.

Islamic humanism in community nursing and primary health

Holistic Islamic teachings significantly inform Muslim healthcare professionals' practice. According to Rahman et al. (2017), Islamic medical care increases ethical deliberations and social interactions, in which religious texts are often used in care delivery. Humanism, while not necessarily a religious philosophy, focuses on making ethical decisions and improving the well-being of humans. As such, Islamic healthcare practices are defined as "treatment with a holistic approach" (Rahman et al., 2017). It is impossible to separate Islam's teachings from Islamic humanism, as the concepts of justice, equality, and dignity are fundamental to Islam and humanism (Leirvik, 2020). At the basic level, being human implies that an individual possesses innate dignity, and equality and justice are critical to dignity (Leirvik, 2020). Hence, traditional Islamic practices are inherently humanistic, as the belief in humankind is also part of the greater belief in God Almighty and the moral duties assigned to humankind (Tan & Ibrahim, 2017). Despite Islamic humanism being more focused on the collective community than the individual, the individual remains an integral part of the collective. Humanistic values are therefore essentially non-negotiable, especially with respect to patient care. Additionally, Islamic philosophy can help resolve important moral and ethical dilemmas for healthcare workers, patients, families, and society in administering patient care. In nursing, the decision-making process is based on a set of guidelines and rules, and Islamic humanistic values, such as maintenance of life, protection of freedom of belief, preservation of honor and integrity, and protection of property, could preside over Islamic patient-centered decisions (Gatrad & Sheikh, 2001). Practitioners' adherence to these principles is emphasized in nursing legal and ethical codes that dictate the standards of practice, and nurses must comply to ensure high-quality care and positive patient outcomes.

Rufaidah Al-Aslamia could also be considered a pioneer for community nursing in Islam, notably because she set up some of the earliest healthcare establishments in history. For example, she treated wounded soldiers through mobile clinical units and assembled a group of nurse volunteers and traveled to various regions to care for the wounded (Bodrick et al., 2022; Cortés-Guiral et al., 2021; Kadioğlu, 2021). That said, she realized the need to dedicate a center to the community, which would cater to community members in need of medical services (Nordin, 2019). Rufaidah built a tent next to the Prophet's residence and invited everybody who needed healthcare assistance to visit. The healthcare center was considered the heart of the community since it hosted soldiers, children, women, and other patients who experienced different ailments (Cortés-Guiral et al., 2021). Rufaidah's focus on healthcare transcended the battlefield when she realized that the community needed a center that was accessible to the sick.

Additionally, Rufaidah studied community diseases, pioneering a sense of clinical research on prevalent health issues in her vicinity. Most notably, she focused on infectious diseases that affected the Muslim community during battles, and her studies provided insights into better disease control and encouraged better management (Al-Rashed et al., 2020). These contributions curbed the spread of diseases during the battles. She was a role model in nursing owing to her ability to promote innovative and beneficial approaches that increased the quality of care at a period when healthcare practitioners did not necessarily understand crucial procedures, risks, and how to manage conditions.

Rufaidah's nursing practice in Madinah and the first Islamic hospitals in Cairo and Baghdad portray crucial insights into the conceptual framework of Islamic healthcare. Contemporary healthcare has only recently seen a shift in focus on culture as a significant element of care (Hoseini, 2019). However, evidence reveals that Islamic healthcare integrated social and cultural beliefs into the care process. As previously mentioned, Islam propagates kindness, equality, justice, and respect for all life (Mohd, 2019). Thus, Islamic care contains humanistic concepts. For instance, Rufaidah offered community care to all injured people during the Battle of Khandaq (Bodrick et al., 2022). Thus, she cared for everyone regardless of their convictions, gender, age, and social status. A contextual framework incorporating humanism would consist of four major multi-dimensional concepts: human, health, environment, and nursing (Hoseini, 2019). The human notion contains the body, spirit, human nature, and instinct (Hoseini, 2019). Meanwhile, overall health is believed to comprise wellness, intellectual health, and transcendence. Additionally, the framework also considers natural and social environments during care delivery. Hence, Islamic holism makes the conceptual nursing framework accommodative and effective for both Muslim and non-Muslim patients.

Conclusion

Islamic healthcare and Islamic nursing have not been exhaustively discussed within the field of nursing philosophy. While extensive literature has appraised Western nursing pioneers and their approaches to patient care, minimal attention has been directed to the fundamental contributions of Islamic care that influenced contemporary Muslim nurses globally. Islam being the second-largest religion in the world, it is expected that Islamic humanism would be widely taken into account to cater for Muslim patients, who make up a significant proportion of healthcare seekers. This has, however, been proven not to be the case. As illustrated by Rufaidah Al-Aslamia, Islam is a way of life that influences an individual's perceptions and behaviors, and Islamic humanism provides guidance in providing holistic care to Muslim patients. This review reveals that Islamic humanism can enrich person-centered care to a level that leads to the development of a care framework ideal for all patients. Integrating Islamic humanism into person-centered care enables practitioners to integrate values and beliefs that are fundamental to the Muslim patient. Rufaidah Al-Aslamia demonstrated this conception in early Islamic care, which entailed holistic features. Rufaidah's historical contributions are valid in contemporary nursing, given that she ensured that the patients' received hygienic care in comfortable and well-ventilated tents. Additionally, the Muslim nursing pioneer delivered care to children and women across Madinah. Islamic humanism therefore also improves nurses' understanding of the concept of "person" from the standpoint of the Muslim patient. This review of Islamic humanism as a nursing philosophy has revealed that its incorporation highlights that Muslim and non-Muslim nurses can benefit from this approach in providing nursing care to Muslim patients.

References

Abu Rabia, R., Hendel, T., & Kagan, I. (2021). Views of Bedouin physicians and nurses on nursing as a profession in Israel: There is more to strive for. *Nursing & Health Sciences*, 23(2), 498–505.

Al-Bar, M., & Chamsi-Pasha, H. (2015). *Contemporary Bioethics: Islamic Perspective*. New York: Springer.

Al-Rashed, A. M., Al Youha, S. A., & Al Safi, S. H. (2020). The history and current status of women in surgery in the Arabian Gulf. *IJS Global Health*, 3(5), e23.

American Humanist Association. (2014, September 15). *A humanist approach to Islam*. https://americanhumanist.org/key-issues/statements-and-resolutions/islam/

American Humanist Association. (2018, November 15). *Humanist common ground: Islam.* https://americanhumanist.org/paths/islam/

Arkoun, M. (2011). The struggle for humanism in Islamic contexts. *Journal of Levantine Studies,* (1), 153–170. https://www.academia.edu/3731409/The_Struggle_for_Humanism_in_Islamic_Contexts_by_Mohammed_Arkoun

Basha, H. (2020). *Archetypes Rooted in Saudi Arabian and Islamic Cultural Traditions.* Edmond, OK: The University of Central Oklahoma

Bodrick, M. M., Almutairi, M. B., Alsolamy, F. S., & Alfayyadh, H. M. (2022). Appraising Rufaidah Al-Aslamia, first Muslim nurse and pioneer of Islamic nursing: Contributions and legacy. *Jurnal Keperawatan Indonesia* [Nursing Journal of Indonesia], 25(3), https://doi.org/10.7454/jki.v25i3.2369

Chao, D., Badwan, M., & Briceño, E. M. (2022). Addressing diversity, equity, inclusion and belonging (DEIB) in mentorship relationships. *Journal of Clinical and Experimental Neuropsychology, 44*(5–6), 420–440.

Cortés-Guiral, D., Mayol, J., & Wexner, S. D. (2021). Diversity in surgery: A historical, international, and contemporary perspective. *Current Surgery Reports, 9*(5), 1–10.

Edgar, S. (2002). The five pillars of Islam in the Hadith. *Studia Antiqua, 1*(2), 71–82.

Gatrad, A. R., & Sheikh, A. (2001). Medical ethics and Islam: Principles and practice. *Archives of Disease in Childhood, 84*(1), 72–75.

Goodman, L. E. (2013). Humanism in Islam. In *Encyclopedia of sciences and religions* (1st ed., pp. 1022–1024). Springer.

Gustafson, C., & Lazenby, M. (2019). Assessing the unique experiences and needs of Muslim oncology patients receiving palliative and end-of-life care: An integrative review. *Journal of Palliative Care, 34*(1), 52–61.

Hasan, E. (2022). Evaluating religious inclusion and belonging. In E. Hasan (Ed.), *Embracing Workplace Religious Diversity and Inclusion* (pp. 49–59). Cham: Palgrave Macmillan.

Hibbert, D., & Al-Dossari, R. R. (2015). Developing enterostomal therapy as a nursing specialty in Saudi Arabia: Which model fits best? *Gastrointestinal Nursing, 13*(3), 41–48.

Hoseini, A. S. (2019). A proposed Islamic nursing conceptual framework. *Nursing Science Quarterly, 32*(1), 49–53. https://doi.org/10.1177/0894318418807944

Hussain, S. (1981). Rufaida Al-Aslamia. *Islamic Medicine, 1*(2), 261–262.

Hussain, M. (2012). *The Five Pillars of Islam: Laying the Foundations of Divine Love and Service to Humanity.* New York: Kube Publishing.

Jan, R. (1996). Rufaida Al-Aslamia, the first Muslim nurse. *Image: The Journal of Nursing Scholarship, 28*(3), 267–268.

Jones, J. L., & Jones, L. L. (2022). A space is a terrible thing to waste: HBCU role in fostering diversity, inclusion, equity, belonging, and liberation. In A. El-Amin (Ed.), *Implementing Diversity, Equity, Inclusion, and Belonging Management in Organizational Change Initiatives* (pp. 234–247). IGI Global.

Kadioğlu, M. (2021). The first female pirate in Islamic history [İslam Tarihinin İlk Kadın Korsanı]. *ALTRALANG Journal, 3*(01), 118–137.

Khan, Y. (2015, November 6). Humanist vs Islamic perspectives on science and the modern world. *The Guardian,* https://www.theguardian.com/science/blog/2015/nov/06/humanist-vs-islamic-perspectives-on-science-and-the-modern-world

Kolmar, A., & Kamal, A. H. (2018). Developing a path to improve cultural competency in Islam among palliative care professionals. *Journal of Pain and Symptom Management, 55*(3), e1–e3.

Leirvik, O. (2020). Islamic humanism or humanistic Islam? *Interreligious Studies and Intercultural Theology, 4*(1), 88–101.

McCance, T., McCormack, B., & Dewing, J. (2011). An exploration of person-centredness in practice. *The Online Journal of Issues in Nursing, 16*(2), 1–9.

McCormack, B. (2003). A conceptual framework for person-centred practice with older people. *International Journal of Nursing Practice, 9*(3), 202–209.

McCormack, B., Dewing, J., & Mccance, T. (2011). Developing person-centred care: Addressing contextual challenges through practice development. *The Online Journal of Issues in Nursing, 16*(2), 1–11.

McCormack, B., & McCance, T. V. (2006). Development of a framework for person-centred nursing. *Journal of Advanced Nursing, 56*(5), 472–479.

Mohd, S. H. (2019). Secular humanism and Islamic humanism – Is there a common ground? *JUSPI (Jurnal Sejarah Peradaban Islam), 3*(1), 33–40. https://doi.org/10.30829/juspi.v3i1.4025

Nordin, M. M. (2019). Keeping communities healthy: The Islamic paradigm. *Journal of the British Islamic Medical Association, 1*(1), 24–28.

Olsson, L., Jakobsson, E., Swedberg, K., & Ekman, I. (2013). Efficacy of person-centred care as an intervention in controlled trials – A systematic review. *Clinical Nursing, 22*(4), 456–465.

Rahman, M. K., Zailani, S., & Musa, G. (2017). Tapping into the emerging Muslim-friendly medical tourism market: Evidence from Malaysia. *Journal of Islamic Marketing, 8*(4), 514–532.

Rassool, G. H. (2000). The crescent and Islam: Healing, nursing and the spiritual dimension. Some considerations towards an understanding of the Islamic perspectives on caring. *Journal of Advanced Nursing, 32*(6), 1476–1484. https://doi.org/10.1046/j.1365-2648.2000.01614.x

Santana, M., Manalili, K., Jolley, R., Zelinsky, S., Quan, H., & Mingshan, L. (2018). How to practice person-centred care: A conceptual framework. *Health Expectations, 21*(2), 429–440.

Tackett, S., Young, J. H., Putman, S., Wiener, C., Deruggiero, K., & Bayram, J. D. (2018, July). Barriers to healthcare among Muslim women: A narrative review of the literature. *Women's Studies International Forum, 69*, 190–194.

Tan, C., & Ibrahim, A. (2017). Humanism, Islamic education, and confucian education. *Religious Education, 112*(4), 394–406.

Wong, E., Mavondo, F., Horvat, L., McKinlay, L., & Fisher, J. (2022). Healthcare professionals' perspective on delivering personalised and holistic care: Using the theoretical domains framework. *BMC Health Services Research, 22*(1), 1–3. https://doi.org/10.1186/s12913-022-07630-1

Part 3

Patient care

12 Dependency

Simon van der Weele

Introduction

Rose is a woman in her seventies, who resides in a group home for people with intellectual disabilities somewhere in the Netherlands.[1] Rose has a severe intellectual disability. She also has been deaf and blind since birth. This means that Rose is unable to express herself verbally or understand verbal language. It also means that she needs assistance with basically every ordinary task in order to get through the day.

When Rose was younger, she could still stand up and walk around. On her best days, she would dance around the group home, hopping and jumping to a rhythm no one else could hear. In those days, Rose still had her own little ways of communicating her wants. When she needed something, she would find her way to an assistant and grab them by the hand. When she was uncomfortable, she would push away whatever it was that bothered her – object or person. But now that Rose is getting older, she has gradually lost these skills. Her arthritis causes pains that make it unbearable to stand or sit up straight, let alone walk around. Rose is only comfortable when lying down, meaning in practice she spends most of her time in bed, where she can often be found restlessly tossing and turning about. She has also become incontinent; she now makes use of a catheter, as well as of incontinence briefs, to make sure she never wakes up in a spoilt bed.

Carl is a nurse employed by Rose's group home, often tasked with taking care of Rose. He has known Rose for about 15 years. Over time, Carl has grown quite fond of Rose. Although caring for her was always difficult, he gradually developed his own ways of finding out her needs and making sure they are met. But as Rose has grown older, Carl finds that caring well for Rose has grown increasingly challenging.

Carl worries that the catheter and incontinence briefs are a cause of Rose's restlessness. Rose tends to pull away when Carl changes her catheter, and frequently tries to maneuver her way out of her briefs, which Carl interprets as resistance. Carl and his colleagues have tried moving Rose to a different bed in the daytime, to offer her different sensations and more of a daily rhythm. But doing so usually aggravates rather than quietens Rose's restlessness. Worst of all, Carl can't be sure how Rose feels about any of this. All she can do is yell when she is in pain, or agitatedly wriggle about underneath her sheets when she is uncomfortable.

Carl's relationship to Rose is one of extreme dependency. Rose's various impairments render her utterly dependent on the care of others to survive, let alone thrive. Yet, caring for Rose is no easy task for Carl, as her impairments also make it exceedingly difficult to determine and fulfill Rose's needs. This dependency causes Carl moral distress. He wants to help Rose live life as comfortable as possible, but also make room for Rose to live her

DOI: 10.4324/9781003427407-15

life in her own way, according to her own preferences. But these preferences are hard to make out. In this way, Rose's dependency gives rise to all sorts of moral tensions.

The example of Rose and Carl may be extreme, but it is an extreme case of a widespread phenomenon. Dependency in nursing care is everywhere, no matter the capacities of the patient or the nature of their condition. There is dependency at the GP's office, in home care, in the cancer ward, at the ICU, and at the hospice. And that means that the moral tensions that dependency gives rise to are everywhere in nursing care, too. Indeed, empirical studies suggest that nurses struggle a great deal when dealing with the dependency of the people they care for, and they experience feelings of guilt, insufficiency, worry, impatience, and powerlessness as a result (Piredda et al., 2020; Strandberg and Jansson, 2003).[2]

In this chapter, I explore the place of dependency in nursing care and how and why it brings moral tensions for nurses. I also discuss how nurses can and do deal with dependency in everyday care practice. I will suggest that dependency is not a problem to be solved, but rather a given to be grappled and tinkered with. I also offer a moral vocabulary to specify this process of tinkering. To make my points, I draw from care theory, as well as from some of my own ethnographic research on care for people with intellectual disabilities. Although I argue that dependency is part of any form of nursing care, my discussion will spotlight situations of extreme dependency throughout. This is to illustrate that nurses find ways of managing the moral tensions caused by dependency even when there is no imaginable way for dependency to be resolved.

Dependency in nursing care

Nursing theorists have long recognized that dependency is part and parcel of nursing care. In fact, nursing care has often been defined as a practice that seeks to bring persons from periodic dependency to full *in*dependence. Victoria Henderson (1964, p. 64) famously regarded nursing as a practice aiming 'to assist the individual, sick or well, in the performance of those activities contributing to health or its recovery (or to peaceful death) that he would perform unaided if he had the necessary strength, will or knowledge'. In other words, she depicted nursing as a response to a person's dependency, typically imagined as a temporary break from full self-reliance, which the nurse was to help restore: for Henderson, the nurse is to 'help [the patient] gain independence as rapidly as possible' (1964, p. 64). Similarly, Dorothea Orem (1959) perceived nursing care as filling up what she called a 'self-care deficit': nurses were to respond to a person's decrease in self-care, by fulfilling the needs this person could no longer fulfill, but also by stimulating and promoting self-care and acts of independence. Hence, these theorists made two claims about the place of dependency in nursing care: (1) nursing care is necessitated by a patient's dependency and (2) the task of the nurse is to curtail this dependency by restoring a patient's independence (Dijkstra et al., 1998, p. 145).

It is difficult to squabble with the first of these claims. Care arises from dependency; this simple fact has been recognized and demonstrated by many care theorists (Kittay, 1999; Noddings, 1984; Tronto, 1993; see also Van der Weele, 2021a). Joan Tronto, for instance, notes how 'care arises out of the fact that not all humans or others or objects in the world are equally able, at all times, to take care of themselves' (1993, p. 145). Care, in its foundation, consists in the act of meeting a need that a care recipient cannot meet alone. It is in this sense that care implies dependency.

The second of these claims requires more explanation, however. Intuitively, restoring a patient's independence may seem an appropriate purpose for the nurse; supporting a patient's autonomy is typically regarded as an important responsibility for nurses (Risjord, 2014). Yet, the example of Rose and Carl suggests that not all nursing care can have the restoration of independence as its primary objective. Some dependency relationships will persist, no matter how skilled the nurse or how receptive the patient. This holds in the care of people such as Rose, but also in many forms of elderly care, psychiatric care, and end-of-life care (where it is finally the moment of death that ruptures the dependency on nursing care, as Henderson herself also noted).

It is therefore important to consider the suitability of recovering independence as an objective for nursing care. I want to mention two of its drawbacks. First, if the nurse must strive, as Henderson put it, to aid the patient in returning to independence as quickly as possible, this leaves nurses working with patients for whom independence is *not* a realistic goal with a highly restricted imaginary of what their profession is about. Surely caring for someone like Rose is a worthy pursuit for any nurse; yet, if that pursuit consists in restoring independence, it remains unclear what good care for Rose might realistically entail.

Second, setting independence as the objective of nursing care risks reiterating the notion that dependency is an unwanted condition best avoided. Nancy Fraser and Linda Gordon (1994) have shown in detail how in Western modernity, dependency has come to be a stigmatized condition, rife with negative connotations. Dependency is associated with psychological weakness and moral failure; it is also perceived as antonymic to the ideals of autonomy, equality, and freedom that feed liberal imaginations of the good life.

Yet as many feminist scholars have pointed out, this aversion toward dependency is both self-deluding and harmful. It is *self-deluding*, as it runs counter to the reality that members of a social species such as *homo sapiens* are inevitably dependent in many facets of life and across significant stretches of their lifespan (Butler, 2010; Engster, 2019; Kittay, 1999); we are, as Alasdair MacIntyre (1999) puts it, 'dependent rational animals'. The upshot is that, as Martha Fineman (2004) observes, full independence is a *myth*, as our sense of independence (even if we have it) presumes and relies on all sorts of socially tolerated dependencies that tend to remain hidden.

The cultural aversion toward dependence is also *harmful*, as cultural prejudice against dependency can turn into cultural prejudice against dependent people (Kittay, 2001, 2011). This may render those who are most dependent, and hence most in need of our care stigmatized and marginalized, even when their dependency is nothing more than the inevitable effect of the inherent vulnerability of the human body (Scully, 2014). Such prejudice might manifest itself, for instance, in limited public interest in meeting the care needs of those who rely on government aid to survive and thrive, or in supporting those who work to provide this care. Surely, no nursing theorist would want to reproduce this particular cultural narrative about dependency.

I doubt Henderson and others wanted to make lofty metaphysical claims about the human condition when they wrote about the nursing profession. Indeed, the notion of the 'self-care deficit' makes sense in the context of temporary illnesses and injuries, in which this deficit is formed by the gap between a patient's current condition and the patient's capacities prior to the onset of the illness or injury in question. This deficit may look different for different patients, but seeking to remedy such a deficit need not entail a denial of ordinary human dependency as such.

Nonetheless, given the many cases in which a dependency relationship will be permanent and in which a 'self-care deficit' will have to be filled up by nurses indefinitely (such as the one of Rose and Carl), the goal of restoring dependency will not do as a general objective for nursing care. Moreover, even in situations when independence *does* appear to be a conceivable outcome of nursing care, the nurse is working precisely when independence is *not* yet reached. Hence, nurses always work under conditions of dependency, with clients being dependent on them.

For these reasons, I think we ought to veer away from any conception of dependency in nursing that regards it as a problem to be *solved*. Instead, I suggest, we should approach dependency as a *given* in any care relationship that needs to be grappled and tinkered with by nurses and patients alike. In such a conception, the moral tensions dependency engenders are not to be undone, but only to be navigated as well as possible.

Moral tensions in dependency relations

To get a sense of what these moral tensions might be, let us look again at Carl's concerns about his care for Rose. I think we can broadly distinguish between two. First, Carl is troubled by a conflict between what he thinks Rose needs and what he thinks she wants. Carl is inclined to interpret Rose's behavior with her catheter and her adult briefs as forms of resistance, but he also believes that both grant her a more comfortable and more dignified everyday life. Second, and relatedly, Carl is troubled by the fact that he has no reliable manner of asserting Rose's wants in the first place. As Rose no longer communicates her needs and wants in her trusted old ways, Carl works under conditions of unremitting uncertainty. All this results in a great sense of inadequacy on Carl's part.

Empirical research suggests that Carl is not alone in experiencing inadequacy in the face of these moral tensions. In a study examining the experiences of palliative care nurses with dependency, Piredda et al. (2020) describe how nurses frequently reported a sense of powerlessness as they grapple with conflicts in what patients (seem to) need and what they (seem to) want. Similarly, in a study about perspectives on dependency of hospital nurses, Gunilla Strandberg and Lilian Jansson (2003) remark that nurses experience feelings of guilt and insufficiency in the dependency relationship with their patients. How might we conceptualize the moral tensions causing these feelings?

Care theorists analyze the moral tensions in dependency relationships in terms of *power*. As Eva Kittay (1999, p. 34) puts it, 'inequality of power is endemic to dependency relations'; insofar as a dependency relationship is formed by a caregiver meeting a need that a care recipient cannot meet herself, power will be distributed asymmetrically by definition. Tronto (1993, p. 145) calls this 'the fact of inequality in relations of care'. According to care theorists, it is this 'fact of inequality' that brings moral trouble to any dependency relationship. This is because dependency renders care recipients vulnerable to the whims of the caregiver, burdening the latter with serious responsibilities.

Tronto (1993) provides a number of concepts to consider this moral trouble. One moral threat for any dependency relationship is what she calls *paternalism*. This threat surfaces when caregivers 'come to accept their own account of what is necessary to meet the caring need as definitive' (1993, p. 145), thus harming the autonomy of care recipients. In their role of caregivers, nurses hold the privileged position of interpreting and defining the needs of those in their care, particularly when the latter are unable to voice these on their own. This position is a primary source of the power they can exert over their patient. (Evidently, the moral tensions that Carl faces essentially revolve around concerns about paternalism.)

A second and connected threat distinguished by Tronto is the threat of *otherness*: the 'treatment of those who need care as inherently different and unequal' (1993, p. 105). In Tronto's estimation, our cultural dislike of inequality and dependency can result in the 'othering' of those who find themselves to be dependent. Such 'othering' leads people who need care to be identified as fundamentally different and reduced simply to whatever happens to be the cause of their neediness – a process that can produce various forms of discriminatory treatment. Clearly, this process of othering can only be conceived as part of a broad cultural pattern, but it is not difficult to imagine how it may (and does) lead to abusive forms of nursing care in specific dependency relations.

It is important to note that the distribution of power in dependency relationships is often more complex than the example of Rose and Carl might suggest. As Kittay (1999) observes, how power is distributed hinges not only on capacity, but also on social status; given the social inequalities produced by attributes like gender, race, and class, it matters who is giving the care and who is receiving it (Raghuram, 2019). Moreover, care recipients can exert powers of their own, for instance 'by the manufacture of false needs or by exploiting the worker's caring, concern, and need for the connection forged through the relationship' (Kittay, 1999, p. 34). Additionally, care recipients may resent their dependency, which they can express through resistance to the care they need or even through abuse of the caregiver herself. In other words, dependency can also bestow caregivers with particular vulnerabilities of their own.[3] The dynamics of dependency relationships are therefore unpredictable, and the onus of navigating them well cannot solely be the caregiver's.

Although inequality is a fact for dependency relations, it need not lead to moral abuse. Kittay (1999, p. 33) helpfully distinguishes between *inequality of power* on the one hand and *domination* on the other. While the first is inevitable in care, it can exist without sliding into the nefarious misuse of power that characterizes the latter, she assures us. The moral task of the nurse (as well as of the patient) thus becomes to navigate the dependency relationship in such a way that inequality is accepted, but domination avoided. This makes, as I suggested above, dependency a given to be grappled with, rather than a problem to be solved. But how can (or should) nurses go about this?

Dealing with dependency in everyday care

The example of Rose and Carl shows that nurses are (or can be) keenly aware of the inequalities that are endemic to any relationship of dependency and of the moral tensions they can bring. Yet, it does not yet show how nurses grapple with these tensions in practice to avoid what Kittay calls domination. I now intend to bring up some more examples of my fieldwork in daily care for people with profound disabilities, to give a sense of how nurses can and do deal with dependency and respond to these tensions – even in the most extreme examples of dependency. In doing so, I also seek to enrich the ethical vocabulary available to talk about the tensions springing from dependency relations. A more extensive version of the analysis I will be presenting, containing more and different empirical material (as well as more methodological detail), has previously appeared elsewhere (Van der Weele et al., 2021a).

I am reporting from an ethnographic study I conducted with my colleagues in 2017 and 2018, on everyday care and assistance in group homes for people with intellectual

Table 12.1 Ways of Dealing with Dependency

Way of Dealing with Dependency	Dependency as a Problem of...	Associated Practices
Agentive goods	Self-determination	Choice, doing things yourself, giving a voice
Equalizing goods	Parity	Participation, reciprocity, affection
Affirmative goods	Self-worth	Praise, confidence

disabilities in the Netherlands (see also van der Weele, 2021b; Van der Weele et al., 2021b; van der Weele and Bredewold, 2021). Our curiosity lay in the ways caregivers looked to somehow manage the asymmetries that we considered part and parcel of their relationship to the residents in their care. We analyzed their practices through Jeannette Pols's *empirical ethics of care* approach (for more, see Pols, 2015; Pols et al., 2018): that is, we approached care practices as attempts to put something 'good' into practice, and we approached these 'goods', in turn, as implicit responses to the moral problems caregivers believe they face (Pols, 2019). By studying how caregivers were handling asymmetries in their care, we expected to learn something about the specific problems these asymmetries bring for them – and about the practices caregivers have turned to in order to grapple with these problems. The group home residents we encountered in our study had diverse support needs, but in what follows, I will focus on those whose dependency can be considered extreme, just like Rose's dependency on Carl. I do so to demonstrate that even in cases where dependency cannot conceivably be resolved or even lessened, caregivers still find creative means of navigating the moral tensions they encounter.

We found that broadly speaking, the care assistants we met had developed three ways of dealing with dependency, each revealed in a set of 'goods' these assistants were pursuing. These sets of goods, in turn, implied three distinctive manners of conceptualizing the moral tensions revolving around dependency (Table 12.1).

The first of these found the expression in what we call *agentive* goods, such as *choice*, *doing things yourself*, and *giving a voice*. Such goods are found in practices that 'try to transfer some of their own "executive powers" to the care recipient in order to provide opportunities to exert agency' (Van der Weele et al., 2021a, p. 4). In this sense, they conceptualize the moral tensions of dependency as revolving around self-determination: agentive goods address the asymmetries in dependency relationships by targeting the care recipient's sense of agency. They are thus a clear response to what Tronto identifies as the problem of paternalism.

Assistants found ways of implementing agentive goods even in situations of extreme dependency. Take the following example, featuring assistant Roline and resident Krista, who does not understand verbal language.

> Roline hands Krista a plastic mug of coffee. She helps Krista hold the mug tightly before Krista brings it to her mouth. I tell Roline that I am astonished: just yesterday, a colleague of Roline's had asked me to help Krista drink, because she ostensibly can't hold her own cup. Roline nods. Krista can drink independently; she just needs some help gripping the mug tightly. It takes longer, but it's worth it: it's important to do things yourself.

For Roline, it is important to 'do things yourself'; her purpose is to return a sense of agency to Krista, even if it takes a lot of time. The example suggests two things. First, agency can be looked for in the smallest of details of everyday life, such as simply holding your own coffee cup. This is a crucial aspect of all practices we observed: they are usually not grand gestures, but rather reveal themselves in minute aspects of ordinary interactions. Second, implementing agentive goods takes attention and time, as caregivers need to explore the margins of a patient's capacities, as well as the extent to which these margins may be stretched.

The second way assistants dealt with dependency was through what we call *equalizing* goods. Equalizing goods are manifest in practices that try 'to balance the dependency relationship by allowing for more equal and diverse interactions to take place between caregiver and care recipient' (Van der Weele et al., 2021a, p. 5). Such practices contain an implicit understanding of dependency as a problem of diminished parity, or what Tronto identified as the problem of otherness: they seek to bring a sense of mutuality to a relationship that can be experienced as lopsided and unidirectional. *Participation*, *reciprocity*, and *affection* are equalizing goods in this sense.

Equalizing goods show in ordinary interactions that somehow disrupt the hierarchical relationship that dependency is thought to establish.

> Care professional Julius has his meal with the residents. He tells me some colleagues bring their meal from home, but he doesn't; he thinks that's improper. I ask him why. 'I am no more than they are,' he answers.
>
> (Van der Weele et al., 2021a, p. 6)

Julius assumes that participating in life with the residents he cares for serves as an equalizing gesture. Eating together becomes an activity that mends the sense of diminished parity he anticipates as a consequence of the dependency relationships he sustains with the residents in his care.

Finally, the third way assistants grappled with dependency was through what we call *affirmative* goods. These are goods that seek to 'sustain a positive self-image in the care recipient' (Van der Weele et al., 2021a, p. 6). They tacitly assume dependency to present a problem of diminished self-worth, which assistants respond to by fostering feelings of confidence and competence amongst residents. Like equalizing goods, affirmative goods appear to respond to what Tronto called the problem of otherness. *Praise* and *confidence* are such affirmative goods.

Lacing everyday care practices with words of affirmation was a habit taken up by many assistants we met. It did not seem to matter to them whether or not the praise was understood. This becomes clear when we look at affirmative goods in relations of extreme dependency, with residents who did not understand verbal language.

> Care professional Jantine explains Linda can eat anything. 'She eats everything, I am not sure she is able to experience flavour. Some residents can't.' Then she turns to Linda. 'Delicious, right, girl? What you don't like to eat still has to be invented.'
>
> (Van der Weele et al., 2021a, p. 7)

In this example, Jantine makes a virtue out of something that can be perceived as a shortcoming, framing Linda's inability to taste her food as something she can take pride in. In doing so, it seems to matter little to Jantine that Linda cannot be aware of the discourse surrounding her eating habits. The example suggests that for these assistants, it is of little importance that the people in their care feel the moral tensions they themselves grapple with. Mitigating the moral tensions endemic to dependency relations is a responsibility they commit to even in cases when it is not obvious that the care recipient is troubled by them.

Overwhelmingly, it was through agentive goods that assistants sought to mitigate the tensions they perceived to reside in dependency relationships. It was also through a vocabulary of autonomy and self-determination that assistants tended to speak of the 'problem' of dependency in conversation with us. Hence, they typically framed the moral tensions brought about by dependency as problems of self-determination or what Tronto would call paternalism. Interestingly, however, they hardly ever brought up parity and self-worth in these discussions – as if they did not think of equalizing and affirmative goods as responses to dependency as such. In other words, assistants seemed to be much less aware of what Tronto called the problem of otherness, even if they were clearly attempting to tackle it in practice. Spelling out these tacit goods thus does not only provide us with alternative conceptualizations of what kind of moral tensions dependency may engender; doing so also allows us to offer an addendum to the moral vocabulary caregivers have at their disposal for trying to navigate the asymmetries that are endemic to the dependency relationship.

Taken together, then, these three sets of goods form an account of how caregivers grapple with the moral tensions around dependency in practice. They also help to articulate what it is about dependency relationships that leads to moral trouble. Finally, they demonstrate that for caregivers, dependency as such is not a problem to be *solved*. After all, they engage in these practices fully knowing that the dependency they seek to manage will not abate or diminish in time. Trailing the practices of these assistants brings home the point that dependency is a given to be grappled with, a project which, like all care, relies on creativity, imagination, and experimentation (Mol et al., 2010; Van der Weele et al., 2021a).

Conclusion

Dependency is an inevitable aspect of nursing care, as it is an inevitable aspect of any care relationship. Whether periodical or permanent, patients will find themselves dependent on their nurse, and this means that every nurse will need to look for ways to grapple with the moral tensions this dependency brings. I have therefore suggested that we best veer away from conceptions of nursing that regard dependency as a problem to be solved, and should rather approach it as a given to be tinkered with.

My ethnographic research in intellectual disability care shows that professional caregivers find manifold creative practices of managing dependency in this way. These assistants mitigate the moral problems dependency may bring as much as they can, without believing that this will resolve the dependency relationship itself. By homing in on care for people with profound disability, I wanted to highlight the fact that they do so even in situations of extreme dependency, in which a return to a degree of independence is virtually inconceivable, and in which the care recipient may hardly be aware of the moral tensions vexing the caregiver. Indeed, Rose's dependency distresses Carl, even though he cannot be sure at all that Rose is distressed in the same way. It is worth asking why these assistants nonetheless put in the hard work of dealing with dependency – is managing the 'fact of inequality' a matter of *dignity*, which can be slighted even when the subject of dignity is seemingly unaware of it (Kittay, 2005)? – but that is a problem for another day.

Some final notes. I have not been able here to do justice to the ways in which nurses might be vulnerable to domination in dependency relationships, a point Kittay (1999, 2001) has reminded us of often. I have also not been able to consider the many authors (both in nursing and elsewhere) who have challenged the binary relationship between dependence and independence, for instance, through a vocabulary of relational autonomy (Gómez-Vírseda et al., 2019; Mackenzie and Stoljar, 2000; Risjord, 2014). It has not been my ambition to reproduce this binary; the agentive goods I have written about exemplify precisely the interplay between dependency and independence that relational autonomy gets at. My purpose here, rather, was to install dependency as a keyword for nursing – which begins by pushing against the objective of independence traditionally thought of as central to nursing care. Indeed, my omissions demonstrate just how much more there is to say about dependency in nursing, and how much we can learn by embracing it as one of our key concepts.

Notes

1 Rose and Carl are pseudonyms, as are all the names of participants I met during my fieldwork in intellectual disability care in the Netherlands mentioned in this chapter.
2 Although I will not thematize it in this chapter, empirical research evidences that patients struggle with dependency, too (Eriksson and Andershed, 2008; Martinsen et al., 2022; Piredda et al., 2015; Strandberg et al., 2003, 2002).
3 Kittay, Tronto, and others rightfully note that the dependency relationship also renders caregivers vulnerable to the social fabric around them, which can be more or less supportive for caregivers to carry out their work. This point has obvious relevance for nurses, who frequently work in institutional contexts that put constraints on their capacity to care as they see fit. Since I focus here on moral tensions for nurses in dependency relationships to their patients, I set aside this issue here.

Works cited

Butler, J., 2010. *Frames of War: When Is Life Grievable?* Verso, London.

Dijkstra, A., Buist, G., Dassen, T., 1998. Operationalization of the concept of "nursing care dependency" for use in long-term care facilities. *Australian and New Zealand Journal of Mental Health Nursing* 7, 142–151.

Engster, D., 2019. Care ethics, dependency, and vulnerability. *Ethics and Social Welfare* 13, 100–114. https://doi.org/10.1080/17496535.2018.1533029

Eriksson, M., Andershed, B., 2008. Care dependence: a struggle toward moments of respite. *Clinical Nursing Research* 17, 220–236. https://doi.org/10.1177/1054773808320725

Fineman, M.A., 2004. *The Autonomy Myth: A Theory of Dependency*. The New Press, New York and London.

Fraser, N., Gordon, L., 1994. A genealogy of dependency: tracing a keyword of the U.S. welfare state. *Signs* 19, 309–336.

Gallagher, A., 2004. Dignity and respect for dignity - two key health professional values: implications for nursing practice. *Nursing Ethics* 11, 587–599. https://doi.org/10.1191/0969733004ne744oa

Gómez-Vírseda, C., de Maeseneer, Y., Gastmans, C., 2019. Relational autonomy: what does it mean and how is it used in end-of-life care? A systematic review of argument-based ethics literature. *BMC Medical Ethics* 20, 76. https://doi.org/10.1186/s12910-019-0417-3

Henderson, V., 1964. The nature of nursing. *The American Journal of Nursing* 64, 62–68. https://doi.org/10.2307/3419278

Kittay, E.F., 1999. *Love's Labor: Essays on Women, Equality, and Dependency*. Routledge, New York.

Kittay, E.F., 2001. When caring is justice and justice is caring: justice and mental retardation. *Public Culture* 13, 557–579.

Kittay, E.F., 2005. Equality, dignity and disability, in: Lyons, M.A., Waldron, F. (Eds.), *Perspectives on Equality: The Second Seamus Heaney Lectures*. Liffey, Dublin, pp. 95–122.

Kittay, E.F., 2011. The ethics of care, dependence, and disability. *Ratio Juris* 24, 49–58. https://doi.org/10.1111/j.1467-9337.2010.00473.x

MacIntyre, A., 1999. *Dependent Rational Animals: Why Human Beings Need the Virtues*. Open Court, Chicago.

Mackenzie, C., Stoljar, N., 2000. Introduction: autonomy refigured, in: Mackenzie, C., Stoljar, N. (Eds.), *Relational Autonomy: Feminist Perspectives on Autonomy, Agency, and the Social Self*. Oxford University Press, New York, pp. 3–31.

Martinsen, B., Norlyk, A., Gramstad, A., 2022. What makes dependency on homecare bearable? A phenomenological study. *Western Journal of Nursing Research* 019394592211353. https://doi.org/10.1177/01939459221135325

Mol, A., Moser, I., Pols, J., 2010. *On Tinkering in Clinics, Homes and Farms*. Amsterdam University Press, Amsterdam.

Noddings, N., 1984. *Caring: A Feminine Approach to Ethics and Moral Education*. University of California Press, Berkeley.

Orem, D.E., 1959. *Guides for Developing Curricula for the Education of Practical Nurses*. Government Printing Office, Washington D.C.

Piredda, M., Candela, M.L., Mastroianni, C., Marchetti, A., D'Angelo, D., Lusignani, M., De Marinis, M.G., Matarese, M., 2020. "Beyond the Boundaries of Care Dependence": a phenomenological study of the experiences of palliative care nurses. *Cancer Nursing* 43, 331–337. https://doi.org/10.1097/NCC.0000000000000701

Piredda, M., Matarese, M., Mastroianni, C., D'Angelo, D., Hammer, M.J., De Marinis, M.G., 2015. Adult patients' experiences of nursing care dependence. *Journal of Nursing Scholarship* 47, 397–406. https://doi.org/10.1111/jnu.12154

Pols, J., 2015. Towards an empirical ethics in care: relations with technologies in health care. *Medicine, Health Care and Philosophy* 18, 81–90. https://doi.org/10.1007/s11019-014-9582-9

Pols, J., 2019. Care, everyday life and aesthetic values, in: Brouwer, J., Van Tuinen, Sjoerd (Eds.), *To Mind Is To Care*. V2_Lab for the Unstable Media, Rotterdam, pp. 42–61.

Pols, J., Pasveer, B., Willems, D., 2018. The particularity of dignity: relational engagement in care at the end of life. *Medicine, Health Care and Philosophy* 21, 89–100. https://doi.org/10.1007/s11019-017-9787-9

Raghuram, P., 2019. Race and feminist care ethics: intersectionality as method. *Gender, Place & Culture* 26, 613–637. https://doi.org/10.1080/0966369X.2019.1567471

Risjord, M., 2014. Nursing and human freedom: nursing and human freedom. *Nursing Philosophy* 15, 35–45. https://doi.org/10.1111/nup.12026

Scully, J.L., 2014. Disability and vulnerability: on bodies, dependence, and power, in: Mackenzie, C., Rogers, W., Dodds, S. (Eds.), *Vulnerability: New Essays in Ethics and Feminist Philosophy*. Oxford University Press, Oxford, pp. 204–221.

Strandberg, G., Astrom, G., Norberg, A., 2002. Struggling to be/show oneself valuable and worthy to get care one aspect of the meaning of being dependent on care - a study of one patient, his wife and two of his professional nurses. *Scandinavian Journal of Caring Sciences* 16, 43–51. https://doi.org/10.1046/j.1471-6712.2002.00053.x

Strandberg, G., Jansson, L., 2003. Meaning of dependency on care as narrated by nurses. *Scandinavian Journal of Caring Sciences* 17, 84–91. https://doi.org/10.1046/j.1471-6712.2003.00213.x

Strandberg, G., Norberg, A., Jansson, L., 2003. Meaning of dependency on care as narrated by 10 patients. *Research and Theory for Nursing Practice: An International Journal* 17, 21.

Tronto, J., 1993. *Moral Boundaries: A Political Argument for an Ethic of Care*. Routledge, New York.

Van der Weele, S., 2021a. Four paradigm cases of dependency in care relations. *Hypatia* 36, 338–359. https://doi.org/10.1017/hyp.2021.10

van der Weele, S., 2021b. Thick concepts in social research: What, Why, and How? *International Journal of Qualitative Methods* 20, 160940692110661. https://doi.org/10.1177/16094069211066165

van der Weele, S., Bredewold, F., 2021. Shadowing as a qualitative research method for intellectual disability research: Opportunities and challenges. *Journal of Intellectual & Developmental Disability* 46, 340–350. https://doi.org/10.3109/13668250.2021.1873752

Van der Weele, S., Bredewold, F., Leget, C., Tonkens, E., 2021a. What is the problem of dependency? Dependency work reconsidered. *Nursing Philosophy* 22. https://doi.org/10.1111/nup.12327

Van der Weele, S., Bredewold, F., Leget, C., Tonkens, E., 2021b. The group home as moral laboratory: Tracing the ethic of autonomy in Dutch intellectual disability care. *Medicine, Health Care and Philosophy* 24, 113–125. https://doi.org/10.1007/s11019-020-09991-y

13 Pain

Levinas and ethics

Lawrence Burns

Introduction

A patient in pain presents the nurse with several challenges. A patient suffering from opioid use disorder presents even more. However, every patient is entitled to the same care even though the patient may have a problematic dependence on the drugs that must be provided to relieve that pain. Emmanuel Levinas calls this "demand for analgesia" a "primordial, irreducible and ethical" demand for medical aid (Levinas, Smith and Harshav, 2000, p. 93). Levinas' only sustained "empirical" reflection on the medical-philosophical significance of pain in a medical context is found in the 1982 paper "Useless Suffering". In that text, we see that the ethical subject's obligation to provide relief of pain is the central tenet of Levinas' phenomenological account of ethical responsibility. Furthermore, Levinas draws an important connection between the caregiver's situated response to the patient's pain and the broader issue of its ethical and social significance. By reflecting on the needs of a patient with a complex history of pain and opioid use, we will be able to elucidate a Levinasian account of the nurse's ethical responsibility to "repair" that pain and to see how this responsibility engages broader ethical and political concerns.

A patient

A patient with the initials D.C. was admitted to the Toronto General Hospital in 2020 for a liver resection. D.C. had a successful surgery with optimal pain management and was discharged into the community. This would appear to be a rather routine case, but for the fact that the patient had an opioid dependence. In fact, it was a medication-induced hepatoma that prompted his admission to the hospital. Caring for such patients is the specialty of the Transitional Pain Service, which was established in 2014 as one of the first such programmes (Ogilvie, 2014; reiterated in Clarke et al., 2018, p. 237).

The details of D.C.'s case were published in a 2021 paper by Salima Ladak, a nurse practitioner and founding member of Toronto General's Transitional Pain Service. Ladak's team included a surgeon, an anaesthesiologist and a psychologist, all of whom were co-authors on the paper. They attribute their success to productive dialogue, motivational interviewing, psychological counselling and flexibility in use of pain medications (Ladak et al., 2021, p. 169). In discussions with D.C., the care team developed a personalized post-surgery pain management plan that took account of several factors: his history of fentanyl and heroin dependence, his methadone treatment and the impaired function of his liver. As part of their personalized plan, the team agreed to accommodate D.C.'s

DOI: 10.4324/9781003427407-16

expressed need for higher doses of some pain medications post-surgery. For example, the availability of his on-demand self-administered fentanyl was increased beyond the standard four-hour dosing schedule and represented six times the standard dose (Ladak et al., 2021, p. 168). These decisions required an open discussion about his previous use of opioids, including previously experienced side effects such as hallucinations while using intravenous ketamine (Ladak et al., 2021, p. 167).

The care team also addressed D.C.'s psychological distress and barriers to care from a holistic perspective. D.C. had disclosed that he had been anxious about pain. As a result, he used heroin the day after his surgery (Ladak et al., 2021, p. 168). An additional problem was D.C.'s fear of stigmatization related to drug dependence. D.C. admitted that the frank discussion of his past fentanyl use elevated his stress and he strongly considered leaving against medical advice (Ladak et al., 2021, p. 168). The fear that D.C. would leave against medical advice and the related concern that he would not adhere to his follow-up care after discharge draw attention to the broader public health harms of opioid dependence. Ladak et al. note that 25–30% of such patients will discharge themselves against medical advice (Ladak et al., 2021, p. 169). Lack of medical care, homelessness and overdose are increasingly problematic outcomes of opioid use disorder that deepen the stigma and further limit the capacity of people to heal and thrive in community.[1]

D.C.'s case is instructive in several ways. First, it illustrates the medical challenge of caring for patients suffering from opioid use disorder. In this situation, D.C.'s health was at stake due to his history of drug use and the risks of surgery. His well-being depended on him receiving a sufficient dose of analgesia; yet, research shows that many patients with opioid use disorder are not given sufficient medication.[2] While it is true that the degree of pain experienced affects the quantum of medication provided, it would be wrong to say that his pain only "mattered" if it was serious or actually occurring. The care team made it a priority to understand all of the patient's existing and anticipated pain, including psychological pain and suffering.

Second, the practical problem of dosing to manage physical pain presupposes the urgent obligation to provide relief. Levinas helps us to articulate the ethical aspect of this responsibility to manage pain. To anticipate, D.C's case helps us to see (i) the unjustifiability of pain and (ii) the nurse's responsibility to "suffer at the other's suffering" in order to repair that pain (Levinas, Smith and Harshav, 2000, p. 94). The pragmatic calibration of the responsive performance in view of an unlimited responsibility is another essential component of this model. In short, the nurses providing medical care bore a necessarily *limitless responsibility* for D.C., while at the same time they had to *set limits* on that response. A limitless obligation, but a limited response, rooted in pragmatic considerations about situated responsiveness. Perhaps a better way to think of it is that providing a justification for the pain would excuse and set a limit (or level of tolerance) that is fundamentally in conflict with Levinas' idea of the "uselessness" of pain.

To explore the ethics of pain management further, we will turn to the analysis provided by Levinas in the next sections. In particular, we can compare the "first of its kind" Transitional Pain Service described above with the "first of its kind" French pain clinic that triggered Levinas' reflections on pain in "Useless Suffering". To that end, it is essential to provide a brief overview of the phenomenological method. Following the overview, we return to his dedicated reflections on pain and the nurse's responsive performance. The case just presented will also be re-examined in light of that elucidation of Levinas' ethics.

Levinas and phenomenology

Emmanuel Levinas was born in Kaunas, Lithuania in 1906. He spent his childhood in a thriving Jewish community and was educated at Russian-language schools. Russian literature inspired his philosophical works in conjunction with his studies in Judaism (Lescourret, 1996, p. 48). At the time of his death in 1995, he left behind a unique body of work that promoted the fundamental importance of ethics in philosophy. Phenomenology was the gateway for Levinas' entry into philosophy, but his mature works also reflect the influence of other complementary lines of thought and unprecedented world events.

In 1928, Levinas travelled to Freiburg in Germany to study phenomenology with its founder, Edmund Husserl, and its heir apparent, Martin Heidegger. These encounters consolidated Levinas' interest in phenomenology and led him to write a number of early commentaries and translations of Husserl's work into French.[3] While Levinas was certainly critical of the phenomenological method over his lifetime, he never abandoned it. In a 1981 interview, Levinas noted that, "It was little by little that the essential truth of Husserl, which I still believe today, emerged into my mind, even if, in following his method, I do not at all obey his school's precepts" (Levinas and Cohen, 1985, p. 30). The influence of phenomenology is vital to understanding Levinas' 1982 paper "Useless Suffering", which is the focus of this elucidation of Levinas' ethical philosophy.

Phenomenology is the study of the structures and function of consciousness. Its guiding principle is that consciousness is always consciousness *of something*; it has intentionality.[4] Any given object of consciousness has a meaning *for the subject* that can be delineated using phenomenological analysis: the "inventory" of all of the actual and possible ways in which the object may be intuited by consciousness constitutes the meaning of the object (Levinas et al., 1996, p. 35–6). The subject is also conscious of itself and of its emotional states, such as its experience of pain. The task of the phenomenologist is to "mine" meaning from phenomena and to refine the field of experience.

Following the path set by Rene Descartes in his *Meditations on First Philosophy*, Husserl suspended (i.e., doubted) the existence of the world to reveal the fundamental necessity of transcendental consciousness (Cottingham, 2017; Husserl and Moran, 2012, p. 111). For Husserl, consciousness was *transcendental* in the sense that the world can only exist inasmuch as it has a meaning for the subject. Levinas described this reduction of the existence of the external world as "a violence done to oneself to find oneself as pure thought" (Levinas, Cohen and Smith, 1998, p. 72). Yet, in a problematic sense, this reduction also caused violence to others within the world. Husserl's method appeared to turn the world and other people into mere "ideas" belonging to the transcendental subject that lacked independent reality.[5] His students Martin Heidegger, Maurice Merleau-Ponty, Levinas and others would radically revise the foundations of phenomenology in different ways to restore the independence of the world and other people, with varying success.

Unlike the other philosophers just noted, Levinas is the only one who envisioned ethics as "first philosophy".[6] In his ground-breaking *Totality and Infinity*, ethical responsibility is described through the encounter with the face of the other who, like the idea of infinity, cannot be contained by consciousness (Levinas and Lingis, 1969, p. 75). The subject of responsibility is called to account for itself by "the widow, the orphan and the stranger" who "face" the subject with their need in a way that challenges the subject's position in the world. Such an event demands action rather than reflection, and while it has biblical echoes, Levinas sought to establish ethical responsibility on a non-religious foundation (Levinas and Cohen, 1985, pp. 23–24).

The transition away from Husserl's phenomenology is especially clear in the phenomenological analysis of pain and its relationship to the other. By focusing on the essay "Useless Suffering" and by contextualizing his account with his earlier reflection on pain and suffering, we will explore how Levinas' ideas help us understand the nurse's responsive ethical obligation to care for the other in the medical context.

"Useless Suffering"

Prior to his landmark work *Totality and Infinity,* published in 1961, Levinas had not yet integrated the face of the other into his phenomenological account of pain and suffering.[7] Emphasis was placed on the passivity of sickness and the experience of being as such rather than the exposure to the other who is positioned as the one who can relieve that sickness.

Beginning with his "Reflections on the Philosophy of Hitlerism" (published in 1934), Levinas viewed pain through the experience of embodiment. He described the "impasse of physical pain" of the one who "experiences the indivisible simplicity of his being when he turns over in his bed of suffering to find a position that gives him peace" (Levinas and Hand, 1990, p. 68). We see the same description of pain and embodiment in his 1947 lectures *Time and the Other*, in which he contrasts the "moral pain" in which the subject preserves its freedom, with "physical suffering in all its degrees [that] entails the impossibility of detaching oneself from the instant of existence. It is the very irremissibility of being" (Levinas and Cohen, 1987, p. 69). The invocation of the other begins to emerge in the 1954 paper "The I and Totality", where Levinas writes that:

> The simultaneity of these two moments – the turning of the 'I can' into a thing – constitutes the mode of existence of the third party. Its existence is health and sickness. It reveals itself concretely in suffering, which is incapable of mastering itself from within, and inflected toward external medication.
>
> (Levinas, Smith and Harshav, 2000, p. 29)

While Levinas used many examples of pain and suffering in his work, he typically uses them to illustrate a broader philosophical claim rather than discuss them as instances of medical care. For example, he describes the experience of being responsible for the other as a kind of wound or pain *for the other* and as a "hemorrhage" of the subject's self-sufficiency (Levinas and Lingis, 1991, pp. 49–50, 74). These ideas help express the way that ethical responsibility takes the subject outside or beyond itself and cannot be reduced to the power of consciousness. In a similar vein, he describes responsibility as being held "hostage" by the other for whom one substitutes oneself (Levinas and Lingis, 1991, p. 112). However, in "Useless Suffering", Levinas focuses on pain disorders in "empirical situations of pain" and uses them to illustrate essential features of ethical subjectivity.

One of the consistent themes in Levinas' writings is the idea that pain is experienced as something that fundamentally resists the intentionality of consciousness. He writes that pain is experienced "in-spite-of-consciousness" as something "unassumable" (Levinas, Smith and Harshav, 2000, p. 91). In other words, pain lacks a conceptual meaning-content: it is gratuitous, having no goal or purpose by means of which it could be justified and it is not something that the subject can control. This is not to deny the physiological function of the nervous system as an "alarm signal" engineered to warn us of dangers to be avoided (Levinas, Smith and Harshav, 2000, p. 95). However, such a "purpose" for pain does not override the fundamental experience of pain as something to be endured "for nothing". In addition to being an excessive object of experience that cannot be grasped, pain teaches about the failure of intentionality itself: "at once what disturbs this order and the disturbance itself" (Levinas, Smith and Harshav, 2000, p. 91). Elsewhere, he calls it "Contradiction *qua* sensation: the ache of pain – woe" (Levinas, Smith and Harshav, 2000, p. 92). The French term here is "*le mal*", which also refers to evil or "a wrong" in addition to woe, pain and suffering.

While Levinas asserts that all pain is useless, passivity, negation, submission, absurdity, etc., he refuses to merely intellectualize this claim. In a somewhat uncharacteristic move, he bases his claim on empirical evidence concerning "pain-illnesses" ("douleurs-maladies"). He writes: "Doubtless this depth of meaninglessness that the analysis seems to suggest is confirmed by empirical situations of pain, in which pain remains undiluted, so to speak, and isolates itself in consciousness, or absorbs the rest of consciousness" (Levinas, Smith and Harshav, 2000, p. 93). He highlights the most serious of these pain disorders, describing them as conditions such as one would find in "medical journals certain cases of persistent or obstinate pain, the neuralgias and intolerable lumbagos resulting from lesions of the peripheral nerves, and the tortures that are experienced by certain patients stricken with malignant tumors" (Levinas, Smith and Harshav, 2000, p. 93). The conditions he enumerates are especially significant in that they are examples of cases where pain is superfluous and serves no "use". The idea is that the disorder becomes the pain itself. Pain does not warn of an impending problem; rather, it is the problem.

The pain disorder examples were prompted by a newspaper article about a new pain clinic that opened at the Cochin hospital in Paris on April 2, 1981. Writing in *Le Monde*, medical journalist Claudine Escoffier-Lambiotte expressed the hope that "the centre should be a model for the treatment/welcome of those who suffer from chronic pain and who find that they are abandoned by medicine today" (Escoffier-Lambiotte, 1981; my translation). The theme that pain patients had otherwise been abandoned by the health care system is certainly consistent with Levinas' extensive reflections on the ethical obligation to care for those who suffer. The abandonment is even more acute in the case of a patient with opioid use disorder who may be stigmatized because of their dependence on pain medication. The Transitional Pain Service described by Ladak is an echo of this Paris pain clinic: both are interventions geared to amplify and respond to the unmet medical needs of vulnerable patients. From a pragmatic perspective, the plight of opioid-dependent patients adds an extra layer of complication that requires even more specialized care. However, the goal is the same: to satisfy the demand for analgesia.

Theodicy

Despite his focus on the extreme cases of pain disorders, Levinas' analysis of pain incorporates the full spectrum of pain as experienced by the subject. In "Useless Suffering", for example, he cites the more transitory expressions of pain such as the "moans", "groans" and "sighs" of patients that provoke responsibility in those who hear them (Levinas, Smith and Harshav, 2000, p. 93). The quantum of pain matters less than its qualitative characteristics: namely, the manner in which it strips freedom from the subject and disrupts the power of consciousness. A foreshadowing of this position is found in the passage from *Time and the Other* cited above, where he invokes "physical pain in all its degrees". The urgency of the responsive performance will be greater if the pain is acute and severe, but it is part of a continuum in which intentionality is "undone" by an experience that exceeds the grasp of consciousness. The best way to understand this proposition is through the radical idea that no degree of pain can be justified, no matter how small.

Levinas invokes the philosophical concept of theodicy to shift from the "empirical" reflection on pain disorders to a more metaphysical question about whether pain can ever be justified in view of a greater plan or secondary purpose. In 1710, the rationalist philosopher Gottfried Wilhelm Leibniz provided his solution to the problem of why there is so much pain and suffering in the world. In his *Theodicy*, Leibniz squarely placed the solution to the problem of evil on the idea of an all-knowing, all-powerful and benevolent creator God. Leibniz famously stated that since everything must happen for a reason, evil had to serve some necessary function. Simply put, out of the infinite number of possible worlds, God had to select the one that was "the best" (Leibniz, 1985, pp. 128–29). In this world, human freedom was at the root of evil, not God. Everything everywhere had its use.

Theodicy endorses a radical acceptance of a totalizing narrative that Levinas explicitly rejects. For Levinas, the perspective of the individual who suffers cannot be redeemed by a historical necessity. Rather than revert to a divine order of things, Levinas seeks good works in the "interhuman" order (Levinas, Smith and Harshav, 2000, p. 94). Human pain is a human problem, and while it cannot be eradicated, it should not be justified. To this end, Levinas introduces a kind of redemption through the reparative action of the nurse who "suffers at the suffering of the other" (Levinas, Smith and Harshav, 2000, p. 94). The second order suffering of the care provider bestows a meaning on the event of suffering that is otherwise meaningless, gratuitous and cruel. Suffering here means more the labour of the nurse on behalf of the patient, not necessarily actual harm. Nevertheless, such harms may occur in the course of patient care (Burns, 2017).

After presenting this redemptive suffering, Levinas goes on to reflect on the great evils of the 20th century that defy any attempt at justification. These include the Holocaust, the Soviet gulags, genocide in Cambodia and the bombing of Hiroshima, among many others (Levinas, Smith and Harshav, 2000, p. 97). For the purposes of this reflection on pain, we will remain focused on the medical context, however, but the medical context certainly has its own political dimensions that open the door to theodicy.

In the medical context, we find an example of theodicy at the same hospital in which the Paris pain clinic was established many years later. George Orwell, a profound thinker of totalizing politics, had his own first-hand experience at the Cochin Hospital in 1929. In the short work "How the Poor Die" (Blair, 2018), we see a striking contrast between the two approaches to pain at the same hospital. Orwell was admitted due to a respiratory infection. Over 15 days, he endured terrible treatment and observed others who received worse care. He likened the hospital to a prison staffed by heartless physicians and nurses who treated patients like specimens. Unlike the patient D.C. who received "motivational interviewing" and had "patient-centred dialogue" at a Toronto hospital in 2021, Orwell was subjected to neglect and indignity. He did not trust his care team and escaped "without medical discharge" as soon as he was well enough. Here, we have a concern about leaving "against medical advice" from a different perspective, namely the need to leave in order to preserve one's health rather than to avoid treatment that would be beneficial.

The treatment he received consisted primarily of cupping and the application of a mustard poultice, both of which were painful yet ineffective. Most patients were subjected to the same treatment regardless of their condition and many died. The food was terrible and there was no privacy in the ward. Despite the limitations of medicine at that time, he held English nurses in higher regard, noting that "at least they don't let you lie unwashed and constipated on an unmade bed, out of sheer laziness. The nurses at the Hôpital X still had a tinge of Mrs. Gamp about them" (Blair, 2018). Mrs. Gamp is a character in Charles Dickens' Martin Chuzzlewit who had a grim reputation as a nurse who laid out the dead and was always "right" about everything. The comic antics of Dickens' character were certainly unwelcome for the patients in 1929 just as they would be today.

For patients suffering from opioid use disorder today, the situation has some similarities to Orwell's. Such patients experience greater stigma and face inadequate care due to misconceptions about opioid dependence. Shame is inculcated in patients such as D.C. who are then torn between the desire to flee and the need to stay under medical care. From a more political perspective, the pharmaceutical industry has intensified the problem of opioid dependence by creating powerful drugs that are readily accessed. Advocating for such patients requires action at the bedside, such as described by Ladak et al., but also political action in the legislature or in the medical profession. The temptation of theodicy makes it easy to think that the political problem known as the "opioid epidemic" is justified by the need to repair the pain of those who suffer (i.e., to be accepted as a "necessary evil" or consequence of the effort to solve a greater problem). However, that too is an illegitimate rationalization that ignores the link between the patient's suffering and the politics of care.

The duty to aid

Through the idea of theodicy, Levinas situates the experience of pain within a larger examination of the pain caused by world events. We may well wonder why it is necessary for him to link the expression of pain by a patient to world-historical events such as the Holocaust, especially given Levinas' well-known reticence towards systematic thinking. Nevertheless, it is the inclusion of social solidarity within the midst of an interpersonal patient encounter that helps us understand pain as an ethical phenomenon. The French term for pain, *le mal*, emphasizes the close connection between the pain that calls for a response from the nurse and the idea of a "wrong" that provokes ethical responsibility. Levinas' invocation of the "interhuman order" helps mobilize the resources of the health care provider in order to give meaning to the patient's pain.

Levinas' reflections on the phenomenology of pain and the ethical response to pain provide helpful guidance for understanding what was going on in the case of D.C. and the broader lessons for nurses. The unique feature of Levinas' analysis is that he adopts a phenomenological perspective on how pain is experienced by the subject but also by the witness to the subject's pain who is called upon to repair the person in pain. In other words, Levinas focuses on how pain is expressed (be it "a moan, a cry, a groan or sigh") and how this expression provokes a therapeutic response in the one who witnesses it in a particular context of action. Advocates for patients with opioid use disorder advise taking the patient's narrative as the best indication of the severity of their pain.[8] Listening to the patient in this way reminds us of Levinas' claim that the face speaks (Burns, 2017).

The expression of pain imposes a moral responsibility on the nurse who cares for the patient – a duty to aid. Moreover, all expressions of pain, whether they be minor or debilitating, convey the fundamental unjustifiability of pain. While pain can be given a meaning in this response, it cannot be justified in itself – this is Levinas' core insight and fundamental teaching. By exploring Levinas' ideas about how pain is experienced by the one who suffers and the nurse who responds to that suffering, we see pain as a disruption of experience that reveals the orientation of philosophy around an ethics of obligation rather than a phenomenological account of being or self-knowledge. Such is the original pragmatic contribution of Levinas' ethics to a rich tradition of phenomenological studies.

Notes

1 See, for example, the Director of the Office of National Drug Control Policy's 2017 memo outlining the importance of using "person-first language" to help eliminate stigma within the federal government. The memo references 2015 data showing that 89% of such patients do not receive treatment services for their disorder and that more Americans die from overdoses than car crashes (Botticelli, 2017, p. 2).
2 In part, the inadequate treatment is due to misconceptions about the effects of chronic opioid use, the impact of opioid agonists and negative stereotypes (Paschkis and Potter, 2015, pp. 28–30).
3 In 1929, Levinas wrote that, "We live under the sign of phenomenology" (Levinas, Cohen and Smith, 1998, p. 38). His Strasbourg dissertation, entitled *Theory of Intuition in Husserl's Phenomenology*, was published in 1930 and was soon followed by his translation of *Cartesian Meditations* and several papers on Husserl and Heidegger.
4 In *Cartesian Meditations*, Husserl describes the "universal fundamental property of consciousness: to be consciousness of something; as a *cogito*, to bear within itself its *cogitatum*" (Husserl, 1977, p. 33).
5 "If transcendental subjectivity is the universe of possible sense, then an outside is precisely – nonsense" (Husserl, 1977, p. 84).
6 "But it must be understood that morality comes not as a secondary layer, above an abstract reflection on the totality and its dangers; morality has an independent and preliminary range. First philosophy is an ethics" (Levinas and Cohen, 1985, p. 77).
7 See Moyn (2005) for an account of how Levinas' integration of the other was shaped by his engagement with the work of Kierkegaard and Rosenzweig.
8 Paschkis and Potter (2015, p. 29) regard a patient's self-report as the best gauge of pain levels. However, as they note, this view is not universally endorsed. See Lipscomb for further discussion of this point (Lipscomb, 2022).

References

Blair, E. (2018) *How the Poor Die*. Available at: https://www.orwellfoundation.com/the-orwell-foundation/orwell/essays-and-other-works/how-the-poor-die/. (Accessed: 30 Jan 2023)

Botticelli, M.P. (2017) 'Changing the language of addiction', Memorandum of the Office of National Drug Control Policy, pp. 1–6. Available at: Changing the Language of Addiction | white-house.gov (archives.gov). (Accessed: 30 Jan 2023)

Burns, L. (2017) 'What does the patient say?: Levinas and medical ethics', *Journal of Medicine and Philosophy*, 42(2), pp. 214–235. Available at: https://doi.org/10.1093/jmp/jhw039. (Accessed: 30 Jan 2023)

Clarke, H. et al. (2018) 'Opioid weaning and pain management in postsurgical patients at the Toronto General Hospital Transitional Pain Service', *Canadian Journal of Pain*, 2(1), pp. 236–247. Available at: https://doi.org/10.1080/24740527.2018.1501669. (Accessed: 30 Jan 2023)

Cottingham, J. (2017) *Descartes: Meditations on First Philosophy (Cambridge Texts in the History of Philosophy)*. 2nd edn. New York: Cambridge University Press.

Escoffier-Lambiotte, C. (1981) 'Le premier centre français de traitement de la douleur a été inauguré à l'hôpital Cochin', *Le Monde*, 4 April. Available at: https://www.lemonde.fr/archives/article/1981/04/04/le-premier-centre-francais-de-traitement-de-la-douleur-a-ete-inaugure-a-l-hopital-cochin_2734492_1819218.html. (Accessed: 30 Jan 2023)

Husserl, E. (1977) *Cartesian Meditations: An Introduction to Phenomenology*. The Hague: Martinus Nijhoff.

Husserl, E. and Moran, D. (2012) *Ideas: General Introduction to Pure Phenomenology (Routledge Classics)*. 1st edn. New York: Routledge.

Ladak, S.S.J. et al. (2021) 'The intersection of harm reduction and postoperative care for an illicit fentanyl consumer after major surgery: A case report', *Canadian Journal of Pain*, 5(1), pp. 166–171. Available at: https://doi.org/10.1080/24740527.2021.1952066.

Leibniz, G.W. (1985) *Theodicy: Essays on the Goodness of God, the Freedom of Man and the Origin of Evil*. La Salle: Open Court.

Lescourret, M.-A. (1996) *Emmanuel Levinas*. Paris: Flammarion.

Levinas, E. and Cohen, R. (1985) *Ethics and Infinity: Conversations with Philippe Nemo*. 1st edn. Pittsburgh: Duquesne University Press.

Levinas, E. and Cohen, R. (1987) *Time and the Other*. 1st edn. Pittsburgh: Duquesne University Press.

Levinas, E., Cohen, R. and Smith, M. (1998) *Discovering Existence with Husserl*. Evanston: Northwestern University Press.

Levinas, E. and Hand, S. (1990) 'Reflections on the philosophy of Hitlerism', *Critical Inquiry*, 17(1), pp. 62–71.

Levinas, E. and Lingis, A. (1969) *Totality and Infinity: An Essay on Exteriority*. Pittsburgh: Duquesne University Press.

Levinas, E. and Lingis, A. (1991) *Otherwise than Being or Beyond Essence*. The Hague: Kluwer Academic Publishers.

Levinas, E. et al. (1996) *Emmanuel Levinas: Basic Philosophical Writings*. Amsterdam: Amsterdam University Press.

Levinas, E., Smith, M. and Harshav, B. (2000) *Entre Nous*. New York: Columbia University Press.

Lipscomb, M. (2022) 'Pain is (or may not be) what the patient says it is – professional commitments: objects of study or sacrosanct givens?' in Lipscomb, M. (ed.) *Complexity and Values in Nurse Education: Dialogues on Professional Education*. London: Routledge, pp. 7–27.

Moyn, S. (2005) *Origins of the Other: Emmanuel Levinas between Revelation and Ethics*. 1st edn. Ithaca: Cornell University Press.

Ogilvie, M. (2014) 'Toronto General Hospital program uses new methods to prevent pain killer addictions after surgery', *The Toronto Star*, 14 November. Available at: https://www.thestar.com/life/2014/11/14/toronto_general_hospital_program_uses_new_methods_to_prevent_pain_killer_addictions_after_surgery.html. (Accessed: 30 Jan 2023)

Paschkis, Z. and Potter, M.L. (2015) 'Acute pain management for inpatients with opioid use disorder: Overcoming misconceptions and prejudices', *American Journal of Nursing*, 115(9), pp. 24–32. Available at: https://doi.org/10.1097/01.NAJ.0000471243.30951.92. (Accessed: 30 Jan 2023)

14 Vulnerability and relations of care

Thomas Foth

Introduction

The SARS-CoV-2 pandemic reveals two forms of vulnerability: one is that we are vulnerable through the shared condition of social life characterized by interdependency, exposure, and porosity; the other is that some people have a greater likelihood of being infected and of dying from the virus as a result of systematic social inequality in our societies that increases the risk for some but not for others. The pandemic highlights a global vulnerability because everyone is vulnerable to the virus and to viral infections that can potentially be transmitted by others – we are vulnerable to being harmed by another. Thus, our social and bodily lives are characterized by interdependency – our body is not enclosed but rather porous. The pandemic reminds us that we are given over from the very beginning of our lives to a world we never had a chance to choose, a world made by others. This dependency on others is the precondition for us being able to develop what Western societies understand as singular beings, individuals, or independent selves. Dependency begins before we are even born, continues through infancy, and into adulthood. Our survival is formed by our environment, social worlds, and intimate contacts with others; this "impressionability and porosity define our embodied social lives" (Butler, 2020b, p. n.p.). According to Butler (2020b), the pandemic shows that what I breathe in contains what another breathes out, and what I breathe out will become part of what another person breathes in. But we also share the air with other beings and living things, and what they touch I may touch, and vice versa. It is this dimension of reciprocal and material modes of sharing that highlights what Butler calls vulnerability. At the beginning of the pandemic, the common perception was that the virus affected all of us without difference. We soon realized, however, that this was a dangerous illusion often used by politicians, and the longer the pandemic dragged on, the more we became aware of how this illusion became a pretext for doing nothing. However, historically every epidemic/pandemic has led to unequal consequences depending on where one stands in a hierarchy of lives. This hierarchy of the value of lives becomes apparent when we realize that Black and Indigenous communities were hit hardest. Socially disadvantaged people find it difficult or even impossible to follow public health preventive measures. The pandemic also highlighted the higher fatality rates of elderly individuals, particularly those living in long-term care facilities with pre-existing medical conditions (Fassin, 2020). The systematic devastation of healthcare systems in many parts of the world has meant that many people did not survive the pandemic and are still dying from the consequences of infection. Early on in the pandemic, nurses identified what they called "vulnerable groups" who were particularly prone to experience the viral infection as a

DOI: 10.4324/9781003427407-17

life-threatening disease, and they called for specific public health responses to focus on these vulnerable groups.

This chapter aims to do more than just draw attention to the inequalities exposed by the pandemic. Using the concept of vulnerability enables us to develop a politico-ethical dimension of care that calls on nurses to become an active part of movements struggling for equality and global responsibility for all beings, humans and non-humans, with whom we share this planet. I argue that only once we recognize our interdependence with even those we have yet to meet and who we do not know will we be able to build a world that will make life possible for all. This interdependence is what unites us because at any moment in our shared vulnerability, we can be deprived of what we depend on. Even if we are able to learn how to live with this particular virus, COVID-19 is only a "dress rehearsal" (Latour, 2020) for what will come – another pandemic, the catastrophe of climate change, global war, the blatant disrespect for lives considered not worthy protecting, etc. – in short, the necropolitical times we are living through (Mbembe, 2003, 2016, 2019b). Thus, here I am not philosophizing for its own sake but am rather issuing a call to action for nurses to stand up and to assume responsibility together with others to create a liveable world (see also Fassin & Harcourt, 2019; Harcourt, 2020).

I begin my considerations with a critique of liberal theories about individualism and how they contribute to our understanding of ourselves as independent and autonomous persons. In contrast to the liberal idea of selfhood and individuality, I develop an ethical perspective of grief and vulnerability based on Butler's work on relational selfhood and social bonds. I will then discuss the deadly consequences of the pandemic for some and how we can understand the social inequalities in our biopolitical societies that systematically increases vulnerabilities for those lives not considered as valuable as others – or what Fassin (2018) calls biolegitimacy. Finally, I will critique paternalism in the way many nurses and nursing associations understand vulnerability and advocacy.

The limits of selfhood and individuality in liberal theory

The liberal concept of person and selfhood can be traced back to philosophers like Thomas Hobbes and John Locke, and later on to the Scottish Enlightenment (Foth & Leibing, 2022). John Locke defined the characteristics of the self through consciousness, memory, and personal identity, which is conceptualized as individual ownership of the self of itself (myself, yourself). This identity stays the same over one's lifetime, and individuals possess "an alleged 'specificity,' a 'genericity' separating them from the animal or the vegetal world" (Mbembe, 2019b, p. 13). Following this line of thinking means that we can securely determine who counts as a person and who does not. Thus, selfhood is about the determination of who is included and who is excluded (see, also, Butler, 1997, 2005; Murray & Butler, 2007). In Hobbes (1996), the social and political world emerged from a state of nature that is inhabited by individuals who find themselves in an infinite war or conflict with one another (Agamben, 2015; Butler, 2009, 2021; Hobbes, 1996). As Butler (2021) points out, in the Hobbesian account, the individual just exists; it has no biography or history, no account of individuation – it is just a given. In this view, we are told "that conflict is the first of our passionate relations," not dependency and attachment (Butler, 2021, p. 30). In Hobbes' account, not only does an individual want what another has or desires the territory on which another lives, but there is only one individual in the game: "self-sufficient, without dependency, saturated in self-love yet without any need for another" (Butler, 2021, p. 31). Feminists have long criticized this version of individualism as a masculine idea of who we are. Following the Lockean or Hobbesian understanding of what an individual is, selfhood must be defined through exclusionary boundaries against what the self is not.

In opposition to the liberal conceptualization of the self, Butler argues, we need a relational understanding of selfhood based on social bonds. Relational understanding of selfhood differs from communitarian or national conceptions of the self because these are still based on the idea of self-sufficiency that disavows dependency and relations with others.

Butler's perspective is based on an ethical obligation, which I have to the stranger I have never met before, whom I do not know, and whose language I do not speak. This refers to an understanding of global interdependency that came to the fore in the context of the pandemic: the breath is mine but at the same time, it is not entirely my own because the air I am breathing "is filled with the exhalations of absent and unknown others" (Butler, 2020a). The virus shows us our interdependency in a particularly scary way because we can no longer be certain about our independent selves. "Life exceeds the person in forms of interdependency that we should all learn to affirm, even though that condition may well seem imperilling at the moment" (Butler, 2020a).

The pandemic has also shown us that death is not confined to distant parts of the world, but is a real possibility closer to home. It forced us to recognize that we share the Earth with others (including viruses) and that this planet is our shared fate. COVID-19 reminds us that we are embodied beings and that our bodies have now been transformed into a giant vector of contamination.

> For we have never learned to live with all living species, have never really worried about the damage we as humans wreak on the lungs of the Earth and on its body. Thus, we have never learned how to die.
>
> (Mbembe, 2019a; 2020a, p. S59, see, also 2020b)

With the onset of colonialism and the appearance of "industrialized" races, death was delegated to others. But over the course of the pandemic, it became clear that delegating one's death to others was increasingly difficult. As Butler points out, Indigenous wisdom has always recognized another dimension of interdependency, which is the relation to land, ancestors, and others. Practices of deforestation, ruthless exploitation of resources, the systematic destruction of water and land is not only an attack on Indigenous communities themselves, but also on the forests, lands, and everything that lives in them that is part of the extended sense of self. Food distribution, treatment of forests, and healthcare are all aspects of global interdependency. So too is the right to cross borders, to receive residence and asylum. "For the most part, we have good reasons to understand dependency as a condition of exploitation, but it can, when recast as interdependency, become a global ethics and politics committed to social equality" (Butler, 2020a).

Relationality, interdependency, and global obligation

In contrast to the idea of selfhood and the individual in liberal thinking, it is important to recognize that the individual is the result of a process of individuation. We are not born as individuals but become one over time. However, we are born into a condition of radical dependency and never grow out of it. I have discussed in a different context that as infants we are given over to someone else (Foth, 2013). We have been touched, moved, fed, changed, and put to sleep prior to acquiring an "I." These contacts create proximity to an Other "I" never chose. We are handled against our will because it happens at a pre-ontological stage, before the I is able to say "I" (Butler, 2005; Foth, 2013; Levinas, 1996). Even in adulthood therefore, we are in need of forms of social and economic support; all human capacities must be supported in certain ways.

For example, we all depend on systems of food preparation and distribution, and the pandemic has highlighted the precarious conditions of those working within the food industries. But this condition of precarity actually highlights a vulnerability that precedes it. It is not that vulnerability can be individualized in the sense of my vulnerability or yours, but rather that vulnerability is part of the relations that connect us to each other and to the infrastructures and institutions we need to continue to live. Once these infrastructures or persons on whom I depend disappear or fall apart, I am vulnerable to being dispossessed, abandoned, or exposed to conditions that may be unliveable. And, according to Butler (2021), "[d]ependency can be defined partly as a reliance on social and material structures and on the environment, for the latter, too, makes life possible" (p. 41). Thus, vulnerability is not a subjective state but part of our shared world and our interdependent lives.

The liberal idea of individualism must be understood as a kind of imaginary that disavows our dependency for a fantasy of self-sufficiency. But with liberalism comes another shortfall – that which makes it impossible to imagine equality other than an equality among individuals. The individual person is the unit of analysis and equality is understood as an individual right, as in the conceptualization of human rights, for example. However, this right does not include the "social obligations we bear toward one another" (Butler, 2021, p. 45). If it is true that we are social beings, then equality must be defined based on the social relations that make us who we are, and equality becomes a collective claim on society. "Whatever claims of equality are then formulated, they emerge from relations *between* people, in the name of those relations and those bonds, but not as features of an individual subject" (original emphasis, Butler, 2021, p. 45). Equality, then, is not about trying to overcome dependency to achieve self-sufficiency, but rather to accept interdependency as the fundamental foundation of equality.

Precariousness, grievable lives, and the biopolitics of the pandemic

Mourning and grievable lives during COVID

The pandemic made clear that economic instability has become part of our way of living and that we accept increasing economic disparities between those who profit from existential crises like this pandemic and those who do not. Even pre-pandemic, many people were forced to work for wages that often did not cover the basic necessities of life. As Lazzarato (2013) demonstrates, debt has become a new form of bondage, a particular moral way to govern that is infinite and endless. Students are perhaps the most striking example of lives lived in profound uncertainty with rent and tuition fee increasing causing food insecurity (Debt Collective, 2020; Lazzarato, 2015). Increasingly, many people are driven by the fear of being the next "new poor" (Kaika, 2012, 2017). And they fear not only economic poverty, for in many parts of the world, people are no longer sure where to live because their homes are systematically destroyed by wars and/or environmental catastrophes. Many are also realizing that the sudden loss of life has become part of our everyday experience, and for many, the pandemic was perhaps the most shocking realization of this reality.

All this insecurity has been accompanied by a systematic dismantling of value systems that underpin liberal democratic societies (see, for example, Brown, 2003, 2015, 2019). The idea and importance of a moral consensus are increasingly being replaced by cost-benefits schemes of values, and life is increasingly construed as a form of successful management and in which precarious lives are often designated as dispensable. How is it possible, we must ask, that so many elderly people died in privately run long-term care facilities, how is it acceptable that so many Black, Brown, and Indigenous people died, how could we sacrifice so many front-line workers, often migrants, who had no alternative to work to survive, etc. If all these lost lives were grievable, it would mean that they would have been recognized as lives equal in value to any other life – lives that cannot be calculated in monetary terms. The thousands of lives that are still being lost to the pandemic underline the systematic dismantling of public health infrastructures and highlight the fact that our neoliberal societies are founded on an implicit unequal evaluation of lives. To mourn these countless deaths means to mark the loss of lives of people I do not know, whose names I do not know, and whose language I probably do not speak (Butler, 2020b). And this also means that if someone else goes through a personal loss, even or especially if that person is a stranger to me, I am connected to his or her grief.

This is a form of violence that is part of what Foucault calls biopolitics or biopower, which finds it acceptable that whole populations can die. These conditions are part of the politics of states and economic systems that treat some groups of human beings as dispensable and replaceable based on a rationale that determines whose life matters. These groups are then defined as vulnerable; as the interventions to address the consequences of the pandemic made explicit, the calculation of acceptable mortality rates in relation to productivity is a metric about the value of life. One might conclude that those hardest hit by the pandemic were populations considered to be on their way to death anyway, lives not worth protecting. However, any policy or institution that increases the risk of dying for some is a form of "death dealing" (Butler, 2020b). Death becomes an acceptable consequence of policies that aim at economic recovery and growth at the expense of vulnerable classes. It is a specific form of eugenic calculation to identify dispensable and replaceable workers in the name of economic recovery in the midst of the pandemic. "This is what biopolitics ultimately is: the government of human beings through their differential exposure to the risk of illness and death" (Lorenzini, 2022).

Biopolitics, biolegitimacy, and the rejection into death

With the notion of biopolitics/biopower, Foucault tried to grasp a new dimension of power that emerged with the onset of modernity when biological processes, understood as that which characterizes human beings as a species, became the decisive object of political decision-making. From that moment onward, biological processes became the central problem that governments had to address, leading to what Foucault called the "nationalization of the biological" (Foucault, 2003, p. 240). This biologic form of power addresses collective phenomena to enhance a population's productive capacities and strengthen its national economies (Lorenzini, 2020, 2022). Thus, the population became a scientific and political problem that biopolitics addressed on a global level by installing regulatory mechanisms aimed at establishing a kind of homeostasis among mortality rates, natality rates, or rates of morbidity. According to Foucault, biopower is "a matter of taking control over life and the biological processes of man-as-species and of ensuring that they are not disciplined, but regularized" (Foucault, 2003, p. 256).

This bio-regulation by the state needs experts outside the administrative-bureaucratic state apparatuses, like public health experts and medical and nursing organizations, but also social security and insurance schemes (see, for example, Foth, 2009; Foth et al., 2015). This dimension of biopower aims to save biological life, or what theorists like Arendt (1994) and Benjamin (1965) call naked life – life understood in its biological or physiological essence. This form of power is what Fassin (2018) terms biolegitimacy – a form of power of *life itself* (see, also, Fassin, 2009); biopolitics is about life that can be quantified and measured in terms of life expectancy and can even be translated into monetary values. Seen from this perspective, every *biological* life is treated "equally" (Esposito, 2020; Hannah et al., 2020).

It is important to understand that this form of power does not work through coercion or oppression, imposed primarily on our lives from the outside. Rather, this form of power is part of our subjectivation or what we are and how we understand ourselves (Lorenzini, 2020). It is a central part of why we voluntarily aim to comply with public health advice, when we try to prevent illnesses through the adoption of healthy lifestyles, and why we often feel guilty if we fail to achieve these healthier lives.

But this productive form of power is only one dimension of biopolitics. The pandemic led to the acceleration of racial inequality, an increase in nationalism, the intensification of capitalist exploitation, and the systematic neglect of the elderly who lived in private long-term care facilities. Hesse and Thompson (2022) describe 2020 as

> the year of the two pandemics: COVID-19 and antiblackness, the former structured as emergent, the latter structured as long-standing, with both exploding into the glare of national and global attention, as much through mass anguish and protesting about these social and political phenomena as through their respective epidemiological and antipolitical/antisocial outbreaks in different places at different times.
> (Hesse & Thompson, 2022, p. 452)

Foucault's concept of biopower is helpful here again because a second dimension of biopower is what he called the racism of the state. This specific form of racism introduces differences into populations by identifying and hierarchically sorting different races in the population, qualifying some races as superior to others. Within a system of biopolitics, killing the Other who is identified as a biological danger to the health of the valuable part of the population becomes tolerable – it is not a question of victory but the elimination of a danger that at the end will strengthen the desired race. Fassin (2009) translates this dimension of biopolitics from Foucault as "reject into death" (p. 52). Thus, in a normalizing society, race or racism makes killing acceptable.

To understand this dimension, we need to broaden Foucault's concept of biopower by what Fassin (2018) calls the dimension of *life as such* – meaning the biographical dimension of life and how it is actually lived and experienced. Seen from this perspective, life is a chain of events between birth and death that is impacted by political or structural violence, or policies around health and the social. Fassin summarizes this perspective as "life which is lived through a body (not only through cells) and society (not only as species)" (Fassin, 2009, p. 48). Thus, life is not only about the mere fact of being alive but rather about the living conditions that allow one to live a social or political life, not just one reduced to the simple biological fact of being alive in physiological sense. Therefore, life comprises two dimensions: the physical/biological life (*life itself*) and social/political life (*life as such*).To comprehend life and to grasp the full meaning of life, we cannot reduce life to biological phenomena despite the fact that in biopolitical societies, the physical-biological life prevails.

As seen in the pandemic, governments argue that physical/biological *life itself* must be protected through the particular responsibility of states. As we have discussed elsewhere, constitutional rights can be suspended in the name of life itself and states of emergencies (Agamben, 1998) are justified in the name of saving biologic lives (*life itself*) (see, also, Larocque & Foth, 2021). Thus, during COVID-19, countries all over the globe suspended public liberties and fundamental rights (including the right to a dignified death) in the name of saving every single life in the "war against the virus" (Haass, 2020). And yet, despite the emphasis on the sacredness of life, we see the elimination of what Zygmunt Bauman (2004) calls surplus or wasted lives. Thus, it is not only about tactics and strategies to control biologic life as in biopower, but also about the question of how human beings are treated and evaluated differently. These are clearly political questions and COVID-19 highlighted dramatically that lives are not evaluated equally. Those human groups considered less valuable will be exposed to higher risk of death – differential exposure to health and social risk is a decisive dimension of biopolitical societies. Biopolitics does not erase racial inequalities in the sense that we all belong to the same biological species, but rather systematically relies on hierarchies of unequal value of lives, leading to a continuous multiplication of vulnerabilities used in the governing of populations. Thus, the virus did not put us on equal footing but, on the contrary, exacerbated the production of differential vulnerabilities and social inequalities that form the basis of our societies.

Nursing, "Vulnerable Groups," and paternalism

Caring for the so-called vulnerable populations has been understood as "inherent to a nurse's role" long before the onset of the pandemic (Roberts & Kreeger, 2019, p. 82). Advocacy for vulnerable populations is part of what nursing organizations define as advocacy. In the context of CVOID-19, the Canadian Nurses Association (CNA) declared that vulnerable populations "are at higher risk for more serious illness, complications and death" (Canadian Nursing Association (CNA), 2022). Florczak (2020) defines being vulnerable as being in a state "of susceptibility to harm, powerlessness and marginality of both physical and social systems" (Adger 2006, p. 268 as cited in Florczak, 2020). The aim of nursing advocacy is to find ways to overcome vulnerability in order to cope or to better develop forms of resilience. Resilience means an ability to absorb some negative event, to be able to adapt to such an event from which one can recover (Webber-Ritchey et al., 2020). Thus, the advocacy of nurses and other healthcare professionals aims to develop "effective and equitable mitigation strategies" and to assist healthcare systems and policies to be "better prepared for future pandemics" (Lemkow–Tovías et al., 2022, pp. 1–2).

I turn again to Butler's work to critique this form of advocacy and nurses' definition or determination of what vulnerable groups are. Based on what I have discussed so far, when we ask if we should preserve the life of a certain group it presumes biopolitical considerations because it asks whose lives count as worthy of preservation – whose life counts as a life. Butler (2021) asks who belongs to the group in need of protection and who belongs to the group that imagines certain lives in need of protection. This dimension is closely related to paternalism. If what I discussed, with the help of Butler, as shared vulnerability or the fact that our social relations depend on an avowed interdependency, the identification of "vulnerable groups" becomes problematic. I do not deny that the discourse around nursing advocacy for vulnerable populations has been important for an ethics of care because once a group is "recognized" as vulnerable, it can make claims for its protection – even though only in the name of life itself. As Butler points out, this claim becomes problematic when we think about to whom this claim is addressed and what group designates itself as in charge to protect the "vulnerable." Furthermore, the ones who see themselves in charge to protect the vulnerable groups are themselves divested of vulnerability through that designation.

Nurses who see themselves as answering an ethical claim to protect and preserve life are actually maintaining a social hierarchy in which, on moral grounds, "the vulnerable are distinct from the paternalistically powerful" (Butler, 2021). It would be paradoxical if a politics of vulnerability could lead to the strengthening of social hierarchies, which I argue must be dismantled.

Related also to this nursing discourse about advocacy for vulnerable populations is the earlier discussion about biolegitimacy. As we discussed elsewhere (Larocque & Foth, 2021), a nursing politics of care is morally legitimated by reference to the suffering body and "takes place at the intersection of the neoliberal political economy and regimes of care. The vulnerable subject ironically has more rights and better chances for healthcare, human rights, and housing when it is diseased than when healthy." The suffering bodies of "vulnerable populations" during COVID have become the foundation of political action, and illness turns into a political and biological condition that determines the social condition. "One could say that the biological life (life itself) becomes the foundation for social recognition" (ibid.).

Conclusion

The pandemic could have led to a radical reimagination for all inhabitants of the Earth regardless of species, race, sex, citizenship, or religion. It could have led to a reinvention of particularly the social. Humanity will never find freedom outside of society and community and never at the expense of the biosphere. If we want to survive, we must recognize that what connects all living things is a shared interdependency, and that all experience a vulnerability because of our dependence on others and on infrastructures to live. We must realize that modernity is an endless war on life. Mbembe (2020b) calls this a new period of tension and brutality, meaning that instead of trying to build a common infrastructure, the vicious partitioning of the planet is accelerating and divisions are becoming more entrenched. Nation states are fortifying their borders and trying to "immunize" themselves against outsiders. The violence against surplus populations is being intensified and it seems that the pandemic life in front of screens and in gated communities intensifies.

Instead of nurses trying to "protect" the *life itself* of populations they paternalistically define as "vulnerable," they should become part of the movements fighting against racism, the production and abandonment of surplus populations, and the increasing efforts of nation states to keep the world at a distance based on theories of immunization and contagion (Esposito, 2012, 2019, 2020). Nursing care ethics should be based on the insight that we all depend on each other, on a shared environment, and on other living things, and that this makes us all vulnerable because we all depend on infrastructures that make life possible. Such a political care ethics would put nurses at the forefront of the fight against the systematic dismantling of social and healthcare systems and the systematic destruction of the environment that we all need to being able to live – what Mbembe

(2020b) calls a universal right to breathe. Such a political care ethics would claim that all lives must be grievable lives because only a life that can be mourned when it is lost is a life that has been considered a life when it was lived.

References

Agamben, G. (1998). *Homo Sacer: Sovereign Power and Bare Life*. Stanford University Press.
Agamben, G. (2015). *Stasis. Civil War as as a Political Paradigm* (N. Heron, Trans.). Stanford University Press.
Arendt, H. (1994). *The Origins of Totalitarianism*. Harcourt Brace Jovanovich.
Bauman, Z. (2004). *Wasted Lives. Modernity and its Outcasts*. Cambridge: Polity Press.
Benjamin, W. (1965). Zur Kritik der Gewalt. In *Zur Kritik der Gewalt und andere Aufsätze. Mit einem Nachwort von Herbert Marcuse* (pp. 29–65). Suhrkamp.
Brown, W. (2003). Neo-liberalism and the End of Liberal Democracy. *Theory & Event*, 7(1), 22. https://doi.org/doi: 10.1353/tae.2003.0020
Brown, W. (2015). *Undoing the Demos. Neoliberalism's Stealth Revolution* (W. Brown & M. Feher, Eds. Vol. Zone Books Near Future). Zone Books.
Brown, W. (2019). *In the Ruins of Neoliberalism. The Rise of Antidemocratic Politics in the West*. Columbia University Press.
Butler, J. (1997). *The Psychic Life of Power. Theories in Subjection*. Stanford University Press.
Butler, J. (2005). *Giving an Account of Oneself*. Fordham University Press.
Butler, J. (2009). The Claim of Non-Violence. In J. Butler (Ed.), *Frames of War. When Is Life Grievable?* (pp. 166–184). Verso.
Butler, J. (2020a). *Judith Butler on the Violence of Neglect Amid a Health Crisis* [Interview]. The Nation. https://www.thenation.com/article/culture/judith-butler-force-of-nonviolence-interview/
Butler, J. (2020b, April 30, 2020). *Judith Butler: Mourning Is a Political Act Amid the Pandemic and Its Disparities* [Interview]. https://truthout.org/articles/judith-butler-mourning-is-a-political-...es/?eType=EmailBlastContent&eId=1f5d0cf8-61f9-41b0-a627-9e45fbeb4e2d
Butler, J. (2021). *The Force of Non-Violence*. Verso.
Canadian Nursing Association (CNA). (2022). *Policy & Advocacy - Vulnerable Populations*. CNA. Retrieved October 09 from https://www.cna-aiic.ca/en/policy-advocacy/advocacy-priorities/covid-19/clinical-considerations
Debt Collective. (2020). How Did We Get Here? Financialization From Haiti to the Household. In *Can't Pay Won't Pay* (pp. 49–71). Haymarket Books.
Esposito, R. (2012). The Dispositif of the Person. *Law, Culture and The Humanities*, 8(1), 17–30.
Esposito, R. (2019). Postdemocracy and Biopolitics. *European Journal of Social Theory*, 22(3), 317–324. https://doi.org/10.1177/1368431019850234
Esposito, R. (2020). The Biopolitics of Immunity in Time of COVID-19: An Interview with Roberto Esposito. *Antipode Online*. Retrieved June 16, 2020, from https://antipodeonline.org/2020/06/16/interview-with-roberto-esposito/?subscribe=success#518
Fassin, D. (2009). Another Politics of Life is Possible. *Theory, Culture & Society*, 26(5), 44–60. https://doi.org/10.1177/0263276409106349
Fassin, D. (2018). *La Vie. Mode d'emploi critique*. Éditions du Seuil.
Fassin, D. (2020). The Dangerous Illusion that We Are All Equal Before the Pandemic [Essay]. *NOMIS*. Retrieved October 04, 2022, from https://nomisfoundation.ch/2020/04/17/the-dangerous-illusion-that-we-are-all-equal-before-the-pandemic/
Fassin, D., & Harcourt, B. E. (Eds.). (2019). *A Time for Critique*. Columbia University Press.
Florczak, K. L. (2020). Vulnerability. *Nursing Science Quarterly*, 34(1), 12-12. https://doi.org/10.1177/0894318420965228
Foth, T. (2009). Biopolitical Spaces, Vanished Death, & the Power of Vulnerability in Nursing. *Aporia*, 1(4), 16–26.

Foth, T. (2013). Understanding 'Caring' Through Biopolitics: the case of Nurses Under the Nazi Regime. *Nursing Philosophy*, *14*(4), 284–294. http://onlinelibrary.wiley.com/store/10.1111/nup.12013/asset/nup12013.pdf?v=1&t=iew4j07b&s=01816fc982b0f749e94c8d0908f90a8d8b181d11

Foth, T., & Leibing, A. (2022). Rethinking Dementia as a Queer Way of Life and as 'crip possibility': A Critique of the Concept of Person in Person-Centredness. *Nursing Philosophy*, *23*(1), e12373. https://doi.org/https://doi.org/10.1111/nup.12373

Foth, T., O'Byrne, P., & Holmes, D. (2015). Health Prevention in the Era of Biosocieties: A Critical Analysis of the 'Seek-and-treat' Paradigm in HIV/AIDS Prevention. *Nursing Inquiry*. https://doi.org/10.1111/nin.12114

Foucault, M. (2003). *Society Must Be Defended: Lectures at the Collège de France 1975–1976*. Picador.

Haass, R. N. (2020). At War With a Virus. *Council on Foreign Relations*. Retrieved November 2, 2020, from https://www.cfr.org/article/war-virus

Hannah, M. G., Hutta, J. S., & Schemann, C. (2020). Thinking Through Covid-19 Responses with Foucault - An Initial Overview. *Antipode Online*. Retrieved December 27, 2020, from https://antipodeonline.org/2020/05/05/thinking-through-covid-19-responses-with-foucault/?subscribe=already#504

Harcourt, B. E. (2020). *Critique & Praxis*. Columbia University Press.

Hesse, B., & Thompson, D. (2022). Introduction: Antiblackness—Dispatches from Black Political Thought. *South Atlantic Quarterly*, *121*(3), 447–475. https://doi.org/10.1215/00382876-9825919

Hobbes, T. (1996). *Leviathan. Revised Students Edition*. Cambridge University Press.

Kaika, M. (2012). The Economic Crisis Seen From the Everyday. *City*, *16*(4), 422–430. https://doi.org/10.1080/13604813.2012.696943

Kaika, M. (2017). Between Compassion and Racism: How the Biopolitics of Neoliberal Welfare Turns Citizens into Affective 'Idiots'. *European Planning Studies*, *25*(8), 1275–1291. https://doi.org/10.1080/09654313.2017.1320521

Larocque, C., & Foth, T. (2021). Which Lives Are Worth Saving? Biolegitimacy and Harm Reduction during Covid-19. *Nursing inquiry*, *n/a*(n/a), e12417. https://doi.org/https://doi.org/10.1111/nin.12417

Latour, B. (2020, March 26). Is This a Dress Rehearsal? *In the Moment - Posts from the Pandemic*. https://critinq.wordpress.com/2020/03/26/is-this-a-dress-rehearsal/

Lazzarato, M. (2013). *Governing by Debt* (J. D. Jordan, Trans.; Vol. 17). Semiotext(e).

Lazzarato, M. (2015). The American University: A Moidel of the Debt Society (J. D. Jordan, Trans.). In *Governing by Debt* (pp. 61–90). Semiotext(e).

Lemkow–Tovías, G., Lemkow, L., Cash-Gibson, L., Teixidó-Compañó, E., & Benach, J. (2022). Impact of COVID-19 Inequalities on Children: An Intersectional Analysis. *Sociology of health & illness*, *n/a*(n/a). https://doi.org/https://doi.org/10.1111/1467-9566.13557

Levinas, E. (1996). Substitution. In A. T. Peperzak, S. Critchley, & R. Bernasconi (Eds.), *Emmanuel Levinas: Basic Philosophical Writings* (pp. 79–95). Indiana University Press.

Lorenzini, D. (2020, April 02). Biopolitics in the Time of Coronavirus. *In the Moment*. https://critinq.wordpress.com/2020/04/02/biopolitics-in-the-time-of-coronavirus/

Lorenzini, D. (2022). The Normativity of Biopolitics. In University of Warwick (Ed.), *Dutch-Belgian Foucault Circle*. Coventry. https://warwick.ac.uk/fac/soc/philosophy/research/biopoliticsdemocracy/texts/lorenzini01/

Mbembe, A. (2003). Necropolitics. *Public Culture*, *15*(1), 11–40.

Mbembe, A. (2016). *politiques de l'inimitié*. éditions la découverte.

Mbembe, A. (2019a). Necropolitics (S. Corcoran, Trans.). In *Necropolitics* (pp. 66–92). Duke University Press.

Mbembe, A. (2019b). *Necropolitics*. Duke University Press.

Mbembe, A. (2020a). *Brutalisme*. La Découverte.

Mbembe, A. (2020b, April 13). The Universal Right to Breathe. *In the Moment - Posts from the Pandemic*. https://critinq.wordpress.com/2020/04/13/the-universal-right-to-breathe/?blogsub=subscribed#blog_subscription-2

Murray, S. J., & Butler, J. (2007). Ethics at the Scene of Adress: A Conversation with Judith Butler. *Symposium: Review of the Canadian Journal for Continental Philosophy*, *11*(2), 415–445.

Roberts, B., & Kreeger, L. (2019). Attending to Vulnerable Populations Through Nurse Advocacy on Boards and in Public Service. *Create Nursing*, (2), 82–86. https://doi.org/10.1891/1078-4535.25.2.82

Webber-Ritchey, K. J., Simonovich, S. D., & Spurlark, R. S. (2020). COVID-19: Qualitative Research with Vulnerable Populations. *Nursing Science Quarterly*, *34*(1), 13–19. https://doi.org/10.1177/0894318420965225

15 Placebo effect and nursing

Daniele Chiffi and Mattia Andreoletti

Introduction

A young boy entered the hospital with headache, nausea and vomit following a head injury. All the pain medications, both over-the-counter and prescription ones, failed to provide any relief. Even several months after the head trauma, the boy was still complaining about the same symptoms. After an intense episode of headache, he was brought again to the ER. There, the doctor prescribed a treatment plan consisting of opioids, including morphine. However, on the second day of hospitalization, the opioids were interrupted and substituted with a saline placebo because of the potential serious adverse effects of opioids on such a young patient, but without the informed consent of the mother. The placebo was administered by two nurses, assuming that the patients' mother was aware of it, and the patients substantially improved. When the patient was discharged, the doctor revealed to the mother that he suspended the opioids and replaced it with a placebo. The mother was furious when she found out about the placebo, and she filed charges of professional misconduct against both the doctor and the nurses. While the medical professional board declined to take a disciplinary action against the doctor, the nursing professional board did against the nurses. The nursing board claimed that the nurses had broken the nursing practice act by giving a patient a placebo without first ensuring that the patient or the patient's surrogate was informed of and gave their consent (Rich 2003). On the one hand, since nurses are those who administered the treatment in practice, they should be aware of all the ethical requirements of placebo administration and check for their compliance. But, on the other hand, the mother would have probably never given their consent for the placebo exposing her son to a real risk. This case, in its simplicity, may be quite controversial and illustrates well the epistemological and ethical tangling of the use of placebos in nursing. The aim of this chapter is to try to untangle the key issues at stake.

For this purpose, epistemological and value-based analyses of the nature of nursing (Edwards 2001; Risjord 2011; Bluhm 2014; Chiffi 2021) may offer a suitable framework for understanding and assessing many aspects of clinical reasoning and practice that are almost always relegated to the medical field. As a way of example, in this chapter, we focus on the contribution that philosophy may provide to the understanding of the placebo effect in the context of nursing interventions. Placebos are indeed widely adopted in nursing practice. For instance, a systematic review (Fässler et al. 2010) has shown that most nurses (51–100%) have used placebos in their clinical practice.

As we are going to argue, the role of nurses in placebo interventions, such as pain management, is paramount as their role is fundamental in triggering the placebo effect. But a correct use of placebos requires a deep understanding of its neuropsychological

DOI: 10.4324/9781003427407-18

basis, as well as of the ethical issues at stake. Hence, in what follows, we briefly expose the recent neuroscientific and psychological findings explaining the mechanisms that regulate the placebo effect. Then, against a purely biomedical perspective on care, we highlight the role of nurses as placebo-enhancers. Finally, we briefly discuss the ethics of the use of placebos in clinical practice.

Placebo effect

Over the last decades, researchers have identified and analysed many different aspects of placebo effects with sophisticated neuroscientific and biological tools that have revealed specific biological and chemical mechanisms at the neurological and cellular levels. Nonetheless, it is largely acknowledged that many things behind the placebo effect remained to be elucidated (Chiffi & Zanotti 2017; Chiffi et al. 2021). The placebo effect is a clear example of a clinical phenomenon that is difficult to be explained just within the classical biomedical model of care, which assumes health to be a simple lack of any disease condition.[1] However, given the intricacies and complexity of the concept of placebo effect, we believe that only a broader framework that goes beyond a strictly medical perspective can contribute to explaining their main distinguished features. In this regard, neuropsychology, philosophy and nursing in particular seem to be the main constituents of such an extended framework for the placebo effect. A philosophical analysis on the placebo effect sensitive to the recent neuroscientific findings as well as to a complete healthcare setting, including nursing interventions, may help us dismantle some of the many obscurities behind such a phenomenon. More specifically, the placebo-enhancing role of the caregiver will be critically discussed.

From a neuropsychological perspective, a critical and comprehensive analysis of the placebo effect should take into account the following psychological mechanisms: (i) *Learning*, ranging from classical conditioning to social learning. This means that previous experience or knowledge about effective treatments lead to substantial placebo responses. In classical conditioning, a natural stimulus is repeatedly associated with an unconditioned stimulus, a process that can occur both consciously and unconsciously, while in social learning, the behaviour of a demonstrator, or its by-products, modifies the subsequent behaviour of an observer (Colloca & Benedetti 2009). (ii) *Expectation* (which is always conscious) is related to the beliefs and goals of an agent, and (iii) an *affect theory*, in which the key role is played by the appraisals as those cognitive evaluations of problematic situations that can integrate different kinds of information usually required for the conceptualization of personal meanings and expected values (Ashar, Chang, & Wager 2017). According to the affective view on the placebo effect, a treatment can produce placebo effect if it is administered in a warm and empathic way. This may result in a number of functions: stress reduction, anxiety reduction, social support. The role of affect emerges clearly in studies on the effects of doctor-patient communication, where there is traditionally a focus on the importance of providing empathy and communicating in a warm and friendly fashion.

From a philosophical perspective, one of the most relevant approaches to the placebo effect is the meaning model (Brody 2000). In the meaning model, the placebo effect[2] is assumed to be the reaction of the body to a signal that belongs to the environment. The environment has some "healing" properties that affect our minds and is acting through them. Therefore, the placebo effect is viewed as a meaning relation, i.e., a semiotic interaction between the mind and the body in a healing environment, which is capable of orienting a patient's construction of meanings in a positive direction. As a result, patients may change their thinking and feeling about their illness or condition. Brody has identified three main factors contributing to this change in the meaning of illness:

> [T]he placebo response is most likely to occur when the meaning of the illness experience is altered in a positive direction. A positive change in meaning occurs when one or more of 3 things happens: The patient feels listened to and receives a satisfactory, coherent explanation of his illness; the patient feels care and concern from those around him; and the patient feels an enhanced sense of mastery and control over his symptoms.
>
> (Brody 2000, p. 650)

Remarkably, all these three elements are essential aspects of nursing care. The therapeutic setting is actually a complex context, as any treatment administered routinely has at least two main components: one pharmacological, the other psychosocial. The first and foremost aspect of the psychosocial context is the patient-provider interaction. For instance, the placebo effect has been recently described as a form of interpersonal healing (Miller et al. 2009). However, most of the scientific literature has focused on the patient-doctor relationship, overlooking the role of nursing professionals, that most of the time are those who administer the treatment and interact with the patients at the time of the administration (Miller & Miller 2015).

Classically, as we have seen, contextual factors related to patient-practitioner relationship, healthcare setting and the characteristics of the treatment, patients and practitioner may interfere with treatments outcomes and placebos (Di Blasi et al. 2001). In nursing, an analogous set composed by more than 20 contextual factors that may enhance the placebo effect has been recently proposed by Palese et al. (2019). These contextual factors range from wearing a professional uniform to adopting a holistic approach, tailoring interventions to patient preferences, and values. However, we hold that not all these contextual factors may have an impact on the placebo effect *per se*. According to the most recent neurophysiological findings, placebo effects mainly depend on the behaviours embedded in clinical rituals, which, in turn, may induce different expectations, attribution of meanings of care and social learning (Benedetti 2009). Rituals serve to express symbolic meanings important to groups of people. Unlike routines, (clinical) rituals are meaningful practices that are motivated to achieve a specific goal and are executed with the active participation of a group of people. The role of rituals in nursing in order to understand the placebo effect is discussed in the next section.

Placebo and nursing

A classical definition of nursing, due to Virginia Henderson,[3] is particularly relevant in order to understand a nurse's responsibilities for the placebo effect. She pointed out that

> The unique function of the nurse is to assist the individual, sick or well, in the performance of those activities contributing to health or its recovery (or peaceful death) that he would perform unaided if he had the necessary strength, will or knowledge. And to do this in such a way as to help him gain independence as rapidly as possible.
>
> (Henderson 1966)

This definition is mainly counterfactual, in the sense that it requires the nurse to formulate a set of hypotheses in an alternative scenario in which the patient possesses all the required cognitive resources and bodily functions to perform some daily activities unaided. Indeed, according to Henderson, the main function of the nurse is to help the patient to enhance and possibly restore an optimal level of independence in performing such activities. In our view, such an optimal level can be fixed once the nurse is able to judge a patient's health potential, i.e., understanding the maximal possibility for an individual to restore independence for self-care (given the actual conditions of the patient). This may provide the ground to justify specific nursing interventions. Unlike medicine, in which the classical main purpose is associated with pathological aspects or with an alteration from a given norm, nursing has the proper role of inducing individuals to make the best in order to regulate their psycho-physical processes (Zanotti & Chiffi 2017; Chiffi 2021).

Some decades ago, Robert C. Connelly made it clear that

> as nursing expands its knowledge of the placebo effect, it can begin to educate patients to the self-care implications of this phenomenon [...] and assisting patients to maximize a positive placebo effect to strengthen self-control over the healing process is an expression of utmost respect for the unique possibilities within each person and the healing environment.
>
> (Connelly 1991, p. 337)

For this reason, the placebo effect may be a key feature in promoting health in the sphere of nursing and the information deriving from the placebo effect may be seen as lying at the very heart of nursing knowledge. Consequently, focusing on the placebo effect may be a suitable way to understand the specific nature of nursing knowledge, as this clinical phenomenon is difficult to handle properly from a strictly biomedical perspective, concentrating on the pathophysiological aspects of disease rather than on the patient's perceptions, emotions and beliefs (Pohlman et al. 2013). In light of this, it follows that proper nursing interventions, unlike medical ones, without a patient's *meaning attribution to illness and to clinical rituals* reinforced by *active participation* in healthcare are not particularly effective. This fundamental aspect of nursing is paramount for analysing the placebo effect, too. Yet, not all contextual clinical factors may be relevant for triggering the placebo effect. Focusing on clinical rituals helps us understand that not all clinical contextual factors associated with a (dummy) treatment are essential for the placebo effect. Only those that are relevant for the understanding and conceptualization of clinical rituals are involved in the placebo effect. This is coherent, as we have seen, with the meaning model and with recent neuroscientific research on the placebo effect. Prior experience of clinical rituals can lead to conditioned responses, reinforced expectations (Colloca & Benedetti 2009) and emotion regulation (Chiffi et al. 2021). Clinical rituals are not to be considered as routine actions executed by nurses lacking any empirical foundation, but as the proper way to vehiculate symbolic meanings (Philpin 2002). Rituals are considered essential components of clinical interventions representing one of the main places where art and science meet one another in nursing (Wolf 2013). For instance, Wolf pointed out that

> Nursing rituals take place in daily nursing practice. They serve many important functions, both practical and social, and distinguish the culture of nursing as some of its more private, hidden work is carried out. Nursing rituals take place in

nurse-to-patient, direct care situations and in nurse-to-nurse situations, and mark transitions into the professional nursing role. Rituals show the sacred and profane of nursing through their performance.

(Wolf 2013, p. xii)

Nurses may thus enhance the placebo effect through clinical rituals or other related factors (e.g., communication, empathy), since they are mainly responsible for the execution of such rituals, even more than medical doctors. This is so because rituals require active participation of all individuals, patients included and attribution of meaning to care. As we have seen, this is a specific and often neglected feature of nursing.

Ethical issues

Placebo interventions come unfortunately with ethical issues.[4] Deception is the most pressing one when placebos are used in a clinical setting. Usually, presenting placebos to the patients as active medications requires utilizing deception, which is widely seen as unethical and, more specifically, violates both the medical and the nursing codes of ethics. Deception indeed undermines the principle of *autonomy* that is one of the core values of contemporary medical ethics (Beauchamp & Childress 2001). Autonomy refers to the ability of patients to make their own decisions. This means that nurses must ensure that patients are informed and have access to all the information they need to make decisions about their medical care. Respect for autonomy is therefore a necessary condition to obtain a patient's informed consent, which by definition calls for accurate disclosure of all relevant information about a medical treatment before the patient decides whether or not to receive it. Deception violates patients' rights to autonomy (and informed consent).

Moreover, the use of placebo can lead to mistrust and therefore undermines the doctor/nurse-patient therapeutic relationship. It is largely acknowledged that trust and good communication are fundamental elements in any therapeutic setting, and it has been proven that they lead to better health outcomes (Chandra et al. 2018). So, if a patient finds out she has been deceived, she could lose trust in her physician. Deceiving patients is therefore not only problematic from an ethical point of view, but it could also have an impact on the clinical practice, leading to worse health outcomes. The main question here is whether placebos can be used without deceiving patients. And the answer is likely to be no. As we discussed above, the placebo effect is triggered by neurophysiological mechanisms which require the deception of the patient. Altering patient expectations also has an impact on the therapeutic benefit of "real" drugs. For instance, it has been observed that patients suffering from postoperative pain respond better to the analgesic effects of opioids medications (e.g., morphine) if they are administered open label (in full view of the subject) rather than by hidden injections (pre-programmed machine infusion) (Price et al. 2008). Hidden injections are therefore less effective and less variable compared to open injections. Likewise, the placebo effect might be either eliminated by a hidden injection or enhanced by an open injection (Amanzio et al. 2001).

One could argue that deceptive placebos are always unethical as lying to patients would infringe on autonomy and trust (see, e.g., Asai and Kadooka 2012). This claim is defended by many bioethicists and endorsed by many professional organizations, such as the American Medical Association (Annoni 2018). According to this view, placebo interventions can be administered only with patient's consent and without lying. However, this position seems to be in contrast to many cases of medical practice, in which lying to patients seems intuitively ethically justifiable. For instance, in some cases by lying, physicians might have a better chance of preserving the patients' life. The predominant view in medical ethics is that in these situations, doctors' responsibilities of *beneficence* and *non-maleficence* may legitimately take precedence over the duty of honesty. But this is also the case for placebo, as their use might in fact improve patients' health.

So, it can be argued that deceptive placebos are occasionally acceptable under certain conditions. The core of the argument is demonstrating that the clinical benefit of placebos clearly outweighs any infringement of autonomy and trust. Supporters of this thesis typically emphasize the therapeutic value of placebo in order to achieve this. In some circumstances, placebos might be very valuable from a therapeutic point of view and as such ethically legitimate. Of course, the validity of this argument depends on the scientific evidence available in support of the efficacy of placebos. The most well-known scientific evidence supporting the value of placebos comes from the pioneering meta-analysis entitled "The Powerful Placebo" (Beecher 1955). Since then, confirming evidence has grown dramatically, and nowadays there is a large consensus regarding the efficacy of placebo for treating psychological symptoms (especially pain). For non-psychological symptoms instead, the evidence is more controversial and there is little agreement in the scientific community (Foddy 2009). In those contexts where evidence of efficacy of placebos is not available, the pro-placebo argument falters.

A responsible use of placebo therefore requires a case-by-case judgement, including considerations on several factors, such as the patient's conditions and the context. So, the decision of the use of placebo cannot be left to the single medical doctor or nurse but it should be made collegially, e.g., in ethical committees or extended healthcare teams, whose members have the expertise needed to carefully weigh up ethical arguments and scientific evidence.

More recently, a few studies have shown the benefits of open-label placebo, that is a placebo administered disclosing it to the patient (Kaptchuk and Miller 2018). However, such evidence is controversial, as it is not clear whether the benefits of open-label placebos can be replicated and in which context. To fully understand the mechanisms underlying open-label placebos, more research is therefore required. So far, the issue of whether and to what extent open-label placebos can be administered to patients without creating doubt or unethically manipulating their expectations in order to increase placebo responses is still up for debate.

Conclusion

In this chapter, we have discussed the placebo effect in the context of nursing. Recent scientific findings have indicated that neurophysiological mechanisms related to the placebo effect (i.e., learning, expectations, affects) seem to be activated in the context of clinical rituals. More than medical doctors, nurses are responsible for performing such rituals, wherein patients attribute meanings and actively participate. Based on literature in healthcare and neuroscience, we have argued that nurses, through clinical rituals, trigger the placebo effect and may enhance its magnitude, inducing significant changes in the patients' well-being. Therefore, understanding the placebo effect in nursing may help nurses to evaluate the health potential of patients for self-care. For this purpose, we believe that specific scientific training on the placebo effect is required to improve the nurse-patient relationship.

In addition, we have discussed the ethical issues usually associated with the use of placebos in clinical practice. As we have seen, placebos cannot be ethically defended *a priori*, but requires case-by-case judgements. With regard to this, a good understanding of the mechanisms that regulate the placebo effect and scientific evidence proving its efficacy is necessary to make a legitimate decision. Given the complexity of combining scientific considerations with ethical analysis, such decisions should be made collectively by all the relevant healthcare professionals.

Let us finally come back to the clinical case we presented in the introduction. On the basis of what we have presented in this chapter we might draw some considerations. First, the choice of suspending opioids and administering a placebo seems to be scientifically and ethically justified. The adverse effects of opioids are well known, and as we have discussed above, the placebo effect is very powerful in pain management. Also considering the young age of the patient, in this case, the ethical principles of beneficence and non-maleficence trump over the principle of autonomy. What about the nurses? Do they bear any responsibility? On our account, as they play a key role in triggering (and enhancing) the placebo effect, they share the responsibility of the medical act. In this specific case though, even if they were aware of the lack of the informed consent of the patient (or the mother), they would have been justified in administering the placebo. Nonetheless, it is worth noting here that no one is suggesting that it is permissible to break the professional ethical codes. But if such codes categorically ban the use of placebos, they can be questioned.

Notes

1 According to a classical definition of "placebo", Adolf Grünbaum (1981) claimed that placebos are treatments whose "characteristic features" do not have therapeutic effects on the target disorder. For a very interesting amendment of Grünbaum's definition, see Howick, 2017.
2 In this model, placebo effect is renamed as "placebo response". The word "effect" echoes biomedical causality relations that need not be invoked by the word "response". Moreover, it has been suggested reframing what is usually called "placebo effect" not just as a "placebo response" but as a particular type of a "meaning response" (Moerman and Jonas, 2002; Moerman, 2002). Nonetheless, we will not use any alternative terminology to refer to the placebo effect in order to avoid confusion. For a refinement of the meaning model sensitive to recent neurophysiological research, see Chiffi et al., 2021.
3 Virginia Henderson's books have been considered as "the 20th century equivalent of those of the founder of modern nursing, Florence Nightingale" (Halloran, 1996, p. 23).
4 See, e.g., Annoni (2018) for a comprehensive review on the ethics of placebo interventions.

References

Amanzio, M., Pollo, A., Maggi, G., & Benedetti, F. (2001). Response variability to analgesics: A role for non-specific activation of endogenous opioids. *Pain*, 90(3), 205–215.

Annoni, M. (2018). The ethics of placebo effects in clinical practice and research. *International Review of Neurobiology*, 139, 463–484.

Asai, A., & Kadooka, Y. (2012). Reexamination of the ethics of placebo use in clinical practice. *Bioethics*, 27(4), 186–193.

Ashar, Y. K., Chang, L. J., & Wager, T. D. (2017). Brain mechanisms of the placebo effect: An affective appraisal account. *Annual Review of Clinical Psychology*, 13, 73–98.

Beauchamp, T. L., & Childress, J. F. (2001). Respect for autonomy. *Principles of Biomedical Ethics*, 5, 57–112

Beecher, H. K. (1955). The powerful placebo. *Journal of the American Medical Association*, 159(17), 1602–1606.

Benedetti, F. (2009). *Placebo Effects. Understanding the Mechanisms in Health and Disease*. Oxford University Press, Oxford.

Bluhm, R. L. (2014). The (dis)unity of nursing science. *Nursing Philosophy*, 15(4), 250–260.

Brody, H. (2000). The placebo response. *Journal of Family Practice*, 49(7), 649–649.

Chandra, S., Mohammadnezhad, M., & Ward, P. (2018). Trust and communication in a doctor-patient relationship: A literature review. *Journal of Healthcare Communications*, 3(3), 1–6.

Chiffi, D. (2021). *Clinical reasoning: Knowledge, Uncertainty, and Values in Health Care*. Springer, Cham.

Chiffi, D., Pietarinen, A.-V., & Grecucci, A. (2021). Meaning and affect in the placebo effect. *The Journal of Medicine and Philosophy*, 46(3), 313–329.

Chiffi, D., & Zanotti, R. (2017). Knowledge and belief in placebo effect. *The Journal of Medicine and Philosophy*, 42(1), 70–85.

Colloca, L., & Benedetti, F. (2009). Placebo analgesia induced by social observational learning. *PAIN*, 144(1–2), 28–34.

Connelly, R. J. (1991). Nursing responsibility for the placebo effect. *The Journal of Medicine and Philosophy*, 16(3), 325–341.

Di Blasi, Z., Harkness, E., Ernst, E., Georgiou, A., & Kleijnen, J. (2001). Influence of context effects on health outcomes: A systematic review. *The Lancet*, 357(9258), 757–762.

Edwards, S. D. (2001). *Philosophy of Nursing. An Introduction*. Palgrave, New York.

Fässler, M., Meissner, K., Schneider, A., & Linde, K. (2010). Frequency and circumstances of placebo use in clinical practice-a systematic review of empirical studies. *BMC Medicine*, 8(1), 1–10.

Foddy, B. (2009). A duty to deceive: Placebos in clinical practice. *The American Journal of Bioethics*, 9(12), 4–12.

Grünbaum, A. (1981). The placebo concept. *Behaviour Research and Therapy*, 19(2), 157–167.

Halloran, E. J. (1996). Virginia Henderson and her timeless writings. *Journal of Advanced Nursing*, 23(1), 17–24.

Henderson, V. (1966). *The Nature of Nursing*. The Macmillan Company, New York.

Howick, J. (2017). The relativity of 'placebos': Defending a modified version of Grünbaum's definition. *Synthese*, 194(4), 1363–1396.

Kaptchuk, T. J., & Miller, F. G. (2018). Open label placebo: Can honestly prescribed placebos evoke meaningful therapeutic benefits?. *BMJ*, 363.

Miller, F. G., Colloca, L., & Kaptchuk, T. J. (2009). The placebo effect: Illness and interpersonal healing. *Perspectives in Biology and Medicine*, 52(4), 518.

Miller, L. R., & Miller, F. G. (2015). Understanding placebo effects: Implications for nursing practice. *Nursing Outlook*, 63(5), 601–606.

Moerman, D. E. (2002). *Meaning, Medicine, and the "placebo effect"*. Cambridge University Press, Cambridge.

Moerman, D. E., & Jonas, W. B. (2002). Deconstructing the placebo effect and finding the meaning response. *Annals of Internal Medicine*, 136(6), 471–476.

Palese, A., Rossettini, G., Colloca, L., & Testa, M. (2019). The impact of contextual factors on nursing outcomes and the role of placebo/nocebo effects: A discussion paper. *Pain Reports*, 4(3), 1–9.

Philpin, S. M. (2002). Rituals and nursing: A critical commentary. *Journal of Advanced Nursing*, 38(2), 144–151.

Pohlman, S., Cibulka, N. J., Palmer, J. L., Lorenz, R. A., & SmithBattle, L. (2013). The placebo puzzle: Examining the discordant space between biomedical science and illness/healing. *Nursing Inquiry*, 20(1), 71–81.

Price, D. D., Finniss, D. G., & Benedetti, F. (2008). A comprehensive review of the placebo effect: Recent advances and current thought. *Annual Review of Psychology*, 59(1), 565–590.

Rich, B. A. (2003). A placebo for the pain: A medico-legal case analysis. *Pain Medicine*, 4(4), 366–372.

Risjord, M. (2011). *Nursing Knowledge: Science, Practice, and Philosophy*. Wiley-Blackwell, Oxford.

Wolf, Z. R. (Ed.). (2013). *Exploring Rituals in Nursing: Joining Art and Science*. Springer, New York.

Zanotti, R. & Chiffi, D. (2017). Nursing knowledge: Hints from the placebo effect. *Nursing Philosophy*, 18(3), e12140.

16 Collectivism, personhood, and the role of patient and family

Ingrid Hanssen

Nurses need cultural competence to successfully promote psychological and physiological well-being in immigrant and ethnic minority patients and bolster their feeling of security and personhood. Questions focused through discussions and clinical examples are as follows:

- Why do some immigrant and minority ethnic patients have other expectations concerning treatment and care than most majority ethnic patients?
- Why do many immigrant and minority ethnic patients' families want to stay with the patient around the clock and be involved in the patient's care?
- Why do some immigrant and minority ethnic patients tend to leave treatment decisions to family members?

Introduction

Humans have migrated all through history, but most likely never on the current scale. The United Nations (2022) estimates that there were around 281 million international migrants globally in 2020. Migration contributes to a more culturally diverse population, which makes cultural competency in healthcare, defined as "the ability of systems to provide care for patients with diverse values, beliefs, and behaviors, including tailoring delivery to meet patients' social, cultural, and linguistic needs" (Debesay, Kartzow and Fougner 2021 p. 2), more important than ever before. Cultural competence is needed if nurses are to succeed at promoting psychological and physiological well-being in immigrant and ethnic minority patients and bolster their feeling of security and personhood.

Culture, personhood, and polis

Wherever we come from, and independent of cultural background, from our very first cry to our last breath, we are part of our soma, polis, psyche, and spirit. In other words, we are a body and a self, as well as a social and spiritual being. However, how we think and act, and what expectations and needs we have, for instance, when ill and when facing death, may greatly differ and is influenced by a variety of aspects. Our upbringing, education, social background, life experiences, personality, psychological get-up, and thoughts about why and how we have become ill will be among the factors that form us as persons and as patients – as well as healthcare providers.

DOI: 10.4324/9781003427407-19

Although our cultural background tends to supply us with religious beliefs – or the lack thereof – attitudes, linguistic patterns, culinary traditions, etc., we all develop these traits in our own unique, individual way. Together, our various characteristics constitute what may be described as our personhood, a concept that Dewing (2008) describes as a human being's fundamental characteristics. Lawrence (2007) sees personhood as a human being's fundamental and social position with his or her values, intelligence, past and present. Others, like Ellis and Astell (2010), define the concept in light of interhuman collaboration and communication. Perhaps one may say that promoting patients' personhood is to help them be their own person, whatever this may mean to them.

Research shows that there is a close relationship between how one experiences and describes illness symptoms and one's understanding of illness aetiology and how one perceives one's situation. Both the healthcare provider and the patient have throughout their lives learned why one becomes ill, who one needs to turn to when ill, and what this person – whether a university-educated physician, a shaman, a priest, or a local healer – may be expected to do to treat the problem. The American professor of medical anthropology, Arthur Kleinman (1984), defines a *healthcare system* as the totality of the relationships between illness, the response to it, the individuals experiencing it, those treating it, and the social institutions relating to it. Every medical system builds on knowledge developed in the society from which it stems together with treatment methods and experts who make use of these methods. How we think about illness and behave as patients are something we learn from early childhood. Tamis-LeMonda, Way, Hughes et al. (2008) hold that "[p]arents transmit values, rules, and standards about ways of thinking and acting, and provide an interpretive lens through which children view social relationships and structures" (p. 183). This transmission of beliefs and practices is a universal parenting goal although "the content of such beliefs and practices varies widely across cultures" (ibid., p. 183). There may also be great differences between members of one and the same ethnic group regarding thoughts on illness, expectations concerning treatment and care, and how one should face death.

Thus, our thoughts about illness, treatment, and cure are heavily coloured by our polis, that is, our family, friends, colleagues, and the larger society. Depending on the medical system they relate to, patients may have a very different understanding of disease and illness aetiologies than do persons trained according to Western biomedicine.[1] This tends to be ignored by – or may even be unknown to – biomedically oriented healthcare providers, and existential personalised meanings associated with illness are generally neglected. It may cause healthcare providers to be presented with symptom descriptions which are foreign, even meaningless, to them. This may lead to serious communicative problems[2] and even erroneous diagnoses (Flores, 2005, Alpers and Hanssen, 2022). Kleinman (1984) points to the importance of objectively eliciting and evaluating patients'

> beliefs and values with respect to their illnesses and treatments and to negotiate with (or translate between) these differing perspectives in the same way an advisor gives expert advice to an advisee, who retains the right to accept, alter, or reject that advice.
>
> (p. 58)

This respect is essential to protect the patient's personhood through acting in a way that makes him or her feel accepted and in good hands.

Interrelationship between body, mind, and spirit

Although life philosophies and religions are closely related in most societies, a person's philosophy of life is not necessarily a religious one. Regardless of whether the life philosophy is based on religious beliefs or not, it holds a holistic understanding of one's existence and expresses something about the purpose of our human life in the world. As opposed to this, Western science – including biomedicine – is guided by "its commitment to a fundamental opposition between spirit and matter, mind and body, and (underlying this) real and unreal" (Scheper-Hughes and Lock, 1987, p. 8). Although this has led to the awesome efficacy of the sciences, it has also led to a materialistic understanding of man where measurable bodily phenomena are seen as truer, or more real, than more mental and spiritual ones – for example, the differentiation between physical and psychological illnesses. Patients hailing from other medical systems may not differentiate between body, mind, and spirit, and may hold a truly holistic view of their health problems, as health, polis, and cosmos are perceived as interrelated. Thus, patients may experience illness and pain as important spiritual or psychosocial aspects of their lives. As an example of this, Koffman, Morgan and Higginson (2008) found that Black Caribbeans tended to see pain as representing a trial or test of faith. "This meaning was associated with confirmation and strengthening of religious belief and loyalty to God" (p. 354).

Zukerman and Korn (2014) suggest that religious beliefs affect our world assumptions directly. Among refugees, for instance, religion tends to create a protective shield that prevents some of the negative effects of extremely negative experiences (Abraham, Lien, Hauff, et al., 2023). Faith in God may furthermore alleviate emotional stress (Tippens, 2017) and is associated with better lipid profiles, lower blood pressure, better immune function, and decreased levels of cortisol (Koenig, 2001; Seeman, Dubin and Seeman, 2003). Moreover, religiosity has been shown to moderate the relationship between self-efficacy and traumatic stress (Israel-Cohen, Kaplan, Noy et al., 2016; Abraham, Lie and Hanssen, 2018). Based on these insights, a main goal of palliative care, for instance, is to relieve suffering caused by spiritual problems (WHO, 1990).

Holloway (2006) claims that while healthcare providers are familiar with the assessment of physical, emotional, and social needs, they may be much less comfortable taking account of a patient's spirituality and religious needs, although they are increasingly required to do so. Todd and Baldwin (2006) point out that there has not been a parallel advancement in the areas of alleviation of emotional and spiritual suffering as has been made regarding physical suffering. If the spiritual factor is not acknowledged, whatever this may entail for the person encountered, this will invalidate other ways of knowing and understanding experiences of illness, death and dying, and thus, invalidate for instance the end-of-life experience of many patients. Healthcare providers therefore need to be sensitive to the beliefs of the individual and also be able to recognise the spiritual needs as expressed by persons who only have a loose affiliation to any particular faith system or who has a humanist spirituality (Holloway, 2006).

Personhood in light of individualism and collectivism

Personhood can be neither perceived as innate nor intuitively obvious as "[t]he Western idea of the 'self' as a whole and independent entity [has] developed over time, and [has been] influenced by particular philosophical, legal, and religious traditions" (encyclopedia.com, 2022). The Reformation caused changes in social and interhuman structures which promoted individual choice, personal freedom, and self-actualisation (Oyserman, Coon and Kemmelmeier, 2002). Independence and trust in oneself have developed into virtues that are so central to the Western character, and its positive aspects taken so for granted, that any other way of perceiving oneself is difficult to imagine (Spence, 1985), and through this, what personhood entails.

Hofstede (1980) differentiates between *individualism* and *collectivism* to enable research on differences between various cultures, and through this, one might add different ways of expressing one's personhood. He defines "individualism" as pertaining to societies "in which the ties between individuals are loose: everyone is expected to look after himself or herself and his or her immediate family" (1991, p. 51). In contrast, "collectivism" pertains to a world view where the group, the "we", is the core element.

The difference between individualism and collectivism influences, for instance, the perception of what it entails to be a moral person. In a "modern" and individualistic society, morality tends to be expressed through compliance to rules rather than through the quality of relationships (Johnstone, 1999). In more "traditional" or collectivistic societies, rather than observing abstract ethical principles, one tends to value friendship, family loyalty, empathy, altruism, and trust. A person must learn to fit in and find his or her role in the society to which he/she belongs, and "[a]utonomy becomes secondary, whereas relationships with others are emphasized, being ends in themselves" (Basu-Zharku, 2011, p. 2).

Whether one is brought up in the one kind of society or the other will influence a person's perception of her/himself in relationship to both family and society. It tends to influence whether a person is prepared to make his or her own choices or whether he or she is prone to leave decisions to others. Thus, there seems to be a relationship between autonomy and the concepts of collectivism and individualism (Hanssen and Tran, 2019, Tamis-LeMonda, Way, Hughes, et al., 2008; Berger, 1999; Triandis, 1995, 1994; Hofstede, 1980).

The depiction of value systems through an individualism–collectivism dichotomy is necessarily a sharp simplification that is theoretically and empirically limiting. Many societies exhibit both individualistic and collectivistic characteristics. Moreover, there is a transitional trend from collectivism to individualism in many urban areas around the world (Cao, 2009), and one may find great differences between members of one and the same cultural group (Hanssen and Tran, 2019). Hence, this dichotomous framework can never be accurate or give a full picture of any society. Even so, I find it useful as a superficial explanatory model on a macro level.

Family care or professional care?

In collectivistic societies, leaving the care of, for instance, aged dependents who need healthcare to professionals, is often perceived as elder neglect (Wallhagen and Yamamoto-Mitani, 2006; Hanssen, Mkhonto, Sengane, et al., 2021). According to, for example, many Asian traditions, children are socialised to care for ageing parents and to experience guilt and shame if they violate this principle (Schwartz, Hurley and Park, 2010; Kucukguclu, Mert and Soylemez, 2018). In 2012, China's 11th Standing Committee of the National People's Congress went so far as to assign the care of older people to the family by law (Wang, Xiao, He et al., 2014). Interviews conducted in the Balkans indicate that seeking professional care is associated with guilt and shame also in European collectivistic societies. A Balkan nurse said that it is my duty as daughter to nurse my parents.... I would probably have tried to nurse my parents as long as possible,... There have to be such institutions [for the elderly] and there is a great need for them, but I think it is right to care for the family's old [oneself].

Not being able to do so,

is very stigmatising. The attitude is that it is totally unacceptable that persons who have nurtured us and cared for us in our younger days and as adults, when the day comes that they need nurturing and nursing care, they are being stowed away. That is perceived as turning one's back on them.

(Hanssen and Tran, 2019)

Thus, to cope with the care of a family member who is ill, handicapped, or suffering from a chronic condition tends to be a question of honour and duty.

When institutionalisation is unavoidable, to be present and to take part in the patient's care is expected by the family, and for many, this is also a cultural obligation (Cioffi, 2006). To be actively participating in the patient's care is in "adherence to collectivist-type value orientations [and] have been shown to promote self-esteem and to help protect against anxiety and depression" (Schwartz, Hurley, Park, et al., 2010, p. 550). It furthermore creates a "support systems, facilitating greater allegiance to family and other social ties" (ibid). In a review study on the needs of immigrant patients' family members, Søyland (2017) found that being there for the patient and for each other "seems to be connected to safety and duty ... The family members needed to be close to the ill person both physically and psychologically" (p. 19). Numerous visitors may also be seen in light of religion as many may see it as their religious duty to visit the sick.

The intense emotional connectedness and reciprocal interdependence between patient and family – called a "symbiotic reciprocal relationship" by Nilchaikovit, Hill and Holland (1993) – is perceived as natural and necessary by members of many collectivistic communities. The patient is surrounded by and cared for by his/her family, with the duty, loyalty, and strong relationship involved in this care. Even so, van Wezel, Francke, Kayan-Acun et al. (2016) found in their Dutch study among female Turkish, Moroccan, and Surinamese Creole immigrant family caregivers that although also the younger generation sees caregiving as an obligation, there tends to be a difference in perception between younger and older family caregivers. "The older ones assume that you yourself must provide the actual care, whereas some of the younger carers indicate that they also interpret the term 'caring' as meaning 'ensuring that good care is provided'" (p. 75). This may be an indication of the gradual shift in many urban areas mentioned by Cao (above), from collectivism to a more individualistic attitude.

The traditional connectedness and loyalty may be seen as both laudable and frustrating by nurses I have interviewed. Many feel that some of these family visitors

do not respect that there in fact are others in the room who are poorly. One must show consideration. A little consideration for others. There is a lot of 'me and mine and my family'. They are tremendously good at supporting their family, but they do not notice much outside its limits.

(Hanssen, 2010, p. 97)

Kim (1994, p. 33) explains this by pointing out that the patient's and family's emphasis on duty, collective welfare, and harmony typically only applies "to the in-group and usually does not extend to out-groups". The intense involvement in the patient care that some families display may contrast strongly with individualistic oriented nurses' propensity to have a dichotomous understanding of nursing through the focus on the nurse-patient relationship. This is both supporting and being supported by the individuating effect of principled nursing ethics. When the focus is on the nurse-patient relationship, the individual patient's rights and needs strongly come to the fore. And vice versa: the fact that these rights and principles are so strongly advocated in the nurses' Code of Ethics steers nurses' focus onto the individual patient. Thus, nursing theory and principled nursing ethics mutually influence each other.

A passive patient role

When the role of one part of the equation – the family – is to be active and caring, the role of the other party – the patient – becomes a more passive one. Based on research among patients, patients' family members, and nurses in India and the United States, Bhanumathi (1983) holds that while collectivistic oriented family members are inclined to take an active part in the patient's care even when in hospital, the patients from these families tend to take a passive patient role. Bhanumathi calls collectivistic societies "passivity centred cultures", while individualistic societies she calls "activity centred cultures". She suggests that our illness behaviour is affected by whether we come from the one or the other. A rather extreme example of a patient adopting a passive patient role is a nurse's story about a young man from Sri Lanka who had "had a fairly serious knee operation". After this kind of surgery, it is crucial that the patient starts moving and using his knee as soon as possible. This patient, however, "only wanted to lie flat in his bed until he was well again. He would not eat, he would not get up, he would not do his exercises, not even do something as simple as to urinate himself. He refused to urinate, and so in the end we had to insert a [urine] catheter. He could not understand why we should nag at him and drag him up everywhere, but especially after this kind of surgery it is very important to start exercising. And then it was: 'No, I do not need that; I do not need to eat; no, I will just stay put in bed'; 'no, I do not need anything'". Then "suddenly one day", after a week or so, "everything changed, and then he was willing to do everything" (Hanssen, 2010, pp. 104–105).

Illness behaviour in any society mirrors the expected patient role. Or, as Kleinman (1984) puts it: "illness behavior includes the perception, affective responses to, congizing, and valuation of the symptoms of disease, along with their communication (verbal and non-verbal)" (p. 75). Hence, while patients with chronic illness in a self-care-oriented culture may "be given maximum encouragement and facilities to overcome their physical impairment", in a passivity-oriented culture, they "may be treated as dependents" (Bhanumathi, 1983, p. 21).

Patient autonomy

For a collectivistic oriented patient, the family's involvement is a natural part of treatment and care. The family may have as much – or more – influence on the patient's therapeutic process than the patient his-/herself, and the family's vigilance and partaking in the caregiving are understood as required to safeguard the patient's best interest and promote his or her personhood. This may be difficult for an autonomy-oriented healthcare provider to accept, as the ideal is for the patients themselves to be directly informed and make their own decisions. Within healthcare, autonomy has become such a preeminent ethical principle that the impression is that this ideal exists independent of specific beliefs and cultural values. Autonomy has become such an integral aspect of our reasoning as healthcare providers that some nurses seem to see the patients' *right* to make their own decisions regarding treatment and care as an *obligation* to do so (Hanssen, 2004, 2010). This understanding comes to a point when Chirkov (2008) holds that "[i]n order to be fully humans we need to be autonomous in our actions" (p. 249). This begs the question: Are persons who have internalised a tendency to be depending on family members' choices and decisions for them less human?

Although autonomy is an innate human ability, this ability can be facilitated or suppressed by upbringing and social expectations. This may not the least be the case regarding women's situation in paternalistic oriented families or cultures. Thus, patients' preparedness to be self-determining may be influenced both by the clinical situation/health state and by their cultural background, that is, how the persons in question perceive what it means to be autonomous. Johnstone and Kanitsaki (2009, p. 409) point out that

> ...some ethnic groups (e.g., Greek, Italian, Chinese, Ethiopian) do not regard autonomy as empowering at all but as isolating and burdensome to patients who are often too sick and too uninformed about their condition to be able to make meaningful choices.

Many nurses seem to find the family's often domineering presence as an exacerbating circumstance that makes them feel more vulnerable, which makes approaching the patient in the presence of family members difficult. The nurses' focus on the individual heightens this feeling, as they only see the patient, and not the family, as their client. Some nurses may even avoid doing things for patients with another cultural background than themselves or to leave everything to the ever-present family members (Hanssen, 2010). It is, however,

> vitally important that nurses do not stereotype people of different cultural backgrounds and assume that 'all immigrants' ipso facto practice traditional life-ways, or that 'all immigrants' ipso facto practice a family-centred (versus an individualistic) model of informed decision-making in health care contexts. Many immigrants to a host country assimilate to the mainstream culture of their new country, and have internalized very effectively the core cultural values of the (new) mainstream culture
>
> (Johnstone, 1999, p. 153)

Summary

The current scale of migration makes cultural competency in healthcare more important than ever. How we think and act, and what expectations and needs we have when ill or facing death may greatly differ and are influenced by a variety of aspects like cultural and social backgrounds, education, and life experiences. Depending on which of the world's many medical systems they relate to, patients may have a very different understanding of disease and illness aetiologies than do persons trained according to Western biomedicine. Moreover, patients hailing from other medical systems than Western biomedicine may have a truly holistic perception of body, mind, and spirit. Thus, illness and pain may be experienced as important spiritual or psychosocial aspects of their lives.

A central theme has been individualism versus collectivism and the strong emotional connectedness between collectivistic oriented patients and their family members. This may lead to many visitors and a wish to take an active part in the care of and decision-making concerning the patient's treatment. For many collectivists, to cope with the care of a family member who is ill, handicapped, or suffering from a chronic condition tends to be a question of honour and duty. Not being able to do so may lead to feelings of guilt and shame. How collectivism may influence the perception of autonomy is also pointed out.

For nurses to successfully promote psychological and physiological well-being in immigrant and ethnic minority patients and bolster their feeling of security and personhood, cultural competency is essential. If not provided with culturally appropriate care, this may cause minority patients to feel insecure or even avoid using available healthcare services.

Notes

1 Many medical systems are several thousand years older than "modern" biomedicine, i.e., Chinese medicine and Indian Ayurveda medicine. Among the multitude of illness, aetiologies found around the world are imbalance between forces or fluids in the body, punishment from God/the gods, possession by evil spirits, loss of soul.
2 Linguistic communication problems, although basic, are not discussed here.

References

Abraham R, Leonhardt M, Lien L, Hanssen I, Hauff E, and Thapa BS. The relationship between religiosity/spirituality and wellbeing among Eritrean female refugees living in Norwegian Asylum Centers. *International Journal of Social Psychiatry*, 2021; 1-10.
Abraham R, Lie L, and Hanssen I. Coping, resilience and posttraumatic growth among Eritrean female refugees living in Norwegian asylum reception centres: A qualitative study. *International Journal of Social Psychiatry* 2018; 64(4): 359–366.
Abraham R, Lien L, Hauff E, Leonhardt M, Hanssen I, and Thapa BS. Trauma exposure and religiosity among Eritrean female refugees in Norway. *EC Phsychology and Psychiatry* 2023; 40-54.
Alpers L-M and Hanssen I. Culturally and linguistically correct and congruent translations of PROMs as basis for communication in health care. *Journal of Intercultural Communication* 2022; 20: 14-21.
Basu-Zharku JO. Effects of collectivistic and individualistic cultures on imagination inflation in Eastern and Western cultures. *Inquiries* 2011; 3(2): 1–5.
Berger J. Culture and ethnicity in clinical care. *Archives of Internal Medicine* 1999; 158(19): 2085–2090.
Bhanumathi PP. Nurses' conception of 'sick role' and 'good patient' behaviour: A cross-cultural comparison. *International Nursing Review* 1983; 24(1): 20–24.
Cao J-X. The analysis of tendency of transition from collectivism to individualism in China. *Cross-cultural Communication* 2009; 5(4): 42–50.
Chirkov VI. Culture, personal autonomy and individualism: Their relationships and implications for personal growth and well-being. Papers from the International Association for Cross-Cultural Psychology Conferences *IACCP* 2008. Grand Valley State University ScholarWorks@GVSU
Cioffi J. Culturally diverse family members and their hospitalised relatives in acute care wards: A qualitative study. *Australian Journal of Advanced Nursing* 2006; 24(1): 15.

Debesay J, Kartzow AH and Fougner M. Healthcare professionals' encounter with ethnic minority patients: The critical inciden approach. *Nursing Inquiry* 2021; 29(2). Doi.10.1111/nin.12421.

Dewing J. Personhood and dementia: Revisiting Tom Kitwood's ideas. *International Journal of Older People Nursing* 2008; 3: 3–13.

Ellis M and Astell A. Communication and personhood in advanced dementia. *Healthcare Counselling & Psychotherapy Journal* 2010; 10: 32–35.

Encyclopedia.com. *Personhood*. 2022.

Flores G. The impact of medical interpreter services on the quality of health care: A systematic review. *Medical Care Research and Review* 2005; 62(3): 255–299. doi:10.1177/1077558705275416

Hanssen I. *Facing Differentness. Ethical Challenges in Intercultural Nursing.* Saarbrücken: VDM Verlag Dr. Müller Aktiengesellschaft, 2010.

Hanssen I. From human ability to ethical principle: An intercultural perspective on autonomy. *Medicine, Health Care and Philosophy* 2004; 7(3): 269–279.

Hanssen I and Tran PM. The influence of individualistic and collectivistic morality on dementia care choices. *Nursing Ethics* 2019; 26(7–8): 2046–2057.

Hanssen I, Mkhonto F, Sengane M, Sørensen AL, Tran PTM, and Øieren H. Pre-decision regret before transition of dependents with severe dementia to long-term care. *Nursing Ethics* 2022; 29(2): 344-355.

Hofstede G. *Culture's Consequences: International Differences in Work-Related Values.* Beverly Hills, CA: Sage, 1980.

Hofstede G. *Cultures and Organizations: Software of the Mind.* London: McGraw-Hill, 1991.

Holloway M. Death as the great leveller? Towards a transcultural spirituality of dying and bereavment. *Journal of Clinical Nursing* 2006; 15: 833–839.

Israel-Cohen Y, Kaplan O, Noy S and Kashy-Rosenbaum G. *Journal of Religion and Health* 2016; 55: 1160–1171.

Johnstone M-J. *Bioethics: A Nursing Perspective.* 3rd ed. Sidney, Australia: Harcourt Saunders, 1999.

Johnstone M-J and Kanitsaki O. Ethics and advance care planning in a culturally diverse society. *Journal of Transcultural Nursing* 2009; 20(4): 405–416.

Kim U. Individualism and collectivism: Conceptual clarification and elaboration In: Kim U, Triandis HC, Kâgitcibasi C, et al. (eds.) *Individualism and Collectivism. Theory, Method, and Applications.* London: Sage, 1994, pp. 19–40.

Kleinman A. *Patients and Healers in the Context of Culture.* Berkley: University of California Press, 1984.

Koenig HG. Religion, spirituality, and medicine: How are they related and what does it mean? *Mayo Clinic Proceedings* 2001; 76: 1189–1191.

Koffman J, Morgan M, and Higginson IJ. Cultural meanings of pain: A qualitative study of Black Caribbean and White British patients with advanced cancer. *Palliative Medicine* 2008; 22: 350–359.

Kucukguclu O, Mert H, and Soylemez BA. Turkish family decision making process for placing a loved on with dementia in long-term care. *International Journal of Caring Sciences* 2018; 11(31): 1722.

Lawrence RM. Dementia. A personal legacy beyond words. *Mental Health, Religion & Culture* 2007; 10: 553–562.

Nilchaikovit T, Hill JM, and Holland JC. The effects of culture on illness behavior and medical care. *General Hospital Psychiatry* 1993; 15: 41–50.

Oyserman D, Coon HM, and Kemmelmeier M. Rethinking individualism and collectivism: Evaluation of theoretical assumptions and meta-analysis. *Psychological Bulletin* 2002; 128(1): 3–72.

Scheper-Hughes N and Lock MM. The mindful body: A prolegomenon to future work in medical anthropology. *Medical Anthropology Quarterly* 1987; 1: 6–41.

Schwartz SJ, Hurley EA, Park IJK, et al. Communalism, familism, and filial piety: Are they birds of a collectivistic feather? *Cultural Diversity & Ethnic Minority* 2010; 16(4): 548–560.

Seeman TE, Dubin LF and Seeman M. Religiosity/spirituality and health. A critical review of the evidence for biological pathways. *American Psychologist* 2003; 58(1): 53–63.

Søyland K. *Kulturelle behov hos ikke-vestlige pårørende til akutt og kritisk syke – en litteraturstudie. [Cultural Needs in Non-Western Family Members of Acute and Critically IllPpatients – A Literature Study]*. Norwegian, Unpublished Master thesis. Oslo: Lovisenberg Deaconal University College, 2017.

Spence D. *Predudice, Paradox and Possibility: Nursing People from Cultures Other than One's Own*. PhD thesis, School of Health Sciences, Massey University, New Zealand, 1985.

Tamis-LeMonda CS, Way N, Hughes D, Yoshikawa H, Kalman RK and Niwa EY. Parents' goals for children: The dynamic coexistence of individualism and collectivism in cultures and individuals. *Social Development* 2008; 17(1): 183–209.

Tippens JA. Urban Congolese refugees in Kenya: The contingencies of coping and resilience in a context marked by structural vulnerability. *Qualitative Health Research* 2017; 27: 1090–1103.

Todd J and Baldwin CM. Palliative care and culture: An optimistic view. *The Journal of Multicultural Nursing & Health* 2006; 12: 2.

17 A hermeneutical agential conception of suffering

Franco A. Carnevale

Johnny's story

NB: Child's name and other details have been modified to protect confidentiality

Johnny is a ten-year-old boy who has been in a pediatric intensive care unit (PICU) for three months. He has a mitochondrial disease, diagnosed in the early years of his life, that has seriously impacted his brain and muscle function. He was first admitted to this PICU three years ago, for the treatment of difficult-to-control seizures that required mechanical ventilation and anticonvulsants. During that first admission, PICU team members noted that he had muscle weakness as well as significant alteration of mental function. Johnny was admitted to the PICU this time because of pneumonia associated with respiratory muscle weakness. Although the pneumonia has resolved with antibiotic treatment, he does not have adequate respiratory function to be weaned from mechanical ventilation. Moreover, his seizures have become difficult to control again – requiring supplemental anticonvulsant medications every few days in addition to his baseline seizure medications. The neurology consultant noted that it is difficult to determine if Johnny's condition is currently 'end-stage' and irremediable. It seems likely, however, that he will not be able to breathe independently again.

PICU team members have had discussions with Johnny's parents about his condition. They asked if life-sustaining measures should be continued or withdrawn. They explained that if mechanical ventilation would be withdrawn, Johnny would most likely die shortly thereafter. If it is decided that his life should be sustained, then it is probable that he would require mechanical ventilation for as long as he lives; that assisted ventilation at home would have to be considered if/when his current condition is stabilized.

These discussions have centered primarily on how much Johnny is suffering, how this suffering could be better comforted, and whether this suffering is so bad for him that it is no longer worthwhile to sustain his life. Whenever the level of sedation is reduced, Johnny frequently grimaces and squirms – which nurses characterize as 'inconsolable suffering'. These signs of apparent suffering tend to subside when high-dose sedation is administered, rendering him essentially unconscious. A team member asked at a case discussion meeting, 'Isn't he better off dead than living this way?'. However, views on how badly Johnny is suffering have differed significantly. Diverse views have arisen between his parents and among PICU team members – interpreting the signs exhibited by Johnny in varying ways. This has led to disagreements about how seriously he is suffering and on optimal ways to comfort him. These disagreements have become conflictual, leading to divisions regarding the goals of care for Johnny.

DOI: 10.4324/9781003427407-20

Introduction

Johnny's story brings questions to light that require urgent consideration. An important question pertains to how to discern the severity of Johnny's suffering, which is crucial toward determining how his care can be optimized.

Understanding and attending to suffering has become a major concern within all the clinical professions, including nursing, championed by contributions from palliative care (WHO, 2020). These advances have highlighted that prolonging life should not be the sole aim of clinical care, arguing that *quality* of life should be optimized while considering ways to maximize the *quantity* or longevity of life, particularly with life-limiting illnesses such as Johnny's mitochondrial disease. Indeed, with 'end-stage' or terminal illnesses where death is anticipated, optimizing quality of life is widely considered a primary goal of care.

Suffering has been related to quality of life, where the relief of suffering has become a focus of palliative care throughout the clinical professions (Anderson, 2014). Indeed, the relief of suffering has become a central criterion for justifying medical assistance in dying (MAiD) in Canada (CCA, 2018). In the face of 'intolerable suffering' that 'cannot be relieved', Canadian legislation recognizes a person's choice to have their life terminated – legally acknowledging that the relief of suffering (even through active termination of life) can supersede the prolongation of life as a goal of clinical care.

The significance of suffering within MAiD legislation is tied to the 'sufferer's' (i.e., person who is suffering) account of the (a) tolerability of the suffering and (b) acceptability of available relief measures. This privileging of the sufferer's voice aligns with a dominant view on the assessment of pain where 'Pain is what the patient says it is' (Lipscomb, 2022). This draws on an epistemological position referred to by some as *first-person authority,* where a speaker's self-attribution is considered more justified than an attribution made by someone else (Davidson, 1984). Recognition of *first-person authority* has helped redress paternalistic practices within the health professions, including nursing, where clinicians have sometimes claimed that they know best what patients are experiencing and which interventions are optimal for them. While the recognition of the epistemic authority of patients' own voices has been important, this leaves patients whose voices are more difficult to hear or understand – like Johnny – in a precarious position. *First-person authority* has to be critically examined to identify persons who may be systemically disadvantaged by this viewpoint, including those who communicate differently or have limited linguistic expressive capacities. Moreover, the 'nature' of suffering experienced by patients may be qualitatively distinctive from the understandings of 'non-sufferers' and may be difficult to convey clearly even by persons without communication differences. We should ensure that the suffering of all people is adequately understood and attended to. Although suffering is a significant focus of concern within the health professions, it remains a phenomenon that is difficult to understand and 'assess' in clinical practice, let alone determine how it can be comforted. Suffering involves existential dimensions of people's embodied experiences that cannot be fully grasped by another (Carnevale, 2009).

Given nursing's commitment to holistic conceptions of health and well-being, it is important for nursing to advance our understanding of suffering.[1] Nursing needs to know how a person's suffering can be optimally grasped or understood as well as comforted.

Within this examination of suffering, I argue that understanding a person's suffering has to be rooted within a foundational conception of human agency. I argue for a shift from an *epistemological* focus on how suffering can be 'assessed' to an *ontological* reimagining of the kind of beings that 'sufferers' are, which shapes their suffering experiences and how they can be understood and comforted.

Drawing on Charles Taylor's philosophical ideas on human agency (Taylor, 1985a), I articulate a conception of human agency for nursing which highlights that persons are self-interpreting moral agents who are continually discerning how things matter in light of the broader sociocultural contexts they navigate (Carnevale, 2021). Given the interpretive 'nature' of suffering – eluding objectification – understanding a person's suffering requires hermeneutical approaches in nursing practice and research. I provide some descriptions of how nursing can imagine suffering within a hermeneutic conception of human agency, which can illuminate ways to attend to Johnny's suffering or other sufferers whose experiences may be difficult to understand and comfort.

Current conceptions of suffering in nursing

Suffering has been a major concern within nursing and other clinical disciplines for some time. Rodgers and Cowles (1997) published a concept analysis of suffering for the period 1987–1994. They identified 56 relevant publications within the disciplines of nursing, medicine, and bioethics. As an output of their analysis, they defined suffering as 'an individualized, subjective, and complex experience that involves the assignment of an intensely negative meaning to an event or a perceived threat' (Rodgers and Cowles, 1997, p. 1048). Themes associated with these three attributes included (a) for *Individualized*: peculiar to the one suffering; unique to each individual; varies from person to person; (b) for *Subjective*: difficult to assess/measure; subjective; must be inferred; and (c) for *Complex*: multidimensional, complex; composite; involves physical, psychological, and interactional aspects; physical pain; psychological distress; loss of autonomy or control; strong religious connotations. Rodgers and Cowles highlighted that suffering involves an intensely negative meaning, associated with destruction of a person and losing one's humanity, where changing this meaning may ameliorate the suffering that is experienced.

In my own conceptual analysis of suffering (Carnevale, 2009), I argued that suffering is an emotion that cannot be evaluated objectively by another person who is not experiencing the suffering. I highlighted concerns about the validity of some decisional models for limiting life-sustaining therapies that aim to prevent suffering. I described *empathic attunement* as an approach toward optimally understanding another person's suffering.

Ferrell and Coyle (2008) further examined, 'The Nature of Suffering and the Goals of Nursing' within their book with the same title, building on Cassell's (1982) earlier work within medicine. For Cassell, suffering is 'experienced by persons, not merely by bodies, and has its source in challenges that threaten the intactness of the person as a complex social and psychologic entity' (Cassell, 1982, p. 639). Cassell argued that suffering can include pain but is not limited to it. Focusing primarily on people living with cancer, for Ferrell and Coyle (2008), suffering involves loss, an intensely personal experience, a range of intense emotions, a loss of control, recognition of one's own mortality, asking the question 'why?', separation from the world, spiritual distress, feeling voiceless and although suffering is not synonymous with pain, it is closely associated with it. Ferrell and Coyle (2008) argued that nurses respond to suffering by identifying its sources and offering presence, construing their engagement in largely existential terms.

Shifting the focus from suffering to the sufferer

The literature described above has highlighted valuable contributions toward understanding the attributes of suffering, how it can be understood, and responses that can help comfort a sufferer. I build on these *epistemological* conceptions of how we can 'know about' a person's suffering by articulating a more foundational *ontological* conception of what it is to be a suffering person or sufferer. Understanding suffering has to be rooted in a broader conception of a person's experiences to adequately grasp how suffering is meaningful for sufferers. Moreover, the literature on suffering implies qualitatively distinctive experiences when contrasted with other health-related concerns such as pain or other symptoms, commonly implying an existential orientation.

Dominant views within the health professions can implicitly perpetuate longstanding Cartesian dualisms that underlie clinical thinking along well-known fault lines (e.g., mind/body, physical/existential) (Benner, 2000). A redressing of these fragmenting dualisms requires the recognition of human experiences as embodied. Embodiment implies an irreducible understanding of human experiences as 'whole body experiences', where thinking, feeling, sentience, and actions are regarded as dimensions of integrated wholes (Benner, 2000). The literature on suffering described above has not explicitly articulated a thoroughly holistic understanding of persons and their experiences, which is necessary for adequately understanding suffering.

Drawing on the work of Patricia Benner and associates (Benner, Kyriakidis and Stannard, 2011), understanding health and illness holistically involves a hermeneutical engagement with persons within their relational context, continually examining part-whole aspects of their experiences (see also Benner in this volume). Benner's hermeneutical conception of nursing practice draws on an ontological recognition of persons – patients as well as nurses – as moral agents, building on Taylor's hermeneutical philosophy (Taylor, 1985a). As moral agents, persons are continually discerning salience – what is particularly meaningful – embedded within relational webs of shared understandings (Carnevale, 2021). According to Taylor (2016), the relational 'embedment' of agents has to be understood in light of surrounding sociocultural contexts, which he has described in terms of *horizons of significance* and *social imaginaries*.[2] These shape the moral order that orients human preferences, choices, and actions. Drawing on these contexts, agents derive morally meaningful *aspirations* for their lives as well as *concerns* when these aspirations feel thwarted (Siedlikowski et al., 2022).

Taylor has articulated how understanding human experiences requires hermeneutical inquiry (Taylor, 1985b). This involves an examination of how human expressions convey meaning – meaning that can only be understood through interpretation. Interpretation involves a 'hermeneutical circle' – within an analysis of 'part-whole' relations – attempting to understand the sense underlying the whole through a serial reading of parts (Taylor, 1985b). Hermeneutical analysis examines a person's experiences holistically in light of their sociocultural contexts, which orient how things are morally meaningful. Persons continuously discern what is at stake within their encounters, striving to clarify which actions are morally optimal.

In short, persons are embodied moral agents embedded within meaningful communities that shape what is particularly salient or significant. A person's sense of worth (and the worthiness of their life) and their agential aspirations and concerns are oriented by shared significations within their community. For example, a person living within a community where disability is regarded as a shared interest where all lives are valued – even disabled ones – may experience better inclusion and personal recognition as a human agent where physical and social barriers are readily mitigated through widely mobilized accommodations. This community embedded conception of agency highlights how human experiences are always relational or social. Social contexts can bolster or thwart human experiences. Likewise, suffering is always a social phenomenon.

Learning from the social suffering literature

Suffering within the nursing and other health disciplines literature has been construed in largely individualistic terms. Kleinman, Das, and Lock (1997) have challenged these individualistic views, through anthropological writings, to introduce the notion of *social suffering*. This literature regards suffering as a social experience, mediated by political, economic, and institutional power. For example, bureaucratic responses can amplify suffering. Policies can 'medicalize' suffering as a phenomenon that requires medical expertise to 'diagnose' and 'treat' which can lead to dehumanizing isolation within medical institutions, where the many difficult-to-communicate dimensions of the sufferer's experiences are unacknowledged, further amplifying isolation and disembedment from the person's community footing.

A promising initiative aiming to redress this problem is the emerging recognition of *compassionate communities* within public health models of palliative care (Abel, Kellehear and Karapliagou, 2018). This idea remains under-recognized within the nursing and healthcare literature. This movement acknowledges that the experiences of persons with life-limiting conditions – and all people for that matter – can be bolstered or thwarted by the degree of compassionate engagement fostered within their communities. Suffering can be comforted by the ways that sufferers and their families are accommodated and supported within their communities, which can include community mobilization within institutions like hospitals or hospices.

Reimagining suffering: optimizing our understanding of the experiences of sufferers

The literature on suffering has highlighted that suffering should be understood within the perspective of persons who are suffering, i.e., sufferers. A sufferer is a self-interpreting embodied moral agent who is embedded within a community of relationships where shared understandings shape what is meaningful within everyday life. A sufferer is a person who is experiencing a significant thwarting of their agential aspirations. This feeling involves an embodied sense of deeply disruptive discomfort – a heightened sentience of malaise. This feeling may be associated with discernable bodily disruptions, but not necessarily so. If it is, the suffering experience is broader than what may be sensed within the affected 'body parts'. Suffering may be rooted primarily in 'non-bodily' disruptions, such as a mental health problem or social isolation, but may be experienced and expressed through bodily manifestations (e.g., elevated blood pressure).

The disruption(s) involved with suffering are rooted in a person's relational web of shared understandings regarding 'the good life'. The significance attributed to features of this disruption is shaped by how things matter in that agent's lived community. These features can relate to diminished mobility, persistent sadness, hunger, imminent mortality, social isolation, persistent pain, or precarious housing, among others. Similar bodily and/or relational disruptions within different contexts may imply distinctive experiences and potential for suffering.

Understanding a person's suffering requires a hermeneutical examination of what that person is feeling, what meanings the person attributes to this feeling, and how the person's relational context affects this feeling in good and bad ways (i.e., What makes the feeling better? What makes it worse?). This hermeneutical examination involves a part-whole analysis of the person's experiences associated with their suffering, interpreted within a 'thick' analysis of the person's sociocultural context (Carnevale, 2020).

A hermeneutical analysis of suffering: a framework for practice

Drawing on the hermeneutical conception of suffering described above, which grounds suffering within an agential view of human experiences, I propose a practice framework that can help optimize how suffering can be understood and comforted (Table 17.1). This framework can be helpful for situations where a person's suffering may be especially

Table 17.1 A hermeneutical framework for understanding and comforting suffering

Ensure a continual part/whole analysis

- Shifting focus (back and forth) from 'within person' to immediate and broader social perspectives

Describe the presenting situation where a person and/or a person's advocate* report a feeling that is particularly problematic that they may refer to as suffering (also look out for unreported suffering)

- Is the feeling continuous or episodic?
- Does the feeling fluctuate in degree of malaise it is causing for the sufferer?
- Note all that is being presented or associated with the reported feeling of suffering, including
  - Verbal utterances
  - Non-verbal bodily expressions
  - Other forms of expression

Identify fluctuations in this feeling

- What contextual changes seem to affect these fluctuations?

Continually question speculations through observation and provisional interpretations

- Verify speculations with the sufferer and anyone who knows that person's experiences well
  - Clarify which
    - (a)   methods provide the clearest expressions of the person's suffering
    - (b)   strategies that may be helpful toward comforting the suffering
- Determine the signification of this suffering for this person
- Identify aspects of this experience that are especially salient
- Identify person's most meaningful aspirations and concerns and how these may be associated with their suffering
- Examine these aspirations and concerns in light of the person's sociocultural context

What is understood regarding

- Approaches to care the sufferer would prefer
- Approaches to care that would optimize the person's *best interests*? (for child/youth or adult whose preferences are unknown)
- Strategies that could help comfort this person's suffering
- Strategies that would most strongly bolster the person's aspirations and address their concerns

Discuss these options with the person and/or their advocate and agree on an optimal plan

Implement this plan and continuously assess the person's suffering and adjust the plan of care through the process described above

*Advocate refers here to an interlocutor with recognized legitimacy to speak on behalf of the sufferer.

difficult to (a) understand (e.g., young children with limited linguistic capacities, people who communicate differently, people with altered mental function) or (b) comfort.

Suffering is a social experience that should be examined hermeneutically through a continuously shifting part/whole focus (i.e., 'part' can refer to an individual person or aspects of a person, while 'wholes' can involve immediate social circles to broader community and societal spheres).

A useful starting point is the presentation of a situation where a person – and/or a person's advocate (i.e., an interlocutor with recognized legitimacy to speak on behalf of the sufferer) – reports a feeling that is particularly problematic that they may refer to as suffering.[3] This feeling may be continuous or episodic – possibly fluctuating in the degree of malaise or disruption that it involves for the sufferer.

Make note of all that is visible or is being presented or associated with the reported feeling of suffering. This can include (a) verbal utterances, (b) non-verbal bodily expressions (e.g., facial expressions/grimaces, movements/positioning of arms and legs, respiratory patterns, sweating), or (c) other forms of expression (e.g., diary, drawings).

While noting expressions potentially associated with suffering, try to identify fluctuations in this feeling and what contextual changes seem to affect these fluctuations. In essence, what is happening that seems to make the suffering better or worse? This can include a change in body position, actions of another person, or change within the physical environment (e.g., sounds, temperature, lighting), among other things.

Hermeneutical inquiry involves a continual questioning of speculations – through observation and provisional interpretations – striving to understand a phenomenon of concern with greater clarity. As a nurse notes all expressions that seem reflective of a person's suffering as well as contextual changes that seem to affect this suffering, the nurse should verify these speculations with the sufferer as well as anyone who knows that person's experiences well. Some speculations may be confirmed and some may be refuted. This will help clarify which (a) methods provide the clearest expressions of the person's suffering and (b) strategies that may be helpful toward comforting the suffering.

This analysis needs to be interpreted in terms of the signification of this suffering for this person (i.e., how does it matter?), to identify aspects of this experience that are salient and in need of timely consideration. This involves an analysis of the person's most meaningful aspirations and concerns and how these may be associated with their suffering. A 'thick' understanding of these aspirations and concerns requires an investigation of the sociocultural context that orients what is meaningful for this person (i.e., what is considered a 'good life' within this person's community?) (Carnevale, 2020). Alterations in various capabilities (e.g., eating, walking, driving) and living with various symptoms (e.g., pain, nausea, fatigue, depression) can have quite different meanings and implications for different persons at different times. This analysis can be informed by conversations with the sufferer and people who know the sufferer as well as consultations with community leaders and key documents that can shed light on how the person's sociocultural context orients their life (e.g., cultural or religious engagements, particular personal or family experiences). This inquiry will generate additional speculations on the sufferer's particularly important aspirations and concerns and how these relate to the significance of the suffering experienced by the person and types of actions that can help comfort their suffering (e.g., if the person lives within a cultural/religious tradition that holds strong convictions about the sanctity of life, then MAiD or euthanasia may be an unlikely option for comforting their suffering).

In addition to promoting an effective way to understand a person's suffering and identify comforting strategies, this hermeneutical agential view of a person's suffering also helps ensure an optimal ethical approach to care. A foundational ethical principle within bioethics is *respect for persons* (Brännmark, 2017). This principle is commonly recognized through respect for a person's autonomy and their right to free and informed consent to care. Sufferers are frequently faced with communication limitations (e.g., because of health problems that affect their communication or mental function capacities or because their suffering is difficult to convey to others) or feeling constrained in the options available to them (e.g., due to contexts with limited adaptations to accommodate their bodily alterations), where treatment decisions may feel 'unfree and uninformed'. In many instances, treatment decisions are made by surrogate decision-makers (e.g., for an adult without the mental capacity required to provide consent or a child/youth who is not legally authorized to provide consent). In these situations, decisions made by surrogate decision-makers should be made as the sufferer would have decided (for adults) or according to the person's best interests (for children/youth). The hermeneutical approach to examining a person's suffering described above can help inform and optimize a surrogate's upholding of *respect for (suffering) persons*, as this process will help surrogate decision-makers better understand (a) what care an adult sufferer would have wanted or (b) what care would optimize the best interests of a child/youth sufferer.

This hermeneutical examination of what the sufferer is feeling will help identify what makes the suffering better or worse – from the sufferer's agential perspective. A nurse can draw on this analysis to generate potential action strategies that can optimize comforting of this suffering (i.e., promoting actions that seem to comfort suffering and minimizing/preventing those that seem to aggravate suffering). The nurse should then develop a plan with the sufferer and/or their surrogate decision-maker(s) that mobilizes actions that will optimize the comforting of suffering in ways that best align with the sufferer's aspirations and concerns. This process involves a careful examination of all that is meaningful for the person who is suffering. For example, the benefits of pain relief afforded by some pharmacological treatments may be superseded by unpleasant secondary effects that can impede other agential aspirations (e.g., striving to feel consciously present in important relational experiences, which may be dampened by sedation caused by some medications).

Remembering that suffering is a social phenomenon, action plans should be mindful of the person's community context. How does the person's community environment aggravate and/or comfort their suffering? Which actions can be mobilized that could optimally comfort the person's suffering? For example, if it is found that social isolation is aggravating a person's suffering, can some community members help redress this problem (e.g., mobilizing the person's neighbors, friends within community organizations like schools for young people and 'houses of worship' or 'seniors' groups for older people)? A 'de-medicalized' view of communities would recognize that they are already inclined to mobilizing in these ways and do not require clinician involvement to promote these types of actions. Sometimes, especially with persons who may be dissociated from community ties or where the situation is unfamiliar or challenging for community members, clinicians can help activate such actions. For example, following the death of a child, some schools may not have experience with attending to grief among children and promoting comforting social spaces for bereaved siblings. Involvement of healthcare professionals with expertise in these areas can help promote a school's capacity to act as a compassionate community.

Revisiting Johnny

Drawing on the hermeneutical framework articulated above, which recognizes sufferers as human agents, I revisit Johnny, his family, and the healthcare team working with them – looking for ways to optimally understand and comfort his suffering.

Johnny is unable to speak but has expressed signs of discomfort, which are considered expressions of suffering by his parents and nurses who care for him. These signs include facial grimaces and repeated movements of his arms and legs, with altered respiratory patterns that sometimes disrupt the ventilator's functions. These signs are noted intermittently, varying in duration and frequency. They are frequently aggravated when a medical procedure is performed on Johnny, such as suctioning his airway or when he is repositioned in his bed. Prolonged or more frequent episodes of these expressions seem to be comforted by a variety of actions, such as diminished 'medical handling', caressing touches or vocal soothing (e.g., repeating reassurances or gently singing a song) by either parent, hearing his favorite recorded music, a particular position on his right side with his arms and legs supported by pillows, administration of a bolus, or increased hourly infusion rate of an analgesic/sedative medication.

In a more private conversation that a nurse had with both parents, Johnny's parents described their reflections on his previous and current suffering experiences. They disclosed that they can sense that some members of the healthcare team are questioning the merits of prolonging Johnny's life. They acknowledge that they think he is suffering a great deal during this hospitalization and has had many bouts of suffering in the past. They have observed that he is always at his worst – in terms of suffering – when he is in a medical setting – even when he is having a routine clinic visit. He grimaces and moans and appears significantly distressed in these situations. They described that when he is home, most of time he does not exhibit these signs that have been associated with suffering. In fact, he usually shows signs of comfort and pleasure such as smiling and 'ooh' sounds when hearing music or stories that he likes or eating/drinking his favorite foods with his parents or his older sister. He likes going to an adapted day program where there are many musical and pool activities. They have heard of other children with neurological problems who live at home with assisted ventilation and can attend day programs. In fact, they had been previously told that this could be a likely progression of his condition. They are asking for the PICU team to consider that his life has meaning – that his life has had and can continue to have many good moments. However, they live in a rural setting where community healthcare services are limited. They anticipate – based on responses to their inquiries – that their local community clinic and Johnny's day program will refuse to provide services for him because he will require assisted ventilation.

Considering Johnny's parents as interlocutors for eliciting and interpreting his agential expression,[4] they have illuminated a broader understanding of his suffering experiences. They have corroborated which signs are effective indicators of Johnny's suffering and have highlighted ways in which his suffering can be aggravated or comforted. The have 'translated' his expressions, so his healthcare team can better understand his agential aspirations and concerns in terms of his known likes and dislikes. They also revealed that his suffering experiences are context-dependent. Optimizing his daily life experiences will require mobilizing accommodations within his community services, so he can return home as soon as possible and return to his favorite activities. With the information that is available, the community clinic and day program systems seem to have excluded children requiring respiratory assistance from their programs. Further analysis should examine the sociocultural context underlying these policies, which seem to imply that some children – with particular forms of disability – do not warrant accommodations. What underlying views and values do these policies reveal and what actions can be taken by whom to promote a more inclusive shift in policy orientation?

Future directions

Despite the advances I have attempted to promote within this chapter, many problems persist and some new ones have been highlighted. I will conclude by outlining some of the highest priority problems that require further research.

More research is needed to examine suffering experiences empirically. A great deal of theoretically oriented literature has helped clarify how suffering can be defined or conceptualized. However, very little is known about what it is like to suffer from the sufferers' own experiences as well as what comforts and aggravates suffering. This research should draw on qualitative research methodologies that are especially effective for examining (a) lived experiences as well as (b) how social contexts affect these experiences (i.e., what makes suffering better or worse). Given the hermeneutic conceptualization of suffering proposed here, hermeneutic or interpretive phenomenology methodologies would be well-suited for this research (Benner, 1994; Montreuil and Carnevale, 2018). Participant-observation is a particularly useful method for examining these socially embedded experiences, especially for realms of these experiences that are difficult to access through interviews.

Such research should prioritize the inclusion of persons or groups whose suffering experiences have been especially under-examined. This includes children as well as persons who communicate differently or have altered mental function.

Future research should investigate how features of community contexts can aggravate or help comfort suffering. This will help inform which 'compassionate community' actions should be mobilized.

Future research should ensure that suffering is understood within the broader perspective of people's overall experiences and how these relate to their agential aspirations and concerns. The identification of ways to comfort people's suffering has to be aligned with what is particularly important or meaningful for them (e.g., deep sedation or analgesia may relieve some suffering-related symptoms but may also suppress conscious capacities to feel experiences that are important for a person). Recognition of sufferers as human agents requires the tailoring of all 'suffering comforting' actions to that person's aspirations and concerns, which can be best understood through the hermeneutical approaches described in this chapter.

Notes

1 Although this chapter is written primarily for a nursing readership, most of the ideas discussed are transferable to other professions.
2 *Horizons of significance* refers to the meaningful context within which the agent resides (Taylor, 1989). Societies elaborate meaningful orders that represent how things matter – the relative order of various 'goods'. Taylor defined *social imaginary* as 'the ways people imagine their social existence, how they fit together with others, how things go on between them and their fellows, the expectations that are normally met, and the deeper normative notions and images that underlie these expectations' (Taylor 2004, 23).

3 Nurses should also look for unreported suffering, where persons may experience suffering that they may be unable to express in ways that clinicians can readily understand.
4 For a detailed discussion of how family members can be communication interlocutors for persons who communicate differently, see Carnevale, Teachman and Bogossian (2017).

References

Abel, J., Kellehear, A., and Karapliagou, A. (2018) 'Palliative Care-The New Essentials', *Annals of Palliative Medicine*, 7(Suppl. 2), pp. S3–S14.

Anderson, R.E. (2014) *Human Suffering and Quality of Life*. Dordrecht: Springer.

Benner, P. (Ed.) (1994) *Interpretive Phenomenology: Embodiment, Caring, and Ethics in Health and Illness*. Thousand Oaks, CA: SAGE Publications.

Benner, P. (2000) 'The Roles of Embodiment, Emotion and Lifeworld for Rationality and Agency in Nursing Practice', *Nursing Philosophy*, 1, pp. 5–19.

Benner, P., Kyriakidis, P.H., and Stannard, D. (2011) *Clinical Wisdom and Interventions in Acute and Critical Care: A Thinking-in-action Approach*. 2nd edn. New York: Springer.

Brännmark, J. (2017) 'Respect for Persons in Bioethics: Towards a Human Rights-Based Account', *Human Rights Review*, 18, pp. 171–187.

Carnevale, F.A. (2009) 'A Conceptual and Moral Analysis of Suffering', *Nursing Ethics*, 16(2), pp. 173–183.

Carnevale, F.A. (2020) 'A "Thick" Conception of Children's Voices: A Hermeneutical Framework for Childhood Research', *International Journal of Qualitative Methods*, January 2020, 19. DOI: 10.1177/1609406920933767.

Carnevale, F.A. (2021) 'Recognizing Children as Agents: Taylor's Hermeneutical Ontology and the Philosophy of Childhood', *International Journal of Philosophical Studies*, 29(5), pp. 791–808.

Carnevale, F.A., Teachman, G., and Bogossian, A. (2017) 'A Relational Ethics Framework for Advancing Practice with Children with Complex Health Care Needs and Their Parents', *Comprehensive Child and Adolescent Nursing*, 40(4), pp. 268–284.

Cassell, E.J. (1982) 'The Nature of Suffering and the Goals of Medicine', *The New England Journal of Medicine*, 8;306(11), pp. 639–645.

CCA: Council of Canadian Academies. (2018) *State of Knowledge on Medical Assistance in Dying for Mature Minors, Advance Requests, and Where a Mental Disorder Is the Sole Underlying Medical Condition* (Final Reports). Ottawa: Council of Canadian Academies. https://cca-reports.ca/reports/medical-assistance-in-dying/

Davidson, D. (1984) 'First Person Authority', *Dialectica*, 38(2–3), pp. 101–111.

Ferrell, B.R. and Coyle, N. (2008) *The Nature of Suffering and the Goals of Nursing*. New York: Oxford University Press.

Kleinman, A., Das, V., and Lock, M.M. (Eds.) (1997) *Social Suffering*. Berkeley: University of California Press.

Lipscomb, M. (2022) 'Pain Is (*or May Not Be*) What the Patient Says It Is – Professional Commitments: Objects of Study or Sacrosanct Givens?' in Lipscomb, M. (ed.) *Complexity and Values in Nurse Education: Dialogues on Professional Education*. Abingdon: Routledge.

Montreuil, M. and Carnevale, F.A. (2018) 'Participatory Hermeneutic Ethnography: A Methodological Framework for Health Ethics Research with Children', *Qualitative Health Research*, 28(7), pp. 1135–1144.

Rodgers, B.L. and Cowles, K.V. (1997) 'A Conceptual Foundation for Human Suffering in Nursing Care and Research', *Journal of Advanced Nursing*, 25(5), pp. 1048–1053.

Siedlikowski, S., Van Praagh, S., Shevell, M., and Carnevale, F.A. (2022) 'Agency in Everyday Life: An Ethnography of the Moral Experiences of Children and Youth', *Children & Society*, 36, pp. 661–676.

Taylor, C. (1985a) "What Is Human Agency?" in Taylor, C. *Philosophy and the Human Sciences: Philosophical Papers 1*. Cambridge: Cambridge University Press, pp. 15–44.

Taylor, C. (1985b) "Interpretation and the Sciences of Man", in Taylor, C. *Philosophy and the Human Sciences: Philosophical Papers 2*. Cambridge: Cambridge University Press, pp. 15–57.

Taylor, C. (1989) *Sources of the Self: The Making of the Modern Identity*. Cambridge, MA: Harvard University Press.

Taylor, C. (2004) *Modern Social Imaginaries*. Durham, NC: Duke University Press.

Taylor, C. (2016) *The Language Animal: The Full Shape of the Human Linguistic Capacity*. Cambridge, MA: Harvard University Press.

WHO: World Health Organization. (2020) *Palliative Care (WHO Fact Sheet)*. World Health Organization (5 August 2020). https://www.who.int/news-room/fact-sheets/detail/palliative-care.

18 Hermeneutic phenomenology, person-centred care, and loneliness

Ken Hok Man Ho and Vico Chung Lim Chiang

Introduction

In '*Being and Time*', Martin Heidegger's conception of 'being-in-the-world' lays a foundation for hermeneutic phenomenology that preserves the ontological possibilities of what it is to be human (Heidegger, 1927/2008). To preserve ontological possibilities is to preserve the multiplicity of being. Simply speaking, this multiplicity of being refers to the multiple interpretations of one's own realities. To preserve ontological possibilities, humans have to delve deeply into their own lived experience, going beyond the dominance of everydayness to bring forth their authentic beings (Heidegger, 1927/2008). These authentic beings are alternative interpretations of reality which are not governed by the dominant logic of the modern technological world. As such, hermeneutic phenomenology provides the philosophical path for professionals to develop thoughtfulness and tact in their professional practice through the development of authentic understanding of the experience of clients, as well as of their own selves (van Manen, 2014). In this book, nursing is considered. Person-centred care has been central to nursing practice and nursing knowledge, and the nursing profession traditionally positions patient's views and experiences as fundamental to nursing care. This approach of care builds around the needs of clients and is dependent on knowing our clients through interacting with them (Fazio, Pace, Flinner, & Kallmyer, 2018). As such, holistically understanding the experience of persons being cared for and their loved ones is significant in person-centred care, which is a way of being in nursing. Nursing practice nowadays is highly directed by the techno-driven health care system and its well-defined biomedical framework of diseases. Yet, this framework may not always relate to the needs of persons when or if the biomedical framework, which is highly disease-focused, dehumanises persons. To this end, we argue that the philosophical notion of being-in-the-world, of hermeneutic phenomenology, is a way for nurses to holistically understand the needs of persons under their care. This perspective recognises the various 'beings' that go beyond the taken-for-granted medical and sociological definitions of disease and illness.

In this chapter, we use the terms person and human interchangeably because Heidegger employed human in his writings. Heidegger did not refer to humans as only having physical and psychological attributes, and this corresponds with the stance of leading scholars in person-centred care (McCormack & McCance, 2017b). Moreover, we will consider loneliness, as a universal human experience and a public health threat. Specifically, we employ Heideggerian hermeneutic phenomenology to explore the loneliness of older persons in residential care homes during the COVID-19 pandemic. This example will illustrate the importance of hermeneutic phenomenology in person-centred

DOI: 10.4324/9781003427407-21

care. First, we briefly describe the philosophical tenets of hermeneutic phenomenology in preserving the ontological possibilities of what it is to be human. Personhood is then considered from the perspective of McCormack and McCance (2017a) and Heidegger (1927/2008) in order to delineate the philosophical importance of hermeneutic phenomenology in person-centredness. Finally, we illustrate how the phenomenological findings of loneliness of older adults in residential care homes uncover the core values of personhood in person-centred care.

Hermeneutic phenomenology: truth as the clearing of Being

In 2017, Ho and colleagues provided a reflection on Heidegger's philosophy in conducting a thematic analysis. Their reflections on Heidegger's approach to truth are insightful. For Heidegger, clearing the Being of beings is the utmost task for hermeneutic phenomenology. Heidegger does not refer to being only as an 'object'. Rather, being carries a broader sense of the interpretation of the structure of reality (Ratcliffe, 2002). Human questions about 'who', 'what', 'where', 'when', and 'how' to interpret a reality. However, Heidegger does not agree that merely providing answers to the structure of reality would allow human to approach the truth. For Heidegger, in order to be able to interpret something as real, as a reality, human has to bear a prior understanding of this realness in order to render sense to 'who', 'what', 'where', 'when', and 'how'. However, humans forget the most important question: what must already be the case for the contexture of beings to be intelligible. This important philosophical question points to the quest of the clearing of Being, the answer to which stands prior to the intelligibility of beings.

In order to answer the question about the contexture of beings, we have to first discuss the way of approaching the clearing of Being. 'Alētheia' (the Greek word for truth) understands truth as unconcealment. This unconcealment is a matter of thought that one's own interpretation of the world is released from everyday taken-for-granted metaphysical representation of 'truth'. This metaphysical representation is the reduction of multiple possible beings into only one dominant being (i.e. the inauthentic being (Heidegger, 1929/2008)). For Heidegger, releasing oneself from inauthentic being develops awareness of everyday taken-for-grantedness, thereby allowing those authentic beings veiled behind to be brought-forth (Heidegger, 1946/2008). However, human tends to go astray in the taken-for-grantedness, losing insight into the other possible beings (Heidegger, 1927/2008). As such, the way to approach the clearing of Being is to uncover the presence of what is already present in unconcealment. It is to make known the not-yet-shown beings out of the dominant being. This is a way to preserve the ontological possibilities of human.

In approaching the clearing of Being, there are two modes of knowing under alētheia, namely 'episteme' and 'techne'. For 'episteme', knowledge is determined by the objects themselves and is unchangeable and permanent. The knowing disclosed within the realm of 'episteme' is propositional truth, in which actuality is a dominant logic to justify what is correct and what is wrong. Actuality views actions as a cause to effect (Heidegger, 1946/2008). The dominance of actuality in modern technological world allures the human to disclose truth as unchangeable and permanent by taking a cause-and-effect relationship as the dominant form of being. As a result, the human clings to taking 'correct' actions to exert desirable effects on things in accord with actuality. For example, during the COVID-19 pandemic, in order to contain the virus and to save life, 'correct' actions include social restrictions. For 'techne', beings are changeable and temporal (Rojcewicz, 2006). The essence envisioned under 'techne' is about the Being veiled behind changing beings. As such, actuality is only one of the many possible beings to be uncovered in the realm of 'techne'. 'Techne' is a mode of knowing for preserving ontological possibilities for what is human. While Being is prior to the intelligibility of beings, Being implies that human must bear a primitive understanding of the world veiled behind the changing interpretations of realities, as beings. Therefore, a way to approach the clearing of Being is to uncover various beings, instead of a singular view, in order to show the presence of what is already present among changing beings. This will lead us back to the primitive understanding of the intelligibility of beings. As such, what is human will be aware that every understanding of beings has a prior structure and understanding of the world, *per se*, it is inevitably hermeneutic. Hermeneutics refers to the process by which 'human interprets and makes sense of experiences … according to his/her per-existing values and ways of seeing the world' (Heidegger, 1927/2008). For Heidegger (1954/2008), hermeneutic phenomenology discloses knowledge in accord with 'techne'. The openness to the Being, the primitive understanding, requires human to reflect on the dominance of actuality for preserving the ontological possibilities of human.

After grasping the way to approach the clearing of Being, the final question will be what Being, as primitive understanding, refers to. Heidegger did not provide a concrete answer to this question, or he was reluctant to do so, leaving it open to readers. This openness is, indeed, necessary because Being is not an objective entity that has a structure to be determined. Being bears presupposed conditions for the intelligibility of beings. According to Ratcliffe (2002), Being can be understood as constitutive teleology. Constitutive teleology presupposes conditions that account for our purposive commitments to interpret, experience, and give meaning to the world and to ourselves with a future directionality 'to be able'. These presupposed conditions are the shared intelligible background of meanings (as primitive understanding), as a familiar world, on the basis of which humans understand who they are and who they are going to be (Ho et al., 2022). As such, humans are being-in-the-world. The ultimate goal of hermeneutic phenomenology is to uncover the constitutive teleology (as Being) through interrogating lived experiences. In the next section, we further delineate the significance of hermeneutic phenomenology in person-centred care through discussing the importance of beings in personhood.

Person-centred care and hermeneutic phenomenology: the importance of Beings

Person-centred care has long been central to nursing practice. It focuses on treating people as individuals, respecting their rights as a person, building mutual trust and understanding, and developing therapeutic relationships (McCormack & McCance, 2017a). This approach to care requires nurses and health care professionals to consider the person first, and then the disease. As such, person-centred care is a global movement for humanising health care systems. It involves endorsing people at the centre of care systems more than categorising people and their health care needs according to the dominant biomedical frame of reference. According to the World Health Organization (2015, p. 5), people-centred care is

> an approach to care that consciously adopts individuals', carers', families' and communities' perspectives as participants in, and beneficiaries of, trusted health systems that respond to their needs and preferences in humane and holistic ways. People-centred care also requires that people have the education and support they need to make decisions and participate in their own care. It is organized around the health needs and expectations of people rather than diseases.

Over the last 30 years, frameworks have been developed to guide the development and implementation of person-centred care. Among these frameworks, the person-centred nursing framework (McCormack & McCance, 2006) and the conceptual framework for integrated people-centred health services (World Health Organization, 2015) have proved relatively popular worldwide. Yet, for McCormack and McCance (2017b), prior to any frameworks, the fundamental philosophical question of what personhood is has still to be solved. This question bears both a philosophical importance and a practical importance for nursing, and hermeneutic phenomenology provides a solid philosophical foundation that sheds light on the core values of personhood.

Personhood is an extremely complex idea. We are not going to explore the concept in-depth. Instead, the following discussion seeks to delineate the relationship between person-centred care and hermeneutic phenomenology, grounded in the question of beings. McCormack and McCance (2017b) advocated that it is inadequate to differentiate a person and an animal merely on the basis of physical and psychological attributes. For example, both persons and animals share the same physical attributes of sexuality and reproduction, sight, hearing, smell, and so on. To the same extent, both persons and animals have various degrees of thought, thinking, and emotions. It is inadequate to differentiate persons and animals based on physical and psychological attributes. More importantly, if we regard persons simply as physical or psychological attributes, patients with particular diseases (e.g., dementia, stroke, and so on) or conditions (e.g., intellectual disability, coma) may not be regarded as a person because they have lost physical or psychological attributes. As such, attributing personhood with mere physical or psychological attributes leads the way to dehumanisation in nursing and health care.

Someone may argue that persons have language, while animals do not. This is controversial because animals do have their own language for communication (e.g., whales). Yet, the nature of language does serve as a starting point to shed light on the difference between a person and an animal. In his *Letter on Humanism*, Heidegger (1946/2008) contrasted humans and animals in relation to language. Heidegger (1946/2008) argued that only man has language as their world, and this world carries ontological possibilities. Animals do not have language as their world. Thus, animals are lodged only in their environment. This environment does not carry possibilities. In fact, human language is not only an instrument for communication. Heidegger (1946/2008) suggested that human languages are embedded in intrinsic webs of meanings (i.e. various beings) and are the house of Being (i.e. constitutive teleology). In other words, when a person speaks or writes, he/she already bears prior understanding of what to be expressed. Through text and speech, expressions carry implicit embedded meanings which show how manifold beings depend upon the cultures and contexts of the message senders and the message receivers. As such, culture, context, and the person form a constitutive teleology that relate the self to the world. How oneself relates him/herself to the world is shown through various interpretations of realities (i.e. beings). These are the possibilities born in human language, and thus language goes beyond a mere instrument of communication in our technological world. However, for animals, language does not bear the possibilities of beings. Animals are stuck in a static environment, and they lack possibilities of being (Heidegger, 1946/2008). For Heidegger (1946/2008), the different natures of human and animal language are a crucial consideration that differentiates, for us, what it means to be a person.

However, if a person does not speak or write, is he/she still a person? While Heidegger (1946/2008) suggested that language is the house of Being, it does not follow that for humans, Being is absent if we do not have language. As our beings are expressed through language, language is a medium for researchers, nurses, and health care professionals to access the beings of our clients. McCormack and McCance (2017b) highlight that the core value of personhood is the recognition of 'being'. It is how the self relates to the world that nurtures the possibilities of beings. As such, even though a person with advanced dementia or someone in a coma is unable to communicate, they still relate in or through their self to the world – that is, in their own thinking, and this nurtures the possibility of being. From the vantage point of being, we link up person-centred care with hermeneutic phenomenology philosophically. This approach highlights possibilities of being that render nurses and health care professionals positive ways of interacting with patients as persons, as humans, even when those patients have suffered the loss of physical and psychological attributes.

McCormack and McCance (2017b) demonstrate the possibilities of being in personhood through describing four core 'modes of being' at the heart of person-centredness: (i) being in relation, (ii) being in a social world, (iii) being in place, and (iv) being with self. We will discuss how hermeneutic phenomenology demonstrates its applicability to person-centred care through the four core modes of beings.

Being in relation

Being in relation is an important attribute in personhood. It describes how oneself is related to others, thereby enabling the development of relationships that have therapeutic benefit. It is important to note that when caring for patients in a person-centred way, nurse-patient relations are only one of the many relationships that need to be considered when considering personhood. Other relationships, such as those between the patient and significant others, also require attention. Grounded in hermeneutic phenomenology, it is more important for nurses and health care professionals to develop awareness about the various possibilities of how oneself relates to others. For example, nurses might ask, how are persons being cared for in relation to significant others and ourselves? However, how do we, as nurses, relate ourselves to the persons being cared by us? On top of functional purposes (e.g., symptoms control or life-saving), how shall we relate our identity, as nurses, to the person being cared for in order to nurture and sustain a therapeutic relationship? This therapeutic relationship requires reflective ability, and this involves knowing selves and others, flexibility, and authenticity derived from reflection on values and the places of the person in the relationship (McCormack & McCance, 2017b). In employing hermeneutic phenomenology in care, Ho et al. (2018) investigated the possibilities of being when migrant domestic workers (MDWs) provided home care to older adults. Their findings showed that MDWs relate their self to older adults as maids or companions. More importantly, there is an understanding that the being of the maid or companion is not static. Instead, it depends on the context of home care, the culture of MDWs, and the history of MDWs business. This shows the importance of developing insight into constitutive teleology amidst the changing beings of maid and companion.

Being in a social context

Persons are beings connected in a social world, and interactions between selves and the social world create and re-create meanings (McCormack & McCance, 2017b). This creating and re-creating of meanings manifest the hermeneutic nature of interpretation because every re-creation of meanings is inevitably influenced by prior understandings towards the social world. McCormack and McCance (2017b) highlight the importance of using narrative approaches to uncover the beings of persons shown by the self in narratives. According to McCormack and McCance (2017b, p. 19), 'narratives are holistic and provide a picture of the person's being in the world and their subjective interpretation of that being'. This stance accords with Heidegger who stated that 'language is the house of being' (Heidegger, 1946/2008). Through narratives, nurses are able to understand how the self of the person being cared for relates to the social context of care. In the example of Ho et al. (2017), through reflecting on the narratives with a social context of global care chain, they successfully uncovered a being of MDWs as commodities.

Being in place

For phenomenology, place has a deep connection with the self. More precisely, it is not that physical place offers phenomenological significance. It is rather the spatial nature of place that offers meanings to persons. In another words, it is about how the self relates to the space offered by a physical place. This is highly important for person-centred care. For example, for the purpose of reminiscence, residential care homes decorate their environment according to the shared memory of older adults. In the PhD dissertation of Ho (2017), he demonstrated how MDWs render different meanings to the home of older adults, either as a place of emotional struggles or as a place of peace of mind.

Being with self

Heidegger's notion of authentic being and inauthentic being allows us to understand how we relate to the self. For Heidegger, humans cling to inauthentic being when they evidence a tendency to create meanings about selves according to everyday taken-for-grantedness. Heidegger emphasised the importance of searching for authenticity. That is, seeking an alternative meaning for the self that does not rely on the standards of contemporary society. This understanding is important for person-centred care because it implies that there is room for nurses to assist persons being cared for to re-create meanings in their life. Meanwhile, nurses can also develop empathy towards persons being cared for by understanding their lost beings in accord with the standards of society. A phenomenological study on the loneliness of older adults in residential care homes during the COVID-19 pandemic showed how older adults lost their continuity of self-identity. This self-identity was grounded in how they functioned in contemporary society, and once lost, this contributed to their emotional suffering (Ho et al., 2022). We will take this study as an example in the next section to illustrate how hermeneutic phenomenology nurtured an authentic understanding of the needs of older adults in residential care homes.

Person-centred care and hermeneutic phenomenology: loneliness during the COVID-19 pandemic

A study 'Implications of COVID-19 on the loneliness of older adults in residential care homes' (Ho et al., 2022) demonstrates how hermeneutic phenomenology allows us, as nurses, to holistically understand the needs of older adults in residential care homes during the COVID-19 pandemic.

Social restrictions were identified as an effective measure to prevent the spread of COVID-19, and these were particularly important when vaccines were unavailable. Social restrictions were applied to many settings, including residential care homes. Although person-centred care has been widely adopted by residential care homes internationally, we did not know how social restrictions influenced the well-being of older adult in residential care homes. Older adults living in residential care homes are generally at risk of loneliness as their social networks shrink, and it was suggested that the lockdown of residential care homes placed older adults at risk of experiencing extreme loneliness. We therefore conducted a hermeneutic phenomenological study to explore the lived experience of loneliness of older adults in residential care homes during the COVID-19 period.

We approached ten residential care homes through the research team's network and seven of them agreed to participate in the study. All seven residential care homes were financially subsidised by the Government of Hong Kong Special Administrative Region, China. Each of the seven residential care homes had around 50–70 residents, and each room was shared by between three to six residents. We recruited people aged 60 and above, who were residents of residential care homes during the COVID-19 outbreak in Hong Kong; and scored 6 or more in the Abbreviated Mental Test (AMT). Staff referred older adults to the research team for eligibility screening.

We performed face-to-face interviews with a total of 15 participants in meeting rooms at the seven residential care homes, without accompaniment by family members or staff of these homes. Each interview lasted between 30 and 60 minutes. Participants were asked to share their significant experiences of loneliness during the COVID-19 period. Follow-up interviews were performed. Data analysis was conducted according to the approach of Max van Manen (2014). Since our focus in the following content is to illustrate how the phenomenological findings of loneliness reveal its significance to person-centred care, readers may refer to the cited paper for details of data collection and data analysis.

Findings include an over-arching theme labelled 'a deprived sense of self-significance in a familiar world contributes to older adult's disconnection with prior commitments', and two other themes: 'from collapse to dissolution of self-understanding' and 'restoring meanings by establishing connections with entities'. Instead of showing how phenomenological analysis reaches these themes, we make use of the thematic findings to illustrate how phenomenological findings enable us to identify the four core beings (McCormack and McCance, 2017b) in personhood. This will assist readers to understand the relationship between hermeneutic phenomenology and person-centred care through the example of loneliness.

A deprived sense of self-significance in a familiar world contributes to older adult's
disconnection with prior commitments

> My daughter care about me. During the lockdown, she phones me everyday. However, I am still lonely. My daughter and I are in two parallel worlds. I smuggled from Mainland China to Hong Kong when I was very young. I built my family on my own and I raised my daughters with my own labour...... The point is that I am the only one to face my Parkinson's [disease]. They cannot solve my problem. I have five roommates here and I am the only one who can still walk and eat. However, I am also the only one who will witness myself becoming one of them.... I hope I will get the coronavirus. I am valueless to society and a burden to my daughters.
>
> (Ho et al., 2022, p. 284)

The above narrative showed the importance of 'being with self' in person-centredness. Yet, it requires readers to delve deeply into the constitutive teleology of the older adult. 'To be functional' was identified as the constitutive teleology, a familiar world, that enabled older adults to make sense of and for themselves. The constitutive teleology of 'to be functional' helped the older adult interpret themselves according to the logic of actuality, implying that they regard themselves as a mean to an end. As such, a functional self is a dominant being in self-interpretation. So what was his (the participant's) function? The answer was that he had a function for his daughters and for his society. However, it was this functional self that had created the issues of loneliness as manifested by 'my daughters and I are in two parallel worlds', and 'I am valueless to society and a burden to my daughters'. These show the older adult unable to connect with his functional self in a way that could sustain self-identity. Breakdown in the continuity of the functional self was discovered, 'I have five roommates here and I am the only one who can still walk and eat. However, I am also the only one who will witness myself becoming one of them'. While the functional self is an inauthentic being as it is in accord with actuality, we also see that the older adult was unable to develop alternative self-interpretation on himself. As such, the older adult experienced a difficulty to be being with self. Once a nurse can develop insight on the disconnection with the self, he/she will authentically understand the rationale for assisting older adults to develop alternative self-interpretations, which is the older adult's real need.

Another participant's narrative from the same theme serves as an exemplar to illustrate 'being in a social context'.

> I expect nothing after the pandemic. I am just seeing the doctor again and again. There will not be any differences. I am not a significant one for others. I am not afraid of getting the disease [COVID-19]. I hope I get it, then everything is ended.
>
> (Ho et al., 2022, p. 284)

The COVID-19 pandemic provided a social context to exacerbate older adult's disconnection with the functional self. More importantly, when the self of the older adult is related to the social context of COVID-19, it continuously re-creates a disconnection with the functional self, reinforcing a pessimistic view of the future of the older adult.

From collapse to dissolution of self-understanding

The following two excerpts illustrated how the loss of meaningful relationships contributes to the dissolution of the self of older adults. These two excerpts show the 'being in relation':

> Group activities are cancelled and my family cannot visit me. The free time is really disturbing. I have nothing to do every day, but my mind is not peaceful. Every piece of information about COVID-19 makes me anxious. Without family and group activities, I keep the anxiety within me. I keep silent and bear it. My impression during the past few months is of loneliness.
>
> (Ho et al., 2022, p. 284)

I have several children but end up to live alone in RCH. This disease [implying COVID-19] further keeps me alone. I don't know what I am for ....

(Ho et al., 2022, p. 285)

During the COVID-19 pandemic, a loss of meaningful interpersonal relationships imposed difficulties for older adults when they could no longer interpret themselves according to long-established patterns of interpersonal relationships. During this time, older adults experienced limited freedom to choose how they should make sense of their identities, and they found themselves unwillingly guided by an unfamiliar world (a world no longer full of meaningful interpersonal relationships). This example highlights the importance of being in relation in person-centredness. Through being in relations, either 'good' or 'bad', the self is revealed.

Restoring meanings by establishing connections with entities

The following excerpt about feeling at home further illustrates 'being in relation' and 'being in place':

My home is here [*the residential care home*]. The nurses are very good. They are concerned about my feeling of being trapped every day. They hug me. They talk with me. They encouraged me to reach out within this home, of course, wearing a mask (laughed). I don't feel anxious here. I feel loved.

(Ho et al., 2022, p.285)

From the above excerpt, we feel the nurturing relationship between nurses and older adult. Nurturing relationships are not based on functionality. Nurses care about older adults. In contrast to the disconnection with meaningful relationships as described above, the residential care home became a home for the older adults. As stated, it is not the physical characteristics of a place that matter. What is significant is the spatial nature of the environment. The above excerpts show that within the space, older adults were enabled to develop alternative self-interpretations because of the nurturing interpersonal relationships facilitated by nurses. As such, within the RCH, older adults feel loved.

Conclusions

In the past few years, the presence of COVID-19 has exaggerated isolation and loneliness in society, and this has been particularly felt by older people who need personal care. The challenges for person-centred care for older people have never been so intense, and it is therefore vital that nurses reflect on and gain more experiences of and insight into the delivery of better aged care. Hermeneutic phenomenology provides a very useful theoretical foundation and practical perspective for nurses to re-consider the needs and beings of their clients. The foundation and perspective of hermeneutic phenomenology can inform and improve the practice of person-centred care, for example when dealing with loneliness. In conclusion, it is the possibilities of beings that render nurses and health care professionals to regard a patient as a person, a human, for caring, even though the loss of physical and psychological attributes of the person.

References

Fazio, S., Pace, D., Flinner, J., & Kallmyer, B. (2018). The fundamentals of person-centered care for individuals with dementia. *Gerontologist, 58*(S1), S10–S19. Retrieved from https://doi.org/10.1093/geront/gnx122

Heidegger, M. (1927/2008). Being and time. In D. F. Krell, & D. F. Krell (Ed.), *Martin Heidegger, Basic Writinigs* (D. F. Krell, Trans., rev ed., pp. 37–88). New York: Harper Perennial Modern Classics.

Heidegger, M. (1929/2008). What is metaphysics? In K. D. F (Ed.), *Martin Heidegger, Basic Writings* (K. D. F, Trans., pp. 90–110). New York: Harper Perennial Modern Classics.

Heidegger, M. (1946/2008). Letter on humanism. In D. F. Krell (Ed.), *Martin Heidegger, Basic Writings* (D. F. Krell, Trans., pp. 213–265). New York: Harper Perennial Modern Classics.

Heidegger, M. (1954/2008). The question concerning technology. In K. D. F (Ed.), *Martin Heidegger, Basic Writings* (K. D. F, Trans., pp. 308–341). New York: Harper Perennial Modern Classics.

Ho, K. H. (2017). The lived experience of foreign domestic helpers in caring for older people in the community : a hermeneutic phenomenological study [Dissertation]. Hong Kong Polytechnic University. Retrieved from https://theses.lib.polyu.edu.hk/handle/200/9128

Ho, K. H., Chiang, V. C., & Leung, D. (2017). Hermeneutic phenomenological analysis: The 'possibility' beyond 'actuality' in thematic analysis. *Journal of Advanced Nursing, 73*(3), 1757–1766. doi:10.1111/jan.13255

Ho, K. H., Chiang, V. C., Leung, D., & Ku, B. H. (2018). When foreign domestic helpers care for and about older people in their homes: I am a maid or a friend. *Global Qualitative Nursing Research, 5*, 1–10. doi:10.1177/2333393617753906

Ho, K. H., Mak, A. K., Chung, R. W., Leung, D. Y., Chiang, V. C., & Cheung, D. S. (2022). Implications of COVID-19 on the loneliness of older adults in residential care homes. *Qualiative Health Research, 32*(2), 279–290. doi:10.1177/10497323211050910

McCormack, B., & McCance, T. (2006). Development of a framework for person-centred nursing. *Journal of Advanced Nursing, 56*(5), 1–8.

McCormack, B., & McCance, T. (2017a). Introduction. In B. McCormack, & T. McCance (Eds.), *Person-centered practice in nursing and health care: Theory and practice* (2nd ed., pp. 1–10). Oxford: John Wiley & Sons.

McCormack, B., & McCance, T. (2017b). Underpinning principles of person-centred practice. In B. McCormack, & T. McCance (Eds.), *Person-centred practice in nursing and health care: Theory and practice* (2nd ed., pp. 13–64). Oxford: John Wiley & Sons.

Ratcliffe, M. (2002). Heidegger, analytic metaphysics, and the Being of beings. *Inquiry, 45*(1), 35–57. doi:10.1080/002017402753556607

Rojcewicz, R. (2006). *The Gods and Technology: A Reading of Heidegger.* New York: State University of New York Press.

van Manen, M. (2014). *Phenomenology of Practice: Meaning-Giving Methods in Phenomenological Research and Writing.* Walnut Street, CA: Left Coast Press.

World Health Organization. (2015). *WHO Global Strategy on People-Centred and Integrated Health Services: Interim Report.* Retrieved from http://apps.who.int/iris/bitstream/10665/155002/1/

19 Why thriving – and well-being – ought to be fundamental goals in nursing

Marit Kirkevold

Introduction

Nursing has traditionally been associated with caring for people and families in need of care due to actual or potential illness or disease that limits their ability to care for themselves. The history of nursing in a modern context is intrinsically linked to hospitals, nursing homes and home care nursing. The so-called nursing process, conceptualized as the fundamental clinical assessment and decision-making process in nursing, highlights this orientation towards disease. Its proposed goal is to identify the patient's health care problems (in some contexts referred to as nursing diagnoses) and plan nursing care to address these problems (Henderson 1982, Häyrinen et al. 2010). Even in encounters with healthy individuals, such as healthy pregnant women, newborns or schoolchildren, a major goal has traditionally been to prevent disease and identify possible deviations from normal physical and/or psychological development (Cowley et al. 2015).

Despite the heavy orientation towards disease and illness in the practice of nursing, health has been proposed as its overarching goal. Henderson's classic definition of nursing from 1978, adopted by the International Council of Nurses (ICN), conceptualizes the goal of nursing in relation to restoring health or promoting a peaceful death:

> The unique function of the nurse is to assist the individual, sick or well, in the performance of those activities contributing to health or its recovery (or to peaceful death) that he would perform unaided if he had the necessary strength, will or knowledge.
>
> (first published in Henderson & Nite 1978, p. 5, 1955 ed.)

Nursing has also subscribed to the World Health Organization (WHO) definition of health from 1948 as "a state of complete physical, mental and social well-being and not merely the absence of disease or infirmity". Although celebrated for its comprehensiveness, recognition of the psychosocial aspects of health and emphasis on subjective well-being, it has been criticized for being unrealistic and unattainable. Furthermore, it excludes people with disease or infirmity from being healthy. This conflicts with the experiences of many people with diseases who report feeling healthy despite their disease or functional disability (Huber et al. 2011).

In line with the positive conceptualizations of health, other positive states have been proposed as relevant for nursing and health care. One such phenomenon is thriving. The purpose of this chapter is to explore the relevance of the phenomenon of thriving as a normative goal for nursing care. In contrast to its antonym, failure to thrive, thriving is

DOI: 10.4324/9781003427407-22

a little-used concept in the health care literature generally and in the nursing literature specifically. To the degree that it is explored, it has been described as ill-defined (Bergland & Kirkevold 2006), and some would consider it a synonym of already established terms, such as health, well-being, flourishing, resilience and quality of life. So why take the trouble to explore its relevance?

Generally, there is a dearth of explorations of positive states and nursing outcomes for people with long-term ill-health conditions and people of old age. Despite recent discussions about the need to reconceptualize the concept of health in order to accommodate people with disease and/or functional disability (Huber et al. 2011), most health care professionals and even people with disease and illness themselves understand health mostly as a state of absence of serious or long-term disease (Leder 1990, Seamon 2018). Furthermore, widening the concept of health might lead to confusion rather than clarification, as the official global definition proposed by the WHO in 1948 has already been criticized for being too wide-ranging and unrealistic. Other established terms, such as resilience and quality of life, are increasingly recognized as important goals and outcomes within nursing and health care. Resilience, although a contested concept (East et al. 2020), is usually conceptualized within nursing as an individual trait or a resource that some people have that contributes to health or mastery of stressful situations, including ill health. Originally conceptualized within child psychology to describe a child's ability to withstand adverse life events and develop normally, it has gradually been adopted in nursing and other sciences within a wide range of contexts (Dahlberg 2015, East et al. 2020). However, with this development, it has increasingly become a less precise and useful concept. Quality of life, a widely used and studied term in the health care literature, also contributes to a focus on positive states or outcomes of health care even in the presence of disease or ill health. However, it is a highly abstract and technical concept that has many different definitions and diverse theoretical and philosophical foundations. Within health care, it is increasingly associated with a disease-oriented discourse supplementing the narrow biomedical focus on treating diseases. It is usually not a concept used by patients themselves to describe their situation. The concept of thriving, however, captures a valued and experience-based phenomenon of relevance to people with ill health (as well as people without health problems). Furthermore, it provides a perspective that supplements existing positive concepts, such as quality of life.

This analysis will take as a starting point the empirical nursing literature describing thriving from the perspective of patients receiving nursing care. The rationale is that I understand thriving first and foremost as a lay term capturing an experience of living a life that one is content with or that is worth living. That does not necessarily imply a "happy life" (a life with strong positive emotions) or a life without struggles. According to the Merriam-Webster dictionary, the term comes from old Norse "þrífast" (Norwegian "å like seg"), which in English would mean something in between "to settle (in)" and to "enjoy" a situation or a place. Following a brief summary of thriving from a patient perspective, I review previous theoretical accounts of thriving in the literature, highlighting the need for a more thorough philosophical account that may contribute to a better understanding of thriving as a viable goal for nursing care.

Descriptions of thriving from the perspective of the people themselves

The phenomenon of thriving has been studied mainly in relation to older people residing in nursing homes. The bulk of the very limited research comes from Norway and Sweden.

The reason for this is unclear. Perhaps it is a language issue, i.e., a failure to use an internationally appropriate or accepted term for the phenomenon referred to by the Norwegian term "trivsel" and Swedish term "välbefinnande". An argument for this explanation is that when a colleague and I tried to publish an article on thriving among nursing home residents in the early 2000s in a recognized international qualitative journal, the editor insisted that we change the term thriving to well-being if she were to publish the paper. As this was a qualitative study focusing on the lived experiences of the old people themselves, and they used the term thriving ("trivsel") rather than well-being ("velvære" in Norwegian), we felt obliged to keep the term in order to capture the experiences of our participants. Furthermore, after reviewing the qualitative literature on well-being at the time, we concluded that well-being could not adequately capture the experiences relayed to us during the in-depth interviews. We therefore chose to keep the term thriving and opted to submit the paper elsewhere (Bergland & Kirkevold 2006). Furthermore, when we reviewed the literature, we found some publications using the term thriving written by English-speaking authors, suggesting that the term was in fact a viable option. We identified three different theoretical accounts that could be relevant to understanding thriving (or nonthriving) among nursing home residents though not limited to this population or to the nursing home context (Bergland & Kirkevold 2001). These accounts will be presented in the next section. However, I will first briefly summarize how thriving is described by nursing home residents.

Exemplar I: Thriving in a Norwegian nursing home

One of the first empirical studies focusing on thriving among people with long-term health problems was published in the early 2000s (Bergland & Kirkevold 2001, 2005, 2006, 2008). The study (with different substudies) focused on how mentally lucid nursing home residents experienced living in a nursing home and what contributed to their thriving (or nonthriving) there. The qualitative, interpretive study included in-depth interviews and participant observation of 26 people in two urban nursing homes. The study was inspired by philosopher Alfred Schütz' phenomenology of everyday life (1967). It highlighted that the participants started from the assumption that thriving in a nursing home was completely different from thriving "at home" (in their previous life). The participants highlighted that thriving in the nursing home depended first and foremost on their own mental attitude. They explained that they had to "want to" or "decide" to thrive in the nursing home because they realized that they had to live there. They could not live at home any longer due to ill health and functional decline. Some of the participants reported a mental attitude (or decision) "not to thrive" in the nursing home, reserving thriving for how they felt about their life before moving to the nursing home. A last group felt ambiguous about thriving in the nursing home. However, they all realized that they themselves had a major impact on whether they thrived, making attitude an essential feature of thriving in this context. Another essential aspect of thriving (or nonthriving) was the relationship and care provided by the nursing home staff. The participants recognized that they could not thrive only by assuming a mental attitude of deciding to do so. In order to thrive, they still depended largely on the quality of relationships with the staff (being treated with respect and care) and the quality of the daily care provided to meet their complex care needs. Lack of respectful treatment and/or inadequate care would undermine their efforts to thrive in the nursing home. Other aspects contributing to thriving included relationships with family and friends, interactions with other residents, ability to participate in meaningful activities, a pleasant environment and ability to make excursions from the nursing home. However, the latter aspects could not compensate for a mental attitude of not thriving, a lack of respectful treatment or inadequate care, as these impacted the core of their daily life in the nursing home. The other aspects added pleasant experiences "colouring" their life in a positive way that to a greater or lesser degree depended on access to these experiences.

Exemplar II: Thriving in an Australian nursing home

In a more recent study (Baxter et al. 2021), 21 nursing home residents in a rural nursing home in Australia were invited to participate in narrative interviews in order to uncover the meaning of thriving from their point of view. Applying a phenomenological hermeneutic method inspired by Ricoeur's (1976) theory of interpretation, the study identified four meanings of thriving: striving towards acceptance of being in a nursing home while maintaining a positive outlook; feeling supported and cared for while maintaining a sense of independence; balancing opportunities for solitude and company while living with others; and feeling a sense of home while residing in an institutional environment. The comprehensive interpretation of the identified meanings was inspired by phenomenologist Gaston Bachelard's Poetics of Space (1964). In this work, Bachelard introduces the opening, entering and/or shutting of physical, metaphorical and symbolic doors to understand the complex relations between geometric spaces and lived spaces and places. Applying this interpretive lens to the meaning of thriving, Baxter et al. (2021) suggest that thriving is related to having options (doors to open and close) and choices (opportunities to open and close doors as desired).

Taking these empirical examples as a starting point, I will summarize three main theoretical perspectives on thriving before moving on to a philosophical analysis of the concept. The theoretical perspectives provide useful insights into the concept but also lay the ground for why a more philosophical account of thriving might add to our understanding.

Theoretical perspectives on thriving

As mentioned above, a previous work (Bergland & Kirkevold 2001) identified three theoretical perspectives on thriving: (a) thriving as an outcome of growth and development, (b) thriving as an emotional state and (c) thriving as an expression of a person's physical state. These theoretical accounts add to the dictionary definition of thriving provided initially.

The theoretical argument that thriving is an outcome of growth and development is developed within psychology. It conceptualizes thriving as one of several outcomes when a person encounters an adverse or traumatic event. From this perspective, thriving is a "better-off" state following an adverse or traumatic event. The better-off outcomes may be new or improved knowledge and skills, increased self-confidence and/or better personal relations, which, in turn, contribute to better or quicker mastery of similar situations in the future. This conceptualization of thriving is closely related to resilience and adaptation but must be differentiated from them, according to Carver (1998). Resilience indicates the ability to withstand the effects of adversity but does not necessarily lead to a better-off situation following an adverse event. It could also lead to a return to the previous level of functioning. Adaptation also indicates the ability to handle difficult situations, but the outcome might vary from a worse-off to an equal-to or better-off state following the event. Both personality factors and contextual factors may influence the likelihood of thriving following an adverse event.

The second perspective on thriving conceptualizes the phenomenon as an emotional state. This theory of thriving is based on a sociopsychological interactionist model in which thriving is the outcome of interactions between an individual and a particular environment (Petersen 1995). This perspective, proposed by the Danish psychologist Petersen (1995), assumes that thriving is the result of a positive balance between a person's expectations and his or her actual experiences in a particular context. Thriving occurs when there are more experiences of expectations being fulfilled, whereas nonthriving (or unhappiness) occurs when expectations tend to not be met. This perspective on thriving implies a cognitive process whereby a person is conscious of his or her expectations and assesses the degree to which the environment can accommodate them. Furthermore, if there is a discrepancy between the expectations and the opportunities in the specific environment, the person must actively or passively adjust the expectations and/or take action to change the environment in order to improve the match and increase his or her thriving.

The last identified theoretical perspective on thriving conceptualizes thriving by starting with its opposition – failure to thrive. This perspective, developed primarily within medicine and health care, focuses on the observed phenomenon that some human beings, particularly newborn and young children and very old people, exhibit signs of failure to thrive, indicated through unexplained weight loss (primarily old people) or inability to gain weight and grow as expected (children). The observed phenomenon is often difficult to explain, as it is usually not related to specific causes that explain the state. In the case of older people, frailty has been proposed as an explanation. However, others have argued that frailty is a state of (physical) vulnerability that may lead to failure to thrive, whereas the latter is the process of losing weight and/or experiencing general ill-being (Bergland & Kirkevold 2001).

As this brief review shows, thriving is conceptualized by the first theoretical account as an outcome of a psychosocial mastery or adjustment process and by the second as a psychological state related to preferences and expectations. The last account focuses on bodily processes. However, none of the theoretical accounts provide a more in-depth understanding of the experience of thriving (or nonthriving) among people with serious health issues and functional decline, such as nursing home residents. Therefore, I will turn next to philosophy to gain a better understanding of the concept of thriving.

A philosophical account of thriving

Although there are other potential philosophical perspectives that could be useful in exploring thriving from a philosophical perspective, e.g., approaches inspired by Martha Nussbaum's philosophy of commitment (Bielby 2021, Nussbaum 2011) or human capabilities theory (Wilson-Strydom & Walker 2015), I choose to apply a phenomenological lens. This is based on my assumption that thriving is an experience-based phenomenon – as was highlighted by the empirical exemplars presented earlier in this chapter. As will become apparent, although I started this work assuming that well-being and thriving are distinct concepts, in the phenomenological analysis that I present below, they merge.

Thriving from the perspective of phenomenology

As shown by both the empirical explorations and the theoretical conceptualizations, thriving is closely related to a positive or suitable relation or match between a person and his or her environment and is also a result of adjusting to a challenge or change in life (Bergland & Kirkevold 2005, 2006, 2008, Baxter et al. 2021). Therefore, I contend that it is not fruitful to explore thriving in general terms. Rather, thriving is best conceptualized in relation to a person's specific environment (i.e., material and psychosocial conditions) or, more precisely, the place in which he or she lives. Furthermore, thriving, similar to health and well-being, can be conceptualized as an absence (Burwood 2018). In the same way that health and well-being can be argued to be the absence of ill-being, thriving can be understood as an experiential state in which nonthriving is absent (Bergland & Kirkevold 2006). These ideas, I contend, are consistent with phenomenological philosophical thoughts. In the following, I will therefore explore these ideas from a phenomenological perspective.

To explore the specific relationship between a person and his or her place in the world, I will draw on the phenomenology of place, specifically as conceptualized by the architect David Seamon (2018) and philosopher Donohoe (2011). Furthermore, I will explore thriving as absence by drawing on the conceptualization of well-being presented by Burwood (2018). These phenomenological conceptualizations help, I contend, to understand the experiences of thriving or nonthriving relayed in the empirical explorations of thriving among residents of nursing homes that I take as a starting point in this chapter.

In his explorations of research on well-being and its relation to place, Seamon (2018) argues that two fundamental principles in phenomenology, human-immersion-in-world and lived obliviousness, are of particular relevance.

He explains human-immersion-in-world as

the phenomenological recognition that human beings are inescapably conjoined with and enmeshed in their world, which here relates to the person or group's sphere of action, understanding and experience, both firsthand and vicarious. That people are always already caught up in and enjoined with their world suggests that the well-being of an individual or group cannot be discussed apart from lived relationships with their worlds, including the places in which they find themselves. In other words, individual well-being and place well-being mutually presuppose and afford each other. In this sense, one might more accurately speak of the well-being-of-person-or-group-in-place.

(Seamon 2018, p. 103)

To elaborate on the meaning of human-immersion-in-world, Seamon draws on the concepts of lifeworld and homeworld. The lifeworld is the taken-for-granted activities, experiences, interactions, etc., that make up our everyday lives and that we share with our fellow human beings. The lifeworld is embodied in that it is through our being in the world with our lived bodies that we experience and act in the world. The homeworld is our most foundational embodied experiences, intrinsically connected to our home, our house, i.e., where we live (Donohoe, 2011). Home, inseparable from the house (i.e., the physical building and area in which we live), is where our most basic understandings of the world emerge. Donohoe (2011) explains it thus:

Home .... [the house in which we live] .... is a space that is intimate and into which we usually only allow those whom we consider friends or acquaintances. The house is where we develop a certain style of acting in the world. In many ways it reflects our character in the way in which it is decorated and arranged. But the house too arranges us, much as any building arranges us, but in a much more fundamental and determinate way.

(Donohoe, 2011, p. 26)

Emphasizing immersion in the world, she continues: "The world and the places we inhabit do not contain our bodies. Body and world are intertwined, making place integral to body and vice versa" (Donohoe, 2011, p. 27). In this way, our lives and the place(s) in which we find ourselves constitute our lifeworld.

At the same time, Donohoe is very clear that the homeworld is not necessarily a "good" world. Many people may experience their homeworld as an unsafe place, a place of domination, abuse or insecurity (Donohoe 2011). Nevertheless, she contends, the homeworld is the foundation for how we live and understand our lifeworld:

Homeworld is the place where my body is most habituated. It is not that the homeworld is thereby found to be ethically superior, it is that any other place is more or less alien by relation to and in constitution with the homeworld. I am not at home when I am bodily uneasy, when my habits do not fit, or when they do not yield the results I expect.

(Donohoe 2011, p. 33)

Donohoe (2011), referring to the philosophy of Edmund Husserl, contrasts homeworld with alienworld. She argues that homeworld and alienworld are "co-relative" and that homeworld is associated with what is "normal", whereas alienworld is what is experienced as "abnormal" (p.32). It is important to note here that normal and abnormal are not meant in a moral sense as "ethically superior" (p. 33) but in terms of "habituated engagement with the world":

experiences of alienworlds make the homeworld more explicit to us in its familiarity. Homeworld in its normality can be so close to us as to be unrecognizable until drawn into relief by an alienworld experience.

(Donohoe, 2011, p. 32)

Seamon (2018) emphasizes that the second relevant phenomenological principle is lived obliviousness. This concept

refers to the recognition that well-being is not typically an explicitly experienced dimension of most people's everyday experiences; rather, life simply unfolds more or less automatically, and one may not be aware of or reflect upon any stressful, untoward or undermining elements of daily living that, to an outsider, might indicate a lack of well-being. For sure, human beings often experience self-conscious moments when, on one hand, they feel positive and hopeful about their lives or, on the other hand, feel negative and wish their life might be better. More typically, however, life simply happens. People 'just get on with things' and don't regularly give self-conscious attention to the lived fact that life might be otherwise.

(Seamon 2018, p. 103)

The concept of obliviousness is closely related to Burwood's idea of well-being as an absence. Burwood (2018) ties well-being closely to health, arguing that health is not merely the absence of suffering but is also "to a large degree an experiential absence of one's body" (Burwood, 2018, p. 133).

Referring indirectly to the principle of obliviousness, Burwood (2018) notes:

The healthy body is the homely and familiar body. This is the body that is mostly compliant with one's wishes and desires and is the means by which we achieve our projects in the world and with others. .... The compliant body's familiarity, normality, and routine contribute to its invisibility, and so this very familiarity may breed forgetfulness. We become lost in our projects, whatever they are and whatever their value or desirability.

(p. 133)

According to Burwood (2018), illness leads to a number of "existential 'conflicts' – with oneself, one's body, one's surroundings, and with others" (p. 133):

What was once familiar or routine becomes agonistic and takes on a distant and uncanny aspect. One's experience of good health, on the other hand, consists largely, though not entirely, in the absence of these conflicts. In good health, one might say, one is at home with oneself, one's body, one's environment, and with others.

(p. 133)

What can these phenomenological insights into human immersion-in-world and lived obliviousness teach us about thriving?

I will turn to this question next.

The qualitative studies that I referred to initially emphasize that the experience of thriving in a nursing home is qualitatively or principally different from thriving in the participants' earlier lives (Bergland & Kirkevold 2006). The participants could not even start reflecting on their current state or experience of thriving without this premise. In that sense, thriving as the participants originally understood the term could be related to the lifeworld and homeworld that they had originally lived in prior to moving into the nursing home. Most residents recognized that they would rather live "at home", i.e., in their previous house, and live the way they used to. However, their failing health and functional decline prohibited this. Therefore, they recognized that it was no longer a viable alternative. In this sense, their failing health and functional decline had led to fundamental changes in their lifeworld and homeworld even prior to their move to the nursing home. However, they still conceptualized thriving primarily as a quality of their previous life. With Seamon, Burwood and Donohoe, one may assume that their lives were characterized by human-immersion-in-(home)world and lived obliviousness as they lived their lives at home.

Research has documented that older people living at home accommodate changes in health and functioning in order to continue their "normal" life. In many cases, the changes are gradual, allowing people to adjust and remain immersed in their usual lifeworld for a long period of time (Søvde et al. 2022). At other times, an abrupt change in health and/or circumstances (e.g., loss of a spouse or serious illness) may "throw" the person into a radical change of his or her lifeworld. Regardless of the nature of the change, studies have shown that an old or ill person's home can change from being the "safe haven" ensuring that one can live the life one desires to an "unsafe place" where insecurity takes over and threatens one's very life (Silverglow et al. 2020). The person's lifeworld changes from the lived obliviousness of the familiar homeworld to an "alien" world where he or she no longer feels "at home" and safe (Donohoe 2011).

This change from feeling "at home" to no longer feeling "at home" in one's own house is significant and can be related to the shift from a sense of thriving to a sense of nonthriving or ill-being (Burwood 2018). Furthermore, as we age, and disease and functional decline appear, the lived obliviousness can no longer be maintained. Rather, the body becomes "dys-apparent" (Leder 1990), present to the self in an unfamiliar and uncomfortable or painful way, threatening the usual immersion-in-(home)world and the ability to conduct everyday projects with little or no conscious attention. The body and lifeworld that were once taken for granted no longer exist, thrusting the person into an "alien" world at home (Fudge & Swinglehurst 2022).

As Burwood explains, referring to Leder (1990) and van den Berg (1966):

> The body resurfaces and imposes itself on us in all its contingency and materiality. These moments of resurfacing of the body are what Leder terms modes of 'dys-appearance' – a term he employs to deliberately emphasise their often insalubrious and alienating nature (1990: 69–99). "The healthy person", van den Berg explains, "is allowed to be his body and he makes use of this right eagerly: he is his body. Illness disturbs this assimilation. Man's body becomes foreign to him" (1966: 66). Deleterious conditions such as illness, pain, and bodily impairment are thus commonly accompanied by a sense of dissociation, in which one's body takes on an uncanny aspect: at one and the same time it presents as close and familiar and as an external reality.
>
> (Burwood, 2018, p. 136)

As body and place are enmeshed, the lifeworld, including the home, becomes foreign. When sufficiently "alien", it may present as unsafe, and thriving at home becomes untenable. This is when old people may come to the conclusion that moving is a better alternative than remaining.

Moving from one's home to a different place, e.g., a nursing home, challenges the principles of human-immersion-in-world and lived obliviousness. Given the inseparability of body and place, moving to a totally new environment thrusts the person into a new lifeworld, or an "alienworld", to use the term originally introduced by Husserl (Donohoe 2011, Seamon 2018). The empirical studies of thriving among nursing home residents underscore this. Nursing home residents participating in the studies highlighted how they had to make a substantial effort to experience "thriving" – although a thriving that was different from the one they had experienced at home. In the Norwegian study, the participants talked about deciding or being determined to thrive (Bergland & Kirkevold 2006); in the Australian study, the participants talked about striving for acceptance, of being in a nursing home while maintaining a positive outlook and feeling a sense of home while residing in an institutional environment (Baxter et al. 2021). These expressions suggest that moving into a nursing home can be understood as a transition from the (lost) taken-for-granted lifeworld to striving to create a new lifeworld out of the "alienworld" that the nursing home is experienced as upon moving there. In this sense, thriving in a nursing home indicates a move from being in an "alienworld" (nonthriving) towards a new "homeworld".

Thriving and well-being as fundamental goals for nursing

The above analysis suggests that thriving in a new context requires a fundamental change in the old person's lifeworld. Furthermore, such a change, while dependent on the active efforts of the person him- or herself, also depends on support from the surrounding context. For an alienworld to become a new homeworld, i.e., the place where human-immersion-in-world occurs, integration into the new world is required. Both the Norwegian and Australian studies highlighted that experiencing thriving in the nursing home depended on the responses of the carers and fellow residents. The Norwegian nursing home residents pointed this out clearly by emphasizing that they could not thrive even if determined to do so unless the carers provided high-quality care to compensate for their functional difficulties and meet their needs. Furthermore, thriving depended on the staff demonstrating caring in the way they met and interacted with the residents. In this sense, it is essential for care staff to promote thriving or moving towards "at homeness" (Silverglow et al. 2020) when frail older people move into a nursing home. This highlights Seamon's (2018) point that well-being or thriving depends on the well-being of the place.

Seamon's argument is supported by a recent, multicentre intervention study in six nursing homes in three countries (Sjögren et al. 2022). The study demonstrates that providing thriving-promoting and person-centred care by doing a little extra for each individual resident, developing a caring environment and assessing and meeting highly prioritized psychosocial needs indeed promote thriving. Furthermore, the involved staff reported that being allowed to work in this person-centred way meant that they were able to meet individual residents' needs and expressed preferences in close family like relationships, understand the residents' rhythms and preferences as the basis of their daily work and do "the little extra" for residents (Vassbø et al. 2019). Working in this way also entailed working towards a collective practice and shared goals in collaborative teams. This thriving-promoting and person-centred approach even promoted the staff's thriving at work.

The approach described above is closely related to the concept of lifeworld-led health care introduced by Dahlberg et al. (2009) and further developed and translated into care practices by Galvin et al. (2020). Together, these approaches represent resources that may acknowledge and support older people's own efforts to thrive in a new environment and promote the thriving of other actors in the same environment, thereby contributing to Seamon's ideal of ensuring the well-being of a place and its inhabitants.

Conclusion

This chapter started by proposing that thriving might be a useful concept for conceptualizing a positive goal for and outcome of nursing for people with ill health and functional decline, specifically older people residing in nursing homes. The analysis provided hopefully contributes to a better understanding of the concept and reveals how a phenomenological perspective may guide nurses to promote thriving in frail older individuals. The analysis even suggests that this approach may promote the well-being of the place in which nursing care is provided, including thriving among the staff.

References

Bachelard G (1964). *Poetics of Space*. New York: Beacon Press.
Baxter R, Corneliusson L, Björk S, Kloos N, Edvardsson D (2021). A recipe for thriving in nursing homes: A meta-ethnography. *Journal of Advanced Nursing*, 77(6): 2680–2688.

Bergland Å, Kirkevold M (2001). Thriving--a useful theoretical perspective to capture the experience of well-being among frail elderly in nursing homes? *Journal of Advanced Nursing*, 36(3): 426–432.

Bergland A, Kirkevold M (2005). Resident-caregiver relationships and thriving among nursing home residents. *Research in Nursing & Health*, 28(5): 365–75.

Bergland Å, Kirkevold M (2006). Thriving in nursing homes in Norway: Contributing aspects described by residents. *International Journal of Nursing Studies*, 43(6): 681–691.

Bergland A, Kirkevold M (2008). The significance of peer relationships to thriving in nursing homes. *Journal of Clinical Nursing*, 17(10):1295–1302.

Bielby P (2021). Beyond surviving to thriving: The case for a 'Compassion towards Thriving' approach in public mental health ethics. *Public Health Ethics*, 14(3): 298–316.

Burwood S. (2018). The existential situation of the patient: Well-being and absence. Chapter 13 in Galvin K. *Routledge Handbook of Well-Being* (1st Ed.). eBook. London: Imprint Routledge. https://doi.org/10.4324/9781315724966, pp. 133–140.

Carver CS (1998). Resilience and thriving: Issues, models, and linkages. *Journal of Social Issues*, 54: 245–266.

Cowley S, Whittaker K, Malone M, Donetto S, Grigulis A, Maben J (2015). Why health visiting? Examining the potential public health benefits from health visiting practice within a universal service: A narrative review of the literature. *International Journal of Nursing Studies*, 52(1): 465–480.

Dahlberg K, Todres L, Galvin KT (2009). Lifeworld-led healthcare is more than patient-led care: The need for an existential theory of well-being. *Medicine, Healthcare and Philosophy*, 12: 265–271. DOI:10.1007/s11019-008-9174–7.

Dahlberg R (2015). Resilience and complexity: Conjoining the discourses of two contested concepts. *Culture Unbound*, 7: 541–557.

Donohoe J (2011). The place of home. *Environmental Philosophy*, 8(1): 25–40. https://www.jstor.org/stable/10.2307/26168058.

East L, Heaslip V, Jackson D (2020). The symbiotic relationship of vulnerability and resilience in nursing. *Contemporary Nurse*, 56(1): 14–22, DOI: 10.1080/10376178.2019.1670709

Fudge N, Swinglehurst D (2022). Keeping in balance on the multimorbidity tightrope: A narrative analysis of older patients' experiences of living with and managing multimorbidity. *Social Science and Medicine*, 292: 114532.

Galvin KT, Pound C, Cowdell F, Ellis-Hill C, Sloan C, Brooks S, Ersser SJ (2020). A lifeworld theory-led action research process for humanizing services: Improving "what matters" to older people to enhance humanly sensitive care. *International Journal of Qualitative Studies on Health and Well-being* 15: 1, DOI: 10.1080/17482631.2020.1817275.

Häyrinen K, Lammintakanen J, Saranto K (2010). Evaluation of electronic nursing documentation—Nursing process model and standardized terminologies as keys to visible and transparent nursing. *International Journal of Medical Informatics*, 79(8): 554–564.

Henderson V (1982). The nursing process. Is the title right? *Journal of Advanced Nursing*, 7(2): 103–109.

Henderson V, Nite G (1978). *Principles and Practice of Nursing* (6th Ed.). New York: MacMillan Publ.

Huber M, Knottnerus JA, Green L, van der Horst H, Jadad AR, Kromhout D, Leonard B, Lorig K, Loureiro MI, van der Meer JWM, Schnabel P, Smith R, van Weel C, Smid H (2011). How should we define health? *BMJ*, 343: d4163 doi: 10.1136/bmj.d4163.

Leder D (1990). *The Absent Body*. Chicago: University of Chicago Press.

Nussbaum M 2011. *Creating Capabilities: The Human Development Approach*. Cambridge, MA: Harvard University Press.

Petersen E 1995. *Trivsel og livskvalitet, krise og samfundsudvikling: en antologi [Thriving and Quality of Life, Crisis and Development of Society: An Anthology]*. Institute of Psychology, University of Aarhus, Denmark.

Ricoeur P (1976). *Interpretation Theory: Discourse and the Surplus of Meaning*. Fort Worth, TX: Texas University Press.

Schütz A (1967). *The Phenomenology of the Social World*. Evanston, IL: Northwestern University Press.

Seamon D (2018). Well-being and phenomenology: Lifeworld, natural attitude, homeworld and place. Chapter 10 in Galvin K. *Routledge Handbook of Well-Being* (1st Ed.). eBook. London: Imprint Routledge. https://doi.org/10.4324/9781315724966, pp. 103–111.

Silverglow A, Lidèn E, Berglund H, Johansson L, Wijk H (2020). What constitutes feeling safe at home? A qualitative interview study with frail older people receiving home care. *Nursing Open*, 8(1): 191–199. doi: 10.1002/nop2.618. PMID: 33318827; PMCID: PMC7729533.

Sjögren K, Bergland Å, Kirkevold M, Lindkvist M, Lood Q, Sandman PO, Vassbø TK, Edvardsson D (2022). Effects of a person-centred and thriving-promoting intervention on nursing home residents' experiences of thriving and person-centredness of the environment. *Nursing Open*, 9(4): 2117–2129.

Søvde BE, Sandvoll AM, Natvik E, Drageset J (2022). Carrying on life at home or moving to a nursing home: Frail older people's experiences of at-homeness. *International Journal of Qualitative Studies on Health and Well-being*, 17(1): 2082125. doi: 10.1080/17482631.2022.2082125. PMID: 35634736; PMCID: PMC9673807.

van den Berg JH (1966). *The Psychology of the Sickbed*. Pittsburgh, PA: Duquesne University Press.

Vassbø TK, Kirkevold M, Edvardsson D, Sjögren K, Lood Q, Bergland Å (2019). The meaning of working in a person-centred way in nursing homes: A phenomenological-hermeneutical study. *BMC Nursing*, 18(45). https://doi.org/10.1186/s12912-019-0372-9

Wilson-Strydom M, Walker M (2015). A capabilities-friendly conceptualisation of flourishing in and through education. *Journal of Moral Education*, 44(3): 310–324.

20 Life and death

Nursing responses to euthanasia

Martin Woods

Vignette

The nurses at Havenlea hospice had always presumed that they would not be involved in any acts of euthanasia or assisted dying (AD) at their place of work, even after medically assisted dying (MAD) had recently become law. However, the management of the hospice announced that they were considering a suitable response in light of the legalisation, and that it was their wish that the nurses discuss their collective professional position regarding any act of euthanasia at the hospice. The nurses decided to hold a meeting to discuss their response and requested two of their number to offer arguments at the meeting that were designed to highlight the philosophical and professional issues involved both in supporting MAD at the hospice and in not supporting it.

Introduction

In recent decades, voluntary euthanasia has been closely associated with physician-assisted suicide (PAS), and more recently, with 'medically assistance in dying' (MaiD). This has been explained as occurring when "…an authorized doctor or nurse practitioner provides or administers medication that intentionally brings about a person's death, at that person's request" (British Columbia n.d.). These medications involve the administration of lethal combinations of drugs (e.g. midazolam, phenobarbital sodium, propofol and rocuronium bromide) to cause the premature death of a requesting individual who in most, but not all cases, is receiving palliative care services. As is generally known, countries such as Belgium, Luxembourg and the Netherlands have passed various forms of euthanasia laws that have now been operational for several years. Indeed, not only has such legislation been passed in these countries but considerably modified as well in recent times. For example, it is now possible to request euthanasia in the Netherlands and Belgium if one is 'tired of life', has a psychiatric disorder or (in Belgium) is a 'chronically ill child' (Thienpont et al. 2015).

However, other nations or states have introduced various forms of euthanasia legislation in recent years as well. These countries include Canada, Spain, Columbia, the state of Victoria, Australia, some US states and more recently, New Zealand. It is also of interest to note that other countries have turned down proposed euthanasia legislation in recent years, e.g., the United Kingdom, where such proposals have been rejected numerous times by the UK Parliamentarians. In any event, of considerable importance is the issue that revolves around the possible implications when considering the actual reasons for AD legislation in the first place. For instance, Canadian legislation relates to an individual being in a

DOI: 10.4324/9781003427407-23

'grievous and irremediable' state. In New Zealand, it is an individual who "experiences un-bearable suffering that cannot be relieved in a manner that the person considers tolerable" (End of Life Choice Act 2019). However, it is pertinent to note that even in those countries that have legally practised acts of medically assisted euthanasia for several years, there are a variety of conflicting opinions about the ethical application of such legislation, especially amongst doctors and nurses (de Bellaigue 2019; Raus, Vanderhaegen and Sterckx 2021).

Euthanasia terminology is therefore important from philosophical and professional positions, and so, perhaps in an attempt for greater clarity, or possibly even to dissuade any possible associations with past misdeeds (Benedict and Shields 2014), there are many variations on the use of word 'euthanasia' within legal or medical literature. Legal dis-tinctions are, after all, very important because the exact wording of each piece of legisla-tion sets the exact boundaries for the practice of euthanasia. Subsequently, terms such as 'assisted dying' (AD), or 'medically assisted dying' (MAD), 'medically assisted in dying' (MAiD), 'physician assisted dying' (PAD) or sometimes 'physician assisted suicide' (PAS) have or are being used. These usages vary at times, but wherever doctors or nurses are legally involved in causing the death of an individual either by the active participation or by a passive act of prescribing life-ending medication that the patient then takes, there is an act of euthanasia (Government of the Netherlands n.d.). It remains to emphasise that in all applications, and especially for ethical and professional purposes, the language of euthanasia is intended to be highly specific to enable transparent application in practice.

The main philosophical/ethical issues of (medical) euthanasia

According to Wilkinson (1990), the term 'euthanasia' may be used to imply the delib-erate killing of another person in at least three distinctive ways, namely by 'voluntary euthanasia', or 'involuntary euthanasia', or 'nonvoluntary euthanasia'. Each term carries significant meaning, and undoubtably with that meaning, certain value-ladened possibili-ties. Obviously, voluntary euthanasia suggests the agreement to the act by the person wishing to die; it is therefore a term that tends to reflect the current state of affairs in those countries that have legalised euthanasia. While involuntary euthanasia strongly suggests situations where the person may not wish to die or has not been able to offer an opinion or consent either way but is 'euthanised' all the same. This type of euthanasia is usually associated with illegal and immoral acts. However, nonvoluntary euthanasia also relates to persons who are 'euthanized' without their explicit consent, but for reasons of, for instance, their lack of mental capacity (as in the case of a person in a persistent vegetative state). Clearly, in all situations, there are elements of either 'passive' or 'active' applications, i.e., by withholding or withdrawing essential life support mechanisms, or by actively administering lethal drugs to cause death (Brassington 2020).

Indeed, an important element of any debate concerning medically assisted euthanasia is the 'killing or letting die' argument, essentially a situation where the end result (death) is the same, but the means (active or passive) are considerably different (Huxtable 2020). Unsurprisingly, this particular argument has created numerous challenges concerning meaning, application and consequences. In brief, there are those who argue that the difference between actively killing another person in an act of euthanasia is not signifi-cantly different from merely allowing them to die through, for instance, the withdrawal or withholding of medical treatment. Others, such as many nurses involved in palliative care practices, generally oppose such an argument by claiming that in the first instance (i.e., killing), the act is a form of malevolence, but in the second instance (letting die), it is a well-established act that aims to promote beneficence through compassionate caring practices (Woods and Rook 2022). Here may be found further evidence of 'double-effect' reasoning, as in an act may be acceptable if the motive (and means) is regarded as 'good' regardless of the consequences (Rodrigues, Crokaert and Gastmans 2018). It should be noted that such arguments may often be combined with 'sanctity of life' versus 'quality of life' positions, i.e., those arguments that either reject euthanasia or support it for different reasons (Singer 1995). In the former case, there is the viewpoint that human life has an absolute value (and therefore must not be prematurely ended by anyone). In the latter case, it is argued that we should promote quality of life rather than quantity, essentially supporting the view that there is a considerable difference between the death of a human organism and the chosen death of a self-aware person (Gluchman 2019; Singer 2018).

As may be implied above, ethics-related terms such as autonomy, beneficence, fairness and freedom to choose tend to predominate in matters concerning the ethical aspects of AD. These terms generally tend to follow moral arguments that are themselves often framed within the commonly used biomedical ethics-orientated 'four principles' approach (Beauchamp and Childress 2019) which still may be seen (often with some modifications) within the frameworks of numerous codes of health care-related ethics, both medical and nursing. It should also be noted that within several public, professional or even philosophical debates on this topic, it is still quite common for the ethical issues relating to the topic to be presented as simple sets of binary arguments. For instance, even a cursory glance at the British Medical Association's (BMA) 'Physician assisted dying survey' (2021) quickly reveals a most noticeable binary divide based largely on interpretations of various competing moral principles. A similar problem undoubtably occurs for nurses who may well interpret their ethical codes in different ways depending upon established personal and professional values. However, mindful of the fact that the little vignette at the start of this chapter presents ethical demands from two 'opposing' nurse presenters at the hospice, it seems reasonable to now present the ethical issues in a generally binary fashion that generally uses a 'moral principles' approach.

Ethical arguments for medically controlled euthanasia

Mindful of the notions of doing what is for the good or benefit of others (beneficence), and in avoiding doing them any harm (non-maleficence), any medical or nursing activity must, by their very nature, have a central focus that is aimed towards these moral aims (Beauchamp and Childress 2019). Thus, in the case of an act of euthanasia, it is necessary to weigh up what 'good' actions are over 'bad' ones within the AD context. Subsequently, it may be maintained that there will always be some people for whom the dying process is an unbearable and highly distressing burden that cannot be relieved by beneficial acts of palliative care and kindness. It follows that some individuals do and will suffer without the services of a physician or a nurse to supply the means by which they might end their suffering by dying prematurely. In short, such people have a very low or even arguably, a non-existent quality of life, *at least from their own perspective*. The desirable medically assisted response is to therefore help them to end that suffering by delivering lethal drugs to cause death. This position is often backed up by an appeal towards the avoidance of the other option of unassisted suicide, which can be a major harm for the individual, their families or community (Conejero, Olié, Courtet, and Calati 2018). Medically sanctioned euthanasia is therefore a lesser harm and should be regarded as an actual 'good' in itself. It should be noted that this explanation suggests that palliative services are not entirely successful in responding to the needs of some dying individuals, regardless of any claims that the palliative services might be adequate. Thus, for morally defensible reasons, if an individual (or possibly another individual?) estimates their own quality of life to be irreversibly poor, then they should have the right to choose to be medically assisted to die, and doctors and nurses should respect a person's desire to live or die and take appropriate action (Singer 1995).

In addition, one of the main ethical arguments in favour of both the introduction of medically controlled euthanasia practices heavily concentrates on the notion of an individual's freedom to choose, and by an obvious connection, with its ethical counterpart, the principle of autonomy. In this instance, an argument is promoted that claims each individual has the autonomous right to be able to choose the circumstances of their own death (via medical assistance). Hence, even though doctors and nurses generally regard their roles as life-enhancing rather than life-ending, they should be supportive of the public's wishes for an opportunity to utilise medical euthanasia if needed (Doyal and Doyal 2001). Besides, any doctor or nurse may legally refuse to participate – based on an application of their own autonomous choice – and may use the 'conscience clause' within the given legislation. That such a legislative clause is deemed necessary in the first place, and its impact on other health care staff and the patient and family when refusing to participate, is, of course, a matter for further debate (see later discussion).

But what about one of the most strident and persistent arguments in favour of euthanasia within any given 'liberal' society, namely the central idea of social equitability and individualised fairness? For instance, is it fair, equitable and just that any individual must go on living when faced with an irreversible decline, 'unbearable suffering' and eventual death, or be able to choose an earlier, less traumatic death by taking lethal drugs that are supplied by a nominated health professional? (Young 2020). In the latter scenario, it is maintained that other suitably qualified doctors or nurses should be the ones to provide the means for death on receiving an appropriate request from such an individual. This is basically an argument that supports the right of others to choose the nature of their own dying circumstances, and thereby to expect appropriate health care professionals (HCPs) to support that right as necessary under the law.

It remains to consider the wider social implications of medically sanctioned euthanasia in society. In regard to social perceptions, and if the poll results are to be accepted (which sometimes they are not), it seems to be the case that overall, there has been widespread public support in countries such as the USA and New Zealand for physician-assisted euthanasia in one form or another (Brenan 2018; Roy 2020). There are a number of arguments in support of these positions, e.g., the general public have a right to AD; it would only be fair to have a properly controlled and regulated system where properly trained and qualified HCPs were utilised to supply the means of death; an alternative such as suicide without medical aid would be far worse, and others. Furthermore, the very existence of legislation allowing AD would provide reassurance and 'peace of mind' for those with a terminal illness and their families and close contacts. Other justice-related arguments in support of medically assisted euthanasia often include the problem of scarce resources and expensive treatments that are not particularly beneficial to a dying individual and might therefore be usefully diverted to those with a chance of adequate survival and some kind of acceptable quality of life (Dobken 2018). This position, and to a degree, previously made arguments, suggests that the right moral decision regarding euthanasia is one that largely suggests a utilitarian focus on outcomes rather than means, and certainly on an act that may provide greater societal benefits (Boudreau and Somerville 2014).

Ethical arguments against medically controlled euthanasia

Doctors and nurses do indeed have to pay strong regard towards patient autonomy, informed consent and freedom of choice, but in doing so, they are heavily obliged to ensure that no breaches of autonomous choice are being enacted in the first place. That is, can they be quite sure that the person asking for euthanasia is indeed making a fully autonomous choice? As may be expected, there are numerous arguments to suggest that such certainty cannot be entirely guaranteed (Hartling 2021). For instance, the patient's judgement may be considered to be affected by pain and suffering, and the benevolent thing to do would be to attempt to respond such suffering by 'being-with' the patient and palliating symptoms (Lipscomb 2014), but not necessarily by euthanising the patient. This response applies in numerous instances where it may be argued that the patient is not able to think or act rationally, and there may not be sufficiently convincing evidence that to want to die prematurely is a rational choice per se. Here, it should be noted that depressive symptoms, hopelessness and other psychological factors have all been suggested when some people feel motivated to request euthanasia.

However, regardless of such concerns, what of the autonomous rights of health professionals, namely that doctors and nurses should be allowed to make autonomous decisions as well? For instance, and in light of various moral or ethical codes that support acts of beneficence and non-maleficence (such as 'first, do no harm'), they may decide *not* to participate, which, according to most euthanasia styled laws around the world, is their right to do so. Such rights are often referred to in any related legislation as a 'conscience clause'. But conscience about what exactly? For instance, there is evidence that in enacting the Canadian MAiD legislation, there are professional and ethical disagreements about what such a clause actually means, and certainly problems regarding both the motives *and* the consequences of conscientious refusal to partake (Brown, Goodridge, Thorpe and Crizzle 2021). Nevertheless, although problematic and certainly not without consequences, the clause is at least available in one form or another to those nurses who wish to maintain, perhaps from a virtue ethics perspective, their moral character and ethical motives rather than meeting the presumed strengths of contemporary bioethical positions that are based on, for instance, abstract principlism or consequentialism (Fowler 2020). This would imply a position of not being involved in killing another individual for whatever motive, means or presumed favourable consequences. Hence, it is sometimes maintained that in the case of palliatively nursing a terminally ill person, the generally accepted and desirable moral response is one that 'neither hastens nor postpones death', instead promoting the relief of distressing symptoms via beneficial acts such as the relief of symptoms and causes of distress, the administration of effective pain relief, and/or sedation, the withdrawal of unnecessary treatments and other measures (Palliative Care Nurses New Zealand n.d.). In short, the moral argument in this instance is that nurses (and doctors) should act out of a desire to promote beneficence and non-maleficence above all other considerations, even against the patient's autonomous desire to die by medical means.

The above discussion raises questions about justice and fairness, but now perhaps from a social rather than an individualistic perspective. This is because it may be argued that the very presence of an AD law, however well intended, may extend beyond individualised decision making towards the involvement of entire socio-cultural groups within society, some of whom may not necessarily share 'western' viewpoints that places individual choice and freedom so highly. In short, the individually orientated notions of freedom of choice and the rights of the individual may actually clash with those of collectivism and shared decision making (Woods 2012). Regardless, there remains an argument at least that certain societal groups may feel intimidated by wider societal attitudes towards the elderly, seriously ill and disabled, and even those who are presumed to be 'tired of living'. In turn, this may lay the groundwork for the notion that AD is always an option that people within these groups should always consider (Florijn 2018). Therefore, the argument goes, not only could euthanasia become more available to various individuals, but by social pressure, actually cause those individuals to respond to family and/or social pressure to choose AD rather than attempting to live on in the face of a terminal illness. It is therefore thought impossible to absolutely ensure that decisions are entirely autonomously made, or that an individual may not covertly at least be succumbing to coercion from one source or another. This, then, could be regarded as a form of harm or maleficence, but it also brings to mind an even greater harm, as in the 'slippery slope' argument. That is, the notion that the originally 'well-meaning' act of ending someone's life because of a terminal illness may end up over time in ending the lives of others *with or without* their permission and for increasingly morally dubious reasons such as the presence of 'chronic' health situations, including significant mental decline. For instance, the Netherlands' high court ruled in 2020 that doctors can euthanise patients with severe dementia without the fear of prosecution (France 24). The trend towards offering euthanasia towards those with chronic health conditions (such as several diseases associated with old age) is certainly the case in at least some countries such as Belgium and/or the Netherlands (Service Public Federal 2020). Subsequently, for some nurses and doctors at least, euthanasia certainly would be 'a bridge too far' because it may easily increase the tendency for some people to feel as if they are indeed 'tired of life' or 'being a burden on others', thus threatening presumed ethical principles that are related to common professional practices (see later discussion). It remains to conclude that, for all the supportive ethical or philosophical arguments about the benefits of euthanasia for individuals and society, there remains a significant and fairly widespread degree of ethical *and* professional unease about its application in practice (Trufin 2021).

Professional concerns

In regard to medical euthanasia, it may be said that many health and medical organisations have positioned themselves against such an act, e.g., the World Health Organization state that a fundamental principle of palliative care is to neither 'hasten nor postpone death' (WHO n.d.); and the World Medical Association (WMA) clearly state that: "No physician should be forced to participate in euthanasia or assisted suicide, nor should any physician be obliged to make referral decisions to this end" (2019). Then again, and even though these bodies seem to offer a reasonably clear position, there are other examples of a few attempts at least to offer the 'middle ground' by perhaps promoting a greater degree 'reasonableness' or 'open-mindedness'. For instance, some have attempted to soften their position in either opposing or supporting euthanasia by claiming that their position is in fact a 'neutral' one that supports individual choice. An example: "…we will neither support nor oppose attempts to change the law" (British Medical Association 2021). Nevertheless, of considerable interest within this chapter is the responses of nursing organisations, although in these instances, both judgement and 'positioning' are often far less transparent. For instance, according to the International Council of Nurses (ICN), nurses are expected to 'promote health, prevent illness, restore health and alleviate suffering' (ICN 2012). As may be seen, in this instance, suitable arguments may be constructed that are both for *and* against nursing involvement in euthanasia. The possible lack of absolute clarity on the issue is compounded further within arguments about the commonly perceived nursing roles to alleviate suffering, preserve dignity, guard the sanctity of life and act with compassion where once again, arguments may be constructed both for and against nursing involvement in euthanasia, e.g., alleviating suffering versus preserving the sanctity of life (Pesut et al. 2020). What definitive advice, then, is offered by national nursing organisations? In the case of the New Zealand Nurses Organisation's (NZNO) code of ethics, which promotes notions of respect, trust, partnership and integrity, and of course, deontological notions of the importance of autonomy, beneficence, non-maleficence, justice and other moral principles (NZNO 2019), the response to the euthanasia issue was: "NZNO has chosen to take a principled approach to AD, and advocate for individuals to have the option or choice of AD" (NZNO n.d.). Thus, this nurses' organisation clearly chose a position of nursing support for an individual's freedom to choose the circumstances of his or her own death, i.e., by promoting autonomy above other principles.

Nevertheless, it may be argued that there remains the equally persistent notion that nurses should promote beneficent acts, especially in support of individual, social or common good (Hussain 2018). Again, this position may include the promotion euthanasia as an overall good, however, it may also suggest the promotion of widespread individual and public trust by avoiding any act that 'harms' (as in prematurely killing) the patient by whatever legally sanctioned means. Obviously, such explanations tend to offer a very simplistic account of a very complex problem because when it becomes apparent that the health of an individual cannot be restored, an even greater emphasis is placed on the alleviation of suffering, and the patient's right to choose to accept or refuse treatments, including euthanasia, that are related to that suffering. Such a situation highlights a constant quandary for nurses as they attempt to negotiate the constant flux between the major ethical principles of benevolence and non-malevolence, and individual autonomy and justice. Hence, there will always remain a significant degree of debate, uncertainty and even heated arguments between nurses about the issue of euthanasia. On the one side of the debate, if it is accepted that a doctor's or a nurse's responsibility is to only respond accordingly to the patient's autonomous choices regarding the circumstances of their own death, then the doctor and/or nurse is committed to an act involving the administration of the lethal drugs. On the other, if the moral premise of caring and commitment to do good is applied to a given patient's terminal situation, then a counterargument might be that a nurse's autonomy to act according to her/his understanding of professional standards and codes is of equal importance. Here perhaps, laid bare, is the challenge of euthanasia, i.e., should a nurse to respond to human suffering and the need for comfort by continuing to promote a better quality of life and care within the dying process that leads to a 'natural death'; or interrupt the dying process by supporting the public's desire for complete autonomic choice in this matter leading to 'assisted' dying?

In response, it may be argued that nurses are most familiar with the dying process, and also with the concept of human suffering, and most certainly with "the value of meeting the needs of others through relationships within particular contexts, and the centrality of caring and the prevention of harm" suggests an ethic of care approach perhaps more than any other (Woods 2011, p. 269). They are quite aware that a dying individual and his or her family may be fearful of the dying process, and although the medical and nursing aims are to minimise such presumed and actual suffering, it has to be accepted that the dying process brings with it inevitable consequences associated with sorrow and grief. Hence, a professional nursing response to euthanasia may be a most complicated affair; nurses do indeed care about responding to an individual's pain and suffering at the end of life and do attempt to respond accordingly, but for some nurses at least, this will never mean ending that life prematurely. Others may choose to respond by taking part in acts of euthanasia, arguing that there will always be some cases at least where efforts to minimise suffering are imperfect, thus promoting the notion that an ethically mindful nurse would take part in an act of euthanasia out of professional duty.

Concluding remarks

There are no quick solutions or resolutions to the issues that constantly swirl around the topic of nursing responses to euthanasia/AD. On the one hand, an argument may be constructed that euthanasia has no part in everyday nursing practices, i.e., it is essentially unsupported by the World Health Organization, the ICN's Code of Ethics, and that it may contradict selected parts of many other nursing codes of ethics and conduct. Indeed, legalities notwithstanding, it may also be argued that euthanasia may be lawful but not ethical. On the other hand, others would no doubt argue that in fact the practice of euthanasia/AD generally supports at least one highly respected aspect of the ICN and other nursing bodies codes, namely the right of individuals to choose their own destinies by means of their own autonomous decision making. It is then maintained that nurses and doctors should respect this wish above all else and assist them in their need for a premature but less distressing death. In the final analysis, there are no simple solutions, and even the law recognises the enormous personal and psychological challenges faced by doctors and nurses when involved with the consequences of such legislation by means of a built-in 'opt-out' or 'conscience clause'. Then again, there are clearly those doctors and nurses who will indeed be and certainly are (e.g., legally in Canada; and possibly illegally in other nations) willing to perform such acts, and to do so arguably from their own interpretations of their philosophical and professional interpretations. It would also seem that there is at least some evidence to suggest that many nurses remain ambivalent about being taking part in an act of euthanasia, and some even take part (van Bruchem-van de Scheur et al. 2008). Later, evidence from Belgium suggests that the roles played by the nurse in carrying out euthanasia could vary considerably, i.e., there is evidence that beyond patient and family support, some Belgian nurses are involved in the entire process of euthanasia and even in the administration of lethal drugs (Jones, Gastmans and MacKellar 2017).

Finally, it seems only fair to conclude this chapter by at least predicting what might have happened at Havenlea hospice after the two nurses presented their significantly differing perspectives on this troubling issue at the staff meeting. If common examples of a typical response from New Zealand hospices at least are to be examined, then after a period of deliberation that involved staff, volunteers, members of the Board and local 'guidance groups', the hospice management might well have put out a brief and clearly pragmatic public statement in a similar style to the following:

[This] Hospice provides compassionate and non-judgemental care to all of our patients. While we do not provide assisted dying services, we do support patients with their palliative care needs, whether they choose assisted dying or not...Assisted dying is a different service from palliative care.

(Mary Potter Hospice n.d.)

Overall, it may be the case that while there may well be those doctors and nurses who are willing to assist in acts of AD, it is also quite likely that there will be considerable numbers of the same who will not participate. This seems most likely in those cases where nurses (and doctors) are involved in palliative and/or hospice-based services, but not necessarily exclusively so. Such is the contentious nature of medicalised euthanasia which does indeed create a substantial schism of opinion between bioethicists, nurse ethicists and undoubtably between HCPs.

References

Beauchamp, T.L. & Childress, J.F. 2019. *Principles of Bioethics*. 8th Edition. New York: Oxford University Press.

Benedict, S. & Shields, L. (Eds.) 2014. *Nurses and Midwives in Nazi Germany: The "Euthanasia Programs"*. New York: Routledge.

Boudreau, J.D. & Somerville, M.A. 2014. Euthanasia and Assisted Suicide: A Physician's and Ethicist's Perspectives. *Medicolegal and Bioethics* 4: 1–12.

Brassington, I. 2020. What Passive Euthanasia Is. *BMC Medical Ethics* 21: 41. https://doi.org/10.1186/s12910-020-00481-7 [16 June 2022].

Brenan, M. 2018. Americans' Strong Support for Euthanasia Persists. *Gallup*. https://news.gallup.com/poll/235145/americans-strong-support-euthanasia-persists.aspx

British Columbia. n.d. Medical Assistance in Dying (MAiD) PINs. https://www2.gov.bc.ca/gov/content/health/accessing-health-care/home-community-care/care-options-and-cost/end-of-life-care/medical-assistance-in-dying#:~:text=What%20is%20medical%20assistance%20in, only%20available%20to%20eligible% 20individuals. [3 February 2022].

British Medical Association. 2021. Physician Assisted Dying. https://www.bma.org.uk/advice-and-support/ethics/end-of-life/physician-assisted-dying

British Medical Association. 2021. Physician Assisted Dying Survey. https://www.bma.org.uk/advice-and-support/ethics/end-of-life/physician-assisted-dying/physician-assisted-dying-survey [4 April 2022].

Brown, J., Goodridge, D., Thorpe, L. & Crizzle, A. 2021. "What Is right for me, Is not necessarily right for you": The Endogenous Factors Influencing Nonparticipation in Medical Assistance in Dying. *Qualitative Health Research* 31(10): 1786–1800. https://doi.org/10.1177/10497323211008843

Conejero, I., Olié, E., Courtet, P. & Calati, R. 2018. Suicide in Older Adults: Current Perspectives. *Clinical Interventions in Aging* 13: 691–699.

de Bellaigue, C. 2019. Death on Demand: Has Euthanasia Gone Too Far? *The Guardian*. https://www.theguardian.com/news/2019/jan/18/death-on-demand-has-euthanasia-gone-too-far-netherlands-assisted-dying. [18 January 2022].

Dobken, J. H. 2018. Physician-Assisted Suicide (PAS)/Physician-Assisted Death (PAD): The Rise of Lifeboat Ethics. *Journal of the American Physicians and Surgeons* 23(4): 121–124.

Doyal, L. & Doyal, L. 2001. Why Active Euthanasia and Physician Assisted Suicide Should Be Legalised. *BMJ* 323(7321): 1079–1080.

End of Life Choice Act 2019. (New Zealand Parliamentary Council Office). https://www.legislation.govt.nz/act/public/2019/0067/latest/DLM7285905.html [16 June 2022].

Florijn, B.W. 2018. Extending' Euthanasia to those 'tired of living' in the Netherlands Could Jeopardize a Well-Functioning Practice of Physicians' Assessment of a Patient's Request for Death. *Health Policy* 122(3): 315–319.

Fowler, M.D. 2020. Toward Reclaiming Our Ethical Heritage: Nursing Ethics Before Bioethics. *The Online Journal of Issues in Nursing* 25(2). https://ojin.nursingworld.org/MainMenuCategories/ANAMarketplace/ANAPeriodicals/OJIN/TableofContents/Vol-25-2020/No2-May-2020/Toward-Reclaiming-Our-Ethical-Heritage-Nursing-Ethics-before-Bioethics.html

France 24. n.d. 'Dying with dignity': Dutch Mark 20 Years of Euthanasia. https://www.france24.com/en/live-news/20220401-dying-with-dignity-dutch-mark-20-years-of-euthanasia [12 April 2022].

Gluchman, M. 2019. Different Approaches to the Relationship of Life & Death (Review of Articles). *Ethics & Bioethics (in Central Europe)* 9 (1–2): 87–97.

Government of the Netherlands. n.d. Euthanasia, Assisted Suicide and Non-resuscitation on Request. https://www.government.nl/topics/euthanasia/euthanasia-assisted-suicide-and-non-resuscitation-on-request [21 May 2022].

Hartling, O. 2021. Euthanasia and Assisted Dying: The Illusion of Autonomy—An Essay by Ole Hartling. *BMJ* 374. https://doi.org/10.1136/bmj.n2135 (Published 09 September 2021).

Hussain, W. (2018). The Common Good. In E. N. Zalta (Ed.), *The Stanford Encyclopedia of Philosophy* (Spring 2018). Metaphysics Research Lab, Stanford University. https://plato.stanford.edu/archives/spr2018/entries/common-good/

Huxtable, R. 2020. On Killing and Letting Die, Acts and Omissions: For and Against the Distinctions, in Contemporary European Perspectives on the Ethics of End of Life Care. *Philosophy and Medicine* 136: 229–241.

International Council of Nurses. 2012. The ICN Code of Ethics for Nurses. https://www.icn.ch/sites/default/files/inline-files/2012_ICN_Codeofethicsfornurses_%20eng.pdf [7 March 2022].

Jones, D., Gastmans, C. & MacKellar, C. (Eds.) 2017. *Euthanasia and Assisted Suicide: Lessons from Belgium*. Cambridge: Cambridge University Press. https://doi.org/10.1017/9781108182799

Lipscomb, M. 2014. *A Hospice in Change: Applied Social Realist Theory*. Abingdon: Routledge.

Mary Potter Hospice. n.d. *Our Response to the End of Life Choice Act*. https://marypotter.org.nz/about-us/eolca/ [7 March 2022].

New Zealand Nurses Organisation. 2019. *Guideline – Code of Ethics*. https://www.nzno.org.nz/Portals/0/publications/Guideline%20-%20Code%20of%20Ethics%202019.pdf?ver=19LQpYx8wspprjbTNt9pWw%3d%3d [16 June 2022].

New Zealand Nurses Organisation. n.d. Guidelines: Professional Challenges – Assisted Dying Position Statement. http://www.nzno.org.nz/Portals/0/Files/Documents/Consultation/2016%2011%2008%20%20Guidelines %20-%20Assisted%20Dying%20Position%20Statement.pdf [8 March 2022].

Palliative Care Nurses of New Zealand n.d. *Position Statement on Assisted Dying (2021)*. https://pcnnz.co.nz/wp-content/uploads/2021/11/Palliative-Care-Nurses-New-Zealand-position-statement-2021.pdf [25 June 2021].

Pesut, B., Greig, M., Thorne, S., Storch, J., Burgess, M., Tishelman, C., Chambaere, K. & Janke, R. 2020. Nursing and Euthanasia: A Narrative Review of the Nursing Ethics Literature. *Nursing Ethics* 27(1): 152–167.

Raus, K., Vanderhaegen, B. & Sterckx, S. 2021. Euthanasia in Belgium: Shortcomings of the Law and Its Application and of the Monitoring of Practice, *The Journal of Medicine and Philosophy: A Forum for Bioethics and Philosophy of Medicine* 46(1): 80–107.

Rodrigues, P., Crokaert, J. & Gastmans, C. 2018. Palliative Sedation for Existential Suffering: A Systematic Review of Argument-Based Ethics Literature. *Journal of Pain and Symptom Management* 55(6): 1577–1590.

Roy, E.A. 2020. New Zealand Euthanasia Vote: Polls Point to 'yes' Amid Campaign of Fear and Doubt. *The Guardian*, 14 October 2020. https://www.theguardian.com/world/2020/oct/15/new-zealand-euthanasia-vote-polls-point-to-yes-amid-campaign-of-fear-and-doubt [25 May 2022].

Service Public Federal. 2020. *Euthanasie – Chiffres de l'année 2019*. https://organesdeconcertation.sante.belgique.be/sites/default/files/documents/cfcee_chiffres-2019_communiquepresse.pdf [25 May 2022].

Singer, P. 1995. *Rethinking Life and Death: The Collapse of Our Traditional Ethics*. Oxford: Oxford University Press.

Singer, P. 2018. The Challenge of Brain Death for the Sanctity of Life Ethic. *Ethics & Bioethics (in Central Europe)* 8 (3–4): 153–165.

Thienpont, L., Verhofstadt, M., van Loon, T. et al. 2015. Euthanasia Requests, Procedures and Outcomes for 100 Belgian Patients Suffering from Psychiatric Disorders: A Retrospective, Descriptive Study. *BMJ Open* 5: e007454. https://doi.org/10.1136/ bmjopen-2014–007454

Trufin, F. 2021. Behind the Scenes of Euthanasia, in *Euthanasia: Searching for the Full Story*, edited by Timothy Devos. Cham: Springer, 93–103.

van Bruchem-van de Scheur, A., van der Arend, A., van Wijmen, F., Huijer Abu-Saad, H., ter Meulen, R. 2008. Dutch Nurses' Attitudes towards Euthanasia and Physician-Assisted Suicide. *Nursing Ethics* 15(2): 186–198. PMID: 18272609

Wilkinson, J. 1990. The Ethics of Euthanasia. *Palliative Medicine* 4(81): 81–86.

Woods, M. 2011. An Ethic of Care in Nursing: Past, Present and Future Considerations. *Ethics and Social Welfare* 5 (3), 266–276.

Woods, M. 2012. Exploring the Relevance of Social Justice within a Relational Nursing Ethic. *Nursing Philosophy* 13(1), 56–65. https://doi.org/10.1111/j.1466–769X.2011.00525.x

Woods, M. & Rook, H. 2022. Exploring Hospice Nurses' Viewpoints on End-of-Life Practices and Assisted Dying. *Journal of Hospice & Palliative Nursing* 24(4): E117–E125. doi: 10.1097/ NJH.0000000000000861.

World Health Organization. n.d. Definition of Palliative Care. http://www.who.int/cancer/ palliative/definition/en/ [25 May 2022].

World Medical Association. 2019. Declaration on Euthanasia and Physician-Assisted Suicide. Adopted by the 70th WMA General Assembly, Tbilisi, Georgia, October 2019. Ferney-Voltaire (FR): World Medical Association; 2019. https://www.wma.net/policies-post/declaration-on-euthanasia-and-physician-assisted-suicide/ [14 March 2022].

Young, J.E. 2020. Agency, Uncertainty and Power: Why People Consider Assisted Dying at the End of Life. A Thesis submitted for the Degree of Doctor of Philosophy at the University of Otago, Dunedin, Aotearoa New Zealand, April 2020.

21 Care and compassion in nursing

Sigríður Halldórsdóttir

Historical belief in nursing as a caring profession and traditional values of 'care' and 'compassion' embodied in the word 'nursing' are worth preserving for future generations of nurses. Although the concepts care and compassion have been used in the nursing literature for more than 100 years, nurses must keep on undertaking a systematic philosophic and scientific investigation into these important constructs. It has been suggested that care is the essence and the central, unifying, and dominant domain that characterizes nursing (Leininger, 1984), that nursing is the art and science of human caring (Watson, 1979, 1985), and that caring is a core value to the profession of nursing (Brilowski & Wendler, 2005; Khademian & Vizeshfar, 2008). Focusing on being exquisite care providers, therefore, seems rather important. However, there appears to be a lack of consensus around how fundamental aspects of care and compassion are defined. The aim of the chapter is, therefore, to undertake a systematic investigation into care and compassion and to explore the discourse in the nursing literature about care and compassion.

Traditional values of care and compassion in nursing

Caring has been at the heart of nursing's identity before its recognition as a profession or discipline and it can be argued that Nightingale's references to the importance of sensitivity to the patient's experience, tender attendance to the suffering patient's needs and to nursing as a spiritual practice, affirm the primal connection between nursing and caring (Smith, 2012). Examining Nightingale's works, Wagner and Whaite (2010) assert that her compassionate view of humanity, her deep spiritual beliefs, and the military nursing experiences in the Crimea played an important role in her growth as a nurse and that these factors also greatly influenced her development of modern nursing practice. The authors conclude that the phenomenon of caring relationships in nursing has been a part of nursing's language since Florence Nightingale began to organize nursing into a profession and have become a dominant topic in nursing's professional literature. There are common and broad themes from nursing's heritage about the nature of nursing. Watson (1985) has pointed out that one of these themes is of caring as the moral ideal of nursing whereby the end is protection, enhancement, and preservation of human dignity as well as the view of humans as valued persons in and of themselves, to be cared for, respected, nurtured, understood, and assisted. Another broad theme is the human being's need for care and compassion and the third theme is helping the receiver of care to grow, even after trauma. Such post-traumatic growth refers to positive, psychological change in a person, following trauma (Bryngeirsdottir et al., 2022). This is not new in the literature.

DOI: 10.4324/9781003427407-24

Meyeroff (1971) asserts that caring is helping another to grow and being present for the other through knowing self and other.

What is care and compassion?

Nursing has traditionally been concerned with not only people's needs for care, but also with caring as a value or principle for nursing action (Gaut, 1983). It has been suggested that care is central to nursing expertise, to curing, and to healing (Benner & Wrubel, 1989). Care and compassion are constructs that have been approached from various perspectives by nursing scholars. In the 1970s, Leininger (1978) identified care as an essential human need for the full development, health maintenance, and survival of human beings in all world cultures. She later identified caring as the essence of nursing and health (Leininger, 1984) and stated that caring "is the unique, major, boundary feature of nursing, and one of its most promising areas of study" (p. 14). Watson has written about 30 books on various aspects of caring. In her first books, she introduced her ideas on nursing as a philosophy and science of caring (Watson, 1979) and a human science and human care (Watson, 1985). Griffin (1983) states that a nurse's activities in relation to a patient may be called caring only because these acts are performed in a certain way, as the expression of emotions and that some of these emotions have an essentially moral component and that it might not be altogether too far-fetched to identify a dominant emotion in caring as a kind of love.

Another nursing scholar who has made an important contribution to the understanding of care is Gaut (1983) who used a philosophical analysis in her development of a theoretical description of the concept of care. While the empirical researcher asks questions that require the explanation of events and causes, the philosopher asks questions that invite conceptual clarification or justification. According to Gaut (1983), care as a concept comes from the Old English and Gothic words, *carian* and *kara* or *karon*. She claims that used as a verb, *carian* means having concern for, or feel interest in; to provide for or look after; to have an inclination, liking or regard and thus be inclined or disposed to; and to have regard for in the sense of fondness or attachment for. Gaut (1983) claims that care is love, concern, and understanding. When used in the grammatical form, caring denotes doing or action. Gaut states that caring, whether used in common word usage or scholarly literature, seems to involve at least three senses: disposition or feeling within the carer, the doing of certain activities regarded as caring activities, or a combination of both attitude and action in which the caring about the other disposes the person to care for another through the doing of certain activities. Gaut claims that the nurse's action must be judged solely on the welfare of the person being cared for. Similarly, Morse et al. (1990) further examined the concept of caring. They were concerned about the lack of conceptual clarity of caring in the nursing literature. They identified five epistemological perspectives: caring as a human state, caring as a moral imperative or ideal, caring as an affect, caring as an interpersonal relationship, and caring as a nursing intervention. A pioneer in nursing ethics, Sister Simone Roach (2002), developed an influential theory of caring, postulating that caring encompasses seven essential aspects, i.e., compassion, competence, conscience, confidence, commitment, comportment, and creativity. She was the lead architect of the Canadian Nurses Association's first code of ethics, and considered caring and the components of it, including compassion, to be moral virtues, an inner motivation to care (Bradshaw, 2016).

Care and compassion as the material for bridge-building between a nurse and a patient

Hartrick (2008) asserts that nurses can make a profound difference in people's health and healing experiences through their 'relational capacity', characterized by authenticity and responsiveness. A caring relationship between nurse and patient is an essential part of the caring process and can be seen as a nurturing way of being with another that encompasses both attitudes and actions (Wagner & Whaite, 2010). The nurse-patient relationship is by many considered the core of nursing and I developed a theory on the dynamics of the nurse-patient relationship from seven studies which involved interviewing former patients (Halldorsdottir, 2008). I theorized that from the patient's perspective, the caring nurse-patient relationship can be described as a "dynamic lived reality characterized by a sense of spiritual connection which is experienced as a bond made of energy" (Halldorsdottir, 2008, p. 3). From the former patients' perspective, there are certain prerequisites for a nurse-patient relationship to develop. They felt that they had trusted and connected primarily with the nurse perceived as caring, competent, and wise, what I later termed compassionate competence (Halldorsdottir, 2012b). I have theorized that nursing therapeutics operates through compassionate competence with the nurse-patient connection as the essence and through which caring energy is flowing. When provided, it can increase the patient's sense of well-being and health which can be summarized as a sense of being empowered (Halldorsdottir, 1996). When it is not provided, patients experience the opposite, i.e., uncaring, which can discourage patients and even disempower them. It is clear from listening to former patients that they do not connect with nurses whom they do not experience as caring and, therefore, trust. This aspect of the nurse-patient relationship needs to be better explored in the nursing literature. Moreover, the fact that some nurses are uncaring and therefore not trusted by patients needs to be discussed in more depth in the literature. Thus, care and compassion are the material for the bridge-building between the nurse and the patient as well as the nurse's competence in connecting with patients. For many of the former patients, this nurse-patient relationship constituted the fundamental difference between caring and uncaring. Compassion, however, was perceived by the former patients as the kind of attitude that makes up compassionate competence.

Care and compassion as an acknowledgement of our humanhood

According to Fromm (2000), there are four basic needs of the human being: the need for connection, care, respect, and knowledge. He contends that the deepest need of the human being is the need to overcome one's own separateness and leave the prison of our own aloneness. He asserts that love, or caring, is an active power in man, a power which breaks through the walls which separate human beings from their fellow humans. Meyeroff (1971) explains that to care for other persons, we must be able to understand those persons and their world as if we were inside it. He emphasizes that in being with another, we must not lose ourselves. We must retain our own identity and be aware of our own reactions to the person. Seeing this person's world as it appears to him- or herself does not mean having that person's reactions to it, and thus we are able to help persons in their world: something they might be unable to do for themselves. A final note about this matter is Watson's (2003) invitation to return to the heart and soul of nursing and to our deep humanity. She has been untiring in pointing out the steadily growing body of empirical evidence which supports the idea that the quality of one's relationship with another person is the most significant element in determining helping effectiveness. She contends that a basic element of high-quality care is the development of a relationship. She asserts that to develop such a relationship, the nurse must first get to know the other person. Watson has always emphasized in her works that the nurse must also examine how she regards other human beings – as objects to be manipulated and treated, or as human beings to be understood and cared for. She contends that nurses attain and promote health and higher-level functioning only if they form person-to-person relationship as opposed to manipulative relationships (Watson, 2003, 2004).

Rediscovering care and compassion as the basis of our existence

How do we see the human being? How do we see the nurse? How do we see ourselves? The themes of the universal interconnectedness and interdependence of all, and the intrinsically dynamic nature of reality are recurrent in mystical thought of many different religious traditions, primarily the understanding that we are not only physical beings but also spiritual beings and deeply connected with others. This means that the moment we come out of our isolated individual existence and begin to care for others, to offer ourselves more to our fellow human beings, we become true to our nature. This also means that we need to develop not only as professionals but also as human beings; we need to grow in care and compassion. My understanding is that care and compassion are born of love and can fittingly be called the citadel of the virtues and that we should make every effort until we attain these important virtues. Care and compassion illuminate us with illuminating energies and nurture practical goodness. When it is authentic, we will be sensitive to the needs of the other and respond with generosity. Moreover, care and compassion must be based on respect and goodwill; then, a bridge is built between people. If respect is missing, you come too close for comfort to the other which can lead to over-familiarity. If care and compassion are missing, you can become too distant, leading to indifference and a wall (Halldorsdottir, 1996). The nature of care and compassion is that it is diffusive, unifying, and transforming. There must be a serious intention to be caring and compassionate. Out of all the various things that clamour for our attention, it may not be easy to prioritize care and compassion. However, basically, care and compassion call us to a radical personal commitment.

The powerful effects of positive emotions like care and compassion

Perhaps we have tended to ignore the power of positive emotions both in the nurse and in the patient. However, now we know that experiencing positive emotions has a hidden value that can directly affect and improve well-being on a day-to-day basis. Fredrickson (2013) is a leading scholar within social psychology, affective science, and positive psychology. She claims that positive emotions build our resilience, the emotional resources needed for coping and broadening our awareness, letting us see more options for problem solving. She refers to studies that show that people feel and do their best when they have at least three times as many positive emotions as negative ones and maintains that positive emotions influence how our brains work and act like nutrients. She also explains the importance of 'micro moments' of positive connection with another and how day-to-day experiences of positive emotions add up to make our physical hearts healthier and more resilient. She, therefore, encourages the cultivation of positivity and compassion to nourish our health and well-being.

Care and compassion and the genuineness of the intention

Listening to former patients on their experiences of care and compassion in nursing (Halldorsdottir, 1996, 2012a, 2012b) has illuminated my perspective on care and compassion as the heart of nursing, fuelled by genuine concern and love (caritas, agape, bhakti), a synthesis of feelings and actions that lead to nursing care deemed by the patient or client as caring. It is my understanding that caring is a force that gives us the motive for action and caring must not only be a matter of words but must show itself in action. Without care and compassion, nursing is incomplete. That said, after having interviewed numerous former patients about care and compassion over the years, it has become clear to me that care and compassion without competence often have limited value for patients. Patients' need for care and compassion is unquestioned. However, the artificial dichotomy between caring and competence found in the nursing literature is most unfortunate, given that nursing is a practical science in which competence is primary, especially from the patient's perspective. One woman whom I interviewed about her experience of caring and uncaring said, "I mean, who would want to go to a dentist who is not competent, however, caring the dentist is, who would want to? I mean the competence is primary for all health professions!" From my perspective, nursing is an autonomous scholarly discipline with its own objectives and specialized service, which I have theorized is provided through the nurse's compassionate competence, i.e., caring, competence, wisdom, attentiveness, communication, and connection, together with self-knowledge and self-development of the nurse (Halldorsdottir, 2012a, 2012b). It is my theory, based on actual patient accounts, that competence administered with care and compassion is the ideal situation and that compassionate competence is the unique contribution of nursing and enhances the well-being of the patient. Using the metaphor of a bridge, a caring encounter may be seen as openness in communication that creates a connection between the nurse and the patient. The caring nurse is skilful, knowledgeable, and committed to the provision of personalized care, and knows how to safeguard the personal integrity and dignity of each person who is a patient (Halldorsdottir, 1996).

Actual patient accounts on the quality of the intention: a few vignettes

Here are a few vignettes which gives important insight into the patient's perspective on the quality of intention we call care and compassion:

FORMER PATIENT: I guess the business of caring is something more than doing duty, that is something that recognized the individuality of the patient, or just seemed to have different kind of intention, that is, where the intention seemed more genuine to comfort.

FORMER PATIENT: There was something in our conversation, which indicated she cared.. about other than that I was a patient in a bed.

FORMER PATIENT: I'm not referring to the mechanics of caring, but in genuinely wishing the patient well, that is wishing the patient speedy recovery. I guess it's having those feelings, I mean it's more than just thinking "wouldn't it be nice if Mary Jones would be able to leave the hospital". It's a feeling tone. I say that because I'm suspicious that people pick up on the feeling tone, so if in fact you're indifferent [and] you just say that, you know, that he or she will be able to leave soon, it's nowhere near as effective and caring as if there really is genuine caring. So, it's a kind of a spiritual dimension to it. It's somehow that it matters, you know, it's almost tangible that it matters to someone that you graduate from the hospital, that you leave … upon your feet.

One former patient answered thus when asked about the fundamental difference between caring and uncaring:

It seems to me primarily *the quality of the intention*, which is a hard thing to specify, you sort of, you feel it, and intuitively, I guess … in the transaction. So, it's not what's done it's the way it's done. … The focus seemed to be on how I *felt*, rather than discharging the responsibility. Not "the patient in room 316 is now done" and I can go back to the next chore and so on. It was more to make sure that I really was o.k.

The discourse on care and compassion in the nursing literature

Much has been written on care and compassion in the nursing literature. What are the key common factors in that discourse? What are the main issues? In an exploratory, cross-sectional descriptive study, using the International Online Compassion Questionnaire, a total of 1,323 nurses from 15 countries completed the questionnaire (Papadopoulos et al., 2016). Most participants (59.5%) defined compassion as "Deep awareness of the suffering of others and wish to alleviate it" but definitions of compassion varied by country. Of participants, 69.6% thought that compassion was very important in nursing and more than half (59.6%) of them argued that compassion could be taught. However, only 26.8% reported that the correct amount and level of teaching are provided. Most of the participants (82.6%) stated that their patients prefer knowledgeable nurses with good interpersonal skills. Interestingly, only 4.3% of the nurses noted that they were receiving compassion from their managers. A significant relationship was found between nurses' experiences of compassion and their views about teaching of compassion.

Von Dietze and Orb (2001) claim that compassion is often considered to be an essential component of nursing care; that is, however, difficult to identify what exactly comprises compassionate care and that compassion is more than just a natural response to suffering; rather, it is a moral choice. Feo et al. (2018), however, claim that the literature on compassionate care has primarily focused on the moral attributes of nurses and their ability to establish meaningful connections with patients and that the literature on fundamentals of care has been split between describing such care as a list of nursing activities and describing it as a complex, multidimensional construct. Durkin et al. (2018) have also asserted that nurses embody and enact compassion through behaviours such as spending time with patients, communicating effectively with them and that patients experience compassion through a sense of togetherness with nurses and compassionate practice is presented by Durkin et al. (2021) as an overarching theme involving three themes: (1) amalgamation of various knowledges and skills, (2) delivery of meaningful actions which alleviate suffering, and (3) meeting individual needs and prevention of further preventable suffering. The expression of compassion by health professionals, they claim, involves the fusion of knowledge and many skills and patients received compassion through the actions of the nurse who alleviated their suffering.

Patient vulnerability

Where is the patient in all this? Hospitals can be very lonely places and it is easy for the patient to get the sense that no one cares – to feel that he or she is just a thing which is being manipulated. To feel genuinely cared for and becoming connected with a wise, caring, and competent nurse changes the experience absolutely and the patient gets a sense of solidarity, an increased sense of security, health, and well-being (Halldorsdottir, 2012a, 2012b). From research findings in psychoneuroimmunology, we now know that the change can indeed be powerful (Halldorsdottir, 2007). Patients' vulnerability in the hospital context is a reality that must be taken into consideration by nurses and other health professionals. Not having a sense of control over yourself or your own situation and feeling often weak in spirit and body makes the average patient feel dependant and defenceless, which means that patients are potentially more deeply affected by health professionals' 'mode of being'. Patients' vulnerability may even be even more pronounced by other factors, such as economic impoverishment, violence, homelessness, alcohol, or drug problem, to name only a few vulnerable groups. Therefore, if meaningful and respectful nurse-patient connections, or for that matter any health care relationships, are to develop with responsible participation of both parties, culture and context must be considered. Furthermore, groups of people that can be perceived as having a degree of responsibility of bringing about their illness or painful situation may be even more vulnerable as patients in that may not be treated as equally dignified human beings as other patients.

Five basic modes of being with another

Riemen (1986) did a very interesting study on patients' experiences of caring and noncaring in the clinical setting. She asserts that being existentially present or available, showing genuine interest in the client as a valued individual by really listening, is considered by clients to be one of the most important aspects of caring. Research on caring and uncaring encounters with nurses and other health professionals from the patient's perspective started with Riemen (1986) and can be seen as a continuation of Nightingale's quest to delineate what nursing is and what it is not (1859/1992). I have postulated, however, that caring and uncaring should not be considered an either/or phenomenon; that there are indeed at least five basic modes of being with another (Halldorsdottir, 2012a):

1. The life-giving (biogenic) mode of being with another, where one affirms the personhood of the other by connecting with the true centre of the other in a life-giving way. *This involves care, compassion, and connection which results in the patient's empowerment.*
2. The life-sustaining (bioactive) mode where one supports and acknowledges the personhood of the other but the life-giving connection does not develop. *This involves care which results in the patient's encouragement.*
3. The life-neutral (biopassive) mode where one does not affect life in the other (neither caring nor uncaring). *This mode of being does not affect the patient.*
4. The life-restraining (biostatic) mode where one is insensitive or indifferent to the other, causing discouragement, developing uneasiness in the other, and negatively affecting existing life in the other. *This involves uncaring which results in the patient's discouragement.*

5. The life-destroying (biocidic) mode of being with another where one depersonalizes the other, destroys joy of life, and increases the other's vulnerability. It causes distress and even despair. It is the transference of negative energy and is often seen in violence. *This mode of being results in the recipients' disempowerment.*

In my conceptualization of the five basic modes of being with another, the basic idea is how a person, who is in a position of power, exercises that power: gives it to the other (empowering mode), shares it with the other (encouraging mode), does not use it (passive mode), misuses it (discouraging mode), or abuses it (disempowering mode).

The life-giving nurses

According to the former patients I have interviewed, the life-giving nurses are very special people (Halldorsdottir, 2008). They seem to be illuminated with the consciousness of spiritual knowledge and seem to be filled with genuine caring. Their thoughts seem to be full of loving-kindness and compassion which spring from love for their fellow human beings. Their cheerful good-willed presence was an element that was extremely important for the patients within the, often, grim reality of the hospital situation. The interesting works by Stithatos (1995a, 1995b, 1995c) have helped me to understand the life-giving nurses. Paraphrasing his words, in them is not bitterness or anger but luminosity and sweetness of a godlike love. They are light because they are virtuous in life, lucid in speech, and wise in thought; they are rich in divine knowledge and 'strong in the wisdom of love'; they are life-giving because through their words they can bring life to those who are in the pit of despair. Through 'the light of their works', they shine before fellow human beings and illuminate them; with the sweet astringency of their words, they brace those who are suffering and by the life present in what they say, 'they give life to those who feel dead'. It seems that the life-giving soul cannot remain static or fixed but aspires to keep on knowing own self and keep on developing and growing. The metaphor of 'a bridge' symbolizes the bond of energy which is perceived by some between heart and heart when a connection has been developed through caring encounters between the life-giving nurse and the patient. It never ceases to astound me to hear former patients tell their stories about the power of the life-giving nurses. They amaze me; they inspire me and impress me. They are dedicated to their hidden spiritual work of nursing and, labourers of care and compassion that they are, they never seem to waver in their love for their fellow human beings.

Here is one former patient's testament where the life-giving nurse's care and compassion possibly saved his life:

> I guess my feeling was, just some relief that I was being cared for. I think in the absence of it I would have felt very alone and very depressed and could well have ... gotten sicker. In fact, it strikes me that it wouldn't take much depression before I became indifferent to whether or not I recovered, and that could easily become a self-fulfilling prophecy. I mean if I didn't have the will to live, I mean the likelihood that drugs would force me to live might be remote, because I was very sick, and without the will, who knows?

Future directions

It is up to nursing as a profession to decide what kind of care and compassion it will work to support for the benefit of the giver as well as the receiver of care. If nurses want to become known as care providers and advocates, however, they must become knowledgeable about care and compassion from the patient's point of view since it is logical to assume that the best source of information about the patient is the patient. It is primarily when care and compassion are studied from the patient's perspective that progress can be made in providing them with the quality of nursing care that can be identified and labelled by them as care and compassion. The way I see it there is a need for care and compassion in today's world especially within health care. I see nursing as the manifestation and the professionalization of care and compassion. To care about a human being in need, and thus caring as a moral ideal, was the origination of nursing. In my opinion, what we need most of all today, to promote the art and science of nursing is compassionate competence, which I see as the essential ingredients of nursing. Care and compassion provide nurses with a vision based on real-life experiences of former patients, a vision that can give nurses metaphorically speaking a goal, a map, and a possibility to direct themselves to a desired end, i.e., increased well-being and health of patients. It gives a vision of nursing practice not of being a mere technology but rather *a mode of being* and *a mode of connecting with the person who is a patient*. I propose that a caring connection with a nurse is a key to a perception of a caring encounter with a nurse from the patient's perspective.

Allowing care and compassion to shape the design of health care organizations means that the idea of prioritizing the nurse-patient relationship should be reflected in all aspects of the organization, from philosophy to work design to individual job descriptions. It might, for instance, be reflected through adoption of departmental philosophies and structure that empower nurses to be caring and compassionate and to develop caring connections with patients. Such emphasis gives directions as to what is important in the education of nurses, what attitudes and skills should be cultivated in nursing students so that the patient is more likely to develop a nurse-patient relationship with them as students and later as nurses. Teaching an ideology of care and compassion necessitates introducing the patient's perspective in nursing education. The interest of nurse researchers and theorists in care and compassion with the nurse-patient relationship in focus has been growing over the last 20 years. However, we still have a great deal to learn about the life-giving nurses, who are, from the patients' perspective, the true experts in care and compassion.

Conclusion

In this chapter, I have analysed care and compassion as constructs and the traditional values of care and compassion in nursing. I have proposed that care and compassion are the material for bridge-building between a nurse and a patient. Moreover, I have claimed that care and compassion are an acknowledgement of our humanhood, and that it is indeed the basis of our existence. Furthermore, I have analysed the powerful effects of positive emotions like care and compassion and given some actual examples of what former patients have told me when I interviewed them. I briefly summarized the discourse on care and compassion in the nursing literature as well as what it is like to be a patient in the health care system. Finally, I claimed that caring and compassion or uncaring are perhaps an oversimplification, and that there are indeed more shades to these human phenomena.

If we turn into the right direction, it is enough to carry on walking

References

Benner P., Wrubel J. (1989) *The Primacy of Caring: Stress and Coping in Health and Illness.* Addison-Wesley.

Bradshaw A. (2016). 'An analysis of England's nursing policy on compassion and the 6Cs: The hidden presence of M. Simone Roach's model of caring'. *Nursing Inquiry*, 23(1), pp. 78–85. Available at: https://pubmed.ncbi.nlm.nih.gov/26059388/

Brilowski GA, Wendler MC. (2005) 'An evolutionary concept analysis of caring'. *Journal of Advanced Nursing*, 50, pp. 641–650. Available at: https://doi.org/10.1111/j.1365-2648.2005.03449.x

Bryngeirsdottir HS, Arnault DS, Halldorsdottir S. (2022) The post-traumatic growth journey of women who have survived intimate partner violence: A synthesized theory emphasizing obstacles and facilitating factors. *International Journal of Environmental Research and Public Health*, 19(14), p. 8653. Available at: https://pubmed.ncbi.nlm.nih.gov/35886504/

Durkin J, Jackson D, Usher K. (2021) 'Compassionate practice in a hospital setting. Experiences of patients and health professionals: A narrative inquiry'. *Journal of Advanced Nursing*, 78(4), pp. 1112–1127. Available at: https://onlinelibrary.wiley.com/doi/full/10.1111/jan.15089

Durkin J, Usher K, Jackson D. (2018) 'Embodying compassion: A systematic review of the views of nurses and patients. *Journal of Clinical Nursing*, 28(9–10), pp. 1380–1392. Available at: https://pubmed.ncbi.nlm.nih.gov/30485579/

Feo R, Kitson A, Conroy T. (2018) 'How fundamental aspects of nursing care are defined in the literature: A scoping review'. *Journal of Clinical Nursing*, 27(11–12), pp. 2189–2229. Available at: https://pubmed.ncbi.nlm.nih.gov/29514402/

Fredrickson PL. (2013) *Love 2.0: Creating Happiness and Health in Moments of Connection.* Avery.

Fromm E. (1956/2000) *The Art of Loving.* Harper Perennial.

Gaut DA. (1983) 'Development of a theoretically adequate description of caring'. *Western Journal of Nursing Research*, 5(4), pp. 313–324.

Griffin AP. (1983) 'Philosophy and nursing'. *Journal of Advanced Nursing*, 5, pp. 261–272.

Halldorsdottir S. (1996) *Caring and uncaring encounters in nursing and health care: Developing a theory.* Linköping University Medical Dissertations No 493. Department of Caring Sciences, Faculty of Health Sciences, Linköping University, Linköping, Sweden. Available at: http://www.diva-portal.org/smash/get/diva2:248040/FULLTEXT01.pdf

Halldorsdottir S. (2007). 'A psychoneuroimmunological view of the healing potential of professional caring in the face of human suffering'. *International Journal for Human Caring*, 11(2), pp. 32–39.

Halldorsdottir S. (2008). 'The dynamics of the nurse–patient relationship: Introduction of a synthesized theory from the patient's perspective'. *Scandinavian Journal of Caring Sciences*, 22(4), pp. 643–652. Available at: https://doi.org/10.1111/j.1471-6712.2007.00568.x

Halldorsdottir S. (2012a) 'Five basic modes of being with another'. In MC Smith, MC Turkel, ZR Wolf (Eds.), *Caring in Nursing Classics: An Essential Resource* (pp. 201–210). Springer.

Halldorsdottir S. (2012b) 'Nursing as compassionate competence: A theory on professional nursing care based on the patient's perspective'. *International Journal for Human Caring*, 16(2), pp. 7–19.

Hartrick G. (2008) 'Relational capacity: The foundation for interpersonal nursing practice'. *Journal of Advanced Nursing*, 26, pp. 523–528. Available at: https://pubmed.ncbi.nlm.nih.gov/9378873/

Khademian Z, Vizeshfar F. (2008) 'Nursing students' perceptions of the importance of caring behaviors'. *Journal of Advanced Nursing*, 61(4), pp. 456–462. Available at: https://doi.org/10.1111/j.1365-2648.2007.04509.x

Leininger M. (1978) *Transcultural Nursing: Concepts, Theories, and Practices.* John Wiley & Sons.

Leininger M. (1984) *Care: The Essence of Nursing and Health.* Charles B. Slack.

Meyeroff M. (1971) *On caring.* Harper & Row.

Morse JM, Solberg SM, Neander WL, Bottorff JL, Johnson JL. (1990) 'Concepts of caring and caring as concept'. *Advances in Nursing Science*, 13(1), pp. 1–14. Available at: https://pubmed.ncbi.nlm.nih.gov/2122796/

Nightingale F. (1859/1992) *Notes on Nursing: What It Is, and What It Is Not* (First edition printed in 1859 in London/commemorative edition 1992). JB Lippincott.

Papadopoulos I, Zorba A, Koulouglioti C, Ali S, Aagard M, Akman O, Alpers L-M, Apostolara P, Biles J. et al. (2016) 'International study on nurses' views and experiences of compassion'. *International Nursing Review*, 63(3), pp. 395–405. Available at: https://doi.org/10.1111/inr.12298.

Riemen DJ. (1986) 'Noncaring and caring in the clinical setting: Patients' descriptions'. *Topics in Clinical Nursing*, 8, pp. 30–36. Available at: https://pubmed.ncbi.nlm.nih.gov/3636032/

Roach MS. (2002) *Caring, the Human Mode of Being: A Blueprint for the Health Professions* (2nd rev. ed.). Ottawa: Canadian Healthcare Association Press. Copy from Archives of Caring in Nursing, Christine E. Lynn College of Nursing, Florida Atlantic University, ARC-005 Sister M. Simone Roach Papers, 1958–2005, used by permission. Available at: https://nursing.fau.edu/uploads/images/Caring%20the%20human%20mode%20of%20being_smallsize-PW.pdf

Smith MC. (2012) 'Caring and the discipline of nursing'. In MC Smith, MC Turkel, ZR Wolf (Eds.), *Caring in Nursing Classics: An Essential Resource Caring in Nursing Classics: An Essential Resource* (pp. 1–8). Springer.

Stithatos N. (1995a) 'On the practice of the virtues: One hundred texts'. In *The Philokalia: The Complete Text* (GEH Palmer, P Sherrard, K Ware (translators), pp. 79–106). Faber and Faber.

Stithatos, N. (1995b) 'On the inner nature of things and on the purification of the intellect (nous): One hundred texts'. In *The Philokalia: The Complete Text* (GEH Palmer, P Sherrard, K Ware (translators), pp. 107–138). Faber and Faber.

Stithatos N. (1995c) 'On spiritual knowledge, love, and the perfection of living: One hundred texts'. In *The Philokalia: The Complete Text* (GEH Palmer, P. Sherrard, K Ware (translators), pp. 139–174). Faber and Faber.

Von Dietze E, Orb A. (2001) 'Compassionate care: A moral dimension of nursing'. *Nursing Inquiry*, 7(3), pp. 166–174. Available at: https://doi.org/10.1046/j.1440-1800.2000.00065.x

Wagner DJ, Whaite B. (2010) 'An exploration of the nature of caring relationships in the writings of Florence Nightingale'. *Journal of Holistic Nursing*, 28(4), pp. 225–234.

Watson J. (1979) *Nursing: The philosophy and science of caring*. Little, Brown.

Watson J. (1985) *Nursing: Human science and human care*. Appleton-Century-Crofts.

Watson J. (2003) 'Love and caring: Ethics of face and hands – An invitation to return to the heart and soul of nursing and our deep humanity'. *Nursing Administration Quarterly*, 27, pp. 197–202. Available at: https://pubmed.ncbi.nlm.nih.gov/13677183/

Watson J. (2004) *Caring Science as Sacred Science*. Lotus Library.

Part 4

Socio-contextual and political concerns

22 Nursing's endless pursuit of professionalization

Denise J. Drevdahl and Mary K. Canales

In a United States (U.S.) county jail, Diana Sanchez, pregnant and in labor for hours, gave birth sans medical supervision or treatment, despite repeatedly informing jail and nursing staff that she was having contractions (Chiu, 2019). Notified that Ms. Sanchez' water broke, the nurse responded that Ms. Sanchez was already scheduled to go to the hospital, so she didn't need medical care (Chiu, 2019). A 2019 lawsuit filed on Ms. Sanchez' behalf alleged that "instead of ensuring that Ms. Sanchez was able to give birth in a safe and sanitary medical setting, nurses and deputies callously made her labor alone for hours" (Chiu, paragraph 2). In an interview after the lawsuit was filed, Ms. Sanchez stated that what hurt more than the pain and suffering she endured was "the fact that nobody cared" (Chiu, paragraph 3). In 2020, Ms. Sanchez settled with the City of Denver, Colorado for $160,000 and with Denver Health for $320,000, twice the amount since they employed the nurses who were deemed "more culpable" (Low, 2020).

Although we would like to believe that Ms. Sanchez' experience was an isolated incident, research on the global mistreatment of women in childbirth suggests otherwise. Recent studies identify the poor treatment women receive during childbirth, including from nurses (Adu-Bonsaffoh et al., 2022; Bohren et al., 2014). These nurses are not who we envision (or hope) nurses should be. One vision of today's nurse is that of the caring and benevolent health care provider (van der Cingel & Brouwer, 2021); yet, Ms. Sanchez explicitly noted that it was the absence of caring that was most distressing (Chiu, 2019). If the nurse is supposed to represent the profession – a profession that promotes the *good* nurse as one who embodies caring, honesty, devotion, and trust, among other virtues (Bell, 2020) – how do we reconcile this portrayal with reports of the *uncaring* nurse?

Image and identity are closely linked as the nursing image that is projected to the world assists in establishing the discipline's identity (Samaniego & Cárcamo, 2013). Today, nursing's professional image and identity are synonymous with care and caring. Although *caring about* engenders notions of concern for the welfare of others, it is not necessarily equivalent to *caring for* – with the latter term viewed as *care work* – that is, "organizing, supervising, or paying for practical care" (Abbott & Meerabeau, 1998, p. 11). We believe that the nurse can *care* for a patient without *caring about* that patient. Although there are legal mechanisms to deal with nurses who physically harm someone, limited attention has been given to nurses who violate nursing's espoused caring image. Nursing rarely acknowledges the existence of nurses who inflict emotional and psychological harm through actions that may be seen as indifferent, unsympathetic, or callous, actions that might also be categorized as racist, classist, homophobic, ableist, or ageist. Preserving a certain picture of nursing has overshadowed the discipline's purpose of protecting the public good.

DOI: 10.4324/9781003427407-26

Modern-day nursing has struggled to create a depiction of nursing such that the occupation is awarded the respect and recognition offered to other occupations in the health sciences, particularly medicine (Godsey et al., 2020; Smith et al., 2021). In seeking this affirmation, agencies and organizations overseeing nursing practice and education have imitated medicine with respect to requiring adherence to competencies, standards, domains, essentials, and similar requirements that supposedly mark an occupation as a credible profession.[1] Competencies and the virtues that undergird them advance a certain image of what constitutes nursing and what it means to be a nurse.

In this chapter, we consider the relationship between competencies and nurses' identity as professionals and raise questions, such as: Is being a nurse freely chosen or do parameters set by the discipline limit who can be a nurse? Why is nursing "obsessed with the idea" of being seen as a profession (Salvage, 1985, p. 89)? What are the consequences of demanding nurses take up certain virtues, such as courage and compassion? What happens if the professed image of nursing is not upheld? We consider these questions and raise others knowing that the answers are, no doubt, elusive, but still worth investigating. We start with an examination of nursing's professionalization project.

The professionalization project

Nursing has spent over a century shaping and reshaping itself, trying to be worthy of the title *profession* – its professionalization project. The discipline appears absorbed with its professional identity in ways that other occupations, especially medicine, are not (Bell, 2020). Windsor et al. (2012, p. 220) asked, "whether or not the promise of the professionalization movement was (and remains) an illusion"? We ask not just if this "promise" is an illusion, but if it is a project worth pursuing?

Discussion of the professionalization project starts with defining what is meant by *profession*. Professions began with the creation of universities and were the label given to those occupations for which an "elite education" was essential (Abbott & Meerabeau, 1998, p. 2). By the 19th century, professions were seen as "superior occupations, requiring intellectual training, a body of expert knowledge, [and] a degree of self-regulation by a professional body" (Abbott & Meerabeau, 1998, p. 3). For centuries, theology, medicine, and law were considered *the* established professions (Fowler, 2015), while the so-called *semi-professions* included occupations such as nursing, social work, and pharmacy (Abbott & Meerabeau, 1998). Given nursing's recent movement into university settings, its relatively short period of required education (sometimes only two years) compared to physician training, its limited theoretical grounding, and its relatively limited amount of autonomy (Manley, 1995), it is not surprising that some still consider it not quite a profession (Abbott & Meerabeau, 1998; Freidson, 2001). Neither nursing education's transition from the hospital to the university, nor the addition of graduate degrees has altered nursing's status within the medical hierarchy. For example, in the U.S., nurse practitioners remain locked in battles with physicians regarding scope of practice, including prescriptive authority (American Society of Anesthesiologists, 2022; Cheny, 2019). These battles reflect how nurses across the globe continue to be viewed as subordinate and subservient to physicians and the health systems in which they work (López-Verdugo, et al., 2021; Teresa-Morales, et al., 2022).

For Hugman (1991), professions are "not types of occupations, but historical forms of controlling occupations" (p. 82); thus, a profession is a mechanism by which power is exerted over an occupation (Hugman, 1991). Beyond Nightingale's early efforts to bring legitimacy and respect to nursing, the modern-day push to professionalize (and control) nursing began in earnest in the early 20th century with the drive for licensure (U.S.) or registration (United Kingdom [U.K.]) (Woods, 1987). Through such efforts, nurses and other interested parties were able to regulate those who they viewed as *unqualified*, as well as the overall supply of nurses (Hugman, 1991). Authority over nursing knowledge was a critical element of early attempts at professionalism, particularly later in the 20th century when nursing education shifted to the university. From Salvage's (1985) perspective, the professionalization project is more about serving nursing's interests – gaining power, autonomy, recognition – than about improving patient care.

Fowler (2015) asserts that "from the earliest moments of the rise of modern nursing, its leaders understood nursing to be a *true* profession" (p. 33) (emphasis added). Why the insistence and need to be seen as a "true profession"? Fowler tells us in a footnote to her *Guide to Nursing's Social Policy Statement*:

> With the status of profession, occupational groups have social prestige, authority, recognition, and financial reward. All this gives them power. That power can be used altruistically to benefit society and be a moral force for good, or selfishly to reinforce monopolistic power elites, restrain other groups, garner excessive wealth, exploit those needing their services and increase political power
>
> (p. 35)

Our sense is that Fowler believes nursing falls within the altruistic use of power. However, we believe that it is not that straightforward and nursing exerts power for altruistic, as well as selfish reasons. Fowler wistfully asks, "is there hope that nursing might take its rightful place among the elite professions" (p. 45)? A few pages later, she answers her own query, proclaiming: "nursing has taken its place in society fully as a profession" (p. 53). Rather than wondering *if or when* nursing will be recognized as a profession (let alone an "elite" one), we should ask if we should even try to be a profession and if so, what do we mean by *profession* and what do we want a profession *to do*? Will being labeled a profession improve patient care? Advance nurses' autonomy? Provide for better working conditions? Make for a better, more caring nurse? It is not a given that attaining professional status assists in meeting any of these goals. What the professionalization project *does* seem to be about is social position. As Titmuss claimed, "professionals are pre-eminently people with status problems" (as cited in Hugman, 1991, p. 8).

The drive toward professionalization and the desire for power within health care institutions and over certain provider groups have fostered machinations that close off nursing to certain groups, such as low-income and racial-ethnic minorities (Goubert et al., 2021). This closure is enacted through a variety of education and licensure regulations. The title *professional* necessitates certain behaviors, knowledge, attitudes, and or virtues, often referred to collectively as competencies. It is these competencies – gained primarily through education – that determine who is allowed into the profession, thus distinguishing between someone who can claim the title *professional* and someone who cannot. As such, the competencies used to demarcate nursing actions constitute an ongoing discourse on professionalism. Much as we question the purpose of professionalization, similar concerns should be raised about competencies. Are competencies about protecting patients' health or protecting nursing's identity and status? What are the links among competencies, professional image, and creating the virtuous nurse? These questions as well as others are taken up next.

Nursing's pursuit of competencies

Nursing's efforts to be seen as a *true elite* profession often mimic medicine. For example, after physicians created medical diagnoses, nurses introduced nursing diagnoses (Gebbie & Lavin, 1974). Once medicine moved to competency-based medical education (ten Cate, 2017), nursing followed suit. The American Association of Colleges of Nursing (AACN) "bold[ly]" stated that the new AACN education essentials "represent academic nursing's best thinking on how to prepare nurses using a competency-based approach to education, *which is similar to how physicians… are prepared*" (AACN, 2021b; emphasis added).

Medicine's shift from process-based to competency-based education was primarily propelled by its desire to be accountable to the public (Carraccio et al., 2002). Nursing's stated reasons for turning to competencies are similar, but nursing education more explicitly focuses on preparing "work ready" graduates (AACN, 2021a, p. 5). From this perspective, nursing competencies are meant primarily to meet potential employers' needs. For many, however, the notion that competency-based education will produce a *practice ready* nurse is preposterous and unachievable. The editor of a U.S. nursing education journal recently wrote that expecting new graduates to function independently in today's complex health care settings, even with the benefit of a residency program, is "unrealistic" and even harmful to new nurses as it sends the message that there is something *wrong* with the individual if they are not ready to function at a high-level post-graduation (Yoder-Wise, 2022, p. 387). Darbyshire et al. (2019) go further: "the term 'work ready' is so teeth-grindingly awful and devoid of shared meaning that its decline cannot come too quickly…We know of no other graduates who are expected to be 'work ready' in the sense that nursing uses it" (p. 1). Creating competencies to meet employers' demands rather than those of the discipline itself (Windsor et al., 2012) echoes points made by Abbott and Meereabeau over 20 years ago when they observed:

> Groups who aspire to professional status are laying themselves open to being controlled by externally-defined standards – a professional discourse which both defines what is to be counted as professional behaviour and targets those who are perceived not to conform to it
>
> (1998, p. 16)

The professionalism discourse both demarcates the outlines of the group and, at the same time, constricts and restricts how the group is *allowed* to function (e.g., when nursing endeavors to satisfy employers). When others outside the discipline label something as nursing or *not nursing,* or as professional or *unprofessional,* it reinforces the idea that a profession is "a construct of domination" (Bell, 2020, p. 2 of 12).

Beyond the issue of *who* competencies are developed *for,* competencies raise other problematic concerns, beginning with differing competency definitions (Lurie, 2012; Windsor et al., 2012). Lack of a standardized definition limits evaluation across competency sets (Larsen & Reif, 2019), while sparse data demonstrating their effectiveness (Carraccio et al., 2002) prompt concerns about whether the various guidelines can be accurately evaluated (Lurie, 2012; Windsor et al., 2012). Multiple authors have questioned the persistent turn to competencies, given the non-existent evidence that they produce highly skilled nurses or improve patient care (Canales & Drevdahl, 2022; Grant, 1999; Pijl-Zieber et al., 2014).

Additionally, competencies often do not lend themselves to being quantifiable. Lurie (2012) doubted that any effort to make competencies "more measurable" would be successful (p. 212), which seems particularly salient, given recent efforts to transform personal values and characteristics into presumably measurable skills. For example, in the U.S., newly graduated nurses are to demonstrate "compassionate caring," "humility," and "empathy" (AACN, 2021a); Province of Alberta, Canada nurses are asked to exhibit "professional presence," defined as "confidence, integrity, optimism, passion, and empathy" (College of Registered Nurses of Alberta, 2021); and U.K. nurses are expected to apply "principles of courage" among others (Nursing & Midwifery Council, 2018). Not only do these *skills* create measurement challenges, but they also "reproduce the predominant traditional, gendered virtue discourse in nursing" (Windsor et al., 2012, p. 218). Historically, this has meant that occupations offering nurturing, personal, and interpersonal interactions (symbolized by nursing's *caring* mantra) have been trivialized or regarded by others (in nursing's case, by medicine) as supportive rather than essential (Davies, 1995). Much as Nightingale deemed only *certain* women as having the requisite qualities to become a Nightingale nurse, the discipline has come full circle such that only certain individuals with specific virtues can be deemed competent, and thus, qualified to be a nurse. Determining achievement of these virtues is another matter. First, the nursing instructor is likely unable to teach nor the nurse manager evaluate if a student or employee is courageous, compassionate, or confident. Even if the virtues could be taught or evaluated, there appear to be limited if any consequences for those deemed lacking courage, compassion, or confidence, thus making moot the entire enterprise.

A final concern is the expectations that are written into competencies with respect to the nurse's *professional* identity. Competencies often include statements about professionalism. In the U.K., the Standards of Proficiency for Registered Nurses include "being an accountable professional" (Nursing & Midwifery Council, 2018, p. 7). In this standard, nurses "act in the best interests of people, putting them first and providing nursing care that is person-centred, safe and compassionate" (2018, p. 7). In the U.S., AACN's competencies for nursing education make it clear that achieving competency is directly linked to professional identity (AACN, 2021b). In AACN's standard on professionalism, once again specific virtues are essential to the practicing nurse, including "integrity, altruism, inclusivity, compassion, courage, humility, advocacy, caring, autonomy, humanity, and social justice" (AACN, 2021a, p. 49). Elevation of virtues over intellectual skills not only underscores caring as the nucleus of nursing practice, but also generates the notion that these *skills* equate to the *good nurse* – that these are skills *required* of the professional nurse. This "gendered, virtue discourse" – that nurses, who are predominantly women, are talked about in terms of being nurturing, courageous, altruistic, compliant – in effect makes theoretical and technical knowledge of secondary concern. It seems that we have not ventured far from Nightingale's dislike of nurses she perceived as "utterly impractical, inconsiderate, untrustworthy, forgetful" (Godden, 2001, p. 288). For Nightingale, it was all about her recruits achieving and maintaining particular "gendered and class-based ideas" than it was about the actual quality of nursing care they delivered (Godden, 2001, p. 290). Image was and remains everything.

While competencies continue to present the nurse as being caring and virtuous, there is concomitant concern among nurses that they are "underutilized and unrecognized for their essential contributions to the healthcare system" (Godsey et al., 2020, p. 809). Generating more competencies that reinforce the gendered virtue discourse only further solidifies this perception rather than changing how nurses are valued or recognized by other health professionals or the public at large. The public's generally positive response to nurses during the COVID-19 pandemic was not related to nurses' degree or which license they held or which accrediting body certified their nursing program. Rather, nurses were lauded for their ability to adapt under dire circumstances, their willingness to *sacrifice* themselves during protective equipment shortages, and their resilience in the face of overwhelming illness and death. These are qualities not only impossible to measure with static benchmarks, but qualities that also underscore the gendered *sacrificial* aspect of nursing. It appears to be a vicious cycle with nursing combating the public's gendered image of the profession while re-inscribing this same identity in its own competency-based guidelines – and then complaining that the public does not recognize the profession for its contributions. Although re-inscription of nursing's gendered past in its current image is troubling, it is only one of many unintended consequences resulting from nursing's competency-based movement.

Unintended consequences

Overreliance on a particular model of education or practice can have unexpected effects (Brightwell & Grant, 2013). One effect is how competencies act as a means of surveillance and enforcement of homogeneity. O'Byrne and Jacob (2019) applied Deleuze's (1990) society of control to HIV prevention. In a society of control, there is a shift from individuals monitoring themselves to a focus on "pervasive and integrated systems that yield desired outcomes" (O'Byrne & Jacob, p. E6). Thus, HIV prevention is not as much about self-surveillance as it is modification of the spaces in which the individual exists, along with "omnipresent and…pervasive observation and monitoring" (O'Byrne & Jacob, p. E6). Today, nursing organizations and accrediting bodies overseeing nursing registration/practice and education, as a society of control, have assumed this surveillance role. This surveillance occurs not just by nursing, but increasingly by "forces of control external to our field" (McIntyre et al., 2020, p. 3 of 8). A recent U.S. example of external supervision is the significant role the Robert Wood Johnson Foundation had in creating the 2010 and 2020–2030 *Future of Nursing Reports* (Kneipp et al., 2022). It is not only those external to the profession; it is nurses themselves – both in education and in practice – who surveil the profession. For example, a recent quality improvement project was conducted in Sweden in which nurse researchers collected data on how well nursing staff used a mandated checklist for patient handovers (Sharp et al., 2019). Improving patient care meant ensuring nurses *followed the rules*, but ignored *why* nurses resisted using the checklist or even if checklists improved patient outcomes. Similarly, nursing education competencies mandate that students meet set expectations and, as a result, students are *never not* being observed. Integrating more patient simulation into nursing education offers yet another way to monitor nursing students' skills, with the omnipotent nursing instructor speaking or watching from a concealed space. Although nursing students are no longer required to live in hospital dormitories and remain single – past strategies intended to keep them virtuous – surveillance of their behavior persists albeit in less overt, yet no less intrusive ways. These examples demonstrate the constant surveillance of nurses, including when done by nurses themselves.

Nurses' activities are standardized and tracked to ensure that they comport with established guidelines, checklists, and the like. Homogenizing effects occur as nursing actions are centralized and monitored through technologies such as electronic medical records.

Ceaseless prompting from the electronic health record consumes the nurse's time and reduces "the complex relationship of patients and nurses to data points" (Dillard-Wright, 2019, p. 5 of 9) that then can be followed and analyzed. The same effects can be applied to practice competencies. Developed to meet demands from health care employers, these mandated systems and structures are instrumental in shaping nursing practice. Dillard-Wright (2019) and St-Pierre and Holmes (2008) claimed that nurses' working conditions are a form of institutional violence based on how nurses' work is ordered and overseen. An argument could be made that practice and education competencies further contribute to institutional violence, given how competencies can be employed to surveil, manage, and discipline nurses and their work.

Another repercussion from the reliance on competencies is making tasks and activities that are observable and measurable the *only* efforts that count as nursing. Devotion to enumerating tasks – what Thorne et al. (2012) called the "task fraternity" (p. 189) – ultimately gives "legitimacy to the enduring invisibility and devaluation of nursing work" (Windsor et al., 2012 p. 213). Darbyshire et al.'s (2019) perspective is that "training" inevitably is about "compliance" rather than about critical thinking, learning, and professional development (p. 2). If one is concerned primarily with mastering behaviors and skills, it then may limit when and how one learns to stand "up to power and status" (Darbyshire et al., 2019, p. 1). The focus on quantifiable, measurable competencies, and being *job ready* "derails central aspects of education like cultivation of the imagination, of esthetic and artistic ability, as well as metaphorical, symbolic and analogical thinking" (Zovko & Dillon, 2018, p. 557). It is ironic that early nurse leaders' extensive efforts to move nursing – metaphorically and physically – from the hospital to higher education, so as to replace training with formal instruction, have come full circle with the turn to competencies and competency-based training. We return to the question of why nursing leaders and employers expect that nurses be *job ready* the minute they graduate? Might this be exactly what employers want: nurses who are too busy honing skills to be asking hard questions, to question authority, to demand change, to make waves? From this perspective, perhaps the empowered, critical thinking nurse is precisely *not* the best employee, while the "courteous, conscientious and quiet" nurse is (Windsor et al., 2012, p. 216). Expecting nurses' "obedience" is a form of surveillance and institutional violence that subordinates nurses' work to the needs of physicians' and health care organizations, while further eroding the ability and opportunity for critical thinking (Bail et al., 2009, p. 1457).

Competencies are built on the assumption that they are essential to becoming a professional, and being a professional nurse means discerning and applying a wide range of knowledge and skills. Substituting this "corpus of knowledge" (Grant, 1999, p. 273) with prescriptive behaviors – with "procedural knowledge" (knowing what to do rather than understanding the processes informing the actions) (O'Connell et al., 2014, p. 2730) – devalues and, in the end, fails to accurately and adequately capture complex human behaviors and actions. A prescriptive behavioral approach limits the attention given to intangibles such as reflective practice, intellectual skills, and experience (Talbot, 2004).

A checklist of competencies will never be able to adequately capture the performance of complex tasks used in nursing (Grant, 1999), especially in today's health care arena where nursing care is provided to hospitalized patients who are sicker than ever, using technology that is more complicated than ever. Benchmarks, designed to measure performance, provide us with information about what people should be able to *do*; they tell us nothing about the steps needed for taking action; for explaining how the nurse moves from an inexperienced doer to the expert critical thinking clinician. The checklist approach, particularly when inscribed as competencies, is binary – one is either competent or one isn't – rather than the reality that competency is always a matter of degree (Talbot, 2004). Competencies also advance the notion that they are the "sole criterion of worth-whileness" (Barnett, 1994, p. 73). Knowledge and understanding are not static; the essence of any practice can never be settled. Attempts to produce a list of competencies are always fated to be incomplete, uncertain, and subject to debate (Barnett, 1994). Once required competencies are established, they become cemented in place; yet, nursing practice always occurs within a particular context – a context that is ever-changing and evolving (O'Connell et al., 2014; Windsor et al., 2011).

What is lost with the endless pursuit of professionalism via competencies are understanding and knowledge, the foundation for all that *doing*. An emphasis on measuring skills, in turn, makes critical thinking and the "intellectual skills integral to nursing work invisible" (Thorne et al., 2012, p. 189). From a competencies perspective, there is no space for "theorizing, philosophizing, and critical deconstruction" (Thorne, et al., 2012, p. 189). Efforts that mirror medicine lead us away from key nursing elements such as nursing theory. Nursing theory tells us what the discipline does, guides its identity, and explains its contract with society; without these perspectives, it leaves nursing with "no purpose other than to support the practice of medicine" (Newman et al., 2008, p. E25). Abandoning nursing theory and focusing on competencies ultimately diminish the "disciplinary uniqueness that is nursing" (Smith et al., 2021, p. 11).

In sum, the turn to competencies may in fact produce the type of nurse the discipline is trying to avoid – someone other than a professional. That is, competency-based curricula or practice "cannot describe what it is to be a professional [as it is] inadequate to describe the higher cognitive skills and the integrated and individual application and structure of complex knowledge, skills and problem-solving necessary for professional performance" (Brightwell & Grant, 2013, p. 109). If competency cannot describe what a nursing professional is, then it is difficult to discern exactly what it *is* describing.

Nursing organizations use competencies and related tools as a means to acquire the status of a profession. To that end, those providing and/or supervising nursing care are monitored to ensure that they are adhering to established criteria. It may well be that these competencies *do* improve patient care (though the results currently are mixed at best), but this does not mean that we should wholeheartedly accept the ideologies and discourses upon which competency-based education and practice are created and recreated. We should always maintain a critical eye on endeavors emerging from professional organizations and leaders, especially when those efforts use competencies as a device to advance nursing's image, social status, and power.

Some concluding thoughts

Salvage's (1985) enumeration of the challenges of the professional project still rings true today: professionalism is divisive through its drive to identify with doctors (e.g., the *Doctor of Nursing Practice* degree; development of nursing diagnoses) and assign the most basic nursing care to carers with much less formal education; professionalism creates a homogenous perspective; professionalism centers on individual rather than on system failures; professionalism fails to challenge the status quo; and finally, professionalism is directed inward at the needs of the professional group, rather than the health system as a whole. To be like those at the top of the professional ladder, nursing achieves its professional status only by keeping the marginalized at the margins (Bell, 2020) – the ultimate form of divisiveness.

Despite these issues, nursing continues to *protect* its image of being a profession; of caring, heroism, servitude, self-effacement, and self-sacrifice (Bell, 2020). To maintain society's trust, nursing reinforces this squeaky-clean, virtuous identity. Competencies are meant to be a mechanism by which nursing's professional identity is inculcated and maintained. Yet, the reality is that there *are* those nurses who do not enact the virtues required by the competencies and thus by the profession. While nurses committing illegal acts, such as illicit drug use or stealing medications for personal use, are penalized, nurses who do not live up to or by the profession's established virtues are rarely, if ever, sanctioned (Papinaho et al., 2022). Consider that at least one of the nurses who ignored Diana Sanchez's cries for help continued to be employed at Denver's county jail several years later (Roberts, 2020). Presumably, Ms. Sanchez's jail nurses met the competencies required for licensure; yet, they still lacked the expected virtues. There may be limited value to competencies if they cannot protect patients in even the most dire circumstances. Nursing has turned to competencies to bolster its image as a profession, but, as Salvage (1985) claimed, nursing has "not examined the negative aspects of professionalism and the greed and elitism with which it is often associated" (p. 91), nor has it considered what to do with the nurse who does not uphold what the profession promotes as the ideal nurse.

In the end, the professionalization project constitutes an act of violence as it maintains a certain picture of nursing, governs who can be a nurse through various education and licensure requirements, and through acquiescence, often keeps nurses silent. Commitment to maintaining the perfect, caring nurse as the ideal limits opportunities for critique. Although nursing positions itself as an agent of change and espouses needing to address pressing issues such as improving health disparities, its fear of not being seen as an authentic and respectable profession prevents the discipline writ large from making waves. For example, the COVID-19 pandemic contributed to nurse burn-out and resignations of epic proportions in the U.S. (Berlin et al., 2022; Padilla, 2022), to which the U.S. nursing organizations responded with webinars on nursing self-care and developing resilience (ANA Enterprise, n.d.), rather than calling for increased salaries and an enhanced role in staffing decisions (Gurley, 2022). These working conditions, as noted earlier, are a form of institutional violence that require redress and, at minimum, demand more than reliance on nursing's professional identity for meaningful change to occur.

The road to professionalization for nursing is paved with competencies, standards, guidelines, essentials, and domains. Our examination of nursing's professionalization project points to professionalization being pursued to gain power and prestige for the discipline itself. Perhaps power and prestige can help nursing improve the public's health. Then again, perhaps not.

Note

1 As there is no globally agreed upon wording for the discipline's *expectations* of a nurse, we use the word *competencies* to stand in for the various terms.

References

Abbott, P., & Meerabeau, L. (1998). *The sociology of the caring professions* (2nd ed.). UCL Press Limited.

Adu-Bonsaffoh, K., Tamma, E., Maya, E., Vogel, J. P., Tunçalp, O., & Bohren, M. A. (2022). Health workers' and hospital administrators' perspectives on mistreatment of women during facility-based childbirth: A multicenter qualitative study in Ghana. *Reproductive Health, 19*(82), 1–11. https://doi.org/10.1186/s12978-022-01372-3

American Association of Colleges of Nursing. (2021a). *The essentials: Core competencies for professional nursing education.* Author. https://www.aacnnursing.org/AACN-Essentials

American Association of Colleges of Nursing. (2021b, April 7). *Bold action taken to transform nursing education and strengthen the nation's healthcare workforce* [Press release]. https://www.aacnnursing.org/News-Information/Press-Releases/View/ArticleId/24807/AACN-Approves-New-Essentials

American Society of Anesthesiologists. (2022, May 31). *Wisconsin governor vetoes dangerous APRN legislation - protects patients in the badger state* [Press release]. https://www.asahq.org/about-asa/newsroom/news-releases/2022/04/wisconsin-governor-vetoes-dangerous-aprn-legislation

ANA Enterprise. (n.d.). *ANA's COVID-19 self-care package for nurses (free).* https://www.nursingworld.org/continuing-education/anas-covid-19-self-care-package-for-nurses/

Bail, K., Cook, R., Gardner, A., & Grealish, L. (2009). Writing ourselves into a web of obedience: A nursing policy analysis. *International Journal of Nursing Studies, 46,* 1457–1466.

Barnett, R. (1994). *The limits of competence: Knowledge, higher education, and society.* Society for Research into Higher Education & Open University Press.

Bell, B. (2020). Towards abandoning the master's tools: The politics of a universal nursing identity. *Nursing Inquiry, 28*(2). https://doi.org/10.1111/nin.12395

Berlin, G., Lapointe, M., & Murphy, M. (2022). *Assessing the lingering impact of COVID-19 on the nursing workforce.* McKinsey & Company. https://www.mckinsey.com/industries/healthcare-systems-and-services/our-insights/assessing-the-lingering-impact-of-covid-19-on-the-nursing-workforce

Bohren, M. A., Hunter, E. C., Munthe-Kaas, H. A., Souza, J. P., Vogel, J. P., & Gülmezoglu, A. M. (2014). Facilitators and barriers to facility-based delivery in low- and middle-income countries: A qualitative evidence synthesis. *Reproductive Health, 11*(71), 1–17. https://doi.org/10.1186/1742-4755-11-71

Brightwell, A., & Grant, J. (2013). Competency-based training: Who benefits? *Postgraduate Medicine Journal, 89,* 107–110. https://doi.org/10.1136/postgradmedj-2012-130881.

Canales, M. K., & Drevdahl, D. J. (2022). A Sisphyean task; Developing and revising public health nursing competencies. *Public Health Nursing, 39,* 1078–1088. https://doi.org/10.1111/phn.13077.

Carraccio, C., Wolfsthal, S. D., Englander, R., Ferentz, K., & Martin, C. (2002). Shifting paradigms: From Flexner to competencies. *Academic Medicine, 77*(5), 361–367. https://doi.org/10.1097/00001888-200205000-00003.

Cheny, C. (2019, February 27). Why physician assistants and nurse practitioners need supervision, say physician groups. *HealthLeaders.* https://www.healthleadersmedia.com/clinical-care/why-physician-assistants-and-nurse-practitioners-need-supervision-say-physician-groups

Chiu, A. (2019, August 29). 'Nobody cared': A woman gave birth alone in a jail cell after her cries for help were ignored, lawsuit says. *The Washington Post.* https://www.washingtonpost.com/nation/2019/08/29/pregnant-woman-diana-sanchez-birth-alone-jail-cell-denver/

College of Registered Nurses of Alberta. (2021). *Scope of practice for nurse practitioners and scope of practice for registered nurses.* https://nurses.ab.ca/protect-the-public/standards-for-rns-and-nps/standards

Darbyshire, P., Thompson, D. R., & Watson, R. (2019). Nursing schools: Dumbing down or reaching up? *Journal of Nursing Management 27,* 1–3. https://doi.org/10.1111/jonm.12730.

Davies, C. (1995). *Gender and the professional predicament in nursing.* Open University Press.

Deleuze, G. (1990). *Postscript on the societies of control*. The Anarchist Library. https://theanarchistlibrary.org.

Dillard-Wright, J. (2019). Electronic health record as a panopticon: A disciplinary apparatus in nursing practice. *Nursing Philosophy, 20*. https://doi.org/10.1111/nup.12239.

Fowler, M. D. M. (2015). *Guide to nursing's social policy statement: Understanding the profession from social contract to social covenant*. American Nurses Association.

Freidson, E. (2001). *Professionalism: The third logic*. The University of Chicago Press.

Gebbie, K., & Lavin, M. A. (1974). Classifying nursing diagnoses. *American Journal of Nursing, 74*(2), 250–253.

Godden, J. (2001). A 'lamentable failure'? The founding of Nightingale nursing in Australia, 1868–1884. *Australian Historical Studies, 32*(117), 276–291. https://doi.org/10.1080/10314610108596165

Godsey, J. A., Houghton, D. M., & Hayes, T. (2020). Registered nurse perceptions of factors contributing to the inconsistent brand image of the nursing profession. *Nursing Outlook, 68*, 808–821. https://doi.org/10.1016/j.outlook.2020.06.005.

Goubert, A., Cai, J. Y., & Applebaum, E. (2021). Home health care: Latinx and Black women are overrepresented, but all women face heightened risk of poverty. The Center for Economic and Policy Research. https://cepr.net/home-health-care-latinx-and-black-women-are-overrepresented-but-all-women-face-heightened-risk-of-poverty/

Grant, J. (1999). The incapacitating effects of competence: A critique. *Advances in Health Sciences Education, 4*, 271–277. https://doi.org/10.1023/A:1009845202352.

Gurley, L. K. (2022, September 12). Largest private-sector nurses strike in U.S. history begins in Minnesota. *The Washington Post*. https://www.washingtonpost.com/business/2022/09/12/minnesota-nurses-strike

Hugman, R. (1991). *Power in caring professions*. Macmillan.

Kneipp, S. M., Canales, M. K., & Drevdahl, D. J. (2022). Philanthropic foundations' discourse and nursing's future: Part II: A critical discourse analysis of RWJF Future of Nursing initiatives. Advances in Nursing in Science, 46(2), 169–187.

Larsen, R., & Reif, L. (2019). Leveling the core competencies of public health nursing to evaluate senior baccalaureate nursing students. *Public Health Nursing, 36*, 744–751. https://doi.org/10.1111/phn.12636.

López-Verdugo, M., Ponce-Blandón, J. A., López-Narbona, F. J., Romero-Castillo, R., & Guerra-Martín, M. R. (2021). Social image of nursing. An integrative review about a yet unknown profession. *Nursing Reports, 11*(2), 460–474. https://doi.org/10.3390/nursrep11020043

Low, R. (2020, August 13). Mother who gave birth in Denver jail, son will receive $480K in settlements. *Fox 31/2 Colorado*. https://kdvr.com/news/problem-solvers/mother-who-gave-birth-in-denver-jail-son-will-receive-480k-in-settlements/

Lurie, S. J. (2012). History and practice of competency-based assessment. *Medical Education, 46*(1), 49–57. https://doi.org/10.1111/j.1365-2923.2011.04142.x.

Manley, J. E. (1995). Sex-segregated work in the system of professions: The development and stratification of nursing. *The Sociological Quarterly, 36*(2), 297–314. https://doi.org/10.1111/j.1533-8525.1995.tb00441.x

McIntyre, J. R. S., Burton, C., & Holmes, D. (2020). From discipline to control in nursing practice: A poststructuralist reflection. *Nursing Philosophy, 21*. https://doi.org/10.1111/nup.12317.

Newman, M. A., Smith, M. C., Pharris, M. D., & Jones, D. (2008). The focus of the discipline revisited. *Advances in Nursing Science, 31*(1), E16–E27. https://doi.org/10.1097/01.ANS.0000311533.65941.f1.

Nursing & Midwifery Council. (2018). *Future nurse: Standards of proficiency for registered nurses*. https://www.nmc.org.uk/globalassets/sitedocuments/standards-of-proficiency/nurses/future-nurse-proficiencies.pdf)

O'Byrne, P., & Jacob, J. D. (2019). The evolution of HIV prevention from discipline to control. *Advances in Nursing Science, 42*(4), E1–E10. https://doi.org/10.1097/ANS.0000000000000268.

O'Connell, J., Gardner, G., & Coyer, F. (2014). Beyond competencies: Using a capability framework in developing practice standards for advanced practice nursing. *Journal of Advanced Nursing, 70*(12), 2728–2735. https://doi.org/10.1111/jan.12475.

Padilla, M. (2022, September 23). The 19th explains: Why the nursing shortage isn't going away anytime soon. *The 19th.* https://19thnews.org/2022/09/19th-explains-nursing-shortage/

Papinaho, O., Häggman-Laitila, A., & Kangasniemi, M. (2022). Unprofessional conduct by nurses: A document analysis of disciplinary decisions. *Nursing Ethics, 29*(1) 131–144. https://doi.org/10.1177/09697330211015289

Pijl-Zieber, E. M., Barton, S., Konkin, J., Awaosoga, O., & Caine, V. (2014). Competence and competency-based nursing education: Finding our way through the issues. *Nurse Education Today, 34*, 676–678. https://doi.org/10.1016/j.nedt.2013.09.007.

Roberts, M. (2020, August 18). Diana Sanchez's horrific jail birth settlement: What you haven't heard. *Westword.* https://www.westword.com/news/diana-sanchez-unattended-jail-birth-settlement-update-and-video-11765451

Salvage, J. (1985). *The politics of nursing.* Heinemann.

Samaniego, V. C., & Cárcamo, S. (2013). The nursing image and professional identity. The future of a construction. *Investigación y Educacíon en Enfermería, 31*(1), 54–62.

Sharp, L., Dahlen, C., & Bergenmar, M. (2019). Observations of nursing staff compliance to a checklist for person-centred handovers–a quality improvement project. *Scandinavian Journal of Caring Science, 33*, 892–901. https://doi.org/10.1111/scs.12686.

Smith, M. C., Chinn, P. L., & Nicoll, L. H. (2021). Knowledge for nursing practice: Beyond evidence alone. *Research and Theory for Nursing Practice, 35*(1), 7–23. https://doi.org/10.1891/RTNP-D-20–00095.

St-Pierre, I., & Holmes, D. (2008). Managing nurses through disciplinary power: A Foucauldian analysis of workplace violence. *Journal of Nursing Management, 16*, 352–359. https://doi.org/10.1111/j.1365–2834.2007.00812.x.

Talbot, M. (2004). Monkey see, monkey do: A critique of the competency model in graduate medical education. *Medical Education, 38*, 587–592. https://doi.org/10.1046/j.1365–2923.2004.01794.x.

ten Cate, O. (2017). Competency-based postgraduate medical education: Past, present and future. *GMS Journal for Medical Education, 34*(5), Doc69. https://doi.org/10.3205/zma001146

Teresa-Morales, C., Rodriguez-Perez, M., Araujo-Hernandez, M., & Feria-Ramirez, C. (2022). Current stereotypes associated with nursing and nursing professionals: An integrative review. *International Journal of Environmental Research and Public Health, 19*, 7640. https://doi.org/10.3390/ijerph19137640.

Thorne, S., Lawler, J., Pryce, A., & May, C. (2012). Reading outside the task fraternity. *Nursing Inquiry, 19*(3), 189. https://doi.org/10.1111/j.1440-1800.2012.00607.x

van der Cingel, M., & Brouwer, J. (2021). What makes a nurse today? A debate on the nursing professional identity and its need for change. *Nursing Philosophy, 22*, e12343. https://doi.org/10.1111/nup.12343

Windsor, C., Douglas, C., & Harvey, T. (2012). Nursing and competencies–a natural fit: The politics of skill/competency formation in nursing. *Nursing Inquiry, 19*(3), 213–222. https://doi.org/10.1111/j.1440–1800.2011.00549.x.

Woods, C. Q. (1987). From individual dedication to social activism: Historical development of nursing professionalism. In: C. Maggs (Ed.), *Nursing history: The state of the art* (pp. 153–175). Croom Helm.

Yoder-Wise, P. S. (2022). The emperor has no clothes and the new graduate is not work-ready. *The Journal of Continuing Education in Nursing, 53*(9), 387–388. https://doi.org/10.3928/00220124–20220805-01

Zovko, M.-E., & Dillon, J. (2018). Humanism vs competency: Traditional and contemporary models of education. *Educational Philosophy and Theory, 50*(6–7), 554–564. https://doi.org/10.1080/00131857.2017.1375757

23 Medicine and nursing through the Advanced Nurse Practitioner lens

Martin McNamara and Wayne Thompson

Healthcare systems are under pressure due to ageing populations, the epidemic of chronic conditions, rising public expectations and the need for cost containment. Advanced Nurse Practitioners (ANPs) comprise one solution to these challenges by increasing access to healthcare, emphasising patient education and disease prevention, and delivering high-quality, cost-effective care across diverse settings.

Nurses and doctors have been formed through their education and training within historically and culturally contingent disciplinary boundaries. These boundaries are becoming more porous, offering the possibility of a richer professional identity for ANPs – and others – that will allow them to realise their full potential. However, current confusion about ANPs' contribution results in their role being underutilised. This situation gives rise to our central question:

What do the discourses circulating in the healthcare system tell us about the professions and disciplines of medicine and nursing – their similarities, their differences and the shifting boundaries between them? Furthermore, how do the structures, relationships and processes that characterise healthcare systems constrain and enable ANPs, and what other ways of being, doing, knowing and relating are possible?

Adopting a systems and discourse analytic perspective, this chapter explores how analysing ANPs' and their medical colleagues' language-in-use helps to address these questions. We applied Gee's (2010) discourse analytic methods and Oshry's (2018) Organic Systems Framework (OSF) to a range of texts, including empirical and theoretical papers, policy documents, opinion pieces and editorials.

We first examined whether, to what extent and in what ways each of Gee's (2010) building tasks of language (Table 23.1) is realised in the texts. This was done by using Gee's six tools of inquiry (Table 23.2) (we embolden these tasks and tools in the chapter). We then examined whether, to what extent and in what ways each of Oshry's (2018) distinctive patterns of systemic relationships and processes is realised in the texts. These patterns of relationships and processes shape how ANPs and medics experience themselves, one another, other members of the system and the system itself.

For Gee (2010), any text represents a discourse. His method of analysis captures debates and discourses swirling about that constitute a particular social reality at a point in time, recognising that this reality is an emerging construction that is always in process. We explore the relationships between discourse and the social realities of the medic and the ANP. The OSF (Oshry, 2018) provides an additional layer of analysis to allow us, first, to investigate how ANPs and medics comprise a system that can be described in terms of its distinctive patterns of relationships and processes, and, second, to illuminate the

DOI: 10.4324/9781003427407-27

Table 23.1 Building Tasks [Adapted from Gee (2011)]

Building Task	Definition
Identities	Using language to enact specific socially situated identities or to project such identities onto others, or to privilege or disprivilege such identities.
Relationships	Using language to create or sustain social relationships or to end or harm them. Any situation whereby the people involved in an event enact and contract with each other.
Politics (the distribution of social goods)	Using language to give or take away social goods or projecting how social goods are or ought to be distributed. Social goods been seen as anything a person or group in society wants and values. Some things (like status, money, love, respect, and friendship) are taken by nearly everyone in society as social goods. Other things are social goods only to small groups.
Sign systems and knowledge	Using language to create, sustain, revise, change, privilege, or disprivilege any language or sign system or characteristic way of knowing the world or making knowledge claims about the world.
Significance	Using language to make thinks significant or important in various ways or to lower their significance or importance.
Activities	Using language to enact specific practices (activities) alone or with others.
Connections	Using language to make things connected or relevant to each other or to make them disconnected or irrelevant to each other.

Table 23.2 Tools of Inquiry [Adapted from Gee (2011)]

Tool of Inquiry	Definition
Situated meanings	Any word or structure in language has a certain 'meaning potential' that is the range of possible meanings that the word or structure can take on in different contexts of use, e.g., 'nursing' in nursing mother or nursing practice or nursing theory. Words have different and specific meanings in the different contexts in which they are used and in the different specialist domains that recruit them.
Social languages	Styles or varieties of a language (or a mixture of languages) that enact and are associated with a particular social identity, e.g., the language of science, medicine or nursing.
Intertextuality	When one text (in this sense) quotes, refers to, or alludes to another text as in 'When John fought with his boss, it was like David and Goliath!' Here my speech (the 'text) has alluded to (made an intertextual reference to) a Biblical text
Figured Worlds	A picture of a simplified world that captures what is taken to be typical or normal – what is taken to be typical or normal varies by context and by people's social and cultural group.
The Big 'D' Discourses	Distinctive ways of speaking and listening and/or writing/reading are coupled with distinctive ways of acting, interacting, valuing, feeling, dressing, thinking and believing. In turn, all these are coupled with ways of coordinating oneself with (getting in synch with) other people and with various objects, tools and technologies.
The Big 'C' Conversations	Debates in society or within specific social groups (over focused issues like smoking, abortion, or school reform) that large numbers of people recognise, in terms of both what 'sides' there are to take in such debates and what sorts of people tend to be on each side.

relationships and processes evident in the texts that characterise the ways in which ANP systems interact with medical systems.

We first provide a background to the ANP role followed by a brief overview of both Gee's (2010) discourse analytic methods and Oshry's (2018) OSF. The principal issues covered are as follows:

- ANP practice is always associated and defined with reference to medicine.
- A hybrid ANP identity which functions with 'one foot in medicine and one foot in nursing'.
- 'Inferior', not advanced, nurse practitioners whose practice is seen as lower quality and 'non-complex' and whose knowledge base and ways of knowing are discursively constructed as having less influence and impact than medical knowledge(s).
- Discursive monopolising of caring and holism evident in discourses such as 'nurses care and doctors cure'.
- Identifying the medical doctor as the 'natural' leader; in fact, an authority figure whose relationship with ANPs is based on concern and control.
- Fear, threat and loss of professional identity characterise doctors' relationships with ANPs.

Brief background to the ANP

There has been a rise in the number of nurses holding advanced nursing practice positions internationally. Advanced nursing practice refers to healthcare services and interventions provided to individuals, families and communities by nurses who have acquired the knowledge to underpin enhanced decision making and clinical competencies that influence patient outcomes (Hamric & Tracy 2019). The first nurse practitioner training programme was introduced in the United States in 1965 by Loretta Ford, a nurse, and Henry Silver, a physician. The concept spread to Canada (1960/1970s), the United Kingdom (1980s) and Australia (1990s). The International Council of Nurses (ICN) (2017) estimates that at least 70 countries have, or are considering introducing, advanced nursing roles. It is no surprise then that discourses concerning advanced nursing practice and nurse practitioners are becoming more evident in medical and nursing journals.

Brief background to critical discourse analysis

James Paul Gee (1948–) provides a critical approach to discourse analysis that is embedded in a theory of language-in-use in culture and society (Rogers et al., 2005; Gee, 2004). Language-in-use is a tool used to design or build things. **Discourse**, according to Gee, refers to ways of combining and integrating language, actions, interactions, ways of thinking, believing, valuing, and using various symbols, tools and objects to enact a particular sort of socially recognisable identity (Gee, 2010). For Gee, discourse analysis

> seeks to balance talk about the mind, talk about the interaction and activities, and talk about society and institutions more than is the case in some other approaches.
>
> (Gee, 2011, p. 5)

Gee (2010) proposes that we continually build, destroy and rebuild our worlds using language in tandem with actions, interactions, non-linguistic symbol systems, objects, tools, technologies and distinctive ways of thinking, valuing, feeling and believing. When speaking or writing, we construct seven areas of reality or building tasks (Table 23.1) giving rise to seven different sets of questions about any piece of language-in-use. When Gee uses the term tools of inquiry, he is referring to '...ways of looking at the world of talk and interaction' (Gee, 2011, p. 12). These tools are relevant to how we, together with others, build **identities** and **activities** and recognise those that are being built around us. They are tools of inquiry in the sense that they lead us as discourse analysts to ask specific sorts of questions about our data (Table 23.2).

Brief background to OSF

Barry Oshry (1932–) provides a framework to observe systems both from the outside – seeing the structure and processes of the whole – and from the inside – listening to the experiences of members within these systems. The OSF (Oshry, 2019) is descriptive and predictive; it provides a conceptual vocabulary for describing relationships and processes within and among systems, offers potential solutions to existing social system problems and opens up avenues for future research. Oshry (2018, 2019) provides a language for describing systems as wholes and his framework allows us to understand and influence a wide range of system phenomena; for example, how, as system members, we experience ourselves, our relationships with others, the systems we are part of, other systems and the relationships among systems. The promise of the OSF lies in its potential to enable us to take more informed actions based on the insights it provides.

A key premise of Oshry's OSF is that while human beings are the most social of social creatures, we are often blind to the workings of the systems of which we are a part. We do not always discern how the structures, relationships and processes of systems affect our consciousness; that is, how we experience ourselves, others, and other systems. This lack of awareness of systems and their workings can result in disempowering scenarios with costs in personal stress, broken relationships, missed opportunities, diminished effectiveness, unrealised potential contributions and destructive behaviours within and across systems. Oshry (1999, 2007, 2018, 2019, 2020) has long been concerned with transforming this system blindness with all of its costs, into system sight with all of its productive possibilities. McNamara and Teeling (2021) show how Oshry's framework was used to introduce healthcare professionals to the new perspectives and possibilities that systems thinking provides.

Applying Oshry's (2018, 2019) ideas to healthcare systems, we can see that some interactions in the system go well, others not so well; we feel close to and work well with some healthcare professionals (contributing to homogenisation in the system) and distant from others (contributing to individuation); we feel cooperative here (contributing to system integration) and competitive there (contributing to differentiation); and we evaluate and judge others. All these interactions are affected by our emotions, including feelings of comfort, discomfort, fear, dislike and love. Oshry (2020) points out that we experience these relationships as highly specific to individuals as if this is who these people really are. However, he argues that when we lift the veil and look beneath the surface of our day-to-day interactions, a very different picture emerges; one that, he suggests, has 'the potential for totally transforming our experiences of ourselves and others, and one that opens clear paths to creating satisfying and productive relationships, creativity and contribution' (Oshry, 2020, p. 13).

Shifting sands, mixing and hybridity

The ANP role disturbs established boundaries within nursing, and between nursing and medicine. For some, the ANP represents a true 'hybridisation' of nursing and medicine (Rashotte, 2005, p. 54), resulting in an integrative and innovative role within the system. For others, notably medics, the ANP is viewed as a threat rather than an opportunity, requiring the imposition of limiting boundaries and other constraints that prevent the ANP role from realising its full potential (Thompson and McNamara, 2022a, b). We show how this disruptive intervention in the healthcare system is constructed and how the relationships and processes evident in the literature characterise the ways in which ANP systems interact with medical systems.

Activities are built by language-in-use such as 'extended', 'expanded', 'advanced' (Laperrière, 2008, p. 395), which has resulted in confusion and ambiguity, and a failure to convey what an ANP contributes to the health system. **Conversations** taking place within the health system focus on whether the foundations of the ANP role are grounded in a nursing paradigm, a medico-nursing worldview or some other healthcare perspective. ANPs are positioned as Oshry's (2018) torn Middles, sliding between nursing and medical identities, creating a conflicted identity for many. Attending to who is contributing to these **Conversations**, some ANPs are clear that 'nursing is the basis for their practice' (Carryer and Adams, 2017, p. 529), whereas others and their health profession colleagues' language-in-use foregrounds the hybridity of a role that functions with 'one foot in medicine and one foot in nursing' (Ulrich, 2010, p. 6).

Conversations highlight ANPs' preoccupation with medicine so that their role and practice are frequently defined with reference to it. Carryer and Adams (2022) consider this association to be antithetical to the essential values of the ANP role as it suppresses differentiation and overidentification with medicine may decrease ANPs' distinctive contribution to the system. By differentiating, ANPs would bring more variety to the system and the system would be richer for it. However, many ANPs employ medical terminology as a **social language**, emphasising 'history-taking', 'diagnostic skills' and 'referral rights' (Paniagua, 2011, p. 383). Enacting this medical identity, ANPs strive for more social recognition and higher status. This 'medicalisation' of the role is recognised by other health professionals whose language suggests that the ANP role has 'lost its nursing and caring identity' (Griffin and Melby, 2006, p. 299). The upshot is that some nurses resist and are 'ambivalent' about the ANP role, using language such as 'nurses who practice in doctors' clothing' to connect the role with a perceived medical identity (Li et al., 2013, p. 356). ANPs are again positioned as Middles, torn between the conflicting identities of medicine and nursing.

In contrast, other ANPs are endeavouring to construct an **identity** for themselves that aligns with nursing. They want society to see them first as nurses and then as advanced practitioners (Burgess and Purkis, 2010). This is evident in language-in-use that emphasises the 'nursing' aspect of the role, such as having 'allegiance to a nursing philosophy of practice' and having skills 'derived from a nursing paradigm' (Carryer and Adams, 2017, p. 529; Lowe, 2017, p. 175). Using the tool of inquiry, **intertextuality**, however, we observe that, when nursing is discussed, commentators often allude to texts that refer to nurses as 'Angels of Mercy' and 'Sex Objects' (ten Hoeve et al., 2014, p. 298). Such references position nurses and nursing as inexpert and less influential than medicine. These texts are products of historical disputes between and among different **Discourses**.

Conversations go beyond the confines of the text itself and feed into and reflect broader **Conversations** taking place in society. These **Conversations** include nursing being identified as a traditional female role and that nurses are less well-educated than other health professionals. Rather than being constructed as professionals who are capable assuming responsibility for their practice and their system, ANPs are instead constructed as Oshry's (2018) oppressed Bottoms, positioned as direct service providers low in the system's hierarchy, constrained to hold others responsible for their condition and that of the whole system, rather than contributing to and shaping the system to the full extent of their education, training and experience.

Geertz (1983, pp. 157–158) suggests that:

> the vocabularies in which the various disciplines talk about themselves to themselves naturally fascinates me as a way of gaining access to the sorts of mentalities at work in them…the terms through which the devotees of a scholarly pursuit represent their aims, judgements, justifications, and so on seems to me to take one a long way, when properly understood, towards grasping what that pursuit is all about.

We now explore these vocabularies and the **Discourses** that ANPs and medics use when talking about themselves, others and the system.

ANPs talking among themselves about themselves and others

Connections are built when ANPs' language connects their identity to partnership and teamwork, foregrounding collaboration as the 'cornerstone' of their role (Thompson and McNamara, 2022a, p. 843). This collaborative model values the integration of the 'diverse knowledge and skills of multiple types of providers' (Stanik-Hutt et al., 2013, p. 498) and constructs the ANP as an exemplar of Oshry's (2018) empowered Top who appreciates the value of distributing responsibility and working with others to shape the system. ANPs make their role relevant and connect it with service improvements by using language such as 'ANPs are in an excellent position to address current (healthcare) shortcomings' (Archibald and Fraser, 2013, p. 270).

Significance is built for collaboration through language-in-use that constructs it as 'critical to establish', suggesting that health services ignore at their peril the benefits of team-working compared to the 'traditional medical hierarchical model of…ineffective teamwork' (Institute of Medicine, 2011, p. 410). **Discourses** are about being certain kinds of people (Gee, 2011) and organisations value health professionals who are cooperative and interprofessional, attributes associated with collaboration and enhanced care. Through a **social language** based on fairness and parity, realised through terms such as 'resisting elitist aspects' and 'commitment to egalitarian power relations' (Burgess and Purkis, 2010, p. 300), ANPs again position themselves as empowered Tops (Oshry, 2018) who support the principle of distributing power and creating responsibility throughout the system. This helps homogenise and integrate a system which would otherwise be over differentiated because of departmental and disciplinary specialisation, and over individuated due to professional power plays. Language-in-use constructs a **figured world** that takes working together to be desirable and necessary for efficient and effective healthcare services. Collaboration enables systems to homogenise and integrate through connectedness and mutual responsibility.

Sign systems and knowledge are constructed by ANPs as they use language to privilege their role over other healthcare roles and build **identities** to persuade co-workers and patients that their role is complex, varied and valuable. ANPs also strive to rid themselves of identities traditionally ascribed to nursing that do not serve their purpose. Language-in-use such as 'better diagnostic skills', 'increased awareness…and a greater impact' (Thompson and Meskell, 2012, p. 204) and 'key players…for a more efficient workforce' (Lowe et al., 2012 p. 682) mark their identity as being effective at 'addressing shortcomings' (Archibald and Fraser, 2013, p. 270). Much of this discussion is ANPs talking among themselves about themselves. Through their talk (Thompson and McNamara, 2022a, b), ANPs position themselves as disempowered Tops (Oshry, 2018) at pains to justify their existence and prove their worth and burdened by arguments based on comparison to, and alignment with, others. They cast themselves as system saviours, sucking up responsibility for the whole system, rather than positioning themselves as independent practitioners with a differentiated and distinctive contribution to make to it.

Connections are established between nursing and a caring function while connecting doctors with a less caring role through language such as 'medics aren't good at the caring piece, psychosocial piece…you'll get the high-powered stuff but you rarely get a lot of detail on the real nitty-gritty, important day-to-day issues' (Begley et al., 2014, pp. 413–414). This language-in-use makes caring relevant to the ANP role but irrelevant for doctors. Nurses use this language to create a simplified **figured world** that constructs nurses as being more caring and holistic than other health professionals. This discursive monopolising of caring and holism by nurses negates the caring and holistic aspects of other professionals' practice. This again positions ANPs as burdened Tops assuming sole responsibility for providing a caring service. This monopolisation of a caring identity arises from **Discourses** wherein the image and identity of nursing are interweaved historically with religious and secular orders. Yet, this identity does not serve the purpose of the ANP because it contributes to the belief that nurses can be caring and kind but at the expense of an identity as a professional practitioner who is educated and knowledgeable and can make a distinctive and significant contribution to transforming the health system. ANPs therefore use language that attempts to create **identities** concerned with 'education, research and policy' (National Council for the Professional Development of Nursing and Midwifery, 2007, p. 3). ANPs now position themselves as Oshry's (2018) empowered Middles, resisting a tendency to get stuck in the middle of others' issues and conflicts to focus instead on how they can best serve the system through a novel, autonomous and distinctive practice.

Medics talking among themselves about themselves and others

Significance, connections and **identities** are built by some medics, with their language-in-use placing certain words and terms to the foreground; for example, indicating that the ANP role is 'lacking' something, provides a 'lower quality of care' and that 'safety issues' arise when independence for the ANP role is discussed (Maten-Speksnijder et al., 2014, p. 51; Hoskins, 2012, p. 1897). Medics are now the burdened Tops, self-identifying as the only professionals that can provide a safe, quality healthcare service. ANPs, however, are constructed as oppressed Bottoms, prevented from becoming all that they have the potential to be. Doubts about advanced nursing practice are made significant through language that constructs ANPs as 'lesser or more narrowly trained' than doctors (Yong, 2006, p. 27), providing services only for patients with simple and non-complex conditions (Power and Phillips, 2017). The phrase 'lesser or more narrowly trained' creates a **situated meaning** that any professional that is not a doctor is identified as inferior. A context is construed that enacts an identity for ANPs that cannot be independent and autonomous but instead requires supervision and management.

Through language that suggests that 'certain tasks are forever to be performed by medicine', a picture is drawn of a simplified and static healthcare world that places healthcare professionals' **identities** in boxes (Carryer and Adams, 2022, p. 36). Epithets such as 'physician extenders', 'midlevel providers' and 'non-physician providers' (Poghosyan et al., 2012, p. 269) diminish the ANP role by signifying it as inferior to medicine and providing a service that is second class. Discursively describing something with reference to lack is problematic, as in 'non-physician'. It constructs an absence or inferiority relative to a dominant referent. Some medics have used this **figured world** and invited others to assume that, while ANPs are highly competent, they cannot care for complex patients and should not be seen as a panacea for healthcare issues (Newhouse et al., 2011). Language such as 'reluctant to accept' (Norris and Melby, 2006, p. 253) and 'ANPs should be supervised' (Nardi and Diallo, 2014, p. 229) builds **activities** for medics whereby they are the overseers of the health service and that any decision in the health system requires their approval. Medics are again positioned as burdened Tops, assuming a 'gatekeeper' function (Irish Medical Organisation, 2017, p. 5), concentrating responsibility in themselves rather than distributing it throughout the system.

This burdened Top identity is reinforced by the language used by Emergency Department clinical directors who suggest that 'ANPs could not match the patient throughput achieved by junior doctors' (Li et al., 2013, p. 356) to link the work of ANPs with decreased efficiency. Such language considers efficiency in absolute terms where numbers are seen as relevant and quality irrelevant. Language such as 'longer consultation times' and 'higher incidence of referrals' (McGlynn et al., 2014, p. 176) creates a **situated meaning** that this is a 'bad thing'. Some doctors use the **big 'D' Discourse** of thinking about a 'good' health service in numbers and hard figures (Li et al., 2013, p. 356) to enact an identity for themselves that is socially recognisable – an element of a get them in and get them out philosophy. Some authors believe that scientific medical knowledge is 'simply the more powerful knowledge' (Beck and Young, 2005, p. 187). Such language is part of a Discourse that enacts a recognisable identity for medics as more erudite than other health professionals.

Relationships are built when medics use language to maintain their superior status in the health system. Medics are burdened Tops assuming responsibility for the ANP system while ANPs positioned as oppressed Bottoms requiring control and supervision. Language-in-use such as 'accepting that nurses should be allowed to undertake certain advanced skills' (Norris and Melby, 2006, pp. 260–261) and identifying physicians as 'natural leaders' (Nardi and Diallo, 2014, p. 229) enacts a relationship with ANPs based on concern and control. The words 'accept' and 'certain' are both used to presuppose that doctors have the final say on what advanced skills the ANP role assumes. This relationship is sustained by language such as 'cannot match' a medic and the 'increased cost' of ANP positions (Li et al., 2013, p. 356). Notions of cost and efficiency are central to the **relationships** being constructed in the language-in-use of medics such as 'ANPs earn as much money as junior doctors and are therefore not a valid alternative' (Markewitz, 2013, p. 23). The **situated meaning** is that even if doctors and ANPs earn the same, it is better to choose the doctor. An imbalanced system is constructed wherein medics are free to pursue their individual goals, whereas ANPs are prevented from individuating and differentiating to become all that they could be.

Language-in-use such as 'decision makers...think of medical solutions to health problems' (Currie et al., 2012, p. 958) builds **connections** between medicine and problem solving, creating an identity for medics as leaders and authority figures. These **connections** are evident in the word 'gatekeeper' to characterise the role of GPs in the health system – a term which indicates control and jurisdiction. The **intertextuality** tool of inquiry shows how this is further accomplished when Irish medical organisations allude to draft policies produced by the Department of Health to argue the case that any expansion of healthcare services should be 'aligned to General Practitioners' (Irish Medical Organisation, 2017, p. 6). By using language such as 'jumped up' (Oxtoby, 2016, p. 448), which positions ANPs as getting above themselves, medics are creating a socially recognisable identity for themselves as defenders against pretenders to their status and power.

Sign systems and knowledge are built by medics' language-in-use such as believing 'that only they could prescribe...they had trained longer than nurses and only they knew the anatomy, physiology, assessment and diagnostic skills, and that nurses couldn't learn or perform them' (Oxtoby, 2016, p. 448) and 'medical ability as a pinnacle of achievement' (Carryer et al., 2007, p. 1824) that confers great authority on the service they deliver and de-privileges the service that other health professions provide. Again, medics act as burdened Tops, sucking up all responsibility convinced that no other professional can 'match their ability' (Li et al., 2013, p. 356). This language presents a **figured world** that invites individuals to assume that medical ability is more important and superior to other health professionals' abilities. Within this figured world, it is taken as typical and normal that doctors would maintain 'professional control over health services' (Street and Cossman, 2010, p. 434).

Sign systems and knowledge are also built by the use of language that de-privileges the ANP role by identifying ANPs as followers and 'not recognised as formal leaders' (Lamb et al., 2018, p. 401). This privileges one profession's body of knowledge and practice over another and accords greater authority to medicine relative to nursing. The **big 'D' Discourse** positions medics as controlling and burdened Tops, while ANPs are positioned as oppressed Bottoms, holding others responsible for their condition. This results in the ANP becoming disempowered and their activities 'constrained by interdisciplinary relationships, organisational culture and role isolation' (Higgins et al., 2014, p. 895).

Concluding remarks

This chapter sets out to reveal discourses circulating in the healthcare system and what they tell us about the professions and disciplines of medicine and nursing – their similarities, their differences and the shifting boundaries between them. We showed how the structures, relationships and processes that characterise the healthcare system constrain and enable ANPs, and that other ways of being, doing, knowing and relating are possible. The chapter alerts healthcare professionals to the ways in which discourses influence opinion and shape identities. While language-in-use represents ANPs as innovative additions to the healthcare system that add value, it also reveals and constructs tensions that impact on and impede their advancement. To support and allow ANPs to advance, we need to be alert to, and challenge, language that positions ANPs as a marginal and contested presence in the health system rather than an important and necessary, even if disruptive, innovation. The value of discourse analysis is that it highlights the need for ANPs to be sensitive to language-in-use, how it shapes them and how they can shape it to better represent their role, the value that it adds to the healthcare system and how it aligns with and complements the roles of other healthcare professionals. In this way, ANPs can become more vocal and visible, assuming a place at the policy table and using their collective voice to articulate the strength and diversity that they bring to the health system. Awareness of language-in-use and how and what it constructs is key to maximising ANPs' potential and strengthening their contribution to healthcare.

References

Archibald, M. M. & Fraser, K. (2013). The potential for nurse practitioners in health care reform. *Journal of Professional Nursing*, 29, 270, 5. https://doi.org/10.1016/j.profnurs.2012.10.002

Beck, J. & Young, M. F. D. (2005). The assault on the professions and the restructuring of academic and professional identities: A Bernsteinian analysis. *British Journal of Sociology of Education*, 26, 183–197. https://doi.org/10.1080/0142569042000294165

Begley, C., Murphy, K., Higgins, A. & Cooney, A. (2014). Policy makers' views on impact of specialist and advanced practitioner roles in Ireland: The SCAPE study. *Journal of Nursing Management*, 22, 410–422. https://doi.org/10.1111/jonm.12018

Burgess, J. & Purkis, M. E. (2010). The power and politics of collaboration in nurse practitioner role development. *Nursing Inquiry*, 17, 297–308. https://doi.org/10.1111/j.1440-1800.2010.00505.x

Carryer, J. & Adams, S. (2017). Nurse practitioners as a solution to transformative and sustainable health services in primary health care: A qualitative exploratory study, *Collegian*, 24, 6, 525–531. https://doi.org/10.1016/j.colegn.2016.12.001

Carryer, J. & Adams, S. (2022). Valuing the paradigm of nursing: Can nurse practitioners resist medicalization to transform healthcare? *Journal of Advanced Nursing*, 78, e36–e38. https://doi.org/10.1111/jan.15082

Carryer, J., Gardner, G., Dunn, S. & Gardner, A. (2007). The core role of the nurse practitioner: Practice, professionalism and clinical leadership. *Journal of Clinical Nursing*, 16, 1818–25. https://doi.org/10.1111/j.1365-2702.2007.01823.x

Currie, G., Lockett, A., Finn, R., Martin, G. & Waring, J. (2012). Institutional work to maintain professional power: Recreating the model of medical professionalism. *Organization Studies*, 33, 937–962. https://doi.org/10.1177%2F0170840612445116

Gee, J. P. (2004). Discourse analysis: What makes it critical? In: Rogers, R. (ed.) *An Introduction to Critical Discourse Analysis in Education*. London, Lawrence Erlbaum.

Gee, J. P. (2010). *An Introduction to Discourse Analysis: Theory and Method*. New York, Routledge.

Gee, J. P. (2011). *How to do Discourse Analysis: A Toolkit*. Oxon, Routledge.

Geertz, C. (1983). *Local Knowledge*. New York, Basic Books.

Griffin, M. & Melby, V. (2006). Developing an advanced nurse practitioner service in emergency care: Attitudes of nurses and doctors. *Journal of Advanced Nursing*, 56, 292–301. https://doi.org/10.1111/j.1365-2648.2006.04025.x

Hamric, A.B. & Tracy, M.F. (2019). A definition of advanced practice nursing. In: M.F. Tracy & E.T. O'Grady (eds) *Advanced Practice Nursing: An Integrative Approach*, 6th Edition, St. Louis: Elsevier, pp. 61–79.

Higgins, A., Begley, C., Lalor, J., Coyne, I., Murphy, K. & Elliott, N. (2014). Factors influencing advanced practitioners' ability to enact leadership: A case study within Irish healthcare. *Journal of Nursing Management*, 22, 894–905. https://doi.org/10.1111/jonm.12057

Hoskins, R. (2012). Interprofessional working or role substitution? A discussion of the emerging roles in emergency care: Interprofessional working in emergency care. *Journal of Advanced Nursing*, 68, 1894–1903. https://doi.org/10.1111/j.1365-2648.2011.05867.x

Institute of Medicine. (2011). *The Future of Nursing: Leading Change, Advancing Health*, Washington, DC, The National Academies Press.

International Council of Nurses. (2017). *International Council of Nursing* [Online]. Available: http://www.icn.ch. [Accessed 17 September 2017].

Irish Medical Organisation (2017). *Submission to the Department of Health on Draft Policies to Enhance Roles for Nurses and Midwives*. Dublin, Irish Medical Organisation.

Lamb, A., Martin-Misener, R., Bryant-Lukosius, D. & Latimer, M. (2018). Describing the leadership capabilities of advanced practice nurses using a qualitative descriptive study. *Nursing Open*, 5, 400–413. https://doi.org/10.1002/nop2.150

Laperrière, H. (2008). Developing professional autonomy in advanced nursing practice: The critical analysis of socio-political variables. *International Journal of Nursing Practice*, 14, 391–397. https://doi.org/10.1111/j.1440-172x.2008.00700.x

Li, J., Westbrook, J., Callen, J., Georgiou, A. & Braithwaite, J. (2013). The impact of nurse practitioners on care delivery in the emergency department: A multiple perspectives qualitative study. *BMC Health Services Research*, 13, 356–356. https://doi.org/10.1186/1472-6963-13-356

Lowe, G. (2017). Nurse Practitioners: Framing their professional identity. *Journal for Nurse Practitioners,* 13, 175. https://doi.org/10.1016/j.nurpra.2016.12.021

Lowe, G., Plummer, V., O' Brien, A. P. & Boyd, L. (2012). Time to clarify – the value of advanced practice nursing roles in health care. *Journal of Advanced Nursing*, 68, 677–685. https://doi.org/10.1111/j.1365-2648.2011.05790.x

Markewitz, A. (2013). Nurse practitioners replacing young doctors: It works, but does it make sense? *European Journal of Cardio-Thoracic Surgery*, 43, 23. https://doi.org/10.1093/ejcts/ezs422

Maten-Speksnijder, A., Grypdonck, M., Pool, A., Meurs, P. & Staa, A. L. (2014). A literature review of the Dutch debate on the nurse practitioner role: Efficiency vs. professional development. *International Nursing Review*, 61, 44–54. https://doi.org/10.1111/inr.12071

McGlynn, B., White, L., Smith, K., Hollins, G., Gurun, M., Little, B., Clark, R., Nair, B., Glen, H., Ansari, J., Mahmood, R., Nairn, R., Balsitis, M., Chanock, D., Mclaughlin, G. & Meddings, R. (2014). A service evaluation describing a nurse-led prostate cancer service in NHS, Ayrshire and Arran. *International Journal of Urological Nursing*, 8, 166–180. http://dx.doi.org/10.1111/ijun.12049

McNamara, M. & Teeling, S.P. (2021). Introducing healthcare professionals to systems thinking through an integrated curriculum for leading in health systems. *Journal of Nursing Management*. 04/2021. https://doi.org/10.1111/jonm.13342

Nardi, D. A. & Diallo, R. (2014). Global trends and issues in APN practice: Engage in the change. *Journal of Professional Nursing*, 30, 228–232. https://doi.org/10.1016/j.profnurs.2013.09.010

National Council for the Professional Development of Nursing and Midwifery (2007). *Framework for the Establishment of Advanced Nurse Practitioner and Advanced Midwife Practitioner Posts*. Dublin.

Newhouse, R. P., Stanik-Hutt, J., White, K. M., Johantgen, M., Bass, E. B., Zangaro, G., Wilson, R. F., Fountain, L., Steinwachs, D. M., Heindel, L. & Weiner, J. P. (2011). Advanced practice nurse outcomes 1990–2008: A systematic review. *Nursing Economic*, 29, 230–50.

Norris, T. & Melby, V. (2006). The Acute Care Nurse Practitioner: Challenging existing boundaries of emergency nurses in the United Kingdom. *Journal of Clinical Nursing*, 15, 253–263. https://doi.org/10.1111/j.1365-2702.2006.01306.x

Oshry, B. (1999). *Leading Systems: Lessons from the Power Lab*. San Francisco, CA, Berrett-Koehler Publishers Limited.

Oshry, B. (2007). *Seeing Systems: Unlocking the Mysteries of Organizational Life*. San Francisco, CA, Berrett-Koehler Publishers.

Oshry, B. (2018). *Context Context Context*. Axminster, Triarchy Press.

Oshry, B. (2019). *The Organic Systems Framework: A New Paradigm for Understanding and Intervening in Organisational Life*. Axminster, Triarchy Press.

Oshry, B. (2020). What lies beneath. *Organisation Development Journal*, Autumn, 38, 3, 11–32.

Oxtoby, K. (2016). Nurse prescribing: 10 years on. *Nurse Prescribing*, 14, 448–449. https://doi.org/10.12968/npre.2016.14.9.448

Paniagua, H. (2011). Advanced nurse practitioners and GPs: What is the difference? *Practice Nursing*, 22, 383–388. https://doi.org/10.12968/pnur.2011.22.7.383

Poghosyan, L., Lucero, R., Rauch, L. & Berkowitz, B. (2012). Nurse practitioner workforce: A substantial supply of primary care providers. *Nursing Economic*, 30, 268.

Power, R. & Phillips, K. (2017). *Not So Minor Injuries*. ANP Regional Conference, 2017 University Hospital Waterford.

Rashotte, J. (2005). Knowing the nurse practitioner: Dominant discourses shaping our horizons. *Nursing Philosophy*, 6, 51–62. https://doi.org/10.1111/j.1466-769x.2004.00199.x

Rogers, R., Malancharuvil-Berkes, E. & Mosley, M. (2005). Critical discourse analysis in education: A review of the literature. *Review of Educational Research*, 75, 365–416. https://doi.org/10.3102%2F00346543075003365

Stanik-Hutt, J., Newhouse, R. P., White, K. M., Johantgen, M., Bass, E. B., Zangaro, G., Wilson, R., Fountain, L., Steinwachs, D. M., Heindel, L. & Weiner, J. P. (2013). The quality and effectiveness of care provided by nurse practitioners. *The Journal for Nurse Practitioners*, 9, 492–500. http://dx.doi.org/10.1016/j.nurpra.2013.07.004

Street, D. & Cossman, J. S. (2010). Does familiarity breed respect? Physician attitudes toward nurse practitioners in a medically underserved state. *Journal of the American Academy of Nurse Practitioners*, 22, 431. https://doi.org/10.1111/j.1745-7599.2010.00531.x

ten Hoeve, Y., Jansen, G. & Roodbol, P. (2014). The nursing profession: Public image, self-concept and professional identity. A discussion paper. *Journal of Advanced Nursing*, 70, 295–309. https://doi.org/10.1111/jan.12177

Thompson, W. & Meskell, P. (2012). Evaluation of an advanced nurse practitioner (emergency care)—An Irish perspective. *The Journal for Nurse Practitioners*, 8, 200–205. http://dx.doi.org/10.1016/j.nurpra.2011.09.002

Thompson, W. & McNamara, M. (2022a). Constructing the advanced nurse practitioner identity in the healthcare system: A discourse analysis. *Journal of Advanced Nursing*, 78(3), 834–846. https://doi.org/10.1111/jan.15068

Thompson, W. & McNamara, M. (2022b). Revealing how language builds the identity of the advanced nurse practitioner. *Journal of Clinical Nursing*, 31(15–16), 2344–2353. https://doi.org/10.1111/jocn.16054

Ulrich, C. (2010). Who defines advanced nursing practice in an era of health care reform? *Clinical Scholars Review*, 3, 5–7. http://dx.doi.org/10.1891/1939-2095.3.1.5

Yong, C. S. (2006). Task substitution: The view of the Australian Medical Association. *The Medical Journal of Australia*, 185, 27–28. https://doi.org/10.5694/j.1326-5377.2006.tb00446.x

24 The promotion of resilience in nursing

Reification, second-order signification and neoliberalism

Michael Traynor

Don't come to me with your problems – learn some resilience. We have a workshop on Thursday.

Introduction

'Resilience' arrived in public discourse in the 2000s and was perhaps first applied to ecosystems on the interface between man-made and natural environments (Stockholm Resilience Centre, 2012). The concern was how such systems might respond to various kinds of disasters. In parallel, its usage proliferated across public policy from town planning to military support (Neocleous, 2013) as a new policy perspective on what had previously been understood as security. Thinking in terms of resilience rather than security acknowledged that adversity, for example in the form of a terrorist attack, was unavoidable and it was how you responded that counted, how you bounced back.

At a similar time, the use of the term as a positive psychological property of individuals started to dominate in self-help and popular psychology. The more serious psychologists worked on ways to detect and quantify it. Their more popular colleagues turned this into simple checklists on websites where viewers could find out their level of resilience and read tips on improving it (see actionforhappiness.org). In the early 2000s, the word went out in the UK that nurses needed to be, or learn how to be, resilient (Gray, 2011). Courses sprang up teaching it, questionnaires proliferated claiming to measure it. The consensus was that nurses, because of the occupational features of their work, were in particular need of it. The arrival of COVID-19 intensified the resilience imperative for nurses, but also exposed its limits.

In this chapter, I would like to review the way that 'resilience' has been promoted among and written about by nurses. I plan to look at the development and deployment of the term by the 'psy' professions (psychology, psychiatry and others). I see the way that resilience has been used as an example of reification and second-order signification. I also want to suggest that the promotion of resilience among the nursing workforce is a characteristic neoliberal project. I end by arguing for the benefits of engaging critically with the questions and issues that the promotion of resilience raises for nursing.

The promotion of resilience among nurses

The term 'resilience' was adopted by child psychiatrists from the mid-1970s onwards in an effort to account for the differences between the ways that different children appeared to be affected by adverse upbringings. I will return to the origins of the term later in this

DOI: 10.4324/9781003427407-28

chapter. 'Resilience' first appears in nursing literature in the early 1990s where it can refer either to patients that nurses might encounter or to nurses themselves. The latter use tends to dominate over time. Here, it denotes a positive personal characteristic on the part of a nurse that authors associate with what they consider to be positive outcomes. These outcomes often concern a comparative lack of psychological distress (Barnett and Marshall, 1992), acceptance of change (Davis, 1991) or, perhaps most commonly, an ability to continue to work in the workplace despite adverse conditions. Writers often describe this from an organisational viewpoint as retention (Scoble, 1991). The second strand of publication focuses on what had up to this time been the main use of the term applying it to vulnerable populations that nurses might be involved with such as the children of alcohol dependent parents (Jack et al., 1994). Articles that draw on research findings to promote resilience among nurses start to become the more frequent. Giordano's *Resilience – a survival tool for the nineties* is an early example of such a publication (Giordano, 1997).

Published articles about resilience among nurses can, in turn, be placed into two categories although there is some overlap: the first comprises accounts of research projects that aim to measure resilience among groups of nurses, sometimes written in collaboration with psychologists and the second takes the form of editorial or feature articles that describe the value of resilience to nurses and exhort them to become resilient or more resilient. They do this by listing apparent features of resilience. Both categories of articles present resilience as an already available solution to a comprehensive inventory of workplace adversities. Authors tend to start by listing contemporary features of nursing work that make it highly demanding. On inspection, we can see these features as having two origins: those that are intrinsic to the work itself and those that are a result of contemporary demographic, economic and political forces. The first type of adversity includes exposure to patient suffering and death and the close relationships that may develop with these patients (Zander et al., 2010, Dolan et al., 2012). The second type, which tends to be described at greater length, includes global nursing shortages and high turnover (Larrabee et al., 2010, p. 82), political change and under-resourcing of public healthcare (Koen et al., 2011), casualisation, staff shortages, bullying, abuse and violence (Jackson et al., 2007). Various authors argue that continued adversity has effects on nurse absenteeism, intention to leave, psychological morbidity and poor patient care. There is a broad assertion across this writing that for a nurse to remain in the nursing workforce is a sign of resilience and that some of those who remain apparently 'thrive' on the adversity they experience. There is also an assumption that a decision to leave nursing can be understood as succumbing to adversity, i.e. a negative consequence, a sign of pathology. The adage that we cannot always change what happens to us but we can change how we respond to events appears often in this literature as an argument for the importance of resilience. In other words, resilience has the advantage of not requiring a challenge to the status quo.

Three critical explorations

I would like to now sketch out three critical explorations of the imperative to be resilient that I have just summarised. These build upon each other as they explore resilience as (i) an example of reification, (ii) a second-order signifier for the good life and (iii) a characteristic neoliberal project.

Reification

Although the term reification was first used by Marx when discussing commodity fetish-ism in Capital (Marx, 1999), it is through the writing of Georg Lukács (1885–1971) and his essay Reification and the Consciousness of the Proletariat (Lukács, 1971) that writ-ers today tend to approach the term. It was later taken up by members of the Frankfurt School and more recently by contemporary thinkers such as Slavoj Žižek (2012). Lukács describes how reification covers over the social processes involved in and necessary to the production of commodities under capitalism by presenting, for example, the monetary price of an object as the expression of an autonomous force, rather than the result of something that has its origin in human labour and is mediated by the relations inherent in commodity exchange (Lijster, 2017). Another example, closer to this consideration of resilience, would be the way that the processes of production give rise to an objectified, measurable understanding of time and the time taken for a worker to produce a product, his 'performance', which is separated from the worker's total humanity and their social context and treated as an autonomous 'thing' (see https://www.marxists.org/archive/lu-kacs/works/history/hcc05.htm). In the same way, to set out to measure the resilience of nurses working in a clinic is to conjure into existence resilience as a pre-existing internal characteristic or private property of those nurses. It avoids understanding the behaviour of these nurses in the clinic and their responses to psychologists' questions as enactments and reflections of social relations in particular, possibly oppressive organisational set-tings and these within wider political and policy contexts. 'Reification is forgetting' as Horkeimer and Adorno stated (Adorno and Horkheimer, 1979, p. 230).[1] For reification to be effective, that is to not draw attention to the social processes of how this 'thing'—resilience here—arrived, the interests of those state-authorised bodies within the psy pro-fessions who make decisions about what to 'measure' in the name of resilience also need to be forgotten and to remain separated from the final resilience 'score' delivered to the worker and manager. The distribution, in both senses, of these scores creates some nurses as 'resilient' and some as 'at risk'. Those who are discovered to be 'at risk' can perhaps be prioritised for targeted intervention of resilience training. The promotion of resilience might masquerade as humanistic and in the best interests of individual nurses, and prob-ably those who promote it believe this, but it actually has worker performance as its real attraction to managers, the maintenance of a stable workforce and reduction of the costs associated with nurse turnover as many resilience researchers in nursing emphasise (Larrabee et al., 2010). I will return to this point later when discussing the drive for re-silience as a neoliberal project.

  To summarise, 'resilience' as predominantly used in studies of and the management of nursing is a label applied by members of the psy professions as an interpretation of how nurses respond to the psy profession's questioning or their behaviour in the workplace, i.e. by leaving or remaining. The application of this label affects a claim for a unified entity that covers over the social relations inherent in the labour market and its politi-cal context. Psychologists are not unaware of this danger (of reification) but tend to see it in terms of construct validity and argue that if a construct's effects can be observed, this suggests that the construct is 'something real' (https://www.psywww.com/intropsych/ch01-psychology-and-science/constructs-and-reification.html). There are exceptions to this assertion, such as the idea of 'pragmatic nihilism', the proposal that psychological constructs can be understood as metaphors that may or may not point to something that actually exists but are nevertheless useful (Fried, 2017). However, such abstract considerations that do arise within psychology tend not to include awareness of psychologists' complicity with political forces and the interests of capital.

Second-order signifier

Following on from the claim that the emergence of resilience into public discourse, or certain sections of public discourse, can be seen as an example of reification, I would like to explore the effects of the use of this specific label, resilience. Psychologists consider concepts such as resilience, along with, for example, gratitude or optimism or introversion as 'constructs' and the ambiguity of that term reflects an uncertainty and debate about what these things called constructs are, alluded to above. Some psychologists ask: are they natural kinds (true things we *discover*), socially constructed kinds (categories we *produce*), or are they pragmatic kinds (being *useful* for something) (Fried, 2017)? A construct or its components may be 'discovered' through the statistical association between responses to sets of questions that psychologists ask their subjects such as about their apparent anxiety and depression (Zigmond and Snaith, 1983) or their 'personality' on five dimensions (John and Srivastava, 1999). Yet, the labels chosen to name these sets of associations are not innocent and often come already with social meaning and connotation that function as persuasion of their existence and legitimacy. Even the self-report inventories devised to measure anxiety, resilience, happiness or personality do not simply ask people to evaluate their lives or themselves but they do so by means of categories that are themselves value laden (Ahmed, 2010) and loaded with connotation. 'Emotional intelligence', for example, is plausible and fascinating because we are already familiar with the generally positively loaded 'intelligence'. Placing 'emotional' before it, though for a moment apparently incompatible, makes us sense the possible limited nature of intelligence and imagine the world as a better place if emotional intelligence were discovered and encouraged to blossom (Goleman, 1995), and psychologists given more funding to investigate it.

The term resilience is already a metaphor for the springiness of certain materials. In the material world, the tendency to return to a prior shape after an application of force could be either useful or problematic. However, psychological resilience is always and only positively loaded. In fact, its positive loading is frequently returned to our interpretation of the natural world. It is good to spring back, to bounce back, to bend but not break and to grow, all as ways to respond to adversities of various kinds, just like the bamboo common in the images on Internet sites selling resilience services (Peoplebuilders, 2022). Here, resilience takes on a cosmic dimension with the hint of Eastern wisdom provided by the bamboo. However before the term became so popular, we might find other words applied by the researchers that we now consider as 'resilience researchers' to the children that were the focus of early studies in the 1970s and 1980s. E. James Anthony, in the introduction to a collection of such work (Anthony and J. Cohler, 1987), runs through something of the lexicon of terms used prior to settling on resilience: competence, psychoimmunity, invulnerability, even the 'Meursault phenomenon' named after the central character in Camus' novel *L'Etranger* who not only appears unaffected by suffering but is almost totally psychologically detached from the world around him. The theoretical model of these practising psy researchers was that protective factors shielded children from the negative effects of adversity in their upbringing. Their challenge, as researchers, was to find out what these protective factors were. The list of terms above describes the working labels that they applied to their attempts to understand these factors. Anthony's positivism, detectable in his introduction alongside his concern for the welfare of the children he treated and studied, is apparent in his claim that differences in the language used by investigators hide the fact that they are all researching the same phenomenon (p. 6). (In Fried's terms, he would understand the construct as of a natural kind, i.e. there all along.) His explanation for the shift of attention among psychiatrists and others from studying vulnerability to examining resilience is their growing unease that medicine tended to concern itself with detecting 'the most miniscule aspects of disease' while showing little curiosity towards questions about good health (page ix). In fact, the protective factors that this body of foundational research appeared to identify were, they believed, the result of an interaction of family, school, neighbourhood and personal characteristics, in other words, an understanding closer to the ecological use of the term resilience than the highly individualised personal aptitude that underlies its current application to nurses.

However, not only is resilience positive, it has history. Human response to adversity is the core material of philosophy and storytelling from Greek myth and ancient religions to modern fiction and film. So something in the term is *recognisable* and that is what gives it its power. When applied to human affairs, we have to interpret resilience, following Roland Barthes, as a second-order signifier (Barthes, 1972) pointing to a 'semiotic myth' in this case about human well-being, human character and a successful way of living. In Barthes' theory of signs and signification 'first-order' signification is similar to Saussure's coupled notions of the *signifier* as the speech sound (De Saussure, 1974)—or for Barthes an image or other signifying practice—and the *signified* as the concept—or for Barthes, an object. Saussure named the combination of signifier and signified as the sign. In second-order signification, the sign as a whole becomes a signifier of what Barthes calls myth.[2]

For Barthes, myth has a number of features and I will mention two of these for the purpose of this argument. The first is that myth is close to what sociologists might describe as 'collective representation' (Barthes, 1977, p. 165) or what Barthes calls 'a type of speech' giving rise to the sense of recognition when contemporary Westerners come across the term resilience. The notion of growing through adversity is so familiar that those promoting resilience do not need to explicitly refer to any particular previous instance in religion or philosophy (this is the 'what-goes-without-saying' or ideology that Barthes refers to (Barthes, 1972, p. 10)). Nevertheless references to Westernised Eastern wisdom (brief quotes from well-known Buddhists) as well as Western religion can be found embedded in overtly 'scientific' psychological discourse:

> … adversity may provide opportunities for the development of important character traits, echoing St. Paul's insight that "suffering produces endurance, and endurance produces character, and character produces hope" (Romans 5: 3–4).
>
> (AuthenticHappiness
> https://www.authentichappiness.sas.upenn.edu/learn/growth)

In Christianity, as referenced above, resilience is hidden in plain sight, the death and transformed resurrection of Christ representing the ultimate bouncing back. The same story of growth through adversity is told in literature from Shakespeare to the terrorist attacks of 9/11 via World War II and Anne Frank's diary.[3]

The second of Barth's features understands myth as inversion. Referring to Marx, Barthes understands myth as overturning culture into nature, turning:

> the social, the cultural, the ideological, the historical into the 'natural'. What is nothing but a product of class division and its moral, cultural and aesthetic consequences is presented... as being a 'matter of course'.
>
> (page 165)

Resilience, whether you have it, or how much of it you have, how long you can work in an underfunded health system has become part of, or evidence of your nature, of your natural character or skills rather than an effect of managerial practices in the workplace in the context of socioeconomic relations. Applying the label 'resilience' to (what has increasingly become) the way that workers respond to questions on a questionnaire not only provides an impression of a unified natural characteristic, discussed above, but also connects a concern with resilience, in however superficial or subliminal a way, with grand narratives of human growth through adversity.

Contemporary use of the term, then, brings along with it this immense connotation. However, it also adds to this the assumption that those who are able to use and promote the term have special knowledge of what makes the good life, of how we should live. If happiness research shows that the happiest people are married, then the finding also acts as a recommendation to get married (Ahmed, 2010). If resilience research has found that resilient people are grateful, humorous and in 'high-quality' relationships (Dutton and Spreitzer, 2014), then we should make new efforts to be grateful, humorous and in high-quality relationships.

Resilience as a neoliberal project

To summarise the argument so far, resilience can be understood as an example of the Marxist concept of reification. Talk of 'resilience' covers over the social relations engendered by the operation of capital, in this case within the context of the healthcare workforce. The label itself also performs a function through its positive connotations with deeply embedded ideologies of individual character that are so culturally familiar that they appear natural. In the final part of this critique, I would like to suggest that there is also a fit between the approaches of the psy professions, that have played a key role in the promotion of resilience, and the individualising force of neoliberalism.

Neoliberalism has been repeatedly described[4] and critiqued to the extent that it risks becoming overused as an explanation for social ills, including cultural atomisation (Giroux, 2019), the economic and psychic insecurities of extreme individualism (Rose, 1999), particularly in Western societies, and the withdrawal and degradation of state welfare (Navarro, 2007). Nevertheless, despite the possibility of over-reliance on the term, neoliberalism has provided a strong supportive milieu for the popularisation and promotion of resilience. Critics of neoliberalism have developed terms such as 'responsibilisation' to describe the:

> ...process whereby subjects are rendered individually responsible for a task which previously would have been the duty of another – usually a state agency – or would not have been recognised as a responsibility at all.
>
> (O'Malley, 2009, p.276)

In the realm of health, the responsible citizen is understood as an individual who avoids risky behaviour and who cultivates healthy practices and lifestyles, including healthy ways of thinking and feeling. The promise is that resilience and happiness lead to or are associated with material success and productivity (Ahmed, 2010).

There are well-established critiques of the psy professions and their place in intensifying an individualism that serves the needs of capital (Rose, 1999). Parker sets out a forceful argument that contemporary psychology is complicit in the oppressions effected by modern states and capitalism: its job has become to adapt people to become productive members of society (Parker, 2007). He argues that psychology not only alienates people from each other but from themselves. He details how successive psychologically developed assessments at school and then in the workplace alienate people from their apparent failure to be fully productive. The nurse has no knowledge of whether they are resilient or not until they receive their resilience score from psychologists.

> Unbearable misery is treated by psychology as if it were a disorder, failure or illness. One of the most destructive aspects of alienation is the separation of people from feelings of misery and anger, either at their own plight or the plight of others. Our own oppression is then turned by psychologists into 'negative thinking'…
>
> (Parker, 2007, p. 4)

Pavón-Cuéllar develops Parker's critique. The psy professions, he argues, have created as a field and topic of study, the interior life of the individual. Their version of this 'interior life' is something fundamentally separated from the rest of the world:

> Biology takes the existence of its object—life, *bios*—for granted. Likewise, the existence of demons or beliefs about demons is presupposed by their systematic study in demonology. The same holds true for other sciences, including psychology, which must assume that there is a psyche somewhere in the world… Without a psyche, why should we have psychological discourse, a discourse about the psyche? The need for psychology can only be justified if the reality of its object is accepted. This psychic reality can take the form of a substance, a force (or kind of life), a parallel world, an independent human sphere, a mechanism, a functional system, a process (or arrangement of processes), a faculty (or set of faculties), etc.
>
> (Pavón-Cuéllar, 2018, p. 320–21)

So when faced with the effects of adversity, whether related to the social deprivation of the parents of children at risk of harm, or to the underfunded and dysfunctional work environment of the nurse, the natural realm where action is to be taken is, for psychology, within the individual psyche. It emerges that it is the individual's responsibility to do work on themselves to build resilience, for example, by developing a sense of humour as some promoters of resilience suggest (Friborg et al., 2003). This focus on individual responsibility rather than on structural causes—and solutions—of adversity locates resilience discourse within neoliberalism and makes the promotion of resilience, if not psychology as a whole, an attractive project for neoliberal governments (Neocleous, 2013). Pavón-Cuéllar and others argue that the problem is not so much that there is really no psyche but that psychology in particular has developed, for various historical reasons, a version of the psyche that stands over and against everything else, i.e. is fundamentally dualistic, albeit that psychology acknowledges somatic effects of mental health problems and, conversely, chemical causes of mental ill-health. The problem is more that individuals have lost their individual internal being when their existence has been alienated from them by capitalism. In Parker's and Pavón-Cuéllar's more emancipatory model, the psyche and the social are continuous and not two separate realms (Frosh, 2003). A notable example of the alienation of emotions by capital and managerialism takes the form of the demands of emotional labour upon many service sector workers (Hochschild, 1983).⁵ The presence of these strong emotional demands and rules of display of emotions characterises nursing work (Smith, 1992) and is frequently given as a reason that nurses need to 'learn' resilience (Manzano García and Carlos, 2012, Mealer et al., 2012, McDonald et al., 2012). In the writing of many nurse researchers, we can find that the individual 'inner' focus of much psychology mingles with the individualism of neoliberalism to result in a misguided acquiescence. The difference between the challenge that is intrinsic to nursing work and that which results from policy decisions is ignored. They argue that the solution to occupational 'adversity' is to be found in the realm of individual action e.g. the need to develop resilience, and though the cause of the adversity is often described in structural terms (bullying, staff shortages), the possibility of structural change is curiously absent from the discussions and recommendations of these researchers. In fact, the possibility of change is sometimes explicitly rejected in nursing research on workforce resilience with the acquiescent claim that 'nurses' occupational settings will always contain elements of stressful, traumatic or difficult situations, and episodes of hardship' (Jackson et al., 2007, p. 7) or in the equally misguided claim that 'it is important to acknowledge that work stress and crises are inevitable and even necessary for the growth and maturity of the individual and to allow them to reach their full potential' (Manzano García and Carlos, 2012, p. 105). Another author considers that understanding resilience among nurses 'would provide hospital managers with useful guidelines for in-service training that won't be threatening and can facilitate growth in professional nurses' (Koen et al., 2011, p. 3). Promoting resilience among nurses is a way, according to many of the authors, of reducing turnover in the nursing workforce, with the promise that nurses can thrive at the bedside for 'extended periods of time' (Mealer et al., 2012, p. 297).

The benefit of engaging with this philosophical question

In this chapter, I have subjected the notion of resilience and its promotion among nurses to critique. This critique suggests that the appeal of resilience to governments and to managers lies in its welcome shift from a focus on problems to something that sounds reassuringly positive. Promoting resilience is an alternative to addressing difficult structural change. The promoters of resilience tell us that when faced with adversity—we might want to call it oppression—we need, simply, to change the way we think about it. I have pointed to the dangers of resilience in terms of the alienation that can result by configuring individual citizens, individual nurses in this case, as responsible for solving problems that are the result of structural arrangements. An examination of the dangers of an uncritical acceptance of resilience discourse can be flipped on its head and become a setting out of the benefits for nursing of a critical engagement with this issue. This has the advantage of requiring us to imagine an alternative.

The question 'What are the benefits?' raises the further question, 'Benefit for whom?' For nursing? It is possible to use the term 'nursing' as an inclusive but imprecise gesture towards a field of academic intellectual work; the global professional organisations of nurses and their trades unions; and the nursing workforce which is itself a highly heterogeneous group of employees that includes so-called front-line nurses, middle and senior managers, senior civil servants and educators. These groups, and subgroups within them, may well have different and conflicting interests despite the fact that an individual may be a member of more than one of these groups, or may travel from one to another during a career. Those who are involved in intellectual interrogations of nursing have, I think, a responsibility to carefully examine and debate claims and projects to do with nursing work and its organisation and engage with the other groups to discuss the results and to continue debate. Sometimes, it can feel that those who have influence over the profession successively and uncritically take up projects such as the Nursing Process, managerialism, evidence-based practice or resilience when these projects appear to offer some professionalising potential or stand for well-defined solutions to complex problems. Dangers and disadvantages need to be made apparent because those who promote these projects tend to only present one side of an argument. Uncritical acceptance can lead us down a road we might later wish we had trodden more carefully. Professional organisations and trades unions are concerned with collectives by their nature. Their work is to develop the profession and protect and advance the working lives of nurses. A critical engagement on their part with the promotion of resilience would enable, and I think largely has enabled, a continued focus on structural problems facing the workforce and avoided the distractions of the often faddish uptake of resilience training. The workforce itself, as mentioned, is diverse. Front-line staff know first-hand how voicing concerns about safety and their own distress at intolerable working conditions can be met by managers (who are themselves under considerable pressure) with the suggestion to attend resilience training. This compounds their distress because they realise that their managers are either cynical, powerless or naïve, or some combination. Since I have started speaking about resilience, I have been approached by or heard testimony from such nurses. Generally, they hear public critiques of the promotion of resilience with a strong sense of recognition. My hope is that this recognition is the first step of a journey towards resistance and away from acquiescence and burnout.

To end, I would like to argue that an awareness of the history and influences on the contemporary call for resilience gives nurses, in all of the groups above, the opportunity to refuse to be drawn onto this ground and to choose alternatives such as collective action to understand the causes of the adversity that they experience and to work for change. Engaging with this critical question, as I have attempted to do in this chapter, enables resistance rather than resilience.

Notes

1 In the Verso edition, the translation of the German Verdinglichung is 'objectification'.
2 The word or image of a rose denotes the flower. Together, they can be seen to connote 'love'. This is, roughly, first- and second-order signification.
3 These literary moments are taken from a search on the literary website Goodreads.com for 'resilience' which brings up (in March 2022) just under 5,000 titles (https://www.goodreads.com/shelf/show/resilience).
4 The rise of neoliberalism, in its most recent incarnation, is generally associated with the election of the new-right governments of Margaret Thatcher in the UK (from 1979) and Ronald Reagan in the US (from 1981). These governments promoted low-tax free-market economies where enterprise is encouraged and the fates of the idle and incompetent stand as lessons to spur on others. Margaret Thatcher introduced the so-called 'internal market' into the UK NHS in the belief that 'competition' would motivate individual clinicians and managers to make their services more efficient and attractive to 'consumers' – patients.

5 Selling resilience to corporations is part of the invasion of capital into the psyche of workers. Corporate coaching does not offer straightforwardly to improve the productivity of the workforce but makes grandiose claims to be part of a global force for good where everyone on the planet has 'the opportunity to live authentically and bring out their personal best' (see https://www.peoplebuilders.com.au/about).

References

ADORNO, T. & HORKHEIMER, A. 1979. *Dialectic of Enlightenment*, London, Verso.

AHMED, S. 2010. *The Promise of Happiness*, Durham, NC, Duke University Press.

ANTHONY, E. J. & J. COHLER, B. (eds.) 1987. *The Invulnerable Child*, New York, The Guilford Press.

BARNETT, R. C. & MARSHALL, N. L. 1992. Worker and mother roles, spillover effects, and psychological distress. *Women & Health*, 18, 9–40.

BARTHES, R. 1972. *Mythologies*, Frogmore, Granada.

BARTHES, R. 1977. *Image, Music, Text*, London, Fontana.

DAVIS, P. S. 1991. The meaning of change to individuals within a college of nurse education. *Journal of Advanced Nursing (Wiley-Blackwell)*, 16, 108–115.

DE SAUSSURE, F. 1974. *Course in General Linguistics*, London, Fontana.

DOLAN, G., STRODL, E. & HAMERNIK, E. 2012. Why renal nurses cope so well with their workplace stressors. *Journal of Renal Care*, 38, 222–32.

DUTTON, J. E. & SPREITZER, G. M. 2014. *How to Be a Positive Leader: Small Actions, Big Impact*, Berrett-Koehler Publishers.

FRIBORG, O., HJEMDAL, O., ROSENVINGE JAN H. & MARTINUSSEN, M. 2003. A new rating scale for adult resilience: What are the central protective resources behind healthy adjustment? *International Journal of Methods in Psychiatric Research*, 12, 65–76.

FRIED, E. I. 2017. What are psychological constructs? On the nature and statistical modelling of emotions, intelligence, personality traits and mental disorders. *Health Psychology Review*, 11, 130–134.

FROSH, S. 2003. Psychosocial studies and psychology: Is a critical approach emerging? *Human Relations*, 56, 1545–1567.

GIORDANO, B. P. 1997. Resilience—a survival tool for the nineties. *AORN Journal*, 65, 1032–1034.

GIROUX, H. 2019. *We Must Overcome Our Atomization to Beat Back Neoliberal Fascism* [Online]. trouthout. Available: https://truthout.org/articles/we-must-overcome-our-atomization-to-beat-back-neoliberal-fascism/ [Accessed 23rd May 2022].

GOLEMAN, D. 1995. *Emotional Intelligence*, New York, Bantam Books.

GRAY, J. 2011. Building resilience in the nursing workforce. *Nursing Standard*, 26, 2012.

HOCHSCHILD, A. 1983. *The Managed Heart*, Berkeley, University of California Press.

JACK, L., HAINES, V. & WEINSTEIN, N. 1994. Children from alcoholic families -- a population at risk. *Journal of School Nursing*, 10, 27–36.

JACKSON, D., FAU - FIRTKO, A. & EDENBOROUGH, M. 2007. Personal resilience as a strategy for surviving and thriving in the face of workplace adversity: A literature review. *Journal of Advanced Nursing*, 60, 1–9.

JOHN, O. P. & SRIVASTAVA, S. 1999. The big five trait taxonomy: History, measurement, and theoretical perspectives. *In*: PERVIN, L. A. & JOHN, O. P. (eds.) *Handbook of Personality: Theory and Research (2nd ed)*. New York, Guilford Press.

KOEN, M. P., VAN EEDEN, C. & WISSING, M. P. 2011. The prevalence of resilience in a group of professional nurses. *Health SA Gesondheid*, 16, 1–11.

LARRABEE, J. H., WU, Y., PERSILY, C. A., SIMONI, P. S., JOHNSTON, P. A., MARCISCHAK, T. L., MOTT, C. L. & GLADDEN, S. D. 2010. Influence of stress resiliency on RN job satisfaction and intent to stay. *Western Journal of Nursing Research*, 32, 81–102.

LIJSTER, T. 2017. 'All Reification Is a Forgetting' :Benjamin, Adorno, and the Dialectic of Reification. *In:* GANDESHA, S. & HARTLE, J. F. (eds.) *The Spell of Capital Reification and Spectacle.* Amsterdam, Amsterdam University Press.

LUKÁCS, G. 1971. *History and Class Consciousness; Studies in Marxist Dialectics.* Cambridge, MA, MIT Press.

MANZANO GARCÍA, G. & CARLOS 2012. Emotional exhaustion of nursing staff: Influence of emotional annoyance and resilience. *International Nursing Review*, 59, 101–107.

MARX, K. 1999. *Capital: A New Abridgement.* Oxford, Oxford University Press.

MCDONALD, G., JACKSON, D., WILKES, L. & VICKERS, M. H. 2012. A work-based educational intervention to support the development of personal resilience in nurses and midwives. *Nurse Education Today*, 32, 378–384.

MEALER, M., JONES, J., NEWMAN, J., MCFANN, K. K., ROTHBAUM, B. & MOSS, M. 2012. The presence of resilience is associated with a healthier psychological profile in intensive care unit (ICU) nurses: Results of a national survey. *International Journal of Nursing Studies*, 49, 292–299.

NAVARRO, V. 2007. Neoliberalism as a class ideology; Or, the political causes of the growth of inequalities. *International Journal of Health Services*, 37, 47–62

NEOCLEOUS, M. 2013. Resisting resilience. *Radical Philosophy*, 178, 6.

O'MALLEY, P. 2009. Responsibilization. *In:* WAKEFIELD, A. & FLEMING, J. (eds.) *The Sage Dictionary of Policing.* London, Sage.

PARKER, I. 2007. *Revolution in Psychology: Alienation to Emancipation.* London, Pluto Press.

PAVÓN-CUÉLLAR, D. 2018. Marxism, psychoanalysis, and the critique of psychological dualism: From dualist repression to the return of the repressed in hysteria and class consciousness. *Theory & Psychology*, 28, 319–339.

PEOPLEBUILDERS. 2022. *Resilience: Lessons from the Bamboo* [Online]. Sydney, Australia, People Builders Pty Ltd. Available: https://www.peoplebuilders.com.au/blog/resilience-lessons-bamboo [Accessed April 7th 2022].

ROSE, N. 1999. *Governing the Soul – The Shaping of the Private Self.* London, Free Association Books.

SCOBLE, K. B. 1991. *Career Resilient Characteristics and Commitment Among Registered Nurses: Predictors of Organizational and Professional Retention.* Columbia University Teachers College.

SMITH, P. 1992. *The Emotional Labour of Nursing.* Basingstoke, Macmillan Education.

STOCKHOLM RESILIENCE CENTRE. 2012. *What Is Resilience? An Introduction to a Popular Yet Often Misunderstood Concept.* Stockholm, Stockholm Resilience Centre.

ZANDER, M., HUTTON, A. & KING, L. 2010. Coping and resilience factors in pediatric oncology nurses. *Journal of Pediatric Oncology Nursing*, 27, 94–108.

ZIGMOND, A. & SNAITH, R. 1983. The hospital anxiety and depression scale. *Acta Psychiatrica Scandinavica*, 67, 361–370.

ŽIŽEK, S. 2012. *Less than Nothing: Hegel and the Shadow of Dialectical Materialism.* London, Verso.

25 Problematizing moral distress, moral resilience and moral courage

Implications for nurse education and moral agency

Pamela J. Grace

Introduction

Singular healthcare professions, and by association their members, cannot on their own resolve the complex problems or poorly conceptualized policies that interfere with human health and wellbeing. Political conditions, social disadvantages and structural injustices tend to be multi-faceted in origin and effect. They often spring from tangled roots, persistent imbalances within a society and historically set trajectories. Thus, resolving them for the most part requires input from various disciplines with their disparate expertise's and, when it comes to policy change, public support.

The inability to practice well, whether a consequence of systemic or local hurdles, system failure, inadequate education, personal factors or some combination, has raised questions about the scope and limits of a professional's responsibilities to ensure good patient care in particular, and good healthcare in general. I recognize that calling a body of practitioners a profession is itself controversial. However, I use this term as a placeholder for those practices that s or still have a measure of autonomy (Grace, 2022, Grace, In Press) in terms of knowledge development, self-regulation and some freedom to enact clinical judgment.

The concepts of moral distress (MD), moral resilience (MR) and moral courage are related to the idea that healthcare professionals have ethical responsibilities toward those served. However, the uncritical acceptance of these concepts when inadequately defined for purpose leads to confusion about the extent of professional responsibilities and thus what is needed to develop the moral agency of nurses – among other healthcare professionals. Here, I explore the scope and limits of these concepts, as well as their underlying logic in relation to how helpful they are for understanding what is required for the development of nurse moral agency, discussed in more detail later.

My foundational assumption is that groups providing the important human service of improving or maintaining human health are involved in offering a "good" and that making choices about how best to accomplish this is possible to varying degrees depending on internal and external constraints. It is these varying degrees that are of especial concern and which are the focus of ethical decision-making in practice. Three particularly salient questions investigated are "to what extent are individuals such as nurses responsible for assuming the risks of ethical action in difficult circumstances, under which conditions and with what sort of preparation?"

Finally, I propose that understood a certain way with limits illuminated and for particular circumstances, the concepts of MD, MR and moral courage may help expose occult barriers to good practice. They, along with insights from psychology, may help

DOI: 10.4324/9781003427407-29

to highlight the nature and range of educational processes needed to develop confidence in ethical decision-making. However, they remain unstable concepts that in the absence of a critical approach to their use may contribute to maintaining a status quo that is rife with injustices. The addition of critical inquiry that exposes the roots of such injustices may help remove the burden of resolution for intractable obstacles from being reliant "entirely on the character of the individual nurse" (Traynor, 2017, p. xi).

Moral distress

The late philosopher Andrew Jameton (2013), who is credited with coining the phrase "Moral Distress" in his 1984 book, *Nursing Practice: The Ethical Issues* (p. 6), notes that in the 1970s and 1980s, nurses sought courses in medical or bioethics, in larger numbers than the intended audience of medical students and physicians, partly because of lack of confidence in their ability to address the everyday problems they faced. "The concept moral distress was thus useful in promoting a more direct discussion of the moral problems nurses were facing" (p. 298). Jameton (1984) defined MD, which he differentiated from moral uncertainty, as arising when "one knows the right thing to do, but institutional constraints make it nearly impossible to pursue the right course of action" (p. 6). He also claimed that "nursing is the morally central health care profession" (p. xvi) because it has retained the values of health and compassion as central to practice. This is unlike medicine which has been more concerned with managing the institutions and technologies of healthcare (Jameton, 1984).

Conceptual ambiguity

The nursing profession, with some exceptions, has adopted Jameton's definition as explanatory of sometimes long-lasting unsettling emotions experienced in ethically conflictual situations where nurses feel powerless. Since Jameton's introduction of MD into the nursing and healthcare lexicon, the concept remains ill-defined and contentious, in part because of its obvious subjectivity. Of the two main definitions, Jameton's view (subsequently revised) – the more narrowly specified – assumes that nurses claiming to experience, or evaluated as experiencing, MD have an understanding of ethics and ethical decision-making (how to conceptualize likely best actions in a given situation). Thus, they can identify accurately that the distress they are experiencing is as a result of ethical judgments that are unable to be enacted – a failure of moral agency. A broader view includes the above as well as an alternative possibility that nurses know something is amiss but are not clear about what is wrong or how they should act (Howe, 2017; McCarthy & Deady, 2008; Morley et al., 2019). Accepting a broader definition of MD, however, does not overcome the problematic nature of MD as a concept that has significant subjective aspects because it still begs several questions. Important questions include:

> What preparation is necessary for nurses to grasp the ethical implications of any action they take as nurses, what knowledge and skills are needed to help nurses' consistently make good decisions and to what extent is the distress experienced complicated by prior life circumstances conscious or subconscious?

as described by Winslade (2017). The latter question self-evidently requires abilities for authentic self-reflection. Monteverde (2016) provides the important suggestion that we emphasize the idea of perception related to MD noting it as "perceived moral distress" (p. 107), thus allowing for normative critiques of the concept as discussed next.

Johnstone and Hutchinson (2015) call for abandoning the concept as proposed initially by Jameton and accepted by nursing scholars and researchers who have focused on MD – the narrow version. Noting that an anchor for one "theory of moral distress is the idea that nurses know what is the right thing to do but are unable to carry it out" (p. 8), they raise three objections. First, no evidence exists to support the validity of nurses' moral judgments in some of the situations where a claim is made that actions were blocked. Indeed, subsequently many of these judgments would be seen as seriously flawed when subjected to an ethical analysis. They note that "rarely are the bases of the nurses' moral judgments revealed, and rarely is it admitted that nurses might be mistaken or misguided in their moral judgments, or that their moral judgments may be just plain wrong" (p. 8). Anecdotally, this can be due to medical information to which the nurse has not been made privy. This may be due to poor communication or a discounting of the nurse's need to know. A second objection is that the professional responsibility of nurses to take other actions after the fact is not admitted. I have argued this point elsewhere (Grace, 2001). This again can be seen as a failure of adequate ethics education for nurses. Professional responsibilities exist for the immediate environment and addressing recurring problems or those having roots in unjust sociopolitical structures. As discussed later, developing MR (given a specified definition) might help alleviate distress and go some way toward addressing it; however, without a critical stance, it will be insufficient to resolve those problems that are the result of deeply seated injustices. Johnstone and Hutchinson's third objection is that the subjective nature of the experience of MD is what the nurse says it is. However, studies in cognitive psychology reveal the ubiquity of errors in human judgment that may affect identification of the locus of a given experience of distress (Peters & Filipova, 2009). The inevitable subjectivity involved renders MD an amorphous concept capturable only by descriptions of events and experiences that have given an agent pause, caused regret and to which they attribute psychological and physical sequelae. As Howe (2017), a psychoanalyst, proposes, "(P)erhaps in analyzing moral distress, greater attention should be given to implicit as well as the explicit source of the feelings of distress" (p. 43). In this sense, Monteverde's (2016) suggestion that we emphasize the idea of perception related to MD is in alignment with Howe's. When the largely subjective nature of experiences of MD is not accounted for, the use of the concept to underlie research or education will be inadequate at best. Further, without more clarity and specificity, research on the concept of MR, proposed as a way to mitigate or manage MD, may also be flawed. Muddiness in one concept when used as a springboard to study or resolve another is obviously problematic.

Moral distress and subjectivity

As examples of the inherent subjectivity of experiences of MD, however defined, and in accord with studies in moral and cognitive psychologies (Doris et al., 2010; Kahneman, 2011), it is likely rare that any distress experienced is attributable purely to the obstructed action or uncertainty about which action is preferred (Carse & Rushton, 2017; Howe, 2017; Johnstone & Hutchinson, 2015). Other possible reasons confounding the perception of distress include subconscious imprinting from past life processes and events, frustration, anger about not being heard, past disempowering experiences, strong identification with the patient or family, disapproval of a patient's lifestyle or other choices and so on.

Morley et al.'s (2019) synthesis of existing literature on MD led to a conclusion that there are three components that make up the necessary and sufficient conditions for moral distress as currently discussed. These are "(1) the experience of a moral event, (2) the experience of 'psychological distress' and (3) a direct causal relation between (1) and (2)" (p. 660), presumably as expressed by the person experiencing the distress. The causal relation from such studies is at least partly subjective and depends on an understanding of the nature of the moral in a "moral event" and an attribution of "psychological distress" to that understanding.

Shortly, I examine in more depth the idea of MR as it relates to nurses and ethical decision-making. First, a little about the obstacle to good practice that arises when people fail to notice the ethical aspects of an issue that has implications for a patient or patients.

Distress associated with patient care problems: the positive spin

The perception that one is experiencing MD – however defined – is generally understood in negative terms. That is, it is taken as problematic for one who experiences it as well as potentially for the person or persons who are the epicenter of the negatively perceived event. However, given the discussion so far, it can be argued that failure to experience moral or other emotional distress when it is warranted is also problematic. It is so because of the likelihood that the patient will fail to have their needs met, or similar situations will recur and remain unaddressed. For example, a patient who has no one to care for her at home is ordered for discharge after major hip surgery. The nurse discharging the patient fails to account for this, and when it is pointed out to him says "it is not my problem" or "others who are sicker needs this bed" and does not request further resources.

Paradoxically, numbness and distancing have been cited as sequelae of unrelieved or repeated MD. Besides the problem of dampened responses to repetitive feelings of powerlessness, evidence suggests that nurses do not always recognize the inherently ethical nature of their work (Grace et al., 2003; Hakimi et al., 2020; Milliken & Grace, 2017; Milliken et al., 2019). Thus, it could be argued that the absence of an experience of some sort of distress in morally problematic situations is also an ethical issue (Howe, 2017). Failure to experience distress in what ought to be distressing situations has been attributed to two disparate sources. One is a failure of nurse education to develop practitioners who understand the commitments of professional responsibility to further nursing goals (Grace, 2018; Milliken & Grace, 2017) and two the numbing effects of repeated unaddressed ethically problematic situations (Chambliss, 1996; Howe, 2017). In the first case, nurses may lack ethical sensitivity – awareness that their actions (including inaction) have ethical implications (Milliken & Grace, 2017). In the second case, repeated unaddressed or unresolved situations annihilate emotional responses to them. Both are problems for basic and continuing nursing education to address.

The concept of MR is starting to emerge and has been proposed as a way to help nurses manage and ameliorate their experiences of MD. Also a somewhat amorphous concept dependent as it is, at least in part, on a person's perception of their ability to bounce back from or resist feelings of distress. Psychological resilience has been subject to philosophical and empirical scrutiny in the psychology literature and has a generally accepted definition. It is conceptualized in the American Psychological Association

(APA) Dictionary as "the process and outcome of successfully adapting to difficult or challenging life experiences, especially through mental, emotional, and behavioral flexibility and adjustment to external and internal demands" (American Psychological Association, 2022).

Resilience

Resilience, in the form of resilience theory and science, entered the psychology lexicon around the 1970s as a result of observations that some children with traumatic backgrounds thrived, while others did not. Much of the subsequent research has also focused on children and characteristics that promote resilience (Masten, 2001, 2018) about which far more remains to be understood. Dictionary definitions of resilience refer to both the characteristics/substance of materials and ask psychological processes. Related to human beings there is some agreement that term means "the action or act of rebounding or springing back... the ability to recover readily from, or resist being affected by a(n emotional) setback or illness" (Brown, 1993, p. 2562). Contemporarily, interest in the potential of this concept to help healthcare professionals counter MD and its effects has grown, leading to the addition of the qualifier "moral". As proposed by Rushton (2016), MR is distinguishable from more general psychological resilience

> in its focus on (1) the moral aspects of human experience, (2) the moral complexity of the decisions, obligations and relationships, and (3) the inevitable moral challenges that ignite conscience, confusion, and moral distress... (it) is defined as the capacity of an individual to sustain or restore their integrity in response to moral complexity, confusion, distress, or setbacks.
>
> (pp. 112–113)

The presence of MR is supposed to be able to help mitigate the experience of MD because it enables the person who failed to act, withstand or rebound back from the emotional and physical sequelae of failing to act. From the psychology literature, factors proposed as contributing to the development of personal resilience generally include: "Maintaining good relationships, having an optimistic view of the world, keeping things in perspective, setting goals and taking steps to reach them, and being self-confident" (Newman, 2005, p. 227). However, Newman (2005) cautions "one individual's strategy for building resilience will likely not be the same as another's ... (it) is an individualized process dependent, in part on each individual's strengths, skills, and experience" (p. 227). Although many researchers believe that certain aspects are amenable to development in persons, it is unclear to what extent and under what circumstances (Fleming & Ledogar, 2008). The recent literature surrounding MR in healthcare professionals strongly favors the idea that it can be developed (Heinze et al., 2021) but given Newman's (2005) cautions individual differences in ability to learn need to be accounted for. Additionally, resilience is not a static process (Flynn et al., 2021); many influences can undermine it.

Demonstrations of resilience, how one knows the person has resilience or has developed resilience, require at a minimum that "both adversity and positive adaptation must be evident" (Fletcher & Sarkar, 2013, p. 14). However, both adversity and positive adaption themselves require further definition. We need to delineate what sorts of, and how much adversity is required and for whom. Subsequently, the question to be asked is "what counts as positive adaptation among different persons with differing abilities"?

Mahoney and Bergman (2002), describing research about positive adaptation, note that it involves a process or "processes by which individuals' attain overall patterns of adjustment that represent unusually favorable developmental trajectories, given their background and available resources" (p. 198). For current purposes, this definition focuses on the individual and what is needed for the individual to thrive at best and survive at worst. However, much of what requires resilience stems from conditions external to the person and these require a different level of redress.

Given research in psychology, consensus about the essential ingredients of resilience is lacking. Moreover, it is unclear how the qualifier "moral" provides clarity about to what extent it can be developed, how it can be developed, how it can be maintained and what purposes developing it would serve. This is especially pertinent related to research in psychology on the human reluctance to counter the directives of authority figures regardless of how obviously misguided or unreasonable (Stangor et al., 2022). I am not discounting the idea that some conception of MR could be helpful in nursing education. Those qualities gleaned from research that are linked to resilience include the ability to self-reflect and reflect on prior actions, persistence and so on.

Criticisms of the use of the term, MR, include that to be measured, it would have to be narrowly defined, and in being narrowly defined, it would likely fail to capture what is needed to develop persons who can overcome MD. Acquiring certain knowledge and skills might go some way to ameliorating sequelae of MD, but does not resolve the underlying conditions that have given rise to MD (in whatever form this is perceived). The essence of resilience, as presented by recent nurse scholars, represents resistance and recovery but not proactivity or prevention. This is in line with dictionary and psychological definitions of resilience.

Thus, the complexity and limitations of the concept belie its easy adoption as an educational or developmental strategy for nurses (Newman, 2005). Later, I argue that the development of nurses' acumen in ethical critique and analysis is critical to the management of obstacles to practice and allows the rightful locus of such obstacles to be exposed.

Sala Defilippis et al. (2019) offer a cogent critique of current definitions of resilience as adopted in nursing that goes part way in reflecting the concerns noted above and supports the necessity for critical inquiry into sources of disquiet in nursing practice. They argue for a different understanding of MR as a virtue that allows a person's sense of integrity (thus power to act ethically) to be preserved and/or developed. Drawing on prior work related to the virtues in nursing, they call for a radical reconceptualization of MR that allows critiques of the status quo. If nursing work is inherently moral work as I and others before me have stressed (Grace, 2018; Sellman, 2011; Yarling & McElmurry, 1986), then nurses have responsibilities not just to practice well in the moment as able but also to address underlying sociopolitical conditions that obstruct good care – albeit collaboratively and with others as needed. This view accounts for the place and role of nurses within the sociopolitical complexity and power structures of modern societies.

Sala Defilippis et al. (2019) offer MR as a character quality (virtue) that enables consistently good actions and allows for the preservation of one's sense of integrity. Their perspective is informed by an Aristotelian notion of virtue as the use of reason and habitual practice to discover the middle ground (the most cognitively sound) between extreme actions (vices). The excessive action is beyond one that would be warranted and thus is foolish and may be risky. A too timid action would fall short of what was required. MR then is posited as the mean between "faintheartedness and rigidity" (p. 1). "The virtue of moral resilience is the character trait, which allows nurses to remain open for compromises with themselves and with the given situation without compromising their own moral integrity" (p. 5). Presumably, developing MR is subject to an educational process. In other words, a differentiation needs to be made between what is needed and possible in the moment, including a compromise of one's own beliefs about a situation (as long as these compromises are not morally serious enough to shake one's sense of integrity), and what requires action after the fact perhaps in collaboration with others. While this goes someway to rectifying the issue of critical evaluation, the question about how to develop nurses' MR even from this expanded perspective remains, given the nature of individual differences as discussed earlier. Traynor (2017), among others, calls attention to the problem that developing nurse resilience in the absence of critical attention to the social and political matrix that is healthcare delivery will not adequately mitigate nurse (or other healthcare professionals) perceived MD.

A type of psychological resilience then, MR as discussed so far, is inadequate to underpin nurse basic and ongoing education or mitigate experiences of MD. It is inadequate because as previously noted, it places the focus of development on maintaining one's psychological stability and ability to persist but is not, by any definition about addressing what ought to be. Traynor's (2017) conception of "critical moral resilience" may provide a more explanatory account of what is needed to develop nurses with realistic conceptions of the scope and boundaries of their role as these occur within sociopolitical contexts and inevitable power imbalances. Critical MR may offer a way to judge the levels and types of courage that can be realistically expected of nurses. One purpose of developing skills in ethical decision-making is to advocate that what one knows in a given situation is conveyed articulately and in a way that facilitates collaboration. This requires a reasonable level of courage as discussed next.

An outcome of skill and experience in ethical decision-making is the ability to judge, at least roughly, the risks and benefits of acting in conflictual situations. Some actions are extremely risky, and a nurse may be willing to undertake them, but they should be understood as supererogatory in nature – that is they are beyond the expectations of nurses generally. As an example, John Welch, a nurse anesthetist, volunteered his services in Sierra Leone in 2014 to help with the Ebola crisis. When interviewed pre-departure, he is noted to have said, "if not me, who?" (CBS News, 2014). Nurses have historically assumed risks greater than expected of the public generally and have done so for all sorts of reasons, including the public good. The next section explores the meaning of moral courage and what it entails for nurses.

Moral courage

As a young UK nurse in my very early 20s, I undertook a temporary position in large psychiatric hospital in the North of England. My goal was satisfy the requirements to practice in the US. While accompanying a small group of patients to recreational therapy, an altercation broke out between an adolescent with personality disorder and an older man recovering from a bout of delirium tremens. The adolescent boy delighted in needling other patients and on this occasion the older man reacted. He raised his fist to take a swing at the boy. I stepped between them and yelled STOP and luckily the older man stopped. Was this foolish or courageous? Would I have done this had I been visiting a pub and a similar altercation occurred ... I don't think so. I do remember thinking, "I have to do something, I am in charge". The weight of my responsibility led to my action.

Was it foolish or courageous? I am not sure. I do know that I have not always spoken up when my words might have made a difference to a patient's trajectory, and I sometimes saw this as a lack of courage. I am also aware that on some occasions I lacked the ability to articulate coherently and cogently what was wrong. As I have argued elsewhere (Grace in Press), this is what led me to further studies in philosophy and to develop a certain level of expertise in ethical decision-making. If nurses have moral responsibilities to their patients beyond that of persons to each other in the course of daily life, how do they go about deciding the boundaries of those responsibilities and what are the limits of so-called courageous action.

My dissertation work married studies in philosophy with nursing education and practice experiences and culminated in a philosophical analysis of advocacy as used in a variety of disciplines. A big insight from this exploration was that actions have to be carefully considered related to the level at which they are directed. Immediate actions that might be too risky or impotent necessitate tackling via a different avenue. In turn, this requires sound ethical judgment.

The late Ann Hamric et al.'s (2015) challenge to healthcare providers is "must we be courageous?" (p. 33). In their discussion, they differentiate supererogatory actions from those required by professional practice. In so doing, they also highlight that institutional hierarchies and injustices are often the cause of a perceived need for courage by healthcare professionals such as nurses. Injustices of this sort oblige different sorts of actions for their redress but first their nature and causes have to be identified. Hamric et al.'s article constitutes a critique of the profession's call for nurses to be courageous when they are at serious risk. They appeal for recognition that there is a typology of courage. Moral courage in terms of everyday practice consists in actions that are taken after a course of deliberation. "The courageous nurse of physician must wisely choose (their) battles" (Hamric et al., 2015, p. 35). More-than-ordinary risks do come with the job, for example, exposure to violent patients, infectious diseases and so on. These risks are generally understood by those who embark on healthcare careers. But demanding courage beyond these risks is unreasonable. The implications of this are that healthcare professionals, including nurses, should receive both the education and support that facilitates moral action while managing and balancing risks to self and patients. Hamric et al.'s critique is well taken and later I offer some recommendations about the sorts of education that will prepare nurses to make wise ethical judgments. However, it is helpful to contextualize recommendations with current definitions of moral courage as they apply to the actions of nurses.

A general definition of moral courage is that it is that "which enables a person to encounter odium, disapproval, or contempt rather than depart from the right course" (Brown, 1993, p. 1827). Lachman et al. (2012) defined "moral courage (as) the willingness to stand up for and act according to one's ethical beliefs when moral principles are threatened, regardless of the perceived or actual risks (such as stress, anxiety, isolation from colleagues, or threats to employment)". From the business literature, "moral courage (is) the ability to use inner principles to do what is good for others, regardless of threat to self (and) as a matter of practice" (Sekerka & Bagozzi, 2007, p. 135).

James Rest's (1984) four-process model of moral action derived from an extensive review of research literature in cognitive psychology and related disciplines provides some insight into the idea of moral courage as character strength. The four interrelated cognitive processes will be familiar to some readers and are "moral sensitivity, moral judgment, moral motivation, and implementation" (Bebeau, Rest & Narvaez; 1999; Narvaez & Rest, 1995). Failure in any of the components is problematic since the aim of a good action for a particular purpose requires all components to work symbiotically. The fourth component most resembles contemporary definitions of moral courage in that it "necessitates working around impediments and unexpected snags. Envisioning and keeping in sight the final goal is vital... These characteristics of perseverance, resoluteness and competence comprise what we call "character" or "ego-strength"" (Narvaez & Rest, 1995, p. 396). However, in terms of moral courage viewed as a sort of virtue, all four components are in play. Without moral sensitivity, an ethical issue would not be noted as such. Without knowledge of circumstances, principles of ethical action and skills in ethical analysis, *moral judgments* would not occur. In the absence of *moral motivation*, the best action would not be initiated and without *moral character* persistence in resolving the problem might cause abandonment of the act when difficulties present.

Moral responsibility and moral agency

As noted earlier, the healthcare professions exist to provide a good. The good is that of furthering individual and societal health from the perspective of the given profession and its historically developed goals. Thus, a professional responsibility to further that good is assumed by members of a profession on entering the profession. Ability and willingness to enact moral agency, even in the face of obstacles, are dependent both on understanding the scope and limits of professional responsibilities and on the know-how and skills to overcome obstacles. Discernment is required about the source of the obstacles and therefore the level at which they should be addressed (micro, meso or macro). As defined earlier, moral agency in nursing and healthcare practice requires knowledge, ability and motivation to identify (clinical and moral judgment) what is required and possess the character and fortitude to enact the best course of action. While a nurse with adequate ethics preparation may have the ability to resolve issues at the micro or immediate practice level, those stemming from institutional (meso) or policy (macro) levels for the most part require intra and inter-disciplinary collaborations. Colleagues and I have taken these ideas and used Rest's four component framework to envision nursing curricula both undergraduate and graduate (post-graduate). We proposed that when persistently anchored by ideas of nursing goals, purposes and perspectives, the four components of moral reasoning allow us to focus on different aspects needed to develop moral agents (Robichaux et al., 2022).

Summary

The concepts of MD, MR and moral courage should not be accepted uncritically and without attention to how they are being used and for what purposes. We must (a professional responsibility) inquire "what precisely is meant by their use, what purposes are supposedly served by using them, and do they allow for critique of extant environments including sociopolitical and structural injustices"? Maintaining good practice in the face of the contemporary complexity of healthcare settings requires ongoing support for nurse moral decision-making and attention to factors both internal and external to the nurse (Lee et al., 2020).

References

American Psychological Association (2022). Dictionary of Psychology: Resilience.

Bebeau, M. J., Rest, J. R., & Narvaez, D. (1999). Beyond the promise: A perspective on research in moral education. *Educational Researcher*, 28(4), 18–26. https://doi.org/10.3102/0013189X028004018

Brown, L. (Ed.). (1993). *The New Shorter Oxford English Dictionary, Volume 2, N–Z*. Oxford: Clarendon

Carse, A., & Rushton, C. H. (2017). Harnessing the promise of moral distress: A call for re-orientation. *Journal of Clinical Ethics*, 28(1), 15–29.

CBS News (October 10, 2014). Boston nurses heads to West African to fight Ebola. https://www.cbsnews.com/boston/news/boston-nurse-heads-to-west-africa-to-fight-ebola/

Chambliss, D. F. (1996). *Beyond caring: Hospitals, nurses, and the social organization of ethics*. University of Chicago Press.

Doris, J. M., & Moral Psychology Research Group. (2010). *The moral psychology handbook*. OUP Oxford.

Fleming, J., & Ledogar, R. J. (2008). Resilience, an evolving concept: A review of literature relevant to aboriginal research. *Pimatisiwin*, 6(2), 7–23.

Fletcher, D., & Sarkar, M. (2013). Psychological resilience: A review and critique of definitions, concepts, and theory. *European Psychologist*, 18(1), 12.

Flynn, P. J., Bliese, P. D., Korsgaard, M. A., & Cannon, C. (2021). Tracking the process of resilience: How emotional stability and experience influence exhaustion and commitment trajectories. *Group & Organization Management*, 46(4), 692–736. https://doi.org/10.1177/10596011211027676

Grace, P. J. (2001). Professional advocacy: Widening the scope of professional responsibility. *Nursing Philosophy*, 2(2), 151–162.

Grace, P. J. (2018). *Nursing ethics and professional responsibility in advanced practice* (3rd Ed.). Jones & Barlett.

Grace, P. (2022). No moral compass: A critique of the goals and methods of contemporary nursing ethics education. In *Complexity and values in nurse education* (pp. 72–95). Routledge.

Grace, P. J. (In Press). An argument for the distinct nature of nursing ethics. In Deem and J. Lingler (Eds), *Nursing ethics: Normative foundations, advanced concepts, and emerging issues* (Chapter 2). Oxford University Press.

Grace, P. J., Fry, S. T., & Schultz, G. S. (2003). Ethical issues experienced by psychiatric/mental health and substance abuse nurses. *Journal of the American Psychiatric Nurse's Association*, 9(1), 17–23.

Hakimi, H., Joolaee, S., Ashghali Farahani, M., Rodney, P., & Ranjbar, H. (2020). Moral neutralization: Nurses' evolution in unethical climate workplaces. *BMC Medical Ethics*, 21(1), 114. https://doi.org/10.1186/s12910-020-00558-3

Hamric, A. B., Arras, J. D., & Mohrmann, M. E. (2015). Must we be courageous?. *The Hastings Center Report*, 45(3), 33–40. https://doi.org/10.1002/hast.449

Hamric, A. B., Borchers, C. T., & Epstein, E. G. (2012). Development and testing of an instrument to measure moral distress in healthcare professionals. *AJOB Primary Research*, 3(2), 1–9.

Heinze, K. E., Hanson, G., Holtz, H., Swoboda, S. M., & Rushton, C. H. (2021). Measuring Health care interprofessionals' moral resilience: Validation of the Rushton Moral Resilience Scale. *Journal of Palliative Medicine*, 24(6), 865–872. https://doi.org/10.1089/jpm.2020.0328

Howe, E. G. (2017). Fourteen important concepts regarding moral distress. *The Journal of Clinical Ethics*, 28(1), 3–14.

Jameton, A. (1984). *Nursing practice: The ethical issues*. Englewood Cliffs: Prentice-Hall.

Jameton, A. (2013). A reflection on moral distress in nursing together with a current application of the concept. *Journal of Bioethical Inquiry*, 10(3), 297–308.

Johnstone, M. J., & Hutchinson, A. (2015). 'Moral distress'–time to abandon a flawed nursing construct? *Nursing Ethics*, 22(1), 5–14.

Kahneman, D. (2011). *Thinking, fast and slow*. Macmillan.

Lachman, V. D., Murray, J. S., Iseminger, K., & Ganske, K. M. (2012). Doing the right thing: Pathways to moral courage. *American Nurse Today*, 7(5), 24–29.

Lee, S., Robinson, E. M., Grace, P. J., Zollfrank, A., & Jurchak, M. (2020). Developing a moral compass: Themes from the clinical ethics residency for nurses' final essays. *Nursing Ethics*, 27(1), 28–39. https://doi.org/10.1177/0969733019833125

Mahoney, J. L., & Bergman, L. R. (2002). Conceptual and methodological considerations in a developmental approach to the study of positive adaptation. *Journal of Applied Developmental Psychology*, 23(2), 195–217.

Masten, A. S. (2001). Ordinary magic: Resilience processes in development. *American Psychologist*, 56, 227–238.

Masten, A. S. (2018). Resilience theory and research on children and families: Past, present, and promise. *Journal of Family Theory & Review*, 10(1), 12–31.

McCarthy, J., & Deady, R. (2008). Moral distress reconsidered. *Nursing Ethics*, 15(2), 254–262.

Milliken, A., & Grace, P. (2017). Nurse ethical awareness: Understanding the nature of everyday practice. *Nursing Ethics*, 24(5), 517–524.

Milliken, A., Ludlow, L., & Grace, P. (2019): Ethical awareness scale: Replication testing, invariance analysis. *AJOB Empirical Bioethics*, 10(4), 231–240.

Monteverde, S. (2016). Caring for tomorrow's workforce: moral resilience and healthcare ethics education. *Nursing Ethics*, 23(1), 104–116.

Morley, G., Ives, J., Bradbury-Jones, C., & Irvine, F. (2019). What is 'moral distress'? A narrative synthesis of the literature. *Nursing Ethics*, 26(3), 646–662.

Narvaez, D., & Rest, J. (1995). The four components of acting morally. In D. Narvaez & J. Rest (Eds.), *Moral development: An introduction* (pp. 385–400). Allyn & Bacon. Narvaez, 7 Rest

Newman, R. (2005). APA's resilience initiative. *Professional Psychology: Research and Practice*, 36(3), 227.

Peters, R., & Filipova, A. (2009). Optimizing cognitive-dissonance literacy in ethics education. *Public Integrity*, 11(3), 201–220. https://doi.org/10.2753/PIN1099-9922110301

Rest, J. R. (1984). Research on moral development: Implications for training counseling psychologists. *The Counseling Psychologist*, 12(3), 19–29. https://doi.org/10.1177/0011000084123003

Robichaux, C., Grace, P., Bartlett, J., Stokes, F., Saulo Lewis, M., & Turner, M. (2022). Ethics education for nurses: Foundations for an integrated curriculum. *Journal of Nursing Education*, 61(3), 123–130.

Rushton, C. H. (2016). Moral resilience: a capacity for navigating moral distress in critical care. *AACN Advanced Critical Care*, 27(1), 111–119.

Sala Defilippis, T. M., Curtis, K., & Gallagher, A. (2019). Conceptualising moral resilience for nursing practice. *Nursing Inquiry*, 26(3), e12291.

Sekerka, L. E., & Bagozzi, R. P. (2007). Moral courage in the workplace: Moving to and from the desire and decision to act. *Business Ethics: A European Review*, 16, 132–149.

Sellman, D. (2011). *What makes a good nurse: Why the virtues are important for nurses*. Jessica Kingsley Publishers.

Stangor, C., Jhangiani, R., & Tarry, H. (2022). Obedience, Power, and Leadership. Principles of Social Psychology-1st International H5P Edition. https://opentextbc.ca/socialpsychology/

Traynor, M. (2017). *Critical resilience for nurses: An evidence-based guide to survival and change in the modern NHS*. Routledge.

Winslade, W. J. (2017). Moral distress: Conscious and unconscious feelings. *The Journal of Clinical Ethics*, 28(1), 42–43.

Yarling, R. R., & McElmurry, B. J. (1986). The moral foundation of nursing. *Advances in Nursing Science*, 8(2), 63–74.

26 Equality, equity, and distributional justice in nursing

Ageism and other impediments

Michael Igoumenidis and Evridiki Papastavrou

Introduction

In the beginning of 2020, Northern Italy was one of the first European areas to face the dire consequences of COVID-19 for health care systems. Among other issues, mechanical ventilation could not be offered to all patients who needed it. In many cases, this meant that health care professionals had to make harsh triage decisions on the use of ventilators that ultimately came down to who lives and who dies. The *New England Journal Of Medicine's* national correspondent Lisa Rosenbaum spoke to physicians about triage practices, but they were reluctant to reveal details, implying that age-based cut-offs were being used to allocate ventilators.[1] The Italian College of Anesthesia, Analgesia, Resuscitation, and Intensive Care (SIAARTI) issued recommendations which acknowledged that an age limit for ICU admission might ultimately need to be set, and were met by wide criticism.[2] Though it may be appropriate to consider stage of life in theoretical decision-making, it is not easy for clinicians to take the actual decision or communicate their rationale to the public.

In developed countries, ethically challenging triage decisions are limited to cases of mass disasters or other emergency situations that put health care systems under extreme pressure. But the fact that direct life and death dilemmas rarely arise does not mean that there are no cases of difficult prioritization, rationing and allocation decisions in everyday practice, or that they are not important. They may lack the dramatic impact of giving patients the chance to live or letting them die, but, in the long run, everyday care decisions lead to great consequences for health outcomes – irrespective of whether clinical professionals perceive existing dilemmas related to these decisions or not. At the microeconomic level, rationing of health resources is more explicit and direct, performed by health professionals, and based on care demands, professional experience, and personal values. At the macro-economic level, decisions are more distant and impersonal, taken by policymakers who are based on economic models, laws, regulations, and abstract principles. In both instances, equity is a central notion. Resources have to be allocated to patients in an equitable manner. Is this task attainable?

In this chapter, we shall try to provide some answers to this question from a practical point of view, reflecting at the same time nursing's moral imperative to promote health equity in the context of the multiple roles played by nurses to promote justice in everyday practice. The COVID-19 pandemic has brought some pressing ethical dilemmas from the background of moral theory and academic lectures to the fore of public health policies and clinical practice. Equity notions and problems of justice have been troubling scholars, academics, and policymakers for a long time, but can the same be said about

DOI: 10.4324/9781003427407-30

clinical professionals or patients? It is important to examine their standpoint, both in the context of the pandemic's pressing circumstances and in their normal routine within health care systems. First, we shall provide a brief theoretical and historical account of equality, equity, and distributional justice. We shall then examine their significance for health services, and the ways in which distributional justice aims at correcting health inequities. Inequities are influenced by a number of factors, where age plays a dominant role, and not only in dramatic triage decisions. We shall briefly mention other factors, but our debate will focus on the issue of age discrimination in resource allocation and the problems it creates, in an attempt to show that equity, in its strict sense, is an unattainable ideal. The COVID-19 pandemic has made this quite clear and shows the need for modesty when proclaiming equity-related goals. The nurses' role and its relation to these goals need to be constantly subject to consideration and re-examination.

Equality, equity, and distributional justice

These concepts are closely interrelated and subject to many different interpretations, which often create confusion as to their significance. The terms "equality" and "equity" are often used interchangeably, even though there are important distinctions between them. Equality is typically defined as treating everyone the same and giving everyone access to the same opportunities. In contrast, equity involves trying to understand and give people what they need, which is not the same for all. Equality can only work if everyone starts from the same place and needs the same things; equity refers to the issue of different starting points and different needs, and aims to compensate for these differences. In Aristotle's words, society should aim at treating equals equally and unequals unequally, in proportion to their inequality.[3] Therefore, the notion of equity transcends the notion of equality.[4] Justice is another closely related notion that is also transcended by equity. Plato had contrasted equity with justice in his *Laws*,[5] arguing that equity, because it is distinct from *strict* justice (which is good), cannot itself be good. In *Nicomachean Ethics* (Bk. V, 1137a, 31–1138a, 2), Aristotle explicitly rejects Plato's analysis, claiming that, although equity is not identical with strict justice, it is, nonetheless, a kind of justice.[6] In fact, according to Aristotle, equity is better as it corrects justice's tendency towards abstractness, impartiality, and indifference.[7] Equity demands justice to be exercised in relation to others, giving prominence to singularity and uniqueness. We can then remark that strict justice corresponds to the notion of equality, whereas equity is related to a different kind of justice that has been described as *fairness*.

Aristotle also separates *distributive* justice from *retributive* justice; the former refers to the fair allocation of wealth, titles, and any other good that can be given to members of a society, and the latter refers to rules and penalties that govern relationships between the members of a society.[8] Distributional justice aims at allocating goods in the fairest way and at correcting situations that are perceived as unjust within societies. Many important thinkers have dealt exhaustively with this issue, asserting that equity can only be achieved through distribution choices. For instance, Hobbes redefined distributive justice as equity, invoked to correct unreasonable adjudications arising from the application of general laws to particular cases.[9] To achieve equity, policies and procedures may result in an unequal distribution of resources, as people possess unequal goods and have unequal needs. In his seminal *Theory of Justice*, John Rawls advocates this view with his egalitarian *difference principle* of justice, which holds that inequalities in the distribution of goods are permissible only if they benefit the least well-off members of society.[10]

Notwithstanding practical difficulties, such as defining the least advantaged members of society in a consistent way,[11] it is clear that the issues of inequity can only be solved by unequal allocation of resources.

We have already discussed the distinctions between equality, equity, and justice in a general manner. Focusing on the context of health, similar distinctions need to be drawn. "Health equity" can be defined as the state in which everyone has the opportunity to attain full health potential and no one is disadvantaged from achieving this potential because of social position or any other socially defined circumstance.[12] "Health inequality" is the term used to designate variations and disparities in the health achievements of individuals and groups; it is a descriptive term that need not imply moral judgement. However, "health inequity" refers to those inequalities in health that are deemed to be unfair or stemming from some form of injustice.[13] In other words, some inequalities, such as defective genes, may be unavoidable and therefore are not generally considered unjust, whereas others, such as socioeconomic circumstances, might be avoided and so are considered inequitable.[14] Principles of distributive justice are used both by policymakers at the macro-economic level and by health professionals at the micro-economic level, so as to compensate as much as possible for health inequalities and inequities, through unequal – but fair – distribution of health care resources.

Health inequalities result from purely medical factors, such as hereditary illnesses or accidents causing injuries. Health inequities are based on non-medical factors, known as *social determinants of health*, such as income, education, neighbourhood and physical environment, employment, social support networks, as well as access to health care.[15] We could say that health inequalities are *differences*, whereas health inequities are *unfair differences*. The factor of age is unique in this regard, standing out as a socio-medical criterion which causes both health inequalities and inequities. In terms of inequality, older people usually have increased health needs, as this is the natural state of affairs; however, in terms of inequity, they often belong to the most disadvantaged members of societies, which leads to extra health problems and demands, or to inadequate coverage of existing demands, as we discuss below.

Ageism within society and health care

To be sure, the issue of ageism cannot be exhausted here, but some important remarks are in order. First of all, there have been various attitudes towards the elderly throughout different ages and societies. There have also been different conceptions and definitions of them; for instance, in ancient Greece, the elderly called *presbuteroi* (elders) somewhat arbitrarily fell between the ages of 30 and 59, and *gerontes* (old men) were those above 60. We also have to bear in mind that, whatever the percentage of the over-60s in antiquity, the certainty is that it was very much lower than today's figure.[16] Before modern medicine, the majority of the population died young, whereas war and political instability also claimed many young lives. Wealthy individuals and aristocrats were more likely to live to an old age, because of their superior diets and resources; yet, there were also underprivileged older people, who had a restricted and passive social role.

In ancient Greece, elders were not respected, unless they had performed some heroic deeds in their youth. The Greek conception of old age was generally gloomy, considering its dark mythological origin: *Geras* (the god of old age) was the son of *Nyx* (night) and *Erebos* (the personification of darkness). In Greek mythology, it is also prominent the underlying theme of elders dethroned by their children, which sets up this practice as an acceptable precedent.[17] Nevertheless, the care of elderly, or *geroboskia*, was a sacred duty. Sons were held responsible for the maintenance of their older parents according to Greek and Roman laws, and severe penalties were imposed on offspring refusing to provide care for them.[18] However, there were no public facilities for the care of older people in general. Ancient Greeks' practices towards older people were a legacy to the next generations, and there was no interest in the poor or the elderly outside the narrow kinship circle.[16] In addition, older people were often perceived as expendables; when the Athenians besieged the island of Keos in the Aegean sea, the Keians voted for all people over 60 years of age to commit suicide by drinking hemlock, in an attempt to preserve the food supply.[19] Practices of disposing parents or the elderly can be found in the myths and in the actual habits of many cultures. For instance, in the past, the Inuits would leave their elderly on the ice to die during famines,[20] whereas in the southern Indian state of Tamil Nadu, the illegal practice of senicide – known locally as *thalaikoothal* – is said to still occur in the name of custom, particularly when the elders themselves think that they have become a burden for their children.[21]

Ageism, defined as prejudice or discrimination on the grounds of a person's age, is thus widely present throughout the history of societies. Still, the elderly gradually gained increased attention in many parts of the world. In the 2nd century AD, the Greek physician Galen was the first to maintain that *gerokomikón* should be a speciality of medicine, aiming to the health of the elderly. His ideas joined with Roman institutions and the charity ideal of the rising Christian religion, and led to the creation of the first *gerokomeia*, hospices for the old. There is no evidence of such institutions in the Western Roman Empire, but they were founded and proliferated in the Eastern Roman Empire, mainly in the Byzantium of the Middle Ages.[22] They have evolved to modern private and public nursing homes for the elderly which are part of many countries' health and social services systems, and indispensable in our aging societies.[23] Yet, this does not mean that they always provide quality care or that they are free of ageist behaviours[24,25]; in fact, one could argue that the whole idea of homes for the elderly is ageist: "The easy solution that the older person exiting from hospitals should go to the supposed safe haven of the nursing home… [is] ageist unless the same suggestions would be made for a comparable person of a younger age."[26] Indeed, younger people with disabilities would never willingly tolerate living in nursing homes, and they would rightfully demand social services and adjustments that enable them to participate in social activities as much as possible.

However, it is true that older people have greater needs that often designate nursing home placement as the only solution. Caregivers' reasons for placement primarily include the need for more skilled care, the caregiver burden, and the elders' dementia-related behaviours,[27] and factors such as hip fracture, reduced mobility, and multiple comorbidities also increase the risk for nursing home admission.[28] In any case, irrespective of whether they live in nursing homes or not, older people tend to have various health problems and functional disabilities which regularly put great strain on health and social care systems. Various studies demonstrate that annual medical expenses more than double between ages 70 and 90,[29] whereas the oldest group (85+) consumes three times as much health care per person as those 65–74, and twice as much as those 75–84.[30] It has been suggested that the association of age with health care costs is a "red herring," as there are analyses where health care expenditures depended on remaining lifetime, and proximity to death, rather than calendar age.[31] Furthermore, age-related losses, including cognitive impairment, falls, fractures, hearing impairments, and dementia, are an even greater driver of costs compared to age.[32] But, in any case, it is beyond dispute that the elderly consume disproportionately large amounts of health and social care resources.

In many countries, particularly where social security systems are weak and private payments for health care is the norm, the elderly may face serious challenges in their efforts to receive the care they need; yet in these countries, this can be true for any age group. Claims of ageism within health care have a sound basis, but only when it comes to particular staff attitudes and behaviours, such as "elderspeak" (infantilizing communication).[25] Apart from that, health care is delivered according to needs, even though elder needs are far greater and more expensive. Societies respect their elders and value their lives. After all, older people are a vulnerable group, yet one where most of us aspire to belong at some point. If ageing is a naturally occurring inequity, in the sense that it gradually deprives people of their physical and social abilities, society is willing to allocate more resources to the elderly, so as to compensate as much as possible for this deprivation. Besides, in terms of intergenerational justice, it is only fair to do so; in the context of *indirect reciprocity*, current elderly population is entitled to receive more health resources from current younger and productive generations, just as the latter will expect when they grow old in their turn, and just as the current elderly did in their past years with their elderly.[33]

In theory, all of the above are potentially correct. In practice, the situation is not as straightforward as it may seem. As discussed in the Introduction, crisis situations, in which anywise finite resources become scarce, constitute an open field for ageism. To be sure, our society will not vote for the elderly to drink hemlock like the Keians had done, but prioritization of some kind is always necessary, as evidenced by the COVID-19 pandemic responses, and age cut-offs are surely factors to consider. However, resource allocation on the basis of recipients' age also takes place during non-crisis periods. One obvious example is the use of QALYs by health policymakers in defining thresholds for specific care interventions; an arguably ageist approach as, other things being equal, the elderly with a shorter life expectancy will be given lower priority.[34] Considering all of the above, we can assert that ageism is an attitude deeply rooted in our society and in our health care systems, leading to behaviours and decisions that have a negative impact on the elderly, on their autonomy and self-conception, as well as on their mental and physical health. Despite methodological concerns,[35] it is well documented that ageism leads to barriers in access or denial of health care services and treatments, with age being the primary factor determining who receives certain procedures and treatments,[36] whereas ageism also exacerbates social isolation and loneliness.[37] And patients' age is only one of the many factors that poses a challenge to the principles of equity and justice in health care.

Nurses' perceptions in relation to health equity and inequity

Up to this point, we have used ageism to show that equity in health is an unattainable ideal, not because moral agents are explicitly ageist, but due to the fact that age-related inequities occur naturally and subtly all the time, probably since the beginning of societies, thus making their mitigation efforts very difficult. As noted above, age is a unique socio-medical criterion to consider when it comes to allocation of health care resources. Eminent philosophers have considered age discrimination in health care as just, such as John Harris with his *fair innings* argument: there is some span of years that we consider a reasonable life, and those who reach the appropriate threshold must consider any additional years a sort of bonus which may be cancelled when this is necessary to help others reach the threshold.[38] Under this view, and in a utilitarian context, ageism may even promote equity. But this is a discussion that falls out of the scope of this chapter. When aiming for justice in the allocation of health resources, there are several other obstacles that do not leave much room for optimism.

Health inequities result from social determinants such as education, neighbourhood and physical environment, employment, and access to health care. In essence, all these factors are related to one's income and social class. Those who can afford to pay for better housing, nutrition and private health insurance surely have better chances to maintain their health. But, for the sake of the argument, let us suppose that we talk about a public health system where income and social class do not matter; patients get care according to their needs, not their ability to pay. This is a universally accepted principle for public systems. Policymakers may consider age as a criterion for health resources allocation, but all the other factors are irrelevant from a macro-economic point of view. Yet policymakers deal mainly with abstract principles and statistics from the comfort of their meeting rooms and offices, whereas health professionals at the micro-economic level have a first-hand view of the effect that their decisions have on specific patients, and tend to get more influenced by their personal feelings, moral values, and beliefs. According to Aristotle's view that we already discussed, they are better situated to deliver equity among patients, as they can correct justice's tendency towards abstractness, impartiality, and indifference.[7] Bearing this in mind, we turn to examining the case of nurses.

Traditionally, nurses are closer to patients than other health professionals[39] and hold a unique position in health care systems. Like all other health professionals, they have to work within the context and the limitations set by policymakers, who try to achieve macro-economic justice by defining what reasonable care is to be expected.[8] In addition, and despite the nursing profession's increasing autonomy, by and large nurses work within an actual context created by physicians, as the latters' therapeutic decisions have a direct impact on the subsequent care which nurses provide. Apart from these influences, nurses allocate their care to patients based on various factors, and their judgement is mainly influenced by the urgency of the patients' clinical condition and the satisfaction of biomedical needs; high priority is given to the clinical tasks that are more visible, whereas relational, social, and emotional needs of patients are of secondary importance.[40] Additionally, there are indications that nurses are influenced by the presence of significant others, the patients' family status as well as the social status.[41]

Prioritization is an important dimension of the nursing care distribution techniques,[42] and this is why nurses admit a feeling of guilt, inadequacy and frustration in situations where the institutional culture or other factors affect decision-making priorities.[43] Let us assume, for the sake of the argument again, that nurses are free from influences and can decide on their own how to allocate their finite resources (i.e. mainly their time and expertise) to patients. Can they do this in an equitable manner? From our perspective, this question is rhetorical. It is true that nurses are in a position to mitigate some health inequities by allocating more resources to the least advantaged, but they do not possess an objective moral compass to do so. Nurses are humans with emotions, and, at the micro-allocation level, professional detachment is not always guaranteed.[44] Absolute justice requires an impossible impersonality, a neutrality fit for judges, not carers.

These considerations do not stop nurses from recognizing the problem of health inequities and taking up appropriate initiatives. The International Council of Nurses (ICN) has advanced nursing's position in tackling disparities through its "fact sheets" on numerous social determinants.[45] National nurses associations have launched social justice projects, involving the promotion of discussions on equity in health care.[46] From their various positioning within institutions, nurses can either promote or resist institutional practices that influence health inequities. Nursing scholars have proposed that feminist practices of critical self-reflection and deepening political consciousness are the first steps towards practical action by nurses to address health inequities.[47] Nurse educators have tried to embed immersive experiences and related assignments in nursing curricula as a strategy towards dismantling health inequities that result from structural racism in health care.[48] Also, nursing researchers have explored nursing professionals' perceptions on health inequities, in an effort to identify and propose specific interventions. Some of the most recent findings are summarized below.

Rooddehghan et al. (2019) attempted to explain the process of the realization of equity in nursing care, by conducting interviews in a sample of 27 clinical nurses in Iran.[49] They point out that participants' main concern in providing equitable care is the *rationing* of nursing care, which could be easier if more resources were available, that is, a better nurse-to-patient ratio. This is related to another problem identified in this study, namely that health systems' structure is inconsistent with equity, hindering the nursing profession from reaching its full potential. Nurses also perceived a "lack of clarity in measuring equitable care," as the concept of equity can mean different things to different people in the context of health and health care. Schneiderman and Olshansky (2020) interviewed 13 registered US nurses beginning their online graduate advanced practice educational programme, who acknowledged their limitations to meeting the health equity goal as they could only address the patient in front of them and not change the whole system to treat everyone fairly. They also proposed that health education is a way to improve health equity since many patients are not aware of how to work with the health care system or how to improve their own health through preventive measures.[50] Rudner (2021) states that nursing is a health equity and social justice movement, but the ability to implement changes to promote these goals depended on and still depends on access to power and resources.[51] In this context, Wilson et al. (2022) interviewed ten elected or politically active Canadian nurses, and found that their nursing education and work equipped them to be capable of engaging in political spheres; more nurses should be inspired and helped to become active politically, as a way to advance public policy related to health inequities.[52]

With regard to age-related health inequities, nurses' views are more ambivalent. Though some ageist behaviours are clearly described as inappropriate and undesirable by nurses and other health professionals, the issue of withholding certain treatments depending on the patient's age creates hard to solve ethical dilemmas; for instance, avoidance of invasive or painful medical treatment can be potentially perceived as compassionate care rather than as undertreatment due to ageist attitudes.[53] When elder patients' quality of life is greatly diminished by their prolonged survival, withholding treatments for them that are offered to younger patients – with far better chances of success – can be considered as sound medical decision-making.[54] Is this discrimination based on naturally occurring differences between the young and the old (health inequalities), or on unfair differences (health inequities)? In many cases, it is indeed difficult for most health professionals, or any person for that matter, to draw the line. Research shows that student nurses hold positive attitudes and perspectives towards older people and on the prospect of caring for them,[55] but nursing education would be improved by incorporating theories of life-course and harmonious aging that could help nurses to understand more aspects of elder treatment, and to detect true ageist bias when it occurs.[56]

Educational and research initiatives on these issues are important, as well as political, social and institutional initiatives. They can help and guide nurses towards mitigating health disparities in many levels, and delivering patient-centred care according to needs. Yet, all the difficulties we described above remain strong. Equity should be respected and dispersed within the nursing profession, but it should also be accepted with its unavoidable limitations in practice, and its imperfect implementation should not discourage those who believe in and strive for it.[4] Realistically speaking, achieving equity is an unattainable ideal, in health care and otherwise. Reducing inequities, however, is a more pragmatic approach. The reasonable goal is not equity; it is the least possible inequity, between patients, and in society as a whole. The most just allocation of resources is the one that is the least unjust.

Conclusions

At first, the COVID-19 pandemic had been described as "the great equalizer" as it seemed to transcend wealth, fame, prestige, and age; everyone was at risk. It soon became evident that this was not the case. Pandemics have the ability to amplify existing health inequalities, disproportionately affecting socially disadvantaged groups, including racial and ethnic minorities and low-income populations.[57] Disparities in social determinants of health result in differential exposure to the virus, differential vulnerability to the infection and differential consequences of the disease.[58] In addition, as we saw in the beginning of this chapter, age disparities result in differential treatment, particularly in pressing circumstances where resources are scarce. The prioritization of ICU beds and ventilators towards the young may have created tensions and moral distress among health professionals,[59] but many social factors have played a much bigger role in deciding who lives and who dies during the pandemic, many of which go unnoticed in everyday clinical routine.

NEJM's correspondent Lisa Rosenbaum proposed to separate clinicians providing care from those making triage decisions. The "triage officer," backed by a team with expertise in nursing and respiratory therapy, would make resource allocation decisions and communicate them to the clinical team, the patient, and the family.[1] Yet, this is similar to what takes place within health care systems anyway, irrespective of pandemics or other crisis situations. Policymakers make resource allocation decisions at the macro-economic level, and health professionals abide to these decisions and make their own micro-economic allocation within clinical settings. The latter can try to provide equitable care, but, in the end of the day, the most important decisions have already been taken, and they can only manage the outcomes of these decisions. The same is true with health inequities in general. Social determinants have already created them at the macro-level; health professionals can only manage them and try to correct them, by use of distributional justice principles, but also influenced by their own personal moral codes, priorities and biases. Equity is a constant dynamic process, not something that can be achieved at some point.

Bearing this in mind, let us return to the current pandemic and conclude with a somewhat optimistic view. It is true that age discriminations have always been present in our societies and that the global spread of COVID-19 virus has amplified these discriminations. In terms of health equity, it was once again asserted that the elderly, among other vulnerable groups, do not receive the same level of preventive or therapeutic care as other, more advantaged members of society. However, in terms of battling health inequalities, humanity has made crucial steps in the right direction. Lockdowns and quarantines disrupted the global economy in unprecedented ways, meeting with strong resistance from many experts and laypersons who disagreed. Governments imposed these measures despite the societal cost, attempting to protect the elderly and other immuno-suppressed individuals. The healthy and the young are also at risk for severe COVID-19 symptoms and fatal outcomes, but this risk is lower by far. Global lockdown was necessitated mainly due to the frailty of the elderly, and they were the first to be immunized when vaccines became available. Society embraced and tried to protect them as efficiently as possible, even though this meant that many people's lives changed for the worse. The pandemic has shown that humanity is willing to challenge the status quo and go at great lengths to protect its members. On this basis, maybe we can gradually learn to promote equity at all levels in more drastic and efficient ways, by caring more for the others. And the nursing profession has a great deal to contribute to this end.

References

1. Rosenbaum L. Facing Covid-19 in Italy — Ethics, Logistics, and Therapeutics on the Epidemic's Front Line. *New England Journal of Medicine* 2020; 382: 1873–1875.
2. Orfali K. What Triage Issues Reveal: Ethics in the COVID-19 Pandemic in Italy and France. *Bioethical Inquiry* 2020; 17: 675–679.
3. Aristotle. *Nicomachean Ethics* [Translated by Kerr Thomson JA]. Harmondsworth: Penguin Classics, 2004, Book V, 1131a.
4. Papastavrou E, Igoumenidis M, Lemonidou C. Equality as an Ethical Concept within the Context of Nursing Care Rationing. *Nursing Philosophy* 2020; 21(1): e12284.
5. Georgiadis C. Equitable and Equity in Aristotle. In Panagiotou S (ed.) *Justice, Law and Method in Plato and Aristotle*. Edmonton: Academic Printing and Publishing, 1987, pp. 159–172.
6. Aristotle. *Nicomachean Ethics* [Translated by Kerr Thomson JA]. Harmondsworth: Penguin Classics, 2004, Book V, 1137a–1138a.
7. Petrilli S. Justice, Fairness and Juridical Perfectibility. *International Journal of Legal Discourse* 2016; 1(1): 1–22.
8. Igoumenidis M, Kiekkas P, Papastavrou E. The Gap between Macroeconomic and Microeconomic Health Resources Allocation Decisions: The Case of Nurses. *Nursing Philosophy* 2020; 21(1): e12283.
9. Olsthoorn J. Hobbes's Account of Distributive Justice as Equity. *British Journal for the History of Philosophy* 2013; 21(1): 13–33.
10. Rawls J. *A Theory of Justice*. Cambridge, MA: Belknap Press of Harvard University Press, 1971, p. 266.
11. Altham JEJ. Rawl's Difference Principle. *Philosophy* 1973; 48: 75–78.
12. NASEM. *Communities in Action: Pathways to Health Equity*. Washington, DC: The National Academies Press, 2017, p. 32.
13. Kawachi I, Subramanian SV, Almeida-Filho N. A Glossary for Health Inequalities. *Journal of Epidemiology and Community Health* 2002; 56: 647–652.
14. Raine R, Or Z, Prady S, Bevan G. (2016). Evaluating Health-Care Equity. In Raine R, Fitzpatrick R, Barratt H, Bevan G, Black N, Boaden R, et al. (eds.) Challenges, Solutions and Future Directions in the Evaluation of Service Innovations in Health Care and Public Health. *Health Services and Delivery Research* 2016; 4(16): 69–84.
15. Marmot M. Social Determinants of Health Inequalities. *The Lancet* 2005; 365: 1099–1104.
16. Finley MI. The Elderly in Classical Antiquity. *Greece & Rome* 1981; 28(2): 156–171.
17. Minois G. *History of Old Age: From Antiquity to the Renaissance* [translated by Tenison S]. Chicago: University of Chicago Press, 1987, p. 44.
18. Parlapani E, Holeva V, Nikopoulou VA, Sereslis K, Athanasiadou M, Godosidis A, Stephanou T, Diakogiannis I. Intolerance of Uncertainty and Loneliness in Older Adults During the COVID-19 Pandemic. *Frontiers in Psychiatry* 2020; 11: 842.

19. Parkin TG. *Old Age in the Roman World*. Baltimore: Johns Hopkins University Press, 2003, p. 264.
20. Battin M. Age Rationing and the Just Distribution of Health Care: Is There a Duty to Die? *Ethics* 1987; 97: 317–340.
21. Chatterjee P. Thalaikoothal. The Practice of Euthanasia in the Name of Custom. *European Researcher* 2014; 87(2): 2005–2012.
22. Musitelli S. Gerokomikón: A Brief Survey of the History of Geriatrics from Creation to the 16th Century. *The Aging Male* 2002; 5(3): 181–196.
23. Cassel CK. Policy for an Aging Society: A Review of Systems. *JAMA* 2009; 302(24): 2701–2702.
24. Konetzka RT. The Challenges of Improving Nursing Home Quality. *JAMA Network Open* 2020; 3(1): e1920231.
25. Williams K, Shaw C, Lee A, Kim S, Dinneen E, Turk M, Jao YL, Liu W. Voicing Ageism in Nursing Home Dementia Care. *Journal of Gerontological Nursing* 2017; 43(9): 16–20.
26. Kane RL, Kane RA. Ageism in Healthcare and Long-Term Care. *Generations: Journal of the American Society on Aging* 2005; 29(3): 49–54.
27. Buhr GT, Kuchibhatla M, Clipp EC. Caregivers' Reasons for Nursing Home Placement: Clues for Improving Discussions with Families Prior to the Transition. *Gerontologist* 2006; 46(1): 52–61.
28. Toot S, Swinson T, Devine M, Challis D, Orrell M. Causes of Nursing Home Placement for Older People with Dementia: A Systematic Review and Meta-Analysis. *International Psychogeriatrics* 2017; 29(2): 195–208.
29. De Nardi M, French E, Jones JB, McCauley J. Medical Spending of the US Elderly. *Fiscal Studies* 2016; 37(3–4): 717–747.
30. Alemayehu B, Warner KE. The Lifetime Distribution of Health Care Costs. *Health Services Research* 2004; 39(3): 627–642.
31. Zweifel P, Felder S, Meiers M. Ageing of Population and Health Care Expenditure: A Red Herring? *Health Economics* 1999; 8(6): 485–496.
32. Hazra NC, Rudisill C, Gulliford MC. Determinants of Health Care Costs in the Senior Elderly: Age, Comorbidity, Impairment, or Proximity to Death? *European Journal of Health Economics* 2018; 19: 831–842.
33. Gosseries A. Theories of Intergenerational Justice: A Synopsis. *Surveys and Perspectives Integrating Environment and Society* 2008; 1: 39–49.
34. Tsuchiya A. QALYs and Ageism: Philosophical Theories and Age Weighting. *Health Economics* 2000; 9(1): 57–68.
35. Salway SM, Payne N, Rimmer M, Buckner S, Jordan H, Adams J, Walters K, Sowden SL, Forrest L, Sharp L, Hidajat M, White M, Ben-Shlomo Y. Identifying Inequitable Healthcare in Older People: Systematic Review of Current Research Practice. *International Journal of Equity in Health* 2017; 16(1): 123.
36. Inouye SK. Creating an anti-Ageist Healthcare System to Improve Care for Our Current and Future Selves. *Nature Aging* 2021; 1: 150–152.
37. Mikton C, de la Fuente-Núñez V, Officer A, Krug E. Ageism: A Social Determinant of Health that Has Come of Age. *The Lancet* 2021; 397(10282): 1333–1334.
38. Harris J. *The Value of Life*. London & New York: Routledge, 2002 (first published 1985), p. 91.
39. Tadd W, Clarke A, Lloyd L, Leino-Kilpi H, Strandell C, Lemonidou C, Petsios K, Sala R, Barazzetti G, Radaelli S, Zalewski Z, Bialecka A, van der Arend A, Heymans R. The Value of Nurses' Codes: European Nurses' Views. *Nursing Ethics* 2006; 13: 376–393.
40. Suhonen R, Stolt M, Habermann M, Hjaltadottir I, Vryonides S, Tonnessen S, Halvorsen K, Harvey C, Toffoli L, Scott PA; RANCARE Consortium COST Action - CA 15208. Ethical Elements in Priority Setting in Nursing Care: A Scoping Review. *International Journal of Nursing Studies* 2018; 88: 25–42.

41. Halvorsen K, Førde R, Nortvedt P. The Principle of Justice in Patient Priorities in the Intensive Care Unit: The Role of Significant Others. *Journal of Medical Ethics* 2009; 35(8): 483–487.
42. Skirbekk H, Nortvedt P. Making a Difference: a Qualitative Study on Care and Priority Setting in Health Care. *Health Care Analysis* 2011; 19: 77–88.
43. Busanello J, Lunardi Filho WD, Kerber NP. Nurses' Production of Subjectivity and the Decision-Making in the Process of Care. *Revista Gaúcha de Enfermagem* 2013; 34: 140–147.
44. Carmack BJ. Balancing Engagement and Detachment in Caregiving. *Journal of Nursing Scholarship* 1997; 29: 139–143.
45. Reutter L, Kushner KE. Health Equity through Action on the Social Determinants of Health': Taking Up the Challenge in Nursing. *Nursing Inquiry* 2010; 17: 269–280.
46. Wilmot S. Social Justice and the Canadian Nurses Association: Justifying Equity. *Nursing Philosophy* 2012; 13(1): 15–26.
47. Pauly BM, MacKinnon K, Varcoe C. Revisiting "Who Gets Care?": Health Equity as an Arena for Nursing Action. *Advances in Nursing Science* 2009; 32(2): 118–127.
48. Garner SL. Building Nurse Upstanders for Health Equity. *Journal of Nursing Education* 2022; 61(7): 417–420.
49. Rooddehghan Z, ParsaYekta Z, Nasrabadi AN. Equity in Nursing Care: A Grounded Theory Study. *Nursing Ethics* 2019; 26(2): 598–610.
50. Schneiderman JU, Olshansky EF. Nurses' Perceptions: Addressing Social Determinants of Health to Improve Patient Outcomes. *Nursing Forum* 2021; 56(2): 313–321.
51. Rudner N. Nursing Is a Health Equity and Social Justice Movement. *Public Health Nursing* 2021; 38(4): 687–691.
52. Wilson DM, Underwood L, Kim S, Olukotun M, Errasti-Ibarrondo B. How and Why Nurses Became Involved in Politics or Political Action, and the Outcomes or Impacts of this Involvement. *Nursing Outlook* 2022; 70(1): 55–63.
53. Ben-Harush A, Shiovitz-Ezra S, Doron I, Alon S, Leibovitz A, Golander H, Haron Y, Ayalon L. Ageism among Physicians, Nurses, and Social Workers: Findings from a Qualitative Study. *European Journal of Ageing* 2016; 14(1): 39–48.
54. Skirbekk H, Nortvedt P. Inadequate Treatment for Elderly Patients: Professional Norms and Tight Budgets Could Cause "ageism" in Hospitals. *Health Care Analysis* 2014; 22(2): 192–201.
55. Neville C, Dickie R. The Evaluation of Undergraduate Nurses' Attitudes, Perspectives and Perceptions toward Older People. *Nurse Education Today* 2014; 34(7): 1074–1079.
56. Dahlke S, Hunter KF. Harnessing Nursing to Diminish Ageism. *International Journal of Older People Nursing* 2022; 17(2): e12417.
57. Mein SA. COVID-19 and Health Disparities: the Reality of "the Great Equalizer". *Journal of General Internal Medicine* 2020; 35(8): 2439–2440.
58. Burström B, Tao W. Social Determinants of Health and Inequalities in COVID-19. *The European Journal of Public Health* 2020; 30(4): 617–618.
59. Hostiuc S, Negoi I, Maria-Isailă O, Diaconescu I, Hostiuc M, Drima E. Age in the Time of COVID-19: An Ethical Analysis. *Aging and Disease* 2021; 12(1): 7–13.

27 Avoiding the triumph of emptiness

The threats of educational fundamentalism and anti-intellectualism in nursing education

Louise Racine and Helen Vandenberg

Introduction

Nurses face the complexities of healthcare environments in a knowledge-intensive society through their disciplinary scholarship and professional practice. The nursing profession began in the mid-1800s as a new form of women's labour, initially styled as an apprentice-style trade rather than an academic discipline (Reverby, 1987). Nursing training was firmly linked to daily life in early 20th-century hospitals, which was often more associated with charity than knowledge-based work. The earliest nursing training schools in Canada enrolled young women for three years, providing room and board in exchange for labour. Students received little formal education, and training focused more on character, obedience, and behaviour than knowledge of medical sciences and related therapeutics. Today, nursing education is provided in higher learning institutions, and nursing schools compete to attract the best and brightest students. Nurses are also in high demand worldwide, a need that has increased due to the COVID-19 pandemic coupled with structural issues that affect nursing recruitment and retention. Nursing schools in universities advertise compelling missions to attract students with promises of world-class education, especially among elite universities (Timmins, Thompson, & Watson, 2022). Although post-secondary education can position nursing students for rewarding careers, navigating the corporate university culture, underpinned by neoliberal ideology, can be perilous for the sustained development of nursing in academia (Darbyshire, 2008; Darbyshire, Thompson, & Watson, 2019; Thompson & Watson, 2006). While nursing schools are eager to serve an increasing number of students and prepare them for the workforce, significant goals like the development of nursing knowledge and values become ancillary (Darbyshire et al., 2019; Morrall & Goodman, 2013; Rolfe, 2016; Thompson, 2009; Thompson & Darbyshire, 2013; Timmins et al., 2022).

In this chapter, we examine the issue of anti-intellectualism in nursing and discuss its impact on the status of nursing as an academic discipline. We utilize John Henry Newman's view of university education as a heuristic means to analyse anti-intellectualism in nursing education. We examine the disciplinary and historical trends that foster an uncritical acceptance of anti-intellectualism in nursing. Our goal is to suggest some areas of reflection to counter anti-intellectual trends and avoid the triumph of ignorance embedded into a culture of educational fundamentalism in nursing (Alvesson, 2013; Perron & Rudge, 2016).

Disciplinary trends

The nature of nursing as a human-centred practice discipline complexifies its relationships with academia as nurses focus on experiential learning. This focus on experiential

DOI: 10.4324/9781003427407-31

learning departs from technical rationality characterizing applied disciplines like engineering, where theory development and testing research applications can be straightforward (Rolfe, 2012a). Rolfe (2012a) points out that corporate universities have failed nursing in the sense that they fail to recognize that the ontological and epistemological requirements of nursing are different from those of pure or applied technical disciplines. Nurses require more than professional training to meet the labour demands of a post-industrialized society. Nurses must be able to make complex decisions about patient/community health using evidence, ethics and consider individual patient needs in various contexts. As a profession and a discipline, nursing demands more than the application of evidence-based knowledge but requires nurses to use holistic, ethical, contextual, and relational knowledge to contribute to the well-being of individuals, families, and communities (Doane & Varcoe, 2021). Nursing requires a pragmatic approach to praxis to improve people's experiences of health, illness, and healing. Pragmatism moves us into what Thorne and Sawatzky (2014) describe as "particularizing the general" to attend to individuals' unique expressions of illness and suffering. Because of its practice features and the view that nursing remains a female-dominated profession, there has been little respect for nursing as an academic discipline by governments, the academy, and, unfortunately, by nursing itself (Darbyshire et al., 2019; Perron & Rudge, 2016; Ryder, Connolly, Kitson, Thompson, & Timmins, 2022; Thompson & Watson, 2006; Timmins et al., 2022).

Nursing's adherence to the diktats of neoliberal corporate culture creates conditions of vulnerability for nursing in higher education (Cuchetti & Grace, 2020; Eisenbauer, 2015; Foth & Holmes, 2016). In addition, nursing's departure from the linearity of technical rationality and its reliance on advanced technology as pedagogical tools may support "disembodied thinking" (Boler, 2002). In its focus on rationality and positivism, Cartesian knowledge underpins biomedical and nursing Western ways of knowing (Doane & Varcoe, 2021). Disembodied thinking means that technology supports digital Cartesianism by separating general knowledge about illness from the particularities of its unique embodied experiences. Technology shapes thought patterns, and a new generation of nurses can miss connecting with the wholeness of the lived experiences of illness (Cuchetti & Grace, 2020). When machines supersede humanity, nurses focus more on computer data, checkboxes, and monitoring devices and can miss vital patient information (Cuchetti & Grace, 2020).

Nursing education is now jeopardized as universities represent profit-generating businesses with students as customers, diluting academic standards and increasing enrolment to generate tuition to supply the labour market. The *McDonaldization* embedded in the corporatization of nursing programmes encourages the domination of fast-food restaurant principles of "standardization, efficiency, and routinization," where grades do not necessarily indicate an enhanced ability to navigate complex healthcare contexts" (Alvesson, 2013, p. 80). These McDonaldization principles contribute to educational fundamentalism by supporting a naive perception of nursing education where the acquisition of credentials and competencies does not reflect the abilities and critical thinking skills required to apply scholarly knowledge in practice situations. For instance, Rolfe (2014) underlines the importance of providing nursing students with the "5Cs of caring: Compassion, competence, communication, courage, and commitment" (p. 1460). Nurses can be taught to be technically competent and skilful, but caring, empathy, ethical, and authentic reflective practice represents more complex attributes or competencies to teach (Cuchetti & Grace, 2020). Rolfe (2014) insists that teaching the art of nursing is best achieved through a broader education with exposure to the humanities and liberal arts, where students learn to develop the moral frameworks that foster compassion, courage, and commitment. When students are only prepared as labourers focused on efficiently completing tasks, they cannot appropriately respond to the suffering of others (Rolfe, 2014).

The unfettered emphasis on filling seats has led many nursing schools to lose sight of their mission to advance and enhance practice (Rolfe, 2012a, 2012b). Willis, Grace, and Roy (2008) underline that the central focus of discipline is to facilitate humanization, quality of life, and healing in living and dying. As extensively discussed by nurse theorists, the central focus of nursing centres on the human experiences of health and illness, including illness generalities but particularities of the individual experiences (Thorne & Sawatzky, 2014). As a result of educational fundamentalism, nurses have become more educated; yet, they often lack the rigorous education to help them develop the knowledge, abilities and morals to maintain quality nursing practice.

Nursing education in the 21st century reflects growing anti-intellectualist trends underpinned by the hegemonic views of neoliberalism. With its worship of technocratic and consumerist ideologies, a neoliberal university culture privileges cost efficiency, work readiness, and standardized exams as the foremost measures of success in nursing education. These measures can lead to anti-intellectualism as students-consumers only desire the end product (e.g., the degree) with minimal involvement with any content reflecting the complexities of actual practice.

Anti-intellectualism in nursing

Anti-intellectualism supports the view that thinking remains in the realm of the elite, far from the everyday realities of rank-and-file nurses. Scholarly advances can hardly thrive in contexts where anti-intellectualism prevails. Anti-intellectualism translates into a disrespectful view of things of the mind, including knowledge of history, ethics, philosophy, and the study of abstract nursing theories. Anti-intellectualism also incurs a disdain for the theorists seen as members of an elitist class dwelling in universities' ivory towers (Balough & Girvan, 2010). In his book *Anti-Intellectualism in American Life,* published in 1963, Richard Hofstadter noted the increased preference for knowledge of practical skills added to a decrease of any taste for cultivated intellectual development. Thompson and Watson (2006) argue that universities are caught in anti-intellectual currents of homogenous mediocrity where the search for knowledge and truth becomes irrelevant and even self-indulgent. Contemporary anti-intellectualism incorporates a business mentality and consumerism favouring predictability, control, replacement of humans by non-human technology, calculability, practicality, and efficiency (Eigenberger & Sealander, 2001; Rolfe, 2012a, 2013).

Educational fundamentalism enforces the need to prepare nursing students for the practical realities of the workforce. As such, researchers often find that students in applied programmes (e.g., business, law, and nursing) have higher rates of anti-intellectual attitudes than students in more abstract programmes (e.g., sociology) (Laverghetta & Nash, 2010). They claim that university recruiters emphasize work readiness and the ability to solve practical problems, issues that perpetuate anti-intellectual attitudes. When the end goal of higher education is to secure a well-paying job, it is not surprising that students expect job training rather than more intellectual pursuits like critical thinking and a critical understanding of health, illness, and suffering in complex and chaotic healthcare environments (Laverghetta & Nash, 2010). Padgett (2021) under-scores that learning involves a transformative endeavour beyond the mere acquisition of motor skills and the accumulation of knowledge. Padgett (2021) underlines that because of the high stakes related to the US national nursing exam (NCLEX) as an indicator of programme quality, students expect nurse educators to prepare them for the exam. This focus on the NCLEX often comes at the expense of exploring more complex questions about context, ethics, and history, knowledge upon which the existence of the discipline depends (Padgett, 2021). While learning should be a process of intellectual and personal maturation, it becomes a process of knowledge acquisition closely aligned to textbooks and standardized tests, leaving little room for developing critical thinking or acquiring knowledge indirectly related to hands-on techniques. Padgett (2021) even contends that standardized tests and the focus on "having the definite right answers" jeopardize nurs-ing education as it does not "prepare students for the uncertainties of clinical practices" (p. 8). Padgett (2021) critiques the influence of student teaching evaluations as a means to evaluate teaching effectiveness. Students' evaluations of teaching and learning remain controversial as they may not reflect the actual quality of teaching but the satisfaction of the students as consumers of higher education (Rowan et al., 2017).

Laverghetta (2018) reports that students with higher anti-intellectualist attitudes score high on academic entitlement, consumerist attitudes, and classroom incivility. Laverghetta mentions that students who hold anti-intellectual beliefs see education as a product and tend to adopt an attitude of entitlement, taking little responsibility for their academic performance. Incivility represents a lack of respect, and overt rudeness that interferes with teaching and learning is becoming a common concern among nursing educators (Butler & Strouse, 2022). Nursing professors are often kept busy satisfying customers rather than wrestling with the pressing questions of the discipline, which could sustain or promote intellectual development (Darbyshire, 2011; Thompson & Darbyshire, 2013; Racine & Vandenberg, 2021; Rolfe, 2012a).

Anti-intellectualism does not represent a significant study area in nursing, but more authors are now discussing the threat of declining nursing standards in nursing educa-tion (Padgett, 2021; Rolfe, 2014; Shields, Purcell, & Watson, 2011; Thompson & Dar-byshire, 2013). For example, Chinn (2014) underlines nurse educators' tendency to no longer emphasize or teach nursing philosophy or theories because fundamental nursing knowledge is viewed as obsolete and not applicable to contemporary nursing practice. Rudge (2013) suggests that nursing activities have been streamlined in health settings to support the managerial delivery model to which nursing education contributes with the standardization of curricula and learning activities. The standardization of nursing edu-cation is often promoted in a context of supposed economic scarcity, where the ultimate goal is a cheaper and more efficient production of nursing labour. That labour quality is an afterthought, as has been observed multiple times throughout nursing's history (Ash-ley, 1976). As Rudge (2011) points out, an anti-intellectual nursing workforce, after all, is likely obedient and docile, which contributes to the "well-run" system.

Neoliberalism in contemporary nursing education

We contend that neoliberalism is the overarching force driving anti-intellectualism and educational fundamentalism in contemporary nursing education. The intense competi-tion for students can support lower academic standards by dumbing down content (Rolfe, 2019) while overselling excellence and world-class education in what Alvesson (2013) describes as a zero-sum game. A zero-sum game whereby large student enrolment, grade inflation, learning deterioration, and increased completion rates likely generate anti-intellectualism (Alvesson, 2013). Students in ballooning class sizes are assessed through modules and multiple choices exams rather than critical reflexive assignments. More students graduate without completing time-consuming and costly activities that encourage examining values, beliefs, debates, arguments, self-expression, or creativity (Holmes & Lindsay, 2018).

The greater number of post-secondary graduates in a neoliberal landscape results in lesser value for university degrees in the labour market (Alvesson, 2013). In their seminal work, *Academically Adrift*, Arum and Roksa (2011) pointed out the failure of higher education to equip students with the necessary skills to succeed in a highly competitive global economy. In their study, Arum and Roksa (2011) reported no meaningful increases in critical measures of student learning among American undergraduate students, and stated that

> in a typical semester, 32% [of students] did not take any courses with more than 40 pages of reading per week. Fifty percent did not take a single course in which they wrote more than 20 pages over the semester
>
> (p. 2)

More disturbing is the fact that "on average, a student in a typical semester spends only 12 and 14 hours per week studying (approximately 50% less than full-time college students did a few decades ago)" (Arum & Roksa, 2011, p. 3). They argue that the primacy of social engagement over academic rigour must serve as a cautionary tale to universities. Nursing and neoliberalism are not strange bedfellows, as the impact of neoliberal ideology on nursing knowledge and practice has been discussed elsewhere (Browne, 2001; Holmes & Gastaldo, 2002; Rudge, 2011). Foth and Holmes (2016) underline that short-term goals, efficiency, fiscal accountability, focus on competency-based education, and objective measurement of these competencies (OSCEs) illustrate the impact of neoliberalism on nursing education. Neoliberal policies encourage nursing schools to conform to the diktats of governmental and external funders rather than resist and risk wholesale downsizing in favour of nursing programmes that are willing to lessen standards and sacrifice the teaching of the mind (Thompson, 2009). We now explain some of the historical events underpinning the development of anti-intellectualism in nursing.

Historical trends

Several long-standing historical and social influences have fostered an uncritical acceptance of anti-intellectualism in nursing. For instance, historian Joann Ashley (1976) argues that nursing has long been hampered in its professional development because of the perceived view that nurses were to be little more than servants to hospitals and physicians. Early nursing students were often utilized as a cheap source of labour and were discouraged from intellectual growth. During the late 1800s, professional nursing training emerged through an apprenticeship model in which students provided labour in exchange for nursing training. Nursing students worked 10–12-hour shifts, learning through repetition, often with short classes provided in the evenings. Due to the sexism of the time and the devaluing of education for women, educational standards were low, and students were denied the professional status granted to medicine. Because nursing was often characterized as a female calling or service, public criticism arose when nurses demanded improved economic and professional circumstances. Though there were a few exceptions in Canada's largest cities, nursing training maintained little connection to higher education centres until the mid-to-late 1900s (McPherson, 1996). The early apprenticeship model of nursing training discouraged a concerted effort to develop nursing knowledge and to methodically improve nursing practices (Ashley, 1976).

Another social phenomenon that hindered the professional development of nursing was the association between nursing and menial women's labour and domestic housekeeping (Ashley, 1976). Because the public knew little of what nurses did, this often left the impression that nurses required little knowledge or medical education. Many early nursing schools emphasized a socialization process more than a formal education (Ashley, 1976). They stressed feminine ideals and the need for obedience, subservience, and knowledge of hygiene. This focus allowed entrepreneurs to create nursing schools of less highly trained nurses or sub-nurses. The cheap mass production of sub-nurses proliferated and was a constant assault on the status of nursing.

According to historian Kathryn McPherson (1996), by the early 20th century, Canadian nurses further differentiated themselves from menial domestic labour by associating their work with scientific management, germ theory, and efficiency. Nursing students were increasingly expected to fulfil several rationalized tasks, including patient record keeping, performing diagnostic tests, facilitating medical treatments, administering medication and nursing therapeutics, monitoring supplies, cleaning and organizing the ward, and patient care, which included patient feeding and hygiene (McPherson, 1996). Though the utilization of science helped to differentiate professional nurses from untrained domestic servants, they tended to utilize the scientific knowledge created by other disciplines rather than taking part in forming their own knowledge base. Nurses thus focused more on the principles of efficiency rather than on scientifically studying and improving nursing practices (Reverby, 1987). In 1932, a national survey of the state of nursing education in Canada called the Weir report provided significant support for nursing leaders to advance educational opportunities for nurses (Mansell, 2004). Moreover, the increasing complexity of medicine created a greater need for more educated nurses. Nursing leaders were convinced that universities were the ideal location for the future of nursing education and began to work towards establishing nursing science to encourage nurses to utilize scientific methods to evaluate nursing practices.

Divisions between the nursing elite and the concerns of rank-and-file nurses further slowed the development of nursing's intellectual growth (McPherson, 1996). Although many elite nursing leaders regularly argued for professionalization as a primary goal, rank-and-file nurses were more concerned with working conditions and employment issues. These divisions meant that while the nursing elite sought improved and standardized nursing education, rank-and-file nurses were often more interested in enhanced pay, hours of work, and stable employment (McPherson, 1996). These differing goals fragmented nursing leadership and led to differing goals for nursing's most significant political organizations. These divisions continue with varying priorities among academic nurses, nursing unions, and nursing registration/regulatory colleges.

Another problem remains that many members of the general public still view nurses as occupational labourers. This perspective makes it difficult to specialize further and enhance nursing knowledge. The general lack of awareness can be seen even in practising nurses, who fail to recognize the vast knowledge required to provide excellent nursing care. Many practising nurses question the need for four-year degrees (three in the UK), insisting that intellectual/research activities are frivolous attempts by the elite to undermine or waste the time of rank-and-file nurses. These divisions demonstrate an uneasy relationship between bedside nurses and the elite's goals of professionalization and intellectual development. The disappearance of nursing history in nursing programmes during the last 70+ years has undermined the pursuit of quality nursing education and professionalization, weakening the benefits that such developments afforded many nurses in the past (Grypma, 2017). Most of today's students are simply unaware of what has been gained or lost, thus making it easier to convince student-as-consumer narratives focused on "student-empowered education" and "edutainment" (Darbyshire, Watson & Thompson, 2018; Thompson, 2009). Such narratives sound appealing but encourage students to stand firmly against improved standards that would look less like entertainment and more like work. Neoliberalism generated the commodification of nursing education in the UK, Canada, and globally and has been reduced to vocational training in environments where true scholarship is rare (Darbyshire et al., 2018). We now turn to John Henry Newman's view of a university education to explore potential avenues to survive educational fundamentalism and anti-intellectualism, which infiltrate nursing education today.

John Henry Newman's view of a university education

Cardinal John Henry Newman (1801–1890), a brilliant English philosopher, has defined a view of a university education that still attracts educators' attention today (Pelikan, 1992). Newman's idea of a university education is profoundly intertwined with his experiences in the Anglican and Catholic faiths, his education at the University of Oxford, and his view about the Enlightenment. The idea of a university education arose to counteract the pragmatic or utilitarian view of knowledge. Instead, Newman believed that the development of abstract knowledge, such as through an understanding of theology, philosophy, Greek, Latin, literature, and history, was a goal in itself (Pelikan, 1992; Rolfe, 2012b).

For Newman, the purpose of a university education was to help students achieve intellectual and personal maturity through the development of the mind. The quest for truth is the optimal goal of a university education. Newman (2015) asserts that truth and knowledge cannot be separated, as knowledge represents the search for truth. Truth resides in "facts and their relations" (p. 39). For Newman, pursuing knowledge for its own sake is a legitimate enterprise, and universities are to teach universal knowledge rather than specialized technical knowledge (Rolfe, 2012b). The notion of relationships between sciences means that truths are partials, and there is a need for multiple truths to illuminate the understanding of the whole. For Newman, knowledge comprises understanding facts in themselves or their relation to other perspectives or contexts. He points out that "knowledge is the apprehension of facts, whether in themselves or in their mutual positions and bearings" (Newman, 2015, p. 39). Newman supports a hierarchy of sciences where some sciences will be more critical than others, but together they will complete each other. Newman believed in the need for a transformative education where students would be exposed to diverse knowledge and not only knowledge to perform a specific technique or task.

Newman (2015) defined two forms of knowledge: one knowledge was based on reason and called "useful knowledge," while the other was based on philosophy and named "liberal knowledge." Newman described two types of education, one philosophical and the other mechanical, serving different goals. Philosophical education supported the acquisition of liberal and general ideas while mechanical education focused on the particular (specific) problems.

(Newman, 2015, p. 83)

Newman recognized the benefits of mechanical or applied knowledge in solving problems while contending that the closer knowledge gets to concrete facts or situations, the less valuable the knowledge would be. For Newman, applied knowledge did not represent an intellectual pursuit of developing reason, critical thinking, and wisdom. Newman did not see applied professional knowledge as liberal knowledge because applied knowledge served practical purposes like the restoration of health but did not translate into what Newman refers to as the "benefit of the soul" (p. 84). Newman (2015) argues, "education is a higher word; it implies an action upon our mental nature and the formation of a character. It is something individual and permanent" (p. 84).

The need to acquire philosophical or liberal knowledge may be what nursing needs to survive and thrive in the corporate university. A heavy focus on standardized tests and practical tasks may turn nursing education into a form of industrial assembly line production. Rolfe (2014) suggests that "our students are woefully undereducated and that many of them are, in fact, hardly educated at all" (p. 1459) and that nursing education is still very much a work in progress.

Discussion

Passionate debates around the interpretation of Newman's idea of a university education exist in the nursing literature (Rolfe, 2012b; Thompson & Watson, 2006; Thompson, 2009; Watson & Thompson, 2010). Myrick (2004) contends that "the original purpose of a university education was designed to foster a desire for right conduct and good things which ultimately cannot be neatly packaged and delivered" (p. 23). Watson and Thompson (2010) support the view of knowledge development for its "own sake," while other scholars believe that nursing scholarship should focus on developing or testing knowledge for clinical practice (Rolfe, 2013; Thorne & Sawatzky, 2014).

We cannot apply Newman's view of a university education to nursing or any other health sciences as it would assert that nursing belongs not to academia but to a vocational school. For Newman, pragmatism does not elevate the mind. However, if we accept the idea of a liberal education as being introduced to multiple sorts of scientific knowledge, then nursing could fit the category. Newman points out that a liberal education broadens the mind and cultivates the habit of the mind. In other words, Newman suggests that the faculty in a liberal university should teach students how to think and theorize about their fields. He emphasizes: "The object of training [students] is to prepare them to assume their roles as citizens by "making them more intelligent, capable, and active members of society" (Newman, 2015, p. 3).

The corporatist view of the university has transformed education into training and directed schools of nursing to become factories for the production of nurses and fulfil "indicators of excellence" (e.g., enrolment, rate of completion, students' satisfaction) influencing teaching and educational outcomes and university rankings (Foth & Holmes,

2016; Rolfe, 2016; Thompson & Watson, 2006). University funding is tied to the achievement of governmental indicators of excellence. Nevertheless, there is no indication that higher rankings translate into improved quality of nursing education (Rolfe, 2016). Although the place of nursing schools within universities varies worldwide, a shared focus on developing competencies for care delivery in disease-oriented health systems characterizes current nursing schools' missions.

Historically, nursing leaders have been sensitive in framing the discipline as innovative and forward-thinking (Nelson & Gordon, 2004). The focus on preparing nurses for "real-world" practice and "tangible outcomes" illustrates nursing educators' attempts to move away from the notion of the ivory tower and elitism associated with high-level thinking. For Perron and Rudge (2016), nursing's attraction to real-world outcomes relates to political economy. Real-world knowledge stems from the politics of ignorance because it implies that other forms of knowledge will be overlooked, subjugated, erased or devalued (Perron & Rudge, 2016). For Alvesson (2013), education fundamentalism supports a mediocrity of academic outcomes to produce "industry-ready" workers by diluting curriculum and standardizing content leading to intellectual emptiness and reducing education to an assembly line model.

We argue that these current trends feed anti-intellectualism and impoverish nursing from its philosophical, historical, and theoretical bases. With a continued focus on practical knowledge, especially via technology like virtual reality and artificial intelligence, is it possible to reverse anti-intellectualism in nursing? Can we reconcile solving so-called "real-world problems" with intellectual, ethical, and humanistic pursuits?

Thriving despite anti-intellectualism: personal and sociopolitical avenues

Rolfe (2019) points out, "there is no simple answer to the problem of market-driven universities" (p. 7). Counteracting anti-intellectualism in nursing education requires that nursing educators create more opportunities for critical thinking. First, undergraduate nursing students can use their personal experiences in the context of history and society to engage in intellectual craftsmanship (Rolfe, 2012b). The convergence of personal experience and self-reflection on practice is critical, given the complexity of healthcare in which future nurses will be engaged. Developing effective critical thinking requires extra time, resources and valuing educators' time and effort to increase the quality of the learning experiences. Technology cannot solve the problems of shrinking resources, decreasing the number of faculty, and increasing classroom sizes. Technology can be used to promote effective interactive activities emphasizing the synthesis of critical thinking and reflection through various quality interactive and engaging activities. High standards must be maintained, such as smaller class sizes, more student and faculty interactions, and a culture of wisdom that fosters more complex ways of thinking (Pesut & Thompson, 2018).

Inspired by Heidegger's work on meditative thinking, Cuchetti and Grace (2020) suggest inserting the notion of intentional authenticity into nursing curricula. Meditative thinking means to account for patient needs and meanings while remaining critical of the impact of technology in nursing care. Cuchetti and Grace (2020) underline the modern tendency to avoid deep thinking to entertain calculative thinking, where thinking activities are superficial and disconnected from one's existence and lived experiences.

Calculative thinking represents the uninterrupted flow of nursing work without a profound consideration of the meaning of life and the ethical and moral choices related to a human-centred practice discipline like nursing (Cuchetti & Grace, 2020). Calculative thinking is made worse by the use of technology and its related digital Cartesianism, which separates thinking from ethics and the bodily experiences of illness and suffering. As such, the uncritical worship of technocratic efficiency devalues nursing as a knowledge-based discipline.

Social and political activism

Social and political activism is the second potential avenue to counteract anti-intellectualism (Tsui, 2000). The recent COVID-19 pandemic and crises within healthcare systems worldwide indicate that social, ethical, historical, and emancipatory knowledges are needed to address the complexity of health and social problems (Kagan, Smith, Cowling, & Chinn, 2009). Gender inequity, social injustice, and racism impact individuals' and populations' health (Kagan, 2014; Racine, 2021), and these issues arise within nurses' everyday practice. These issues cannot be easily solved through clinical pathways and atheoretical empirical research but can be addressed through acquiring a hermeneutics of practice integrating reflexivity and action. Kagan (2014) points out that "nurses must live within a constant process of critical analysis" (p. 324). Nursing theorizing is needed to address the social, cultural, and economic constructions affecting health (Kagan, 2014; Karnick, 2013; Thorne, 2015; Thorne, 2016).

Praxis-oriented educational opportunities are strategies that promote intellectualism and knowledge development. Social and political consciousness can be developed and nurtured through experiential knowledge like student-led health clinics. Praxis-oriented education counteracts corporate university culture, where thinking activities are made "more and more difficult, less and less necessary" (Rolfe, 2019, p. 7).

Conclusion

In this chapter, our goal was to examine the factors underlying anti-intellectualism in nursing education. We believe that neoliberal technocratic business culture will continue to challenge knowledge development in nursing, and likely jeopardizes the survival of nursing in modern universities. We do not believe nursing fully adheres to Newman's view of the purpose of liberal university education as he advocates for liberal rather than applied knowledge. However, Newman's ideas about the purposes of liberal education might support nurses in fostering the development of ethical and reflective practice, intentional authenticity, meditative thinking, and emancipatory knowledge to face complex social and healthcare issues and refocus on the central unifying focus of nursing as a humanistic and artful science and practice. The survival of nursing in academia resides in valuing the ontology, epistemology, and axiology of nursing while being cautious of the triumph of ignorance enabled by the McDonaldization of programmes, the overreliance and uncritical use of technology, and the worship of financial efficiency. Neoliberalism, educational fundamentalism, and anti-intellectualism contribute synergistically to isolating nursing from its foundations and examining the complexities of patients' lived experiences and nursing care delivery in various healthcare contexts.

References

Alvesson, M. (2013). *The triumph of emptiness: Consumption, higher education, & work organization.* Oxford Press.

Arum, R., & Roksa, J. (2011). *Academically adrift: Findings & lessons for improvement.* University of Chicago Press.

Ashley, J. (1976). *Hospitals, paternalism, and the role of the nurse.* Teachers' College Press.

Balough, R.S., & Girvan, R.B. (2010). Examining the existence and extent of anti-intellectual attitudes and behaviors among university students. *Sociological Points, 5–17.*

Boler, M. (2002). The new digital Cartesianism: Bodies and spaces in online education. *Philosophy of Education, 331–340.*

Browne, A. (2001). The influence of liberal political ideology on nursing science. *Nursing Inquiry, 8*(2), 118–129. https://doi.org/10.1046/j.1440-1800.2001.00095.x

Butler, A. M., & Strouse, S. M. (2022). An integrative review of incivility in nursing education. *The Journal of Nursing Education, 61*(4), 173–178. https://doi.org/10.3928/01484834-20220209-01

Chinn, P.L. (2014). Nursing theories for the 21st century. *Advances in Nursing Science, 36*(1). https://pubmed.ncbi.nlm.nih.gov/24469083/

Cuchetti, C., & Grace, P. J. (2020). Authentic intention: Tempering the dehumanizing aspects of technology on behalf of good nursing care. *Nursing Philosophy, 21*(1), e12255. https://doi.org/10.1111/nup.12255

Darbyshire, P. (2011). The business of nurse educators in troubled times. *Nurse Education Today, 31*(8), 723–724. https://doi.org/10.1016/j.nedt.2010.12.006

Darbyshire, P. (2008). 'Never mind the quality, feel the width': ? The nonsense of 'quality', 'excellence' and 'audit' in education, health and research. *Collegian, 15*(1) 35–41. https://doi.org/10.1016/j.colegn.2007.11.003Darbyshire, P., Thompson, D., & Watson, R. (2019). Editorial: Nursing schools: Dumbing down or reaching up? *Journal of Nursing Management, 27*(1), 1–3. https://doi.org/10.1111/jonm.12730

Darbyshire, P., Watson, R., & Thompson, D.R. (2018). How universities win gold in the Muttleyfication of learning. *Nurse Education Today, 71*, 105–106. https://doi.org/10.1016/j.nedt.2018.09.005

Doane, G.H., & Varcoe, C. (2021). *How to nurse. Relational inquiry in action.* (2nd ed). Philadelphia: Wolters Kluwer.

Eigenberger, M. E., & Sealander, K. A. (2001). A scale for measuring students' anti-intellectualism. *Psychological Reports, 89*(6), 387–402. https://doi.org/10.2466/pr0.2001.89.2.387

Eisenbauer, E.R. (2015). An interview with Dr. Barbara A. Carper. *Advances in Nursing Science, 38*(2), 73–82. https://pubmed.ncbi.nlm.nih.gov/25932816/

Foth, G., & Holmes, D. (2016). Neoliberalism and the government of nursing through competency-based education. *Nursing Inquiry, 24*(2), 1–9. https://doi.org/10.1111/nin.12154

Grypma, S. (2017). Historically-informed nursing: The untapped potential of history in nursing education. *Quality Advancement in Nursing Education, 3*(2). https://doi.org/10.17483/2368-6669.1099

Hofstadter, R. (1963). *Anti-intellectualism in American life.* New York: Vintage.

Holmes, D., & Gastaldo, D. (2002). Nursing as a means of governmentality. *Journal of Advanced Nursing, 38*(6), 557–565. https://pubmed.ncbi.nlm.nih.gov/12067394/

Holmes, C., & Lindsay, D. (2018). "Do you want fries with that?": The McDonaldization of university education—some critical reflections on nursing higher education. *SAGE Open, 8*(3), 1–10. https://journals.sagepub.com/doi/pdf/10.1177/2158244018787229

Kagan, P.N. (2014). Afterword. In P.N. Kagan, M.C. Smith, & P.L. Chinn (Eds.), *Philosophies and practices of emancipatory nursing. Social justice as praxis* (pp. 321–326). New York: Routledge.

Kagan, P.N., Smith, M.C., Cowling, R.W., & Chinn, P.L. (2009). A nursing manifesto: An emancipatory call for knowledge development, conscience, and praxis. *Nursing Philosophy, 11*, 67–84. https://doi.org/10.1111/j.1466-769X.2009.00422.x

Karnick, P.M. (2013). Nursing theory: The neglected essential. *Nursing Science Quarterly, 26*(2), 130–131. https://doi.org/10.1177%2F0894318413477210

Laverghetta, A. (2018). The relationship between student anti-intellectualism, academic entitlement, student consumerism, and classroom incivility in a sample of college students. *College Student Journal, 52*(2), 278–282.

Laverghetta, A., & Nash, J. K. (2010). Student anti-intellectualism and college major. *College Student Journal, 44*(2), 528–533.

Mansell, D. J. (2004). *Forging the future: A history of nursing in Canada.* Thomas Press.

McPherson, K. (1996). *Bedside matters: The transformation of Canadian nursing, 1900–1990.* Toronto: University of Toronto Press.

Morrall, P., & Goodman, B. (2013). Critical thinking, nurse education and universities: Some thoughts on current issues and implications for nursing practice. *Nurse Education Today, 33*(9), 935–937. https://doi.org/10.1016/j.nedt.2012.11.011

Myrick, F. (2004). Pedagogical integrity in the knowledge economy. *Nursing Philosophy, 5*(1), 23–29. https://doi.org/10.1111/j.1466-769X.2004.00164.x

Nelson, S., & Gordon, S. (2004). The rhetoric of rupture: Nursing as a practice with a history? *Nursing Outlook, 52,* 255–261.

Newman, J.H. (2015). *The idea of a university.* Aeterna Press.

Padgett, S. M. (2021). "He just teaches whatever he thinks is important": Analysis of comments in student evaluations of teaching. *Nursing Inquiry, 28*(3), e12411–n/a. https://doi.org/10.1111/nin.12411

Pelikan, J. (1992). *The idea of the university. A reexamination.* Yale University Press.

Pesut, D., & Thompson, S. (2018). Nursing leadership in academic nursing: The wisdom of development and the development of wisdom. *Journal of Professional Nursing, 34*(2), 122–127. https://doi.org/10.1016/j.profnurs.2017.11.004

Perron, A., & Rudge, T. (2016). *On the politics of ignorance in nursing and healthcare: Knowing ignorance.* Routledge.

Racine, L. (2021). Racialization in nursing: Rediscovering Antonio Gramsci's concepts of hegemony and subalternity. *Nursing Inquiry, 28*(2), e12398–n/a. https://doi.org/10.1111/nin.12398

Racine, L., & Vandenberg, H. (2021). A philosophical analysis of anti-intellectualism in nursing: Newman's view of a university education. *Nursing Philosophy, 22*(3), 1–14. https://doi.org/10.1111/nup.12361

Reverby, S.M. (1987). *Ordered to care. The dilemma of American nursing, 1850–1945.* Cambridge University Press.

Rolfe, G. (2012a). Fast food for thought: How to survive and thrive in the corporate university. *Nurse Education Today, 32*(7), 732–736. https://doi.org/10.1016/j.nedt.2012.03.020

Rolfe, G. (2012b). Cardinal John Henry Newman and 'the ideal state and purpose of a university': nurse education, research and practice development for the twenty-first century. *Nursing Inquiry, 19*(2), 98–106. https://doi.org/10.1111/j.1440-1800.2011.00548.x

Rolfe, G. (2013). Thinking as a subversive activity: Doing philosophy in the corporate university. *Nursing Philosophy, 14*(1), 28–37. https://doi.org/10.1111/j.1466-769X.2012.00551.x

Rolfe, G. (2014). Editorial: Educating the good for nothing student. *Journal of Clinical Nursing, 23*(11–12), 1459–1460. https://doi.org/10.1111/jocn.12556

Rolfe, G. (2016). A sacred command of reason? Deceit, deception, and dishonesty in nurse education. *Nursing Philosophy, 17*(3) 173–181. https://doi.org/10.1111/nup.12124

Rolfe, G. (2019). Carry on thinking: Nurse education in the corporate university. *Nursing Philosophy, 20*(4). https://doi.org/10.1111/nup.12270

Rowan, S., Newness, E. J., Tetradis, S., Prasad, J. L., Ko, C.-C., & Sanchez, A. (2017). Should student evaluation of teaching play a significant role in the formal assessment of dental faculty? Two viewpoints. *Journal of Dental Education, 81*(11), 1362–1372. https://doi.org/10.21815/JDE.017.093

Rudge, T. (2011). The 'well run' system and its antinomies. *Nursing Philosophy, 12*(3), 167–176. https://doi.org/10.1111/j.1466-769X.2011.00495.x

Rudge, T. (2013). Desiring productivity: Nary a wasted moment, never a missed step. *Nursing Philosophy, 14*(3), 201–211. https://doi.org/10.1111/nup.12019

Ryder, M., Connolly, M., Kitson, A.I., Thompson, D.R., & Timmins, F. (2022). A critical discussion regarding scholarly development of the nursing profession. A call to action. *Nurse Education Today, 110*, 1–4. https://doi.org/10.1016/j.nedt.2021.105249

Shields, L., Purcell, C., & Watson, R. (2011). It's not cricket: The ashes of nursing education. *Nurse Education Today, 31*(4), 314–316. https://doi.org/10.1016/j.nedt.2010.12.015

Thompson, D. (2009). Is nursing viable as an academic discipline? *Nurse Education Today, 29*(7), 694–697. https://doi.org/10.1016/j.nedt.2009.03.007

Thompson, D. R., & Darbyshire, P. (2013). Is academic nursing being sabotaged by its own killer elite? *Journal of Advanced Nursing, 69*(1), 1–3. https://doi.org/10.1111/j.1365-2648.2012.06108.x

Thompson, D., & Watson, R. (2006). Professors of nursing: What do they profess? *Nurse Education in Practice, 6*(3), 123–126. https://doi.org/10.1016/j.nepr.2006.03.001

Thorne, S. (2015). Does nursing represent a unique angle of vision? If so, what is it? *Nursing Inquiry, 22*(4), 283–284. https://doi.org/10.1111/nin.12128

Thorne, S. (2016). Editorial: PhD without the Ph? *Nursing Inquiry, 23*(4), 281–282. https://doi.org/10.1111/nin.12169

Thorne, S., & Sawatzky, R. (2014). Particularizing the general: Sustaining theoretical integrity in the context of an evidence-based practice agenda. *Advances in Nursing Science, 37*(1), 5–18. https://doi.org/10.1097/ANS.0000000000000011

Timmins, F., Thompson, D. R., & Watson, R. (2022). Editorial: Is the nursing faculty keeping up or slowly drowning? *Journal of Advanced Nursing, 78*(6), e80–e81. https://doi.org/10.1111/jan.15205

Tsui, L. (2000). Effects of campus culture on students' critical thinking. *The Review of Higher Education, 23*(4), 421–441. https://doi.org/10.1353/rhe.2000.0020

Watson, R., & Thompson, D.R. (2010). Continuing professorial development. *Nursing Education in Practice, 10*(6), 319–321. https://doi.org/10.1016/j.nepr.2010.02.004

Willis, D. G., Grace, P. J., & Roy, C. (2008). A central unifying focus for the discipline: Facilitating humanization, meaning, choice, quality of life, and healing in living and dying. *Advances in Nursing Science, 31*(1), E28–E40. https://doi.org/10.1097/01.ANS.0000311534.04059.d9

Part 5
About care

28 Who knew? Towards a sociology of ignorance in nursing

Amélie Perron

Introduction

In September 2020, a media story broke out when a licenced practical nurse, Dawn Wooten, exposed migrant neglect and abuse in a detention centre overseen by Immigration and Customs Enforcement (ICE), an agency under the United States Department of Homeland Security (DHS) (Treisman, 2020). Through a whistleblower complaint, Wooten described gross neglect in the care of detained migrants in the Irwin County Detention Center (ICDC). The ensuing media storm focused on one aspect of Wooten's complaint: an abnormally high rate of hysterectomies and other invasive procedures performed on unsuspecting, uninformed and/or unwilling detained women by a gynaecologist later identified as Mahendra Amin, who treated the women at nearby Irwin County Hospital (ICH). Stories reported many women treated by Amin came back confused and anguished after having undergone invasive procedures they did not understand or consent to (O'Toole, 2020). Some were shocked to learn they would never conceive after the procedure. A review of medical records by the Associated Press (Merchant, 2020) revealed no evidence of mass hysterectomies but found significant abnormalities in how Amin diagnosed and treated medical problems, his ritual tendency to perform unnecessarily invasive or aggressive procedures, and the consent process. ICE, ICDC, and ICH denied all allegations and stopped responding to queries once investigations were launched. Following an 18-month investigation, a bipartisan Senate report was released in November 2022 (Permanent Subcommittee on Investigations, 2022). It detailed the results of a review of statements by key witnesses and of medical records, identifying multiple organisational and individual failures that facilitated the abuse of the women and impeded corrective actions to protect them. The 108-page report answers critical questions about how key DHS, ICDC, and ICH actors influenced the availability of knowledge about the abuse.

Using the aforementioned example, this chapter engages with the sociology of ignorance (SoI), a philosophical and sociological field of study concerned with 'non-knowledge'—that is, information that is not identifiable, retrievable, or intelligible. From this perspective, ignorance encompasses the ways and the things we do not know, cannot know, or refuse to know, with manifold implications in the social world. I hope to make this 'unknown' perspective better 'known' in nursing, given its ability to illuminate issues that both involve and impact nurses.

Shifting our gaze to ignorance

This chapter valorises an unusual concept in nursing: ignorance. Unusual, not because it is rare or unheard of, but because it is typically discussed as a personal, clinical, or legal

DOI: 10.4324/9781003427407-33

problem. Ignorance is usually understood as a void, a gap to be filled with knowledge, because this lack of knowledge creates 'problems'. For the past 25 years however, ignorance has increasingly garnered attention as an entity deserving the same consideration as knowledge, as both ignorance and knowledge enter a dynamic relation that shapes what we know and do not know. New analyses of ignorance in women's studies, anthropology, sociology, political science, and philosophy have made evident its potential in critical analyses of social, historical, and political phenomena, leading to the emergence of a sociology of ignorance (SoI) and the interdisciplinary field of 'ignorance studies' (Gross & McGoey, 2015).

Ignorance scholars are concerned with the way non-knowledge organises the social world, examining the processes through and by which it can be deployed, harnessed, or perpetuated, and its effects—positive or negative—in diverse social and institutional contexts. Analyses have examined the twin process of making and unmaking ignorance through historiographies, economic modelling, anthropological studies, and policy development, noting how for every piece of knowledge generated, there is a parallel growth of ignorance. This has been emphasised by scientists across disciplines, tasked as they are to find answers to pressing questions but also to challenge previous findings in continuous processes of confirmation-refutation. As Firestein (2012, p. 21) contends: 'The known is never safe'.

The SoI forces a shift away from visible or tangible 'knowns' to the spaces of purported epistemic emptiness that lie between. While dominant discourses take it as fact that we form knowledge societies in knowledge economies, ignorance scholars propose that we instead appreciate ignorance as the main driver of social and political life. Phenomena such as forgetfulness, secrecy, deceit, taboo, confidentiality, censorship, tradition, denial, avoidance, or uncertainty pervade our worlds, and involve, one way or another, the impossibility or the refusal to acquire, hold, or share knowledge—that is, each induces a form of ignorance. Consequently, Ungar (2008) challenges us to position ignorance as the starting point of sociological analyses, arguing that ignorance is the norm, while knowledge is the exception. This implies understanding the prevalence but also the practical and productive value of ignorance for diverse actors in different contexts.

The generation or perpetuation of ignorance in any social space may be accidental or wilful. Smithson (2008, p. 209) notes that ignorance 'is an essential component in social relations, organisations and cultures. People are motivated to create and maintain ignorance, often systematically'. There has been in recent years a growing focus on *strategic* ignorance, 'the investigation of the multifaceted ways that ignorance can be harnessed as a resource, enabling knowledge to be deflected, obscured, concealed or magnified in a way that increases the scope of what remains unintelligible' (McGoey, 2012, p. 1). Ignorance may indeed represent an attractive strategy to manage situations where information (i.e., knowledge) is deemed cumbersome, undesirable, or risky (McGoey, 2019; Roberts, 2015). The SoI favours a 'practice-based' view of knowledge and knowledge management as contextually and relationally produced (Tsoukas & Vladimirou, 2001). Institutional attitudes grounded in inquisitiveness, responsiveness, or uncertainty may prompt a decision to inform oneself (i.e., acquire knowledge) while indifference, disbelief, defensiveness, contempt, or resistance may lead one to dismiss certain data or testimonies (i.e., maintain personal or organisational ignorance) and uphold the status quo. As such, ignorance can be socially or institutionally practised through inaction, oversight, and denial of information that challenges certain discourses or systems of thought (Essén et al., 2022; Perron & Rudge, 2016). The SoI helps distinguish the tactics, strategies, structures, etc., that mobilise knowledge and non-knowledge towards preferred social or institutional outcomes.

In nursing, as elsewhere, ignorance is usually characterised as a problem; for example, nurses who ignore care standards or laws guiding their practice expose themselves and patients to significant risks. We have yet to explore, as a profession and a discipline, how ignorance is more than a problem that must be fixed; rather, we should see ignorance as a full-fledged actant (Latour, 2005) in clinical, professional, and education systems. This chapter continues previously undertaken work (Perron & Rudge, 2016) to engage nursing with ignorance studies, and to uncover how such analyses can support our understandings of ignorance as a feature of nurses' clinical and organisational lives.

A discussion of ignorance sits squarely in the realm of nursing philosophy, especially given our many decades of reflections about what nursing is and, relatedly, what constitutes (or should constitute) 'nursing knowledge'. It is generally recognised that nursing scholars (almost exclusively white and in Western institutions) have endeavoured for six decades to articulate and formalise the disciplinary foundations of nursing, and to ensure these are 'knowable' and recognisable in/as authoritative nursing texts. However, in formulating what counts as nursing and nursing knowledge, we inevitably formulate what does not; that is, we necessarily leave other perspectives and insights out of our collective consciousness. This sets limits on how nurses expand the realm of their reflections and investigations and, by extension, how they will (or not) develop a sense of their professional, political and ethical identity and situate themselves in broader socio-political systems. Simply put, nursing's sense of 'what it is' is as much influenced by what is missing from its knowledge base than what nursing 'knows' about itself.

Galison (2004) suggests that intellectual engagements with ignorance are a matter of antiepistemology—not as a form of 'bad' epistemology but as a distinct branch of philosophical thought, interested in

> the study of non-knowledge or the art of how knowledge is deflected, covered and obscured... antiepistemology asks after its shadow: the nature of non-knowledge, and the political and social practices embedded in the effort to suppress or to kindle endless forms of ambiguity and ignorance.
>
> (McGoey, 2012, p.3)

Thinking about non-knowledge is no mere task: how can we 'know' what we 'do not know'? How can we grasp what eludes us? Gross (2007) captures this puzzling question when he states that 'non-knowledge or ignorance refers to a realm that escapes recognition' (p. 748). As such, paying attention to ignorance means that we must first recognise its manifold manifestations that have come to be understood as (and labelled) something else.

Ignorance pervades nurses' lives. Not because nurses are wildly ignorant, but because healthcare systems are rife with people, tools, policies, discourses, and practices that sustain both individual and organisational ignorance. According to the SoI, ignorance must be understood as any circumstance where the generation or flow of knowledge is impeded, resulting in states of non-knowledge. Understanding ignorance as a situation wherein 'not all can be known' or 'knowledge cannot be transmitted' allows us to grasp how circulating ignorance shapes nurses' lives. Nurses navigate ignorance daily due to the clinical, technological, and socio-relational nature of their work and its associated uncertainties (the 'things' we cannot know). For example, three decades ago, Smith (1992, p. 134) observed that 'the complexity of healthcare may make it intrinsically unpredictable: we may never be able to know what we would like to know'. Like other care providers, nurses must contend with the limits of our knowledge, for example, about disease processes and patient suffering. Patients themselves are a source of 'unknowing' when they neglect to provide information (e.g., health status, use of substances, over-the-counter medication or supplements, risky practices), whether this is inadvertent (forgetting) or purposeful (concealing).

Confidentiality constitutes a key instance of ignorance in healthcare. A knowledge-limiting device, confidentiality simultaneously mobilises clinical, administrative, and legal discourses and processes that place restrictions on what can be known about a person and that define circumstances under which these restrictions are breached. Nurses use discretion to determine the appropriateness of sharing patient information with other clinicians, public health authorities, child welfare services, or law enforcement, thus positioning themselves as effective mediators of ignorance. Breaching this secrecy requires compelling reasons, and nurses mobilise various knowledge registers and arguments to justify their decision (e.g., public safety, professional deontology, risk management). Confidentiality is therefore one example of the moral use of ignorance, deliberately harnessed for virtuous reasons. Privacy and patient information protection laws are mundane features of nurses' practice contexts that sanction wilful, strategic forms of (moral) ignorance in societies that uphold citizen's rights to privacy and self-determination as social values.

Omission constitutes another ordinary feature of healthcare systems deserving special consideration. Omission refers to the act of excluding something or someone, or to not doing something that should have been done. In contemporary analyses of ignorance, it refers to the accidental or wilful exclusion of facts, knowledges, or 'knowers'. The most commonly discussed form of omission in nursing describes situations wherein nurses do not record certain information (e.g., interventions, patient preferences, errors in care) which impacts what can be 'known' about their activities and may influence the perceived quality or value of their care (Stevens & Pickering, 2010). Omission may also result from poorly designed documentation systems that fail to record key patient data and/or clinical activities, which can lead to important blind spots in care provision (Bowman, 2013). Away from immediate care activities, ignorance by omission can also result from the exclusion of nurses from decision-making bodies. A striking example occurred during the pandemic, as nurses, though consistently described as the 'backbone' of pandemic management, were glaringly excluded from, or barely represented in, COVID-19 task forces in many countries (Perron, 2022). Their critical public health (preventative) role of testing, contact-tracing, and vaccinating disappeared as public discourses focused on nurses responding to surges in intensive care units. Media reports perpetuated this ignorance through narrow descriptions of 'pandemic nursing': nurses were seldom consulted on risk management, resource allocation, care delivery, or lockdown impacts, featured instead in stereotypical ways emphasising nurses' pandemic-related victimisation and distress (Perron, 2022). These forms of exclusion powerfully constrain the public's and decision-makers' understandings of nurses and their work, perpetuating systemic ignorance about the full scope of their expertise and contributions.

Exclusions of sources of knowledge are powerful epistemic decisions not necessarily based on reason or logic: they may instead reflect unspoken social and political arrangements that determine whose voice 'counts' and whose does not—who can be considered a legitimate knower in a particular instance and who cannot. Far from being exhaustive, these examples provide some glimpses into how everyday social, professional, and political activities hinge on forms of ignorance that we have come to call something else (for other examples, see Perron & Rudge, 2016). Once we overcome strict adherence to terminology, we can catch ignorance 'in the making' or 'at work' in a wide range of decisions and interventions whose epistemic value is often underappreciated. This allows us to gain additional insights into complex cases involving nurses, such as the one described earlier.

Revisiting the case

At first glance, the ICE story is a case of medical abuse perpetrated against migrant women made extremely vulnerable by state-sanctioned programmes of capture, detention, and deportation, a situation publicly exposed by a nurse whistleblower. I suggest that the case has implications with regard to ignorance in several respects. Though it is impossible to provide a thorough account of each of these, I will review some ways ignorance plays out, and how nurses feature (or not) therein. Due to limited space, I focus on two aspects: ignorance produced in care administration of detained migrant women; and ignorance embedded in the investigative report.

Ignorance produced in care administration of detained migrant women

Ignorance was a powerful feature of the administrative structure governing the medical care provided to the migrant women. All administrations involved (ICE, ICDC, and ICH) justified their inaction by consistently claiming they were unaware of any medical abuse until Wooten's public disclosure. Yet, many conditions were in place that precisely ensured administrators would remain ignorant of certain problems. For starters, a general hands-off approach characterised ICE's hiring and oversight processes, as officials did not conduct a background check to vet Amin before referring ICDC detainees to him. Yet, a simple internet search would have sufficed to learn of Amin's entanglement in multiple lawsuits for malpractice and fraud, several of which were pending when he was hired. Amin was not board-certified in obstetrics-gynaecology; yet, no review mechanisms were in place to ensure he met clinical, ethical, and legal standards of care (ICE and ICDC claimed no responsibility to assess the care of off-site medical providers, only to provide detainees with 'access' to care). Administrators emphasised that ICDC medical staff had no responsibility in ensuring detainees sent to ICH received appropriate care, in a language they could understand and based on free and informed consent. Yet, there was no consideration of ICDC nurses' ethical and legal obligations should detainees reveal to them—as they did—problems with Amin's care. There was also no review of the procedures to which ICDC detainees were subjected, which would have revealed disproportionate rates of invasive and aggressive interventions. It seems ICDC's complaints mechanisms were also faulty: though the migrant women recalled submitting grievances to ICDC and ICE, conveying their concerns to ICDC staff, or requesting second medical opinions, these grievances somehow did not reach the appropriate persons to look into the matter. Finally, despite yearly site inspections by ICE being mandatory, none were carried out in ICDC for several years during Amin's contract. Systemic conditions were therefore in place to hinder the identification and communication of critical information to investigate irregularities and trigger corrective actions. Unsurprisingly, the report repeatedly (almost ritualistically) underscores how ICE and ICDC officials were 'unaware' of Amin's inappropriate care and the women's complaints, though it is clear no system was in place to effectively seek and collect such information, amounting to what sociologists of ignorance call 'wilful blindness' on the part of both administrations.

In thinking about the case's relevance to nursing, one might simply recall it was brought to light thanks to a licenced practical nurse. Extensive accounts exist about nurse whistleblowing, which effectively disrupts patterns of ignorance surrounding organisational wrongdoing (Perron et al., 2020). However, nurses were far more involved in this case, namely by contributing to the making and masking of problems in the women's care. For example, current and former nursing staff reported that ICDC care staff knew about complaints against Amin, though this was not documented in the women's records and not relayed to administrators, thereby furthering organisational ignorance about the abuse. Reports point to some ICH and ICDC nurses also contributing to women's ignorance by not answering their questions about Amin's diagnoses or treatment-related decisions. While some nurses did answer the women's questions, others further undermined the consent process by requesting consent at inappropriate times (e.g., minutes before anaesthesia) and, in some cases, pressuring women into accepting certain procedures—elements brought forth by Wooten, former nursing staff and some of the migrant women, but that could not be recollected by some nurses interviewed during the investigation. Reports from former nursing staff also indicated that some ICDC nurses obstructed the flow of accurate information by shredding some of the women's medical requests that were deemed 'too repetitive', and entering false information (e.g., vital signs) in certain patient charts. In other words, nurses were pivotal actors in the facilitation, stagnation, or obstruction of knowledge regarding the migrant women's needs and concerns, as their actions contributed to ignorance in both the detained women and the detention centre more broadly.

Ignorance embedded in the investigative report

The Senate Subcommittee's comprehensive report is an authoritative resource establishing multi-level failures in DHS, ICE, ICDC, and ICH policies and procedures. While the report disrupts certain epistemic arrangements (e.g., practices of accidental or wilful ignorance) that allowed the medical abuse to occur unchecked, it also rests on particular epistemic devices (e.g., witness accounts; nursing notes from patients' medical records) that provided the Subcommittee with the knowledge it sought and determined its understanding of the case. The treatment of this evidence during the investigation and *also* in the rendition of the analysis (i.e., the written report) seems straightforward; however, an ignorance framework helps identify clues regarding investigators' differing assessment of the trustworthiness of their sources. One particular aspect lies in the characterisation of some accounts as unsubstantiated but not others. In particular, the report warns that it was not possible for investigators to assess the accuracy or veracity of some of the migrants' and nurses' allegations of mistreatment, which creates doubts about these witnesses' trustworthiness. Conversely, key administrators' multiple statements to the effect they were 'unaware' of medical abuse are never accompanied by similar caveats, despite the possibility it may be in their interest to conceal their knowledge thereof. This difference signals the Subcommittee's concern about the validity of *claims* of wrongdoing but not about *claims to ignorance* regarding the wrongdoing, thereby discursively assigning a higher level of epistemic legitimacy to institutional agents and officials compared to the migrants and concerned nurses.

Assessing the validity of claims is a crucial part of an investigation. A key verification tool at the investigators' disposal were institutional forms and documents, as evidenced by the report's extensive references to ICDC documents and medical records. Interestingly, other parts of the report simultaneously suggest issues with these same documents, for example, regarding problematic recording of migrants' health status and concerns, and the insertion of inaccurate, incomplete, or fabricated information in medical records (both described as being carried out by nursing staff). The report indicates that investigators found no evidence of document destruction or fabrication of clinical data, though it does not specify how this was assessed, and it does not consider that such evidence is likely impossible to secure. It appears investigators took the lack of evidence to mean that document tempering simply did not occur—a reflex critiqued by many sociologists of ignorance examining the impacts of documentation alteration or omissions in the production of ignorance (Gross & McGoey, 2015). As a result, the report signals potential breaches in the quality of ICDC documentation while simultaneously upholding its soundness as a source of reliable information. In other words, while concerns are raised about the quality of ICDC records, these concerns are implicitly set aside as this documentation is also used to cast doubts about the accuracy or veracity of migrants' and nurses' claims, a powerful epistemic move by investigators who make critical decisions about the legitimacy of both witnesses and documents as sources of information.

Overall, the Subcommittee's report appears as a thorough, comprehensive, and airtight document about institutional and medical practices that facilitated gynaecological abuse of detained migrant women. However, an ignorance perspective requires us to consider both what the report includes and what it leaves out. One aspect in which the report stands apart from earlier analyses of the case is the lack of reference to the context created by state and federal migration control policies and detention systems, spurred by longstanding racial segregation and division in the country. While numerous analyses and commentaries by academics, policy experts, politicians, and advocates drew parallels between the treatment of the migrant women and the U.S.'s history of racism, exclusion, and eugenics, the report makes no reference to such, and the words race and racism do not appear in the report. This absence implicitly suggests that considerations of race and racism in the treatment of the migrant women were irrelevant to the investigation.

So what? Why ignorance matters

The SoI is not about ignorance for ignorance's sake. As Mikulak (2021, p. 827) observes, 'simply identifying moments of ignorance and filing them away in our collective understanding as 'knowledge gaps' obscures how ignorance is not simply an absence of knowledge, but an epistemic practice in its own right'. The above discussion reflects multiple manifestations of ignorance in the form of omission, denial, oversight, unawareness, and forgetting, to name just those. The case therefore hinges on a porous knowledge/ ignorance boundary, revealing complex, overlapping and sometimes intertwined epistemic arrangements that allowed medical abuse to occur. Here, I wish to highlight three aspects laid bare by the SoI: ignorance alibis for those in powerful positions; the power to sidestep and discursively erase certain issues; and nursing's involvement in truth games in practice, regulation, and research.

Ignorance alibis

Mills (1997), McGoey (2019), Sullivan and Tuana (2007), Smithson (2008), Perron and Rudge (2016), and Mikulak (2021) are just some of the scholars who have examined how certain groups induce ignorance in others or resist knowledge (i.e., self-induced ignorance) to create a socio-political advantage. For example, for several years, migrant women had expressed concerns about Amin, which were not investigated. Failure to heed such warning signals points to human and non-human factors (Macrae, 2014) that operate as ignorance-inducing devices. These are built into policies (and *lack* of policies), practices, and cultures that organisations use to run their operations, secure contracts, protect their reputation, and avoid liability. The SoI helps problematise the benefit of remaining ignorant of certain facts, as displayed by ICE, ICDC, and ICH officials.

As McGoey (2020) contends, 'The privilege of *not* asking questions is not shared by society's most vulnerable and exploited people' (italics in original). Ignorance in social systems is often assumed to be a bottom-heavy problem typically characterising low-level employees or lay individuals. McGoey (2019) disputes this view, arguing it is in fact a top-heavy issue that facilitates the maintenance of power relations: 'the cultivation of strategic unknowns remains a resource—perhaps the greatest resource—for those in a position of power and those subject to it' (McGoey, 2012, p. 1). This is evidenced in the case, where top government, prison and hospital officials displayed extensive ignorance about Amin's criminal background, troubling practices at ICDC and ICH facilities, and women's complaints. Given their documented inability and unwillingness to learn critical information about irregularities, it seems these officials knew 'what not to know' to avoid liability, thereby positioning their ignorance not as a failure, but as a political achievement (McGoey, 2019).

Discursive erasure

The Subcommittee's investigation and report were not meant to question migrant detention and deportation structures. They appear to be *only* about medical mistreatment of detained migrant women; thus, the report focuses mainly on Amin (the abusive figure) and institutional failures ('contributive' elements) as factors *detached* from race-based discrimination and policies, as opposed to them being *products* of these. Given its recency, it is unclear how the report fits in broader debates on healthcare practices as conduits for mistreatment of (racialised) persons. However, ignorance about racism as a driver of abusive systems restricts what can be 'known' about the migrant women's victimisation, and it limits discussions on the reforms needed. This poses a serious antiepistemological problem: for example, where migration control policies are concerned, analyses that omit to recognise structural racism work to

> assum[e] the immigration system's racial innocence (Murakawa and Beckett 2010). Under such assumption, it is extremely difficult, if not impossible, to challenge the system itself and propose transformative change: If the system is innocent, one can only critique the practices.
>
> (Liao et al., 2021)

In other words, ignorance induced through the discursive avoidance of certain issues (e.g., racism) leads to disingenuous corrective measures that maintain harmful dynamics of power and exclusion. Such measures are not meant to disrupt entrenched assumptions about gender, race, and class, but in fact reproduce them and fix them in seemingly neutral devices (see, for instance, the report's recommendations). These devices uphold rigid social arrangements predicated on their built-in inability to fully see themselves for what they are (Mills, 1997; Sullivan & Tuana, 2007)—that is, their ability to successfully ignore their most harmful effects.

Nursing's truth games

As mentioned earlier, despite the comprehensiveness of the Subcommittee's report, some gaps persist that are of particular interest to nursing. The report suggests nurses played multiple, and sometimes conflicting, roles in the women's situation, for instance, by making discrete decisions about which information they conveyed (or not) to them and for what purpose (e.g., to uphold or pressure the consent process), which information they documented (or not) in medical records, or which concerns they relayed (or not) to designated authorities. Despite the report identifying serious breaches in nursing care and documentation, nursing regulators have not expressed an intention to conduct a review which might provide additional insights into nurses' participation in abusive practices and systems. Nursing academics have not picked up on the story either: only one nursing publication refers to the case (Dickman & Chicas, 2021), using it only as a springboard for a discussion on the political determinants of health and health equity. This confirms our profession's documented tendency to avoid discussing nursing's participation in unethical or illegal acts (see, for instance, Foth, 2013; Symenuk et al., 2020). Nursing organisations often limit themselves to issuing position statements condemning nurse participation in patient rights violations without further involvement in socio-political debates. Despite having access to nurses' places of employment, nursing regulators do not investigate possible participation of nurse clinicians and managers in abuse. Finally, nurse researchers still tend to stay away from critical analyses of nursing's troubling history with unethical and abusive practices. All these elements point to a trend of evasion—a powerful producer of ignorance—rather than reckoning. This entails epistemological and ontological ramifications through the restriction of what can be known about our profession and discipline, the compounding of our collective ignorance, and the skewing of our professional identity.

Conclusion

This chapter provides a brief and practical introduction to the SoI to make ignorance 'thinkable' in nursing and healthcare. As ignorance is not a mere collection of deficits or voids, we cannot treat it as a vacuum to be filled with science or education. As a core feature of what makes the social 'work', ignorance always involves some productive outcome. Ignorance studies aim to examine the nature of these outcomes and what they accomplish socially and politically.

Still today, nurses are often thought as having little power to influence healthcare policies. Yet, they are actively engaged in power/knowledge processes, meaning they partake in institutional 'truth games' through their privileged position in handling, transmitting, or circumventing knowledge that can inform decisions and practices, with deep ramifications for patients, organisations, and the broader public. Nursing cannot sidestep reflections informed by ignorance studies: it must actively unpack nurses' role as both knowledge and ignorance brokers. This is essential given increasing awareness of nursing's participation (inadvertent or purposeful) in systems of injustice—including epistemic injustice. As epistemic agents, nurses continuously manage the boundaries between ignorance and knowledge, which helps them achieve various outcomes in patient care, social relationships, and organisational governance (Perron & Rudge, 2016). Their epistemic work can both maintain and subvert dynamics of power and associated subjectivities. For example, we may be familiar (and perhaps more comfortable) with the discursive positioning of nurses in states of victimhood, but we have yet to fully reckon with our power to victimise, or passively let care systems victimise, certain individuals.

The SoI offers a different approach to nursing philosophy. It brings us to more seriously identify and problematise what *isn't there* in nursing; to re-examine certain aspects of nurses' work that are misunderstood, invisible, forgotten, censored, or complacently overlooked, to delineate their reasons for being and their ramifications. Analyses of this sort offer new perspectives on certain 'truths', thereby revitalising nursing enquiry. Importantly, they help understand nursing issues not just as social, historical, legal, or political 'things' but also as *epistemic phenomena*; that is, phenomena that rest on particular (anti)epistemic arrangements and differing divisions of epistemic labour.

Acknowledgements

I wish to emphasise the intellectual influences and friendships of Prof. Trudy Rudge, Dr. Virginia Mapedzahama and Prof. Sandra West. I also wish to recognise the works of Feminist, Indigenous, and Race scholars who have paved the way for ignorance studies, and whose contributions are paradoxically (and ironically) under-recognised and under-cited in the writings of many sociologists of ignorance.

References

Bowman S. (2013). Impact of electronic health record systems on information integrity: Quality and safety implications. *Perspectives in Health Information Management, 10*(Fall), 1c.

Dickman, N.E., & Chicas, R. (2021). Nursing is never neutral: Political determinants of health and systemic marginalization. *Nursing inquiry, 28*(4), e12408. https://doi.org/10.1111/nin.12408

Essén, A., Knudsen, M., & Alvesson, M. (2022). Explaining ignoring: Working with information that nobody uses. *Organization Studies, 43*(5), 725–747. https://doi.org/10.1177/0170840621998720

Firestein, S. (2012). *Ignorance: How it drives science.* New York: Oxford University Press.

Foth, T. (2013). *Caring and killing. Nursing and psychiatric practice in Germany, 1931–1943.* Göttingen: V&R Unipress.

Galison, P. (2004). Removing knowledge. *Critical Inquiry, 31*(1), 229–243.

Gross, M. (2007). The unknown in process: Dynamic connections of ignorance, non-knowledge and related concepts. *Current Sociology, 55*(5), 742–759.

Gross, M. & McGoey, L. (2015). *Routledge international handbook of ignorance studies.* London: Routledge.

Latour, B. (2005). *Reassembling the social: An introduction to actor-network-theory.* New York: Oxford University Press.

Liao, W., Ebert, K., Hummel, J.R., & Estrada, E.P. (2021). The house is on fire but we kept the burglars out: Racial apathy and white ignorance in pandemic-era immigration detention. *Social Sciences, 10*(10), 358. https://doi.org/10.3390/socsci10100358

Macrae, C. (2014). Early warnings, weak signals and learning from healthcare disasters. *BMJ Quality & Safety, 23*(6), 440–445.

McGoey, L. (2012). Strategic unknowns: Towards a sociology of ignorance. *Economy and Society,* *41*(1), 1–16.

McGoey, L. (2019). *The unknowers: How strategic ignorance rules the world*. London: Zed Books.

McGoey, L. (2020, Sept 7). The philosopher's ignorance (with a Response by Slavoj Žižek). *The Philosophical Salon*. https://thephilosophicalsalon.com/the-philosophers-ignorance-with-a-response-by-slavoj-zizek/

Merchant, N. (2020, Sept 18). More migrant women say they didn't OK surgery. *Associated Press.* https://apnews.com/article/georgia-us-news-immigration-97f7ee007d0ec241f9401092cc7ea939

Mikulak, M. (2021). For whom is ignorance bliss? Ignorance, its functions and transformative potential in trans health. *Journal of Gender Studies, 30*(7), 819–829. Doi: 10.1080/09589236. 2021.1880884

Mills, C. (1997). *The Racial Contract*. Ithaca, NY: Cornell University Press.

O'Toole, M. (2020, Oct 22). 19 women allege medical abuse in Georgia immigration detention. *Los Angeles Times*. https://www.latimes.com/politics/story/2020-10-22/women-allege-medical-abuse-georgia-immigration-detention

Permanent Subcommittee on Investigations. (2022). *Medical mistreatment of women in ICE detention*. Available at https://www.hsgac.senate.gov/imo/media/doc/2022-11-15%20PSI%20 Staff%20Report%20-%20Medical%20Mistreatment%20of%20Women%20in%20ICE%20 Detention.pdf

Perron, A. (2022). Hypervisible nurses in the covidicene: Reclaiming the scripts of personhood and agency. In Dillard-Wright, J., Hopkins-Walsh, J. & Brown, B.B. (Eds.), *Nursing a Radical imagination: Moving from theory and history to action and alternate futures* (pp. 95–108). Abingdon: Routledge.

Perron, A. & Rudge, T. (2016). *On the politics of ignorance in nursing and healthcare: Knowing ignorance*. London: Routledge.

Perron, A., Rudge, T. & Gagnon, M. (2020). Hypervisible nurses: Effects of circulating ignorance and knowledge on acts of whistleblowing in health. *Advances in Nursing Science, 43*(2), 114–131.

Roberts, J. (2015). Organizational ignorance. In M. Gross & L. McGoey (Eds.). *Routledge international handbook of ignorance studies* (pp. 361–369). London: Routledge.

Smith, R. (1992). The ethics of ignorance. *Journal of Medical Ethics, 18*, 117–118, 134.

Smithson, M. (2008). Social theories of ignorance. In R.N. Proctor & L. Schiebinger (Eds.). *Agnotology: The making and unmaking of ignorance* (pp. 209–229). Stanford: Stanford University Press.

Stevens, S., & Pickering, D. (2010). Keeping good nursing records: A guide. *Community Eye Health, 23*(74), 44–45.

Sullivan, S. & Tuana, N. (Eds.) (2007). *Race and epistemologies of ignorance*. Albany, NY: SUNY Press.

Symenuk, P., Tisdale, D., Bourque Bearskin, D.H. & Munro, T. (2020). In search of the truth: Uncovering nursing's involvement in colonial harms and assimilative policies five years post truth and reconciliation commission. *Witness: The Canadian Journal of Critical Nursing Discourse, 2*(1), 84–96. https://10.25071/2291-5796.5

Treisman, R. (2020, Sept 16). Whistleblower alleges 'medical neglect,' questionable hysterectomies of ICE detainees. *NPR*. https://www.npr.org/2020/09/16/913398383/whistleblower-alleges-medical-neglect-questionable-hysterectomies-of-ice-detaine

Tsoukas, H., & Vladimirou, E. (2001). What is organizational knowledge? *Journal of Management Studies, 38*(7), 973–993. https://doi.org/10.1111/1467-6486.00268

Ungar, S. (2008). Ignorance as an under-identified social problem. *British Journal of Sociology, 59*(2), 301–326.

29 Self-sacrifice in nursing
Taboo or valuable reality?

Inge van Nistelrooij

Introduction

What has always struck me, in the decades of conversations with nurses and other-care professionals providing daily care,[1] is the discrepancy between talks about 'balance' and talks about 'meaningful care'. On the one hand, nurses often tell themselves and each other to 'keep a balance', meaning that they should not cross the professional boundaries of their contractual responsibilities, alternate wisely between other-care and self-care, and generally restrict one's work to one's paid hours and tasks. On the other hand, when nurses get the opportunity to tell more about their work, they often mention meaningful moments that made their work worthwhile, when they felt they 'really made a difference' to another person or other persons. These moments were often 'out of bounds', meaning: unpaid, unregistered, after work-hours or during breaks, undemanded and unexpected, and something one could neither do often nor turn into a rule for all professionals. They even could be the source of inconvenience or tensions with colleagues. Simultaneously, however, these moments were often understood, so the nurses stated, as 'what nursing is all about'. The discrepancy between these experiences ('balance' vs 'out of bounds') was rarely discussed, although the sense that they were connected was almost tangible.

As a moderator of moral deliberation, a care ethicist and care researcher, I started inquiring into these latter moments and experiences. I started from the nurses' belief that they are at the core of practices of care and I have called them 'self-sacrifice' (Van Nistelrooij, 2015). I must be explicit here: *it was I who called it that way*, nurses nor other-care professionals used this term, nor have they easily agreed with me when I spoke about my research (although eventually, they sometimes did). Still, I believe that nurses *show* (not state) how caring practices are not adequately framed when framed as a 'balance' and fail to be adequately represented when compared to any other professional practice that involves mutual exchange and contractual obligations (and limits). Caring does not fit in this kind of construction; rather, it resembles a gift, an offer, a sacrifice, not only of time and energy, but ultimately also of one's self. Care exceeds a paid service, for instance. One puts one's heart in it, so to speak. For caring is responding to needs, and needs are developing, changing, fluctuating. This makes for a practice that requires one to be responsive, flexible, permeable by another, and at times, I believe, sacrificing the self.

Philosophy can be of help to look at the particularity of caring practices and the particular self-understanding of caregivers that stems from these practices. One philosopher who has written extensively on self-understanding that arises and develops in practices, as well as in the wider institutional and political context in which these practices take place, is Paul Ricoeur (1913–2005). By drawing upon his work, I argue for an uncommon

DOI: 10.4324/9781003427407-34

self-understanding for carers that emphasizes connection and entanglement, rather than separation and individualism. Reframing our self-understanding in this way may help to revalue self-sacrifice. I conclude that this is more adequate to understand the core of care practices and professionals, than a claim to 'keep one's balance'. But first, let me explain a bit more on how I came to think of 'sacrifice in care' in the first place.

A question arising in professional nursing care

In the past, I have been working as an ethics trainer in various care facilities, like nursing homes, care for people with intellectual disabilities, hospitals, hospices, and organizations for homecare. The context of this work was limited to the Netherlands and Belgium, North-Western European countries with a capitalist economic system and neoliberal ideology. In this work, I did not operate as an 'ethics expert', but rather as an 'ethics facilitator' (see Walker, 1993), starting from the premise that ethics shows itself in how people act together in relational caring practices. This view is firmly rooted in care ethics, a recent branch of feminist ethics (see Gilligan, 1982; Noddings, 1984, 2015; Tronto, 1993, 2013; Kittay, 1999, 2019; Walker, 2007; Leget, Van Nistelrooij & Visse, 2017). As a care ethicist, I never considered myself an expert in the questions that arise in care practices, but as a facilitator to deliberate on these questions with the experts in the situation, being the people meeting each other and working together in everyday practices of care. Today, I am still thoroughly convinced that ethics is a practice that verbally and non-verbally takes place among people. So ethics is not something happening in meetings, being written in books, or developed by academics. Rather, ethics goes on 'in between' people who act, talk, narrate, and experience together. When people act, talk, or narrate about their experiences, they often implicitly or explicitly express some idea of what a 'good life' means to them. By looking or listening closely, and inquiring into their actions or experiences, one may discover these ideas that lead their actions and experiments, ideals that people aim for, struggle to accomplish, or regret not being able to achieve. This is what ethics is about. People involved in practices, therefore, make moral choices and have ethical reasons for their actions, and 'ethicists' are the facilitators for making their deliberations explicit. That is what I aimed to do. I found myself inspired by collective deliberations where people got to know each other and themselves and what mattered to all those involved in cases that we discussed and considered. Together, we gained a shared understanding of moral goods in particular cases, situations, and also in policy that impacted them.

In these ethics training sessions, I soon started to notice that one topic was a recurring theme. That was the topic of 'professional boundaries': how far do I have to go or get involved?, what are the boundaries of what patients and clients can ask/demand of me?, and: how can I safeguard my personal health by drawing boundaries and communicate about them to my patients and clients as well as my manager? The problem that was put on the table was often something like this:

> Care is boundless, there is always more to be done, there are always more needs than can be met. I have become a caregiver because meeting the needs of others is what motivates me. Often those with the most dire needs (who may be the ones suffering in silence) for me are the most important persons to care for. They also may get under my skin. However, there are pitfalls which I must navigate. On the one hand I am personally affected by their needs and may take these needs, their looks,

their calls, home with me. This can be really burdensome and wear me out. Extra hard is the awareness that what they really need cannot be met within the limits of the available personnel, time and means. On the other hand, if I try to focus upon my tasks according to my job description and try to limit or protect myself, by shutting myself off from needs, I feel that I fail as a caregiver. Then I do not only fail my patients (or clients), I also fail myself. In brief, my responsibility exceeds my job description; I cannot meet my own standards of good care; and I often struggle to do the things that I find meaningful about my job. The alternative would be to work late. Or to work as a volunteer (e.g. in hospice care) where I can meet my goal: to care well, in a personally attuned way. But I think this should be the essence of my paid job.

Many caregivers have voiced this insight in similar ways. It was a struggle felt by them and during the COVID-19 pandemic things got worse. What struck me was that in these wordings, caregivers seemed to voice something specific about care. Something that requires a certain kind of logic that is counter-intuitive in Western culture today. I decided to turn to philosophy for insights and understandings of this other logic, for which I eventually turned to the French philosopher Paul Ricoeur. Below, I elaborate on how his work is helpful, what insights he brought, and how these insights also resonated and gained recognition in my meetings with care professionals.

The foundational question of relational identity

When involved in the deliberations mentioned above, care professionals often discussed the professional boundaries of their work. They expressed the experience of struggling with these boundaries: doing too little or doing too much, neither gave them the feeling of caring well, both for others and for themselves. The often expressed, well-meant advice would be something like: 'You should not take your work home with you', 'You should try to keep a balance between other-care and self-care', or 'You should really limit your feelings of responsibility'. You should, you should, you should. Often, the persons addressed with this well-meant advice, at this point started to look very unhappy, disappointed, or confused. What was it that they did wrong? What they expressed seemed to have back-fired. But still, they felt that there was no other way of being a caregiver. Some backed down, others muttered in protest for a while, stating that it had nothing to do with balance and boundaries, but with how they felt, with the person in need and ..., before they fell silent.

These muttered protests actually get recognition from the view of relationality offered by Ricoeur (1992, 2005). For these protesters questioned the view of being a caregiver which indeed centers about balance and boundaries and the view that care is about carefully guarding what 'I should' do. In other words: they questioned whether an 'I' can be that clearly demarcated in caring and if one's self-interest, self-care, the time and effort one spends on oneself can be seen as being on a scale with others, weighed against and brought in balance with the interests, care, time, and effort spent on them. And if that is so, how come that caregivers often feel that they also let down *themselves*, when they stop caring for others and turn to themselves? In brief, they expressed the idea that the self and others are not that clearly demarcated.

Ricoeur proposes to think about 'who' we are in terms of narratives. He suggests that we have a narrative identity. This means that throughout our lives, we tell stories about who we are and in this narrating activity we construct, reconstruct, and co-construct our identity. This makes our identity evolving rather than the same, fluid rather than fixed, and variable, for our narratives on who we are, what and who 'belongs' to us, vary over time. The story that a person tells at 16, at 40, and at 86 will probably not be the same. What is more, our identities weave together the stories that we have heard about ourselves and stories designed by ourselves which we consider to be 'true' about who we are. For instance, in telling about ourselves we integrate stories that have been told about us, on how we were conceived and born, on how parents and others responded to our birth, and the stories in which our existence was embedded from the first moment, like family legends and family names. Part of these stories consists of interactions with others and our own (re)actions, as well as interactions between the public and the private: we are citizens from the moment of our inscription in public records, as well as family members from the moment that others started to fantasize and tell stories about us, long before we could say 'I' (Ricoeur, 2005). In other words, there is not a 'real' identity 'out there' about which we narrate; there is only this narrating and re-narrating identity in which we simultaneously find out and make sense of who we are.

The ambivalence of this latter phrase is intentional. It reveals that we live in the dialectic of passivity and activity. Our *passivity* refers to what is 'given' to us, so things that we 'find out', or in the midst of which we find ourselves. Our existence, its relational network and its context are given to us and so are the time and place of it, even on a daily basis, with all its ups and downs. Our *activity* is what we do ourselves, that is, our 'making sense' of our existence and its ups and downs, which is also something that we do on a daily basis, implicitly or explicitly. This is typical of Ricoeur: he does not prefer to depict things in a one-sided way. In this case, this means: he does not depict human beings as either passive ('receivers of life') or active ('makers of life'), but he keeps both elements together and develops an idea of human being in the dialectic and infinite movement back and forth between them. This is important to keep in mind, as it enriches our understanding of ourselves. It also means that his idea of what humans are (his ontology) is interwoven with his ethics. For if human beings exist in the dialectic of passivity and activity, human beings can never be held solely responsible for their lives (as there is much that they have not decided on, but rather given to them), and neither can they be held for passive receivers of life, who rather helplessly 'have to deal' with it (as they also make choices and decide about their lives). Other philosophers have tended to one of these extremes, and have either chosen for an understanding of communitarianism in which personal responsibility fades, or for an understanding of rational morality in which the context is marginalized (the philosophy of Kant, primarily), but Ricoeur creates this dialectic position that reconciliates the extremes. The bottom line of this dialectic 'two-sidedness' is that human beings are neither too responsible nor too irresponsible. They are always partly 'moral actors' who can make decisions, choose between right and wrong, or give direction to their lives, as well as partly determined by others, by time and place, by circumstances, which they passively 'receive'.

In this way, the 'selves' of human beings cannot be characterized by boundaries or singularity, like in modern ideas of 'subjectivity', nor are these evaporated in more radical communitarianism. To Ricoeur, human beings are co-constructed by others and others are part of their selves, as the title of his main book – *Oneself as Another* (1992) – expresses. There is no self-other-dichotomy. To make this more concrete: we could see ourselves as persons who *have* relations (or patients, or clients), but that immediately defines ourselves also as *being* relational (Van Nistelrooij *et al* 2017). For if I *have* parents, I *am* a daughter. If I *have* patients, I *am* a caregiver, etc. Therefore my identity is built up by and composed of my relations. And my active role in this composition is to decide about what I internalize or not, include or exclude from my narrative. I cannot decide my family lineage, name, legend, but I can decide about my living up to, ignoring or going against them (Ricoeur 2005, pp. 193–195). As such, the self has not created itself, but it does decide about the meaning and purpose of its life: 'By narrating a life of which I am not the author as to existence, I make myself its coauthor as to its meaning' (Ricoeur, 1992, p. 162). Amidst the circumstances in which the self passively finds itself (happiness or tragedy), the self actively searches for meaning and new direction.

The foundational idea of care as attuning, liminal practice

The foundational idea of dialectics rather than dichotomies from Ricoeur's work also plays an important role in how he looks at practices. This might seem very abstract, but Ricoeur makes it concrete when he discusses care, which he calls 'solicitude'. In various works, he considers what happens between those involved and he emphasizes the relation between giver and receiver and what happens there, in the 'space in-between'. Look, for instance, at this quote on sympathy:

> In true sympathy, the self, whose power of acting is at the start greater than that of its other, finds itself affected by all that the suffering other offers to it in return. For from the suffering other there comes a giving that is no longer drawn from the power of acting and existing but precisely from weakness itself. This is perhaps the supreme test of solicitude, when unequal power finds compensation in an authentic reciprocity in exchange, which, in the hour of agony, finds refuge in the shared whisper of voices or the feeble embrace of clasped hands
>
> (Ricoeur, 1992, p. 191)

What Ricoeur expresses here is this idea of moving back and forth between acting and passively receiving the experience of being affected. Through what happens, power shifts and weakens, capabilities are affected, giving becomes receiving, and receiving becomes giving. Ultimately, what is left is not an exchange or transfer of goods, but a sharing of goods in a 'shared whisper of voices or the feeble embrace of clasped hands'. What Ricoeur does here, is the following: he undermines the classic categories of 'self' and 'other' (again). Instead of creating an opposition or dichotomy he sheds light on a third term: the relationship itself. There are not two, but three poles: the self, the other, the relationship. This is a dynamic pole that cannot be discerned from the outside, but can be experienced by those involved.

The relationship can be considered the 'liminal space' where things (such as time, energy, commitment, and care) are neither here nor there, but experienced by both *in their interaction*. Ricoeur (2005) makes the distinction between reciprocity and mutuality, and sacrifice is a form of mutuality in his view (Ricoeur, 2005, pp. 229–233; see also Van Nistelrooij, 2015). Reciprocity indicates commercial exchange, where the act of payment means the end of mutual obligations. This is visible from the outside and can be discerned by others. Mutuality, however, is an experience of those involved *in* the relationship. It transcends the exchange as a form of recognition of each other and the connectedness between them. In the act, more is given than care; there is a gift, a generosity, or sacrifice that is meaningful on both sides. Both are involved as human beings. Instead of a gain on the one side and a loss on the other, this mutuality is an expression of self-realization *in* the interaction. This means that the self of the caregiver *as caregiver* is realized as meaningful, as purposeful, as is the self of the recipient *as recipient*, in the mutual recognition in interaction.

What is relevant to our topic here, is that many activities in the past did not have a 'price tag', which also meant that they were not bound to time or place. They were no part of commercial exchange and considered to be 'without price', 'unpayable', and transcending any monetary value. Ricoeur draws upon historical research that, for instance, shows how in historical France 'teachers, physicians, and midwives are remunerated by payments that oscillate between gifts and salaries. Even 'honoraria' do not exclude polite or courteous gifts' (Ricoeur, 2005, p. 240). These were given and received in the awareness that the goods were 'without price', that no price could be set or paid. In other words, the gifts given and received (development, health, a healthy baby) were bigger than a remuneration could express. Ricoeur argues that nowadays we still know about the pricelessness of some goods that can never be part of commercial exchange, like 'security, responsibilities, duties, and honours', 'moral dignity', 'integrity of the human body, and the non-commercialization of its organs, to say nothing of its beauty, or that of gardens and flowers or the splendour of natural landscapes' (Ricoeur, 2005, p. 237).[2] This idea directly opposes the idea that any activity or demand is only worthwhile when it does give a 'return on investment' or 'pay off'. And as such it speaks to self-sacrifice in care.

Ricoeur's 'little ethics' of living a good life, with and for others, in just institutions

In the previous section, it already becomes clear that Ricoeur's ontology, so his view of what being (human) is, is linked to his idea of ethics and 'what to do morally'. That is, that doing good to another is not simply beneficial to this other alone, but is mutually beneficial. In order to elaborate on this idea, his dialectical ethics brings us even closer to the idea of 'self-sacrifice' and what this could entail for caregiving practices.

Ricoeur has considered the various branches of ethics and has brought them together in a dialectical movement. This means that rather than choose for one kind of ethics and reject another, he valued more than one ethics and brought them together in a dynamic and fruitful tension. As such, he reconciled three ideas of ethics: Aristotelean teleological ethics, Kantian deontological ethics, and practical virtue ethics. Aristotelean teleological ethics revolves around the central idea of a 'good life' that gives purpose, sense and direction to life; Kantian deontological ethics centers around norms that forbid evil, and practical virtue ethics is where practical knowledge is developed on what to do in this particular situation. I will explain this further.

Ricoeur's first and primary question of ethics is the question of the 'Good Life'. This is not a question that can be answered once and for all. Rather it is the 'image that each of us has of a full life' and that is the 'ultimate end of our action' (Ricoeur, 1992, p. 172). It is our idea of 'living well' that is 'the very object of the ethical aim' (idem). It is neither fixed, like contained in a thing, nor arbitrary, as it draws upon collective moral ideas. But it can neither be determined for all, rather it is the idea of a good life that each of us has of what a good life is and what purposes are meaningful to pursue. Teleological ethics means that that act or practice is good, that strives to meet these goals (telos is purpose or goal). Each has an idea, a personal goal, of what a good life might be and one makes decisions and plans for the pursuit of that good life (and remember: one is never solely responsible, nor is one not irresponsible for these ideas and decisions).

The second part of the motto takes us to the interpersonal level: a 'Good Life' is connected to living 'with and for others'. A Good Life, Ricoeur suggests, is unthinkable without others. As his studies of identity have made clear, others are part of me and I am part of others; there are no clear-cut boundaries between us; rather, we are interwoven. Therefore, a good life in the literal sense includes others. But also look at the careful juxtaposition of 'with and for'. There is a careful dialectic here between what one receives and gives, what one passively undergoes, but also what one does for another in reaching out. Not only is every life lived *with* others, otherwise one would not come into being nor survive the early years. It is also lived *for* others: one cannot withdraw from others without harming the self. Nor can one be self-centered, as living requires also to act on behalf of others. In a view where human interconnectedness or interwovenness stands central, happiness and goodness can only be mutual.

And finally Ricoeur includes the socio-political level when he states that such a life can only be lived in 'just institutions'. These institutions, to Ricoeur, are more characterized by common mores than by constraining rules (1992, p. 194) and as such they are part of the ethical aim (1992, p. 201). In institutions, the opposition between the individual and society is transcended, as the institution only exists when individuals accept their roles and act according to them. So here, again, there is a dialectic movement between the individual and the collective levels.

In ethical terms this means that Ricoeur has built a dialectical movement between Aristotelian telos, Kantian obligation, and (again Aristotelian) virtue ethics. This is how his argument unfolds: the primary question is that about the good life that gives purpose to my life (which is never individual, but always interconnected with others). That is the first that needs to be answered. After that, my idea of the Good Life, the projects that I develop in its pursuit, need to pass through the sieve of the deontological norm, preferably negatively formulated. Deontology offers us the prohibitions of evil and harm, like, for instance, the biblical Ten Commandments: 'you shall not lie', 'you shall not kill', 'you shall not steal', 'you shall not inflict pain', etc. These negative norms, prohibitions, and taboos, are the touchstones for my (intended) actions in order to decide if I am morally allowed to pursue them.

And thirdly, we must invent actions that fit with particular situations, persons and circumstances. In practical situations, the norms can conflict. For instance, when a person is in despair about their health condition and one has knowledge about the diagnosis, a general obligation of honesty ('you shall not lie') is in conflict with the prohibition to inflict harm. This problem cannot be solved by looking at norms alone, Ricoeur argues, as they conflict and seem irreconcilable in the concrete relationships and concrete responsibilities that one faces. Here, on this practical level, exceptions need to be made regarding certain norms and on behalf of others, as is required by the idea of the 'Good Life'. These exceptions are invented by practical wisdom, according to Ricoeur's famous ethical guideline:

> Practical wisdom consists in inventing conduct that will best satisfy the exception required by solicitude, by betraying the rule to the smallest extent possible.

This, then, is his ethics: one cannot find any kind of ethical action; this is guided by a dialectical movement that starts with the vital question of the good life; the answer to this question must pass through the sieve of the moral norm; and when these conflict in concrete circumstances, practical wisdom must find a course of action that is inspired by the ethical aim and in which the norm is trespassed to the least possible extent. Returning to the example of telling the truth to the dying mentioned above (Ricoeur, 1992, p. 269;

see also Van Nistelrooij, 2015, pp. 228–229), practical wisdom leads to not following the naïve solicitude of the first position of the dialectic (not telling the truth as that would make the patient unhappy), nor bluntly and uncaringly follows the deontological logic (one shall not lie, under no circumstances). Rather, practical wisdom helps to develop a practice of critical solicitude that has been tested against the norms of respect and the conflicting prohibitions of lying and of adding harm. Then a course of action can be found that is as honest as possible, in a caring way.

Conclusion

Ricoeur's idea of interwovenness and his focus upon the 'in-between' help to completely reframe the conventional negative idea of self-sacrifice in care. It denounces the possibility of demarcating the self of the caregiver, the idea that underlies the conviction that caregivers should separate themselves from patients and clients from time to time in order to recuperate. Instead, Ricoeur's view of interwoven human being and interhuman practices turns self-sacrifice into a matter of connection, not separation or individuality. Therefore it is not a diminishment of the self, but rather a form of self-realization. Second, his centrality of the ethical idea that gives sense and meaning to a person's life, makes the 'good life' turn inescapably around other persons. Therefore, an appeal to take care of oneself or of one's boundaries, misses the caregiver's conviction that this cannot be done *apart from* caring for the other. And finally, since the personal, interpersonal practical, and the political levels are connected in 'living a Good Life, with and for others, in just institutions', caregivers, who believe that their personal 'good life' depends upon others, will have a hard time to be understood by colleagues, friends, families, and society as a whole, as long as they are characterized by capitalism and neoliberalism and their core idea of individualism. I believe that the nurses that I heard speaking about meaningful care that was 'out of bounds' expressed a vital core of care. I believe that those who advised them to 'limit themselves' did not understand their understanding of themselves as interwoven, nor of care as being about interwovenness and connectedness. These nurses expressed that self-sacrifice, with the purpose of caring with and for depending others, to them remains the core of nursing care. It could be a powerful counternarrative for our society as well.

Notes

1 For the sake of readability, I will write 'nurses', with the intention of including all those who provide daily care professionally. I therefore ignore the distinction made in, for instance, the Netherlands between 'nurses' and 'care aids', the latter meaning lower educated caregivers, who perform less technical nursing procedures, and primarily give general daily care like washing, dressing, helping with toilet visits, and changing beds.
2 It must be said, however, that human organs have increasingly been commercialized nowadays, for instance, in commercialized surrogacy and commercial organ trade for transplants.

References

Gilligan, C. (1982) *In a Different Voice. Psychological Theory and Women's Development.* Cambridge, MA: Harvard University Press.
Kittay, E.F. (1999). *Love's Labor. Essays on Women, Equality and Dependency.* New York: Routledge.
Kittay, E.F. (2019). *Learning from My Daughter. The Value and Care of Disabled Minds.* Oxford: Oxford University Press.

Leget, C.J.W., Van Nistelrooij, A.A.M. & Visse, M.A. (2017) Beyond demarcation: Care ethics as an interdisciplinary field of inquiry. *Nursing Ethics*, 26(1): 17–25. https://doi.org/10.1177/0969733017707008

Noddings, N. (1984) *Caring. A Feminine Approach to Ethics and Moral Education.* Berkeley: University of California Press.

Noddings, N. (2015) Care ethics and "caring" organizations. In: Engster D. & Hamington M. (eds.), *Care Ethics and Political Theory*, Oxford: Oxford University Press, pp. 72–84.

Ricoeur, P. (1992) *Oneself as Another.* Chicago, IL: The University of Chicago Press.

Ricoeur, P. (2005) *The Course of Recognition.* Cambridge, MA: Harvard University Press.

Tronto, J.C. (1993) *Moral Boundaries: A Political Argument for an Ethic of Care.* New York: Routledge.

Tronto, J.C. (2013) *Caring Democracy. Markets, Equality, and Justice.* New York: New York University Press.

Van Nistelrooij, I. (2015) *Sacrifice. A Care-Ethical Reappraisal of Sacrifice and Self-Sacrifice.* Leuven: Peeters Publishers.

Van Nistelrooij, A.A.M., Visse, M.A., Spekkink, A. & De Lange, J. (2017) How shared is shared decision-making? A care-ethical view on the role of partner and family. *Journal of Medical Ethics*, 43: 637–644. https://doi.org/10.1136/medethics-2016-103791

Walker, M.U. (1993) *Keeping Moral Space Open: New Images of Ethics Consulting.* The Hasting's Center Report, Vol. 23, No. 2, pp. 33–40. Garrison: The Hastings Center.

Walker, M.U. (2007) *Moral Understandings. A Feminist Study in Ethics.* Oxford: Oxford University Press.

30 Is there a personal responsibility for health?

M. Murat Civaner

A dialogue in the times of COVID-19

Lisa: Sometimes I can't keep my anger towards patients quiet!

Daphne: What's wrong?

Lisa: So many people are dying in intensive care, there are so many warnings, so much training, but people are still hesitant to get vaccinated. A patient just came in -- again, Covid... And he hasn't been vaccinated. He is 62 years old and has heart disease. I inevitably asked him the reason: he had heard a lot of rumours, what if he had a heart attack after vaccination, etc. These people are incapable of making a simple loss/benefit calculation! Don't they realise that they are harming themselves and others?

Daphne: Unfortunately... They are not few... Especially the anti-vaccine people. It is even more strange that there are nurses and doctors among them. I really don't understand...

Lisa: Well, I'm not in the mood for understanding actually. We shouldn't provide services to such people. Lock them all up on an island; let them do whatever they want! If they don't want anything from medicine, at least they shouldn't harm others. Or, I don't know, impose extra taxes on them, prevent them from leaving the house, etc.

Daphne: It's not that simple, is it? Aren't we obliged to provide services to everyone? And besides, everyone has a right to services?

Lisa: Okay, but what can I do? Should we force them to be vaccinated?

Daphne: Of course, they cannot be forced. But are their decisions not to get vaccinated fully informed? Can it be called an autonomous decision if it is based on the wrong reasons? We need to respect autonomous decisions, but not misinformed decisions, right?

Lisa: But following your point of view, do we have to accept that almost all patients who are obese, who smoke, who do not wear helmets, who are drug addicts, who do not use condoms and have STDs are not responsible at all? Don't patients also have a responsibility towards their health? Must we let them live as they please despite all the public education, warnings, etc., let them behave recklessly, and when their bodies deteriorate, someone will try to restore them out of altruism anyway! I don't think this is fair. I think we should only have an

---

DOI: 10.4324/9781003427407-35

Daphne: obligation to provide services to those who have done their best and still get sick.

Daphne: What I'm trying to say is that we shouldn't be so presumptuous when we hold responsibilities to people. Is it right to blame people without knowing what conditions they live in and why they do what they do?

Lisa: Perhaps that's true... But you know, I'm not so tolerant when their behaviour harms others...

Daphne: I hadn't thought of it that way... But if there is such a criterion as harming others, then we have to talk about what we understand by harm. For example, would someone who goes into a hypoglycaemic coma because he doesn't take his medication properly be harming those who love him? Or, even (smiling), if you get cancer because you smoke, won't your loved ones be sad? Should you be held responsible if you go ahead knowing that?

Lisa: I think I understand what you're saying. Maybe we should limit it to infectious diseases?

Daphne: But even then, I think it's important to determine the right share of responsibility. Besides, what then? Do we impose sanctions? Which sanctions don't violate the right to health?

Lisa: Hmm... It's something to think about. You have an ethicist friend if I recall correctly?

Daphne: Yes, but to be honest, it is often difficult to understand what they are saying. I had a consultation recently, and he talked and talked and talked... In the end, either I didn't understand what I was supposed to do or he didn't have a clue!

It is often argued that people have responsibilities over their health, including promoting self-health, providing healthcare workers with appropriate information, and adhering to agreed treatment plans. However, if there is such a responsibility, what are the grounds for it? How should its scope be determined? To whom does such a responsibility exist? In case of failure to fulfil that responsibility, what kind of sanctions could be implemented? Undoubtedly, the guiding values for justifiable answers to those questions are human rights, the right to health, patient rights, and professional moral values. Yet, we cannot easily reach a consensus because of the moral tension deriving from various conflicting values. Such tensions, which can be encountered almost every day, may become more pronounced and negatively affect service delivery, especially in extraordinary situations such as pandemics. Indeed, many studies are showing that nurses may think that the diseases of the patients are the result of their fault and may have negative attitudes towards them accordingly (Snelling, 2015). This chapter deals with those questions by analysing the premises behind the personal responsibility discourse.

The conditions of moral responsibility

What are the conditions for moral responsibility? First of all, it should be noted that the concept of responsibility requires at least two parties. For example, on an island where there are no others, one cannot claim the existence of a general responsibility because defining a duty towards oneself is entirely up to one's voluntary choice based on one's values. Of course, the individual may feel sorry for not taking care of her health, may have regrets, etc.; however, the fact that she will feel bad as a result of her behaviour does not necessarily constitute a justification for having a responsibility towards herself. The idea that the individual has a responsibility towards herself is based on those who love her or those who may be affected by her behaviours in a broader sense; it is based on relations with others beyond that person. For example, the International Council of Nurses (ICN) states that nurses should lead a healthy lifestyle as part of a responsibility to patients to provide a proper quality of service: "Seek a work-life balance, ongoing personal growth, and maintain a healthy lifestyle" (ICN, 2022). It can also be argued that this idea of personal responsibility for health has a religious basis that is independent of obligations to other people. For example, in Islam, a person is responsible for taking good care of the body given to her by God. However, here again, another party is taken as a reference. We are a whole that comprises our personality and body. The brain is not a separate machine inside the body; it is continuously changing along with the other parts by interacting mutually. To think otherwise would be a dualistic and baseless claim.

As explained above, "responsibility towards oneself" is a misconception. Therefore, for one's behaviour to give rise to responsibility, that behaviour must affect others. However, in this case, the fair attribution of responsibility depends on the fulfilment of certain conditions. Moral responsibility involves "attributing certain powers and capacities to that person, and viewing her behaviour as arising (in the right way) from the fact that the person has, and has exercised, these powers and capacities" (Talbert, 2022). Based on this definition, it can be argued that several conditions must come together for responsibility to occur. The first of these is that the person must be competent. In other words, the person must have the capacity to comprehend the meaning of the phenomenon that she encounters/experiences and to distinguish good from bad (ability to understand). In addition, the person must be able to choose the good and say no to the bad in the face of that situation (ability to will). The combination of the ability to understand and the ability to will indicates that the person is capable of making rational decisions. For example, when a ten-year-old girl is touched inappropriately by an older man, she can understand that this touch is different from the affectionate touch she is used to, but she may not know what to say or how to ask for help to stop or avoid that behaviour in such a situation. The girl in this example has the ability to understand, but not the ability to will, and therefore cannot be said to act with free will. The existence of free will is, as is well known, the first condition for holding an agent morally responsible.

The second condition is that the person has sufficient knowledge and sufficient comprehension of that knowledge (epistemological condition) to decide what to do in the face of the phenomenon in question. Only a person who has sufficient, accurate, and complete knowledge about reality and who also comprehends that knowledge, in other words, who is not only informed but also "enlightened" by comprehending and evaluating the information given, can make an autonomous decision. This is the same reason why simply reading and signing informed consent documents do not necessarily mean that the patient is adequately informed. Without knowledge and comprehension, it cannot be said that the person's decision is autonomous, and therefore the claim that she is responsible for the actions she takes in line with this decision will be highly controversial. The phenomenon of vaccine hesitancy, which has become more widespread today, especially during the COVID-19 pandemic, is a good example of this decoupling of information and "enlightenment". In today's so-called "post-truth world", the individual has difficulty making a decision and may postpone deciding due to the loss of trust in medicine as a societal institution, media, and policy-makers in general. Indecision is exacerbated by the anxiety of not being able to access information on facts in the pandemic in particular, and the effect of misinformation spread by conspiratorial theories. The loss of trust in science and medicine, the main reference for facts, leaves the person unguided in an unfamiliar area and might cause them to lose their common sense. To accuse the person experiencing vaccine hesitancy as "ignorant" or "selfish" without understanding the dynamics influencing and affecting them means overlooking their inability to make autonomous decisions.

Assuming that the person has the competence to make a decision and is sufficiently enlightened, it will be necessary to determine what action options are open to her in order to determine whether she is responsible or not, and if she is responsible, to what extent. Because, as is well known, each individual is born, grows, and lives under different conditions. For this reason, both in the development of her personality and in her actions, in addition to her biological characteristics, the environment that surrounds her, and continuously dialectically interacts with her, is also determinative. A person's health is determined by the combination of social determinants of health such as education level, income level, nutrition, housing conditions, working conditions, the air she breathes, her father's occupation, social class, and the political atmosphere, as much as her genetic structure (Hart, 1997). WHO states that social determinants of health depend on inequalities, which, in turn, affect the level of health (WHO, 2022):

The conditions in which people are born, grow, live, work and age (...) are shaped by the distribution of money, power and resources at global, national and local levels. The social determinants of health are mostly responsible for health inequalities, i.e. the unfair and avoidable differences in health status seen within and between countries.

As Marmot emphasises, "poor social factors may produce poor health" (Marmot, 2004). Likewise, Daniels et al. state that inequalities affect the choices open to people and therefore their health: "Some of these [inequalities] occur at the societal level, where income inequality patterns the distribution of social goods, such as public education, thereby affecting patterns the access to life opportunities which are in turn strong determinants of health" (Daniels et al., 2004). These relationships can be exemplified in almost every health problem. For example, chronic health problems such as obesity, diabetes, and hypertension are closely linked to many factors such as low income, unemployment, psychological problems, the level of preventive and promotive health services, and how the food industry is audited. At this point, it can be claimed that a person's lifestyle also affects her health; therefore, she may get sick because she eats poorly, does not go to the doctor for medical check-ups, and does not exercise. Yet, lifestyle is only one of the determinants of health, and lifestyle itself depends significantly on the other determinants mentioned above. For example, when an individual has limited access to primary healthcare or an unemployed individual has the chronic diseases mentioned above, blaming them for eating poorly, not exercising, not avoiding a stressful life, etc., means overlooking how health is determined. For this very reason, the ICN states that (ICN, 2022):

Nurses recognise the significance of the social determinants of health. They contribute to, and advocate for, policies and programmes that address them. (...) Nurses promote an environment in which the human rights, values, customs, religious and spiritual beliefs of the individual, families and communities are acknowledged and respected

> *by everyone. (…) Nurses advocate for equity and social justice in resource allocation, access to health care and other social and economic services*

The extent to which lifestyle "choices" such as smoking, lack of exercise, poor diet, and stress are the result of freely made choices is highly debatable. The autonomy of each person is one thing, the options for action open to that person are another; therefore not all autonomous individuals make decisions under the same conditions. Moreover, none of us can make rational decisions all the time. Human actions are significantly influenced not only by thoughts but also by emotions and communication. Add to all this the factor of chance/coincidence (misfortune or opportunity), one can see how human actions are determined in complex processes.

The fact that a person is capable of making a decision, that she is sufficiently enlightened, and that the behaviour that is considered to be "right" is among the options open to her still does not sufficiently justify a person's moral responsibility for that behaviour. Further, it is one thing to define what a person should and should not do, and it is quite another to assign fault entirely to her when she does not do what she is supposed to do or does what she should not do. Here it would be appropriate to refer to the concepts of "inattentiveness" and "deliberateness". We do not perform each of our actions by thinking through their possible consequences and intending these consequences to occur (deliberateness). In other words, an action of ours that leads to a negative result may also occur because we do not pay attention and act inadvertently, without knowing or intending the consequences (inattentiveness). It is questionable how much of our actions are intentional and how much are the result of inattention. Especially when taking into consideration that human beings do not always act rationally, that they act with their emotions, habits, values, etc., and that inconsistent/eclectic behaviour is also a human characteristic, it becomes difficult to attribute deliberateness to individuals with reference to a moral rule and thus to attribute all the fault to the individual.

For the reasons explained above, the idea that "the individual is in control of her own destiny", an idea rooted in the liberal understanding that sanctifies the individual, remains simplistic in explaining the phenomenon of illness. Assuming that a person knows that X, Y, and Z adversely affect health and attributing responsibility without knowing what determines the health of that person leads to a judgemental error. Such an approach can be likened to the "blame culture" that configures malpractice as "the last person who touched the patient is the one to blame" (Civaner, 2011). However, it would not be fair to blame people directly and completely for getting sick by overlooking all determinants, and it would prevent us from building a sufficiently robust argument. Instead of placing the whole responsibility on a single person by pointing a finger, it is necessary to understand the factors that are effective in the formation of the problem. To determine what the factors are and their degree of influence, their place in the causal network should be determined. The extent to which that kind of analysis is possible is highly debatable. At the very least, however, we should bear in mind that when determining personal responsibility for health, one can only be held morally responsible for behaviour that occurs within the realms of free will.

Responsibility towards whom?

It has already been mentioned above that responsibility by definition cannot be towards oneself; it requires another party. To which parties can responsibility be attributed in the context of personal responsibility for health? At the outset, the person's relatives may come to mind. However, asserting that a person has a responsibility to her loved ones and relatives to protect her health and to seek medical assistance when necessary would mean attempting a moralistic intervention from outside into the private life of the person.

In addition, it can be argued that people have responsibilities towards the state. However, it should not be overlooked that the responsibilities of the individual are not towards the state but towards society, which is the reason for the state's existence in the first place. The state is not a moral subject in itself; it is merely an apparatus, created by society for the social benefit of all. Recognising it as a moral subject and defining moral obligation towards it prepares a slippery slope towards totalitarian arguments. To recognise that the *raison d'être* of the state is the common good does not mean, for example, that the social credit system in China could be justified because it aims at a "better society". The policies to be implemented for the common good must be formulated by the active participation of the society in the decision-making and audit processes; otherwise, the common good is determined not by all those who will be affected by those policies, but by the minorities who have somehow gained the authority to determine what is good or beneficial for the majority. Today's world and history have shown many times that this method has been abused for the benefit of the few and has caused great inevitable suffering.

There is no personal responsibility for health towards companies either, as there is none towards oneself, one's relatives, and the state. Since companies by their very nature aim at profitability, not human health, the responsibilities that can be defined to them can only be defined on an economic basis, not on a moral one. In fact, they can only be mentioned as customer obligations such as paying the bills promptly. These expressions relate to what kind of financial responsibilities the patient has in a legal contract established with companies in a buying-selling relationship. It is extremely difficult to defend this type of relationship, which is completely contrary to the nature of healthcare, even at the legal level. In particular, the attempt to define responsibilities such as protecting personal health and appropriate use of healthcare resources to reduce costs/increase profitability of companies should be strongly opposed, as it would be immoral.

In that case, the parties for which the person may have responsibilities include healthcare workers, patients, and society in general. Some of these responsibilities, such as sharing relevant health information with healthcare workers, and adhering to agreed treatment plans, are prerequisites for the success of medical treatment rather than patient responsibilities. However, it seems that promoting self-health, respect for the health and well-being of others, and the appropriate use of healthcare resources in the public sector can be defined as responsibilities towards the mentioned parties:

- "If I know I can't make my appointment, I should contact NHS staff beforehand to let them know I will be late, or to cancel or rearrange the appointment to a time that suits me better. This means that they can offer the appointment to someone else who needs it" (NHS Scotland, 2019).
- "I should only use accident and emergency (A&E) departments in cases of severe injury and in emergencies" (NHS Scotland, 2019).
- "Patients should be aware of costs associated with using a limited resource like health care and try to use medical resources judiciously" (AMA, 2022).

- "Be aware of and refrain from behaviour that unreasonably places the health of others at risk" (AMA, 2022).
- "Patients are responsible for respecting the property and rights of others" (UNC Health Center, 2022).

Responsibilities exemplified above can be counted under personal responsibility for health on the grounds of preventing the waste of resources and thus respecting the right of others to receive care. When healthcare resources are wasted, it will make it difficult for others to access the care they need. In theory, then, it could be argued that there is a responsibility "to avoid wasting healthcare resources needlessly and recklessly" towards other members of society.

Theory and practice

Although we accept this in theory, can it be argued that such responsibilities exist in today's world dominated by a liberal understanding? A brief history may help to give a more complete answer to the question. With the development of welfare states and social rights after World War II, many services started to be provided by the state, free of charge and based on needs. Healthcare services were also provided in this fashion, and priority was given to the provision of primary care, and to protecting and promoting health. However, with the worldwide oil crisis in the late 1970s and the transition of socialist countries to capitalism in the early 1990s, neo-liberal policies began to be implemented in many countries. In this framework, healthcare services provided through national health systems started to be privatised. It was claimed that the centralised management of the state was cumbersome and inefficient, that the quality of service would improve with the application of competition and profitability criteria in medicine, and that healthcare services should be run just like any other business. With the projects developed and financially supported by the World Bank, healthcare services were provided by cost-effectiveness criteria. According to the new system, the state should only pay for certain services to a certain level, and citizens should pay out of pocket for the rest. These policies, which have been implemented in many countries for nearly 30 years have increased inequalities and unnecessary expenditures while decreasing access to needed services, contrary to what was claimed. Nevertheless, the commercialisation of healthcare is continuing with other models such as public-private partnerships. Another effect of this liberal transformation, which covers basic public services such as education, energy, transport and communication as well as healthcare, is the increase in individualisation in societies where the majority of people rapidly lose their rights to basic needs. Pumped with the help of the media and the consumption culture, both this liberal understanding and the ability to consume have become the dominant values, and values such as social solidarity, bearing burdens together for the common good, and altruism are being eroded.

One of the reflections of that transformation in healthcare is the dissolution of the social contract between the patient, who is now positioned as an ordinary consumer in an ordinary market, and the healthcare worker, who has become a contracted worker of an enterprise that prioritises profitability in that market. Once healthcare services become a commodity that is bought and sold under free market conditions, the availability and accessibility of the services will depend on market dynamics and the individual's ability to pay. Patients, as customers, are "free" to purchase the services they wish, as much as they can afford. Just as in a liberal society an individual is "free" to buy the television of her choice, or throw it away and buy a new one, she cannot be accused of wasting the healthcare service she has purchased. On the contrary, as a consumer, she will be praised for contributing to the market economy; therefore, as long as she can pay for it, she will be a valuable member of society. In such circumstances, it becomes extremely difficult to argue that an individual has responsibilities towards other members of society. It may even be argued that such responsibility will continue to exist, but perhaps only in the case of infectious disease epidemics. However, this responsibility can only be based on individual values rather than social ones. In liberal societies where everyone is seen and forced to live as an island, individual freedoms are recognised as the most important value to be protected and the limits of individual freedoms are drawn by the individual freedoms of others. Therefore, it can be argued that the individual has a responsibility to wear a mask or be vaccinated in epidemics only on the grounds of not violating the individual freedoms of others rather than a common value that respects every individual as a member of the community. Also, although the responsibility for the life and health of others is theoretically based on intersecting liberties, it is highly questionable to what extent it can be put into practice, as experienced in the COVID-19 outbreak. In today's liberal world that blesses individualisation (so that the individualisation is in the degree of "atomisation"), blaming individuals for not respecting the freedoms of other individuals is both contradictory in itself and it has been experienced that it will not be a remedy in practice. Therefore, there is no solid basis for defining this kind of responsibility in terms of ethics.

Responsibility and sanctions

The concept of responsibility must always include a moral or legal sanction; therefore, if a responsibility towards one's own health can be defined, this section will discuss whether a sanction can be imposed when that responsibility is not fulfilled. One of the first sanctions that comes to mind is to restrict access to healthcare services for the person who does not fulfil her responsibility. In addition, financial sanctions such as paying higher premiums have also been suggested. For example, according to a study conducted in the USA, 53% of the participants think it is "fair" to ask people with unhealthy lifestyles to pay higher insurance premiums than people with healthy lifestyles (Steinbrook, 2006). China's social credit system has a similar approach to unhealthy behaviours (Liang and Chen, 2022). These kinds of sanctions assume that a person's actions are entirely self-determined and do not consider extrinsic factors. Moreover, restricting to access needed services would be contrary to the fundamental right to health. Fundamental human rights are prerequisites for the enjoyment of other rights and cannot be conditionalised because of their very nature. As a matter of respect for human dignity, fundamental rights must be respected unconditionally, regardless of the characteristics of a particular person (ICN, 2022):

> *Human rights are inherent to all persons, regardless of nationality, sex, national or ethnic origin, colour, religion, language, or any other status. (...) Nurses value health care as a human right, affirming the right to universal access to health care for all.*

Furthermore, such a practice means valuing people's lives using criteria other than medical criteria. Considering people who obey certain moral rules, who watch what they eat, who do not commit crimes, who are considered to be useful to society, etc., as more valuable than others will lead to discrimination. Yet, the rules of professional morality impose a duty on nurses to provide services without prejudice and discrimination: "Provide people focused, culturally appropriate, care that respects human rights and is sensitive to the values, customs and beliefs of people without prejudice or unjust discrimination" (ICN, 2022). Once the logic of this idea of non-medical criteria and conditional human rights is accepted, there will be a slippery slope that could lead to not providing liver transplantation to those with alcohol addiction, not providing antiretroviral therapy to HIV+ patients infected by unprotected sexual intercourse, or even not providing services to those injured in traffic accidents because they do not wear a seat belt; it would be so difficult to reach an understanding of where to draw the line.

The proposal to "restrict access to healthcare services" is unacceptable as it does not take into account the web of causality that determines our actions, it is contrary to fundamental rights, and it would lead to discrimination. However, can it be claimed that "The foundations of duty to care towards those who do not fulfil their responsibilities" remains valid? It is accepted that the obligation to provide service will cease in certain circumstances, for example, when healthcare workers are subjected to violence while providing healthcare and the patient's condition is not urgent. This is because violence directly affects the nurse herself and thus the service to be provided to other patients negatively. However, the patient's failure to fulfil her responsibilities regarding her own health does not affect healthcare workers or others, except in infectious disease epidemics, so the duty to care continues to exist. In epidemics, the reasons that undergird the obligation to provide service, such as being the best knower, respecting the right to health, and the duty of non-discrimination, remain valid. The nature of the nursing profession, which is especially care-oriented, is also another reason. Even in today's mechanised medicine, the member of the healthcare team who is closest/remains close to the human being is the nurse. A caring, understanding, compassionate, tolerant, and supportive approach is exactly what patients need. ICN also emphasises these values: "Values in nursing are those ends sought by both the profession and in nurse-patient relationships. These include, for example, health, dignity, respect, compassion, equity, inclusivity" (ICN, 2022).

At this point, it can be argued that nurses have the right to conscientious objection. ICN defines conscientious objection as follows (ICN, 2022):

> *Refusing to participate in required action, or seeking exemption from participation in classes of interventions (e.g. abortion, gender reassignment surgery, organ transplantation) that threaten a person's sense of moral integrity. It also includes the refusal to participate in an action or intervention perceived to be inappropriate for a specific patient or it ignores the patient's wishes.(...) In such cases, the nurse "must facilitate respectful and timely action to ensure that people receive care appropriate to their individual needs.*

As can be seen, determinants of one's own health, such as lifestyle, are not among the grounds for a healthcare worker's conscientious objection. In addition, continuity of service must be ensured in case of conscientious objection. Health professions are a social structure and should be carried out by respecting professional values and rights related to health, not by personal feelings. Blaming a patient for causing extra work, wasting resources, etc., will mean mixing personal feelings with the profession. In such a case, healthcare workers should be aware of their feelings and question their basis.

Conclusion

Sometimes, patients may be blamed for not doing their best to prevent their illnesses, and it is thought that there should be a price for reckless behaviour. In this chapter, it was aimed to evaluate whether this idea is justifiable in terms of health-related rights and professional morality. First, it was emphasised that to be able to define such a responsibility, conditions such as the person's decision-making competence, the level of comprehension of the relevant information, and the context surrounding her should be adequate to allow her to fulfil her responsibility. Based on this, it was argued that the idea that "the person holds her own destiny in her hands" is erroneous, that health is determined by a wide variety of factors, and therefore it would not be fair to fully blame a person for getting sick.

In the next section, the question of "To whom responsibility is owed" was taken up, and the idea that the individual, in the context of healthcare, has a responsibility towards herself, her relatives, the state, and companies were rejected. In theory, it is possible to argue that there is a responsibility to avoid wasting healthcare resources needlessly and recklessly owed to health professionals, patients, and society. However, the dominance of liberalism in today's world, the erosion of social values, individualisation and commodification of healthcare render this argument invalid. As for the case of infectious disease epidemics, where the life and health of other individuals are also at stake, solid moral grounds for respect and care for others have disappeared in the liberal world. Moreover, even when it is accepted that an individual has a responsibility for her own health, no sanction can be justified given the commitment to protecting rights related to health and professional ethical values.

To avoid misunderstanding, it should be emphasised that this chapter does not claim that individuals are not responsible for their actions. However, as bio-psycho-social beings, human beings are involved in complex networks of causality, so their actions are determined not only by themselves but also by the conditions surrounding them. It is very difficult to determine to what extent a person can be morally held responsible for her actions within these conditions just by looking from the outside; therefore it is not fair to judge a person accordingly. Such an assessment of moral responsibility is only possible under conditions where the requirements of the right to health are fulfilled, appropriate conditions are provided for everyone in terms of the social determinants of health, and people are properly informed. People's sense of responsibility towards each other cannot be realised only through legal compulsions aiming to protect individual freedoms. Realistic solutions can only be discussed and grounded where social values such as solidarity and altruism are nurtured and grown further by sharing the benefits and losses altogether as a society, and where all parties can participate in decision-making and audit processes. In the absence of such conditions, the most appropriate approach would be to err on the safe side, rather than simply judging and blaming individuals or attempting to analyse them one by one. Rights related to health and professional values would always provide better guidance on the way ahead.

References

American Medical Association. (2022) *Patient Responsibilities*. Available at: https://www.ama-assn.org/delivering-care/ethics/patient-responsibilities (Accessed: Aug 9, 2022).

Civaner, M. (2011) '"Healthcare-caused harm", instead of "Malpractice"' *Turkish Archives of Pediatrics*, 46, 6–11.

Daniels, N., Kennedy, B. and Kawachi, I. (2004) 'Health and inequality, or, why justice is good for our health', in S. Anand, F. Peter, and A. Sen (eds) *Public Health, Ethics, and Equity*. New York: Oxford University Press.

Hart, N. (1997) 'The social and economic environment and human health', in R. Detels, W.W. Holland, J. McEwen, and G.S. Omenn (eds) *Oxford Textbook of Public Health*. Oxford: Oxford University Press.

International Council of Nurses. (2022) *The ICN Code of Ethics for Nurses, 2021*. Available at: https://www.icn.ch/system/files/2021-10/ICN_Code-of-Ethics_EN_Web_0.pdf (Accessed: Aug 9, 2022).

Liang, F. and Chen, Y. (2022) 'The making of "good" citizens: China's Social Credit Systems and infrastructures of social quantification' *Policy & Internet*, 14, 114–135.

Marmot, M. (2004) 'Social causes of social inequalities in health', in S. Anand, F. Peter, A. Sen (eds.) *Public Health, Ethics, and Equity*. New York: Oxford University Press.

NHS Scotland. (2019) *The Charter of Patient Rights and Responsibilities*. Available at: https://www.gov.scot/binaries/content/documents/govscot/publications/advice-and-guidance/2019/06/charter-patient-rights-responsibilities-2/documents/charter-patient-rights-responsibilities-revised-june-2019/charter-patient-rights-responsibilities-revised-june-2019/govscot%3Adocument/charter-patient-rights-responsibilities-revised-june-2019.pdf (Accessed: Aug 9, 2022).

Snelling, PC. (2015) 'Who can blame who for what and how in responsibility for health?' *Nursing Philosophy*, 16, 3–18.

Steinbrook, R. (2006) 'Imposing personal responsibility for health' *New England Journal of Medicine*, 355, 753–756.

Talbert, M. (2022) *Moral Responsibility*. Stanford Encyclopedia of Philosophy. Available at: https://plato.stanford.edu/entries/moral-responsibility (Accessed: Aug 9, 2022).

UNC Health Center. (2022) *Patient Rights & Responsibilities*. Available at: https://www.nashunchealthcare.org/patients-visitors/patient-rights-and-responsibilities/ (Accessed: Aug 9, 2022).

WHO. (2022) *Taking Action on the Social Determinants of Health*. Available at: https://www.who.int/westernpacific/activities/taking-action-on-the-social-determinants-of-health (Accessed: Aug 9, 2022).

31 Care and its entanglements

Holly Symonds-Brown, Harkeert Judge,
and Christine Ceci

This chapter begins from Moser's (2006, p. 376) observation that if you want to understand what something is, ask 'what it is made to be and how it emerges.' Or another way to frame this would be to say that this is a chapter about care and its entanglements within infrastructural relations. By infrastructural relations we reference what Star (1999) described as the 'boring' things of care – guidelines, institutional protocols and practices, ways to organize space and time and bodies, and the forms of life that become possible therein. The idea we attend to here is that 'care' doesn't just happen, and is not only, or perhaps even primarily, an effect of knowledge, values or ethical thinking. Rather, as Alam and Houston (2020) argue, 'care' circulates, preformed and prefigured, carrying along with it surplus and often unacknowledged normativities, via often unnoticed infrastructural arrangements.

This is a view of care that differs from many traditional nursing approaches to care where care is framed as a task or an affective concept, something usually delivered from nurse to patient. In contrast, considering entanglements of care is about looking for the relations through which care is produced, how it travels and how it is shaped within relations, and how these arrangements and relations have world-making effects. Part of the significance of this form of analysis lies in Tironi and Rodríguez-Giralt's (2017, p. 92) observation that 'there are always other versions of care. Different institutional entanglements, different bodies, different sufferings will bring to bear different modes of caring, being cared for and encountering care.' This means, perhaps rather obviously but we would argue not taken seriously enough, that care is not the same everywhere; it is specific and precarious with different effects, possibilities and limitations. So rather than simply an exercise in philosophical thinking, we think that this idea about care and its entanglements with infrastructural relations has a practical purpose for nursing, in part because as Pols (2018, pp. 58–59) argues, attending to specificities enables one to learn from different practices, 'to scrutinize and learn from differences rather than ignore them.' Opening up taken-for-granted ideas about care, and its practices, helps to de-naturalize these arrangements to show their classifying and arranging forces, their normativities, and thus turn our gaze to a material politics of care.

So in this chapter, we take care as a practice, specifically a world-making practice through which different versions, arrangements and relations of 'care' make or bring about different worlds. To help make the entanglements of 'care' within infrastructural relations more visible, and in a way that reflects our philosophical practice of theorizing from empirical instances, we tell some stories about how 'care in the community' is accomplished, or not, for people living with dementia at home. And in telling these stories we draw on Callon's (2008) writing about prosthesis and habilitation as examples

DOI: 10.4324/9781003427407-36

of distinct scripts that may be embedded in technologies of care and enacted through infrastructural relations, bringing about different subject positions as well as configurations of care. The stories come from Holly's ethnographic study of the relations between day programs and home for people living with dementia and their families, and show something of how infrastructures 'shape' care and how these shapes matter – notably for Holly's participants are effects that play out in terms of shaping who people are, where they can go and what they can do.

Strategies to provide 'care'

We start by positioning day programs as a health technology, with health technologies understood as extending beyond traditional medical devices to 'include physical objects, procedures, social interventions, and health care systems' (Timmermans & Kaufman 2020, p. 584). Technologies such as these involve strategies intended to produce societal transformations in their ability to establish new social relationships and stabilize certain orderings of everyday life according to their particular rationales (Schillmeier & Domenech 2010). For example, day programs appear in the *Dementia Strategy for Canada* (2019) in a shaded text box titled 'Respite Care':

> Adult day programs can bring respite to caregivers, as they provide an opportunity for the person living with dementia to participate in activities and socialize with others in ways that do not require the usual caregiver to be present.
>
> (Public Health Agency of Canada (PHAC) 2019, p. 40)

Day programs, as a strategy to provide care, are designed based on representations of what 'could be.' Within these strategies, particular ideas of care are made manifest and work to both organize and produce relations between materially distinct elements (Law & Mol 1995). For instance, here we are presented with particular ideas of individuals, community, care, dementia and space. These are not just ideas existing only in policy or in the heads of families or health and social care planners. They are material and held 'in-tension' with each other through organizing activities like strategies (Cooper & Law 1995, p. 245). These 'intentions' materialize as interventions in the form of health technologies, such as day programs.

However, health technologies such as day programs do not simply exist on their own. Rather, they are built into existing practices and networks (Star 1999), and as they merge into assemblages of overlapping and entangling technologies, people, materials and objects, their logics overlap and interfere with each other as they work out terms of connection and flow (Farias & Blok 2016). Work started by Star in the 1990s has led to an ecological understanding of infrastructure as something more than the materials and structures that other things run on (Star & Ruhleder 1996). Her work examined the invisible work, interstices and precarity of infrastructure, and she and others have since re-visioned infrastructure as a set of practices and relations that structure and enact our world. No longer understood as a simple backdrop, Simone (2015, p. 375) argues that infrastructure comes with 'specific trajectories of impact,' producing people and lives as it provides specific possibilities for acting and interacting. This force and effect of infrastructure organizes people's lives in particular ways (Berlant 2016; Simone 2015), determining, for example, 'who can circulate easily and who should stay put' (Rodgers & O'Neill 2012, p. 402).

The politics of infrastructural relations are fluid and shifting but it is these sociotechnical relations, and their specific effects, that make up everyday life and care (Star 1999; Suchman 1999). So if we want to think about everyday life and care in the community, we need to look for the specific material relations that are enacted through health technologies such as day programs and their broader infrastructural effects. As noted above, the idea we attend to here is that 'care' circulates via such infrastructural arrangements, distributing various activites and relations, shaping spaces and subject positions generating material effects.

Classifying forces of care in the community

Our first story involves Jan and Louise. Jan is a 90-year-old man recently diagnosed with dementia. In an effort to plan ahead for the possible changes that dementia might bring, Jan and his wife Louise left their longtime home and moved across town to an apartment. At the same time, after becoming lost one day in the city, Jan had stopped driving. With this move and the change in driving, a change in everyday routines occurred. Louise noted that Jan was often 'just sitting' on their couch all day. This lack of activity and the increasing issues with memory concerned her, and she felt she had 'to pull more people in' to help her and Jan adjust to the changes. Soon after the move, Jan and Louise decided that getting Jan back to his regular exercise routine would be good for him – but this now required some support. Jan, we should mention, is a lifelong gymnast. A series of community care referrals led to a home care case manager being assigned to Jan and Louise. During the first home visit, the case manager organizes her assessment of Jan in light of his diagnosis of dementia, and her strategies prioritize her knowledge that caregivers such as Louise are at risk of becoming 'burdened.' This is something to prevent so she arranges for three hours a week of in-home respite and for Jan to be placed on the waiting list for one day a week at the day program.

Rather than considering either the day program, the case manager or Jan and Louise as static, pre-existing entities that come together and affect each other, we can understand each as continually becoming through their relational materiality. For example, the case manager's assessment practices bring the day program into relation with Jan, whose identity is now configured primarily as a person with dementia. Louise's identity is also, at least temporarily, re-configured – no longer a concerned partner seeking opportunities for Jan, she emerges as a caregiver whose risk of care burden might be mitigated, at least for a time, through association with the day program. A generalized intervention alters specific and local relations and arrangements that are themselves also not static but tentative and fluid, resulting in different effects from these entanglements over time (Gan & Tsing 2018).

The day program itself, as a health technology, sits in relation to the larger care infrastructure understood as 'care in the community.' Much of this infrastructure involves invisible work of classification standards, and structured networks of communication that work to divide expertise and responsibility and to institute the spatialization of care in taken-for-granted ways (Langstrup 2013; Star 1999). As Timmermans and Kaufman (2020) explain, established health technologies often go unnoticed as they become ingrained within 'systems' of care, creating infrastructural paths of 'what comes next.' Formal system practices work to organize people, materials and space into discrete service-based units, each with specific need-based criteria that build on each other, and in so doing, forming new identities for people and a sort of stepwise path to institutional care.

Within these administrative logics, the sequencing of low to high-intensity community care services makes sense, but within the 'forms of life' that it creates, other effects are made possible. For example, through this established path-making, the formal health system translates the desire for a place to exercise generated by Jan and Louise, based on a lifetime of interest and ability, into a need for a certain service: respite care. That is to say, while a place for a gymnast to do gymnastics does not logically translate into forms of respite care, a diagnostic label of dementia makes Jan and Louise's request for a leisure activity easy to translate into a health-related concern, one that can fit within classifications of need to be addressed by the formal system rather than the general community.

For the formal system, dementia is often talked about as a problem of care sustainability, whether that be for families or for health systems. This problematization of dementia makes the day program, a specific technology of respite and structured activity, a good 'match' for Jan and Louise. And as Bowker and Star (1999) argue, classification systems have a 'material force,' generating material effects on those categorized. With this translation of Jan's need for exercise, the spaces of care and arguably life are defined for Jan; paths bounded to the home or other controlled spaces are deemed most appropriate for someone with dementia. With this 'material force,' other places in the community, such as the local recreation center located five kilometers from Jan and Louise's home, or the seniors' activity center in which the day program is located, are made invisible. Thus, through its participation in the classification practices of care infrastructure, the day program works to bring Jan and Louise into relation with other people and places, producing particular material ways of living within their community.

For people living with dementia and their families, day programs emerge to tell a particular story about care. This story organizes particular material differences between home and institution and between caregivers and people living with dementia. Through these relations, respite as a specific form of care emerges, one that might be effective at relieving caregiver strain and sustaining people outside of longer-term institutional care. Fundamental to this form of care is a material form of physical distancing required between an identified care 'giver' and care 'receiver.' The pre-existing day program spaces offer a sort of ready-made template, or what Star (1999) would describe as an 'installed base,' from which the care infrastructure of home and institution could be extended into the community. The goals of rehabilitation already present within these programs work to shape the expectations of what could be done in these spaces. So while new ideas of quality of life for people living with dementia extend beyond the caregiver's psychological status, the material distinctions of space and care are embedded in the design of day program. Ultimately, this design works in relation to specific arrangements to shape the practices and subject positions available for people using them.

(Re)configuring family arrangements

Following our key line of thinking, if we want to understand how day programs work as 'care' in the community, we need also to understand what materializes through the configurations that form in the relations between day programs and specific family care arrangements. López-Gómez (2015) offers arrangements as a useful ecological and symmetrical tool for showing the diversity and precarity of how lives are configured and practiced in relations with health technologies. In his study on telecare services for older adults, López-Gómez found the effects of reconfiguring arrangements are often overlooked when new forms of care are added into already existing routines. These effects included new subjectivities, forms of agency and relations with space. Callon (2008) offers additional ideas on arrangements, suggesting that configurations with technology can act as 'agencements' to make particular kinds of actions and ways of being an 'individual subject' possible. The template of who an individual 'is' can be built into technologies in a way that affects the configuration of the arrangement and distributes agency in particular ways (Callon 2008). And along with the agency that configurations enact are the subjectivities that are made possible. As Moser (2003) emphasizes in her studies of life with disability, the importance of attending to how arrangements enact agency lies in the different subject positions and the versions of life that they make possible.

We can see these effects for Jan, a lifelong gymnast seeking a place to exercise, when he begins attending the program one day a week. The program is located in the basement of a community senior center overlooking a beautiful park and duck pond. At the program, he sits at one of three tables with six other people. Initially Jan tried to circulate, changing his seat each time he attended the program but after a few months he can be found sitting in the same spot each time as staff direct him to his table. Jan, who according to Louise, 'never plays games' now spends most of the day at the table while staff lead the group through a daily activity routine of discussions, games, crafts and chair-based exercise. When visiting Jan at the program, Holly hears the group talking about what is next on the schedule – 'there's a walk coming up so we better get to it,' says one woman. Holly asks Jan if the walk is outside and he says with a frown, 'no, it's just inside.' The staff start walking with a few people from one of the tables and soon almost everyone joins them walking in circles around the small main space of the room for about ten minutes.

Sociotechnical arrangements of health technologies enact configurations that shape how an individual is conceived and how they act for themselves. Callon's (2008) ideas on such configurations can be helpful here. Callon identifies that often social policies are based on approaches to sociotechnical arrangements that are themselves based on ideas of either prosthesis or habilitation. These different modes guide the distribution of agency across the arrangement. Callon explains that within a prosthesis configuration, individual agency is embedded in material devices and procedures designed around the idea of an individual who has a barrier or deficit that needs repair. The arrangements are configured to restore access to all resources by enacting a disciplined version of agency that helps to conform the person to norms of expected activity.

With Jan's program and his family arrangements, agency is enacted within a configuration of prosthesis. Jan is centered as a person with dementia who has deficits that require support from space, materials and people in a way that enables him to participate in a 'normal' way within a community space. Within this disciplined agency, Jan is extended in his abilities but also made to conform to universal ideas of what he should and can do. In line with active ageing discourses, Jan can go out of the home and be 'active' and social with others, but because of his dementia, a defined space, planned activities and close supervision by staff is needed to make this happen. While prosthesis approaches to care can be helpful and necessary, they often ignore the webs of relations and attachments in which people exist, creating asymmetries and mismatches between people served and those designing the services (Callon 2008; Peine & Moors 2015).

For Jan and Louise, the arrangements of their home and life are kept separate from those at the program. While Louise values a specific kind of care for Jan, one that connects with his interests and keeps him interactive with the world, the care she experiences is vaguer, and often, the details remain unknown. Jan's interests from home, his book, puzzles, and plants are invisible at the program. In fact, his athletic ability and independence at home are erased and replaced with a subject position of 'being at risk.' He is defined as the deficit, and this definitional action is so strong that the barriers to his inclusion in the community do not get addressed. López-Gómez (2020) argues that the ongoing care and maintenance of the arrangements of daily life are affected in a variety of ways when new services are added in and that there is a sort of violence inherent in the omission of this from design and evaluation.

Configuring prosthesis and habilitation

Our second story is about Wes and Margaret. Wes started using the day program when he was first diagnosed with dementia, and several years later, Margaret decided to join him there as she no longer needed 'time away' from Wes and wanted more social inter-action for herself. At the program, they usually sit at a table together. Sometimes Wes is called on to play the piano for sing-a-longs, and Margaret enthusiastically attempts every craft presented, while Wes sits back and watches or takes short naps in his chair.

Using Callon's (2008) ideas again, the same day program comes into relation with a different family arrangement, and other types of configurations emerge over time. Like Jan, the program began as a prosthetic type arrangement for Wes, extending his ability to participate in the community away from Margaret's supervision. This arrangement aligned with the other services that worked to extend and repair Wes's cognitive abilities so he could get dressed, bathe, and move around the house. These services were not designed for Wes particularly, but were instead scripted by providers with an idea of what a universal form of an older adult male should do in daily life and what a caregiver like Margaret needs to cope. But over time, a different orientation to Margaret and Wes evolved, and a configuration of both habilitation and prosthesis has come about. Callon explains that habilitation focuses on rearranging the world to allow for the network of relations necessary for an individual to act. In contrast to prosthesis which has the effect of extending the abilities of individuals, this approach assumes an interactive view of an individual. Here, people exist in relation to the world and can be seen to have capacity for productive interactions with it.

Holding things together

The first impression on meeting Wes and Margaret is one of precarity. On Holly's first home visit, she stood on the doorstep for five minutes after ringing the doorbell, hearing a voice and bumping sounds coming closer to the door. She also noticed the red peeling paint of the front door, worn stucco and crumbling concrete of the front step, yet a freshly cut lawn. During the visit, Wes and Margaret seemed physically unstable as they lurched around their house, holding on to furniture and railings as they went. Holly felt like she might need to 'catch' them at any moment, but they appeared non-plussed by their travels around the home, moving with a sort of haphazard yet loosely choreographed tempo. They tell Holly they have walking frames, but that they leave these outside on the driveway as it is too difficult to carry them up the three stairs into the house. This pragmatic idea makes sense as it is difficult to imagine either of them even using stairs, let alone with a walker. There is a disorganized quality to the home visits, with one of them usually being in bed on Holly's arrival, requiring a long waiting time on the doorstep, or a long time sitting alone in the front room hearing sounds from elsewhere in the house.

At the program, Margaret and Wes usually arrive looking a bit disheveled. Margaret's shoes are worn and have pieces of the sole hanging off the side, their walkers are often wet, or the wheels are covered in mud from the front path or from being left outside. To see them only as they enter the program, one would think that they have come in from a storm. Thirty minutes later, it seems a different Wes and Margaret materialize sipping their coffee and playing rummy tile; they appear less threadbare and more present, propped up by the new relations and objects their surroundings provide – the coffee, the card game, the other people.

Opposing prosthesis's take on individuals' needing specific compensatory mechanisms to act in a defined way, habilitation draws in interactive ideas of agency. Within socio-technical relations that are flexible and accommodating, with the right interactive type of supports, people can come to be self-managing 'agents.' While an initial impression of Wes and Margaret is one of precarity, there is a sort of durability enacted within the material supports of the day program, enabling their interaction with each other and the world. Within this configuration, Wes and Margaret are not passive agents but interact with the technologies like walkers, railings, home care, and day programs in ways that work for them, and ways that stabilize their arrangement. These configurations of habilitation and prosthesis are not mutually exclusive (Callon 2008), and there are aspects of both present within the day program's configurations of Wes and Margaret's arrangements. There remains a disciplinary script of activities and use of space at the program, but also an acknowledgment of Wes as a product of a network of social and material relations requiring attention. Wes is acknowledged as having memory problems that need compensation, and he is also seen to exist in relation to his attachments. For example, one day after lunch, it is 'sing-along' time and Wes is the guest organ player – he gets up out of his chair with a rocking motion – 'one, two, three, oof!' – and shuffles with his walker over to the organ. A staff member stands with Wes at the organ and asks him to start with 'Roll out the Barrel.' Wes hums a bar of the song to himself then begins playing by ear. The group sings along smiling.

While sing-a-long time is only held once a week, it is in these moments at the program that Wes is enacted in this web of relations that recognize his attachments and his needs for support as an 'individual' who can take action and play an active role within a social setting. And as Moser (2005) notes, this idea of active agency is both a common feature and a bug of normalizing orderings that guide interventions for people with disabilities. From the policy level to the practice level, there is a promotion of supports that can enact a person living with dementia in these presumed 'normal' active ways. This 'ideal' of active/normal agency materializes in practices that emphasize activity and engagement as central goals in programming for people living with dementia, reflecting the types of subject positions that formal health planners seek to maintain and account for through the day programs. For Moser (2005, p. 668), this 'order of the normal' is, in fact, limiting in that it promotes the norm of a subject who is self-contained and centered, and ignores the actual distributed nature of agency as an achievement of many things working together.

Tinkering and durability

One morning at the program drop off time, Wes is helped off the bus by the driver. As Wes hums a song to himself, the driver grabs his walker and sets it up for him, then guides Wes to the front door of the seniors' center. He then returns to help Margaret. The driver escorts them into the entrance where a staff member is waiting. The bus driver confirms with the staff member that Wes and Margaret actually have a pass to ride the bus, and tells her they did not have it with them today but he brought them along anyway. The staff member says she will investigate, ensure that their pass is up to date and ask Wes and Margaret's son to attach the pass to their walkers. In Wes's chart, communication logs also track concerns about times when staff noted his clothing was inappropriate for the weather, he was missing his walker, had bruises on his face from a suspected fall, or arrived late. When asked about what she would do in these cases, the manager says, 'Oh, I just get in touch with the family to make sure everything is okay, and if it sounds like there are issues of needing more supports, I may call home care to ask for them.'

From a distal perspective, or perspectives that highlight defined effects and outcomes (Cooper 1992; Cooper & Law 1995), a day program is a fixed, finished and bounded space. Yet in attending to Wes's attachments, the 'seams' of the day program become less tightly adhered and partial contact points emerge between his home, Margaret, his son and other formal services. The lost bus pass points to a potential breakdown of the network, which then makes visible some of the infrastructure's organizings. The almost invisible relations between the bus driver and day program staff smooth the way for Wes and Margaret to have simple transitions between spaces of the home and the program. Again, as with Jan, the day program as technology no longer stands alone but sits in relation to the other technologies of transportation and home care. These relations are contingent and temporary (Cooper & Law 1995) and similar to Margaret's shoes, it seems that it could all fall apart, but it does not. In Wes and Margaret's story, there are cracks and less than ideal circumstances evident in the clutter, the dirty walkers, family conflict, and the confined isolated space of their lives. There is not a set path of connection that is solid and predictable, but instead, much of the care that the day program provides is that of tiny adjustments and monitoring of Wes and Margaret, their equipment, their shoes, which requires ongoing relations between the program, family members, bus drivers and home care. All of this facilitates Wes and Margaret's ability to have a 'social outing' three days a week together, a shift from the program's previously defined script of merely being a respite space. This arrangement is about care, and the relations within it make room for tinkering. In small ongoing ways, the day program accounts for Margaret and Wes, they are seen, monitored and their interests are occasionally engaged. Within these arrangements, the day program offers something to both Wes and Margaret – moments of enjoyment, social contact, space away from home together.

Learning from different practices

Returning once again to Moser's (2006, p. 376) observation that if you want to understand what something is, ask 'what it is made to be and how it emerges,' we can see from a proximal analysis (Cooper & Law 1995) of the entanglements of day program 'care' with two different family arrangements, that day programs, like other health technologies, have a range of specific and local configuring effects. The proximal analysis brings relations and materials into view, as well as their adjustments and readjustments. There are many intentions at work within these configurations – 'in-tension' are held, for example, inherited ideas of rehabilitation, normalizing discourses of independence, and a narrowing range of subject positions available to people living with dementia and families. In our stories, the program's configuring effects on agency varied within the specific arrangements, at times working as prosthesis, and at others, habilitation.

The 'care' that emerged in these arrangements was not something that happened only between people, a perspective that would cover over the practical tensions encountered as specific 'forms of life' were made out of social-material relations (Berlant 2016). What often goes unnoticed in care – guidelines, protocols and practices, norms and systems of classification, ways to organize space and time and bodies – had much to do with the constitution of everyday life for Jan and Louise, and Wes and Margaret. Some things were brought together, others were pulled apart, simultaneously generating openings and closures, inclusions and exclusions (Lancione & McFarlane, 2016). Our argument is essentially that it matters which openings and which closures and for whom. For Jan, the classifying forces of infrastructure generate a 'fit' that was not there; for Wes and Margaret, material arrangements configure a space of supported agency. In each case, day programs cannot be thought as 'simple locations' of containment, but rather as a configuring health technology-in-practice and an actor within socio-material arrangements. Working to try to unravel the tensions present among these different versions of 'care' in the community opens opportunities for consideration about what goods are at stake in how such 'care' exists, and which goods we want to strive for.

References

Alam, A & Houston, D. 2020, 'Rethinking care as alternate infrastructure', *Cities*, vol. 100, 102662, doi: 10.1016/j.cities.2020.102662.

Berlant, L. 2016, 'The commons: Infrastructures for troubling times', *Environment and Planning D: Society and Space*, vol. 34, pp. 393–419.

Bowker, G. C., & Star, S. L. 1999, *Sorting Things Out: Classification and its Consequences*, Cambridge, MA: The MIT Press.

Callon, M. 2008, 'Economic markets and the rise of interactive agencements: From prosthetic agencies to habilitated agencies', in T. Pinch, & R. Swedberg (eds.), *Living in a Material World: Economic Sociology Meets Science and Technology Studies*, Cambridge, MA: The MIT Press, pp. 29–56.

Cooper, R. 1992, 'Systems and organizations: Distal and proximal thinking', *Systems Practice*, vol. 5, pp. 373–377, doi: 10.1007/BF01059829

Cooper, R., & Law, J. 1995, 'Organization: Distal and proximal views', *Research in the Sociology of Organizations*, vol. 13, pp. 237–274.

Farias, I., & Blok, A. 2016, 'Introducing urban cosmopolitics: Multiplicity and the search for the common world', in A. Blok & I. Farias (eds.), *Urban Cosmopolitics: Agencements, Assemblies, Atmospheres*, New York: Routledge, pp. 1–22.

Gan, E., & Tsing, A. 2018, 'How things hold: A diagram of coordination in a satoyama forest', *Social Analysis*, vol. 62, no.4, pp. 102–145. doi:10.3167/sa.2018.620406

Lancione, M., & McFarlane, C. 2016, 'Life at the urban margins: Sanitation infra-making and the potential of experimental comparison', *Environment and Planning A: Economy and Space*, vol 48, no. 12, pp. 2402–2421. doi :10.1177/0308518X16659772

Langstrup, H. 2013, 'Chronic care infrastructures and the home', *Sociology of Health & Illness*, vol. 35, no. 7, pp. 1008–1022. doi: 10.1111/1467–9566.12013

Law, J., & Mol, A. 1995, 'Notes on materiality and sociality', *The Sociological Review*, vol. 43, no. 2, pp. 274–294. doi: 10.1111/j.1467–954X.1995.tb00604.x

López-Gómez, D. 2015, 'Little arrangements that matter. Rethinking autonomy-enabling innovations for later life', *Technological Forecasting & Social Change*, vol. 93, pp. 91–101. doi: 10.1016/j.techfore.2014.02.015

López-Gómez, D. 2020, 'What if ANT wouldn't pursue agnosticism but care?', in Blok, A., Farías, I., & Roberts, C. (eds.), *The Routledge Companion to Actor-Network Theory* (1st ed.), New York: Routledge, doi: 10.4324/9781315111667

Moser, I. 2003, *Road Traffic Accidents: The Ordering of Subjects, Bodies and Disabilities,* PhD dissertation, Universitetet i Oslo.

Moser, I. 2005, 'On becoming disabled and articulating alternatives: The multiple modes of ordering disability and their interferences', *Cultural Studies,* vol. 19, no. 6, pp. 667–700. doi: 10.1080/09502380500365648

Moser, I. 2006, 'Disability and the promises of technology: Technology, subjectivity, and embodiment within an order of the normal', *Information Communication and Society,* vol. 9, no. 3, pp. 373–395. doi:10.1080/13691180600751348

Peine, A., & Moors, E. H. 2015, 'Valuing health technology-habilitating and prosthetic strategies in personal health systems', *Technological Forecasting & Social Change,* vol. 93, pp. 68–81. doi: 10.1016/j.techfore.2014.08.019

Pols, J. 2018, 'Care, everyday life, and aesthetic values: About the study of specificities', in J. Brouwer and S. Van Tuinen (eds), *To Mind is to Care,* Rotterdam, NL: V2, pp. 42–61.

Public Health Agency of Canada. 2019, *A Dementia Strategy for Canada: Together We Aspire,* viewed 29 June 2022, https://www.canada.ca/content/dam/phac-aspc/documents/services/publications/diseases-conditions/dementia-strategy-brief/dementia-strategy-brief.pdf

Rodgers, D., & O'Neill, B. 2012, 'Introduction: Infrastructural violence: Introduction to the special issue', *Ethnography,* vol. 13, no. 4, pp. 401–412.

Schillmeier, M., & Domenech, M. 2010, *New Technologies and Emerging Spaces of Care,* Farnharm Surrey: Ashgate.

Simone, A. 2015, 'Afterword: Come on out, you're surrounded: The betweens of infrastructure', *City,* vol. 19, no. 2/3, pp. 375–383. doi: 10.1080/13604813.2015.1018070

Star, S. L. 1999, 'The ethnography of infrastructure', *American Behavioral Scientist,* vol. 43, no. 3, p. 377. doi: 10.1177/00027649921955326

Star, S. L., & Ruhleder, K. 1996, 'Steps toward an ecology of infrastructure: Design and access for large information spaces', *Information Systems Research,* vol. 7, no. 1, pp. 111–161. doi: 10.3917/rac.009.0114

Suchman, L. 1999, 'Critical practices', *Anthropology of Work Review,* vol. 20, no. 1, pp. 12–14. doi:10.1525/awr.1999.20.1.12.

Timmermans, S., & Berg, M. 2003, 'The practice of medical technology', *Sociology of Health & Illness,* vol. 25, no. 3, pp. 97–114.

Timmermans, S., & Kaufman, R. 2020, 'Technologies and health inequities', *Annual Review of Sociology,* vol. 46, no. 1, pp. 583–602. doi: 10.1146/annurev-soc-121919-054802

Tironi, M., & Rodríguez-Giralt, I. 2017, 'Healing, knowing, enduring: Care and politics in damaged worlds', *The Sociological Review,* vol. 65, pp. 89–109. doi: 10.1177/0081176917712874

32 Rethinking holism

Expanding the lens from patient experience to human experience

Jason A. Wolf, Mustafa M. Bodrick, and Freda DeKeyser Ganz

Introduction

Nursing practice involves attending to patients from diverse backgrounds and who ascribe to a wide variety of worldviews. For this reason, nursing professionals need to appreciate the implication of individual experiences on their interaction with patients. Holism is a longstanding philosophy of human experience, having been upheld since the 1700s (Schofield, 2021). The concept entails conceptualizing the individual as part of a larger environmental system that shapes his or her perspective on various subjects. In the context of nursing care, holism emphasizes the integration of social, spiritual, cultural, biological, as well as psychological perspectives in each interaction with patients. While the notion of holism has been acknowledged since the 1700s, its application in nursing calls for a careful rethinking of the philosophy with the aim of expanding it to incorporate the larger human experience as a model of each patient's experience with the healthcare system and environment.

Nursing philosophy context and definitions of holism, human experience, and patient experience

A nursing philosophy serves to guide a nurse when engaging in the care of patients, families, and communities. According to Watson (2018), a nursing philosophy is a concise statement that lists the nurse's ethics, beliefs, and values. It may also include their motivation for being in the nursing profession. A comprehensive nursing philosophy should cover aspects such as how the nurse views patient care, patient advocacy, education, and practice. It may also incorporate ethical elements on providing excellent care to patients. In the clinical setting, a nursing philosophy will guide nurses in their practice and enable them to make ethical choices when administering care, advocate for the rights and needs of their patients, uphold the principles and values of nursing, and commit themselves to a lifetime of learning and growth. There are many nursing philosophies that nurses can either adopt or modify to fit their worldview. This essay focuses on one such philosophical stance: holism; and explores the related appraisals on rethinking holism in relation to patient experience and human experience.

Appraising the definition of holism

Holism is a philosophical approach applied in healthcare that advocates for healing the whole person and considering how the clinical environment and community context influence human experience (American Holistic Nurses Association, 2021). By adopting

DOI: 10.4324/9781003427407-37

this perspective, holistic nursing has the potential to improve the quality of care, achieve improved health outcomes, and remove barriers to care (American Holistic Nurses Association, 2021). This approach to nursing practice is particularly valuable in healthcare environments where care is fragmented, provided in silos, and lacks explicit coordination. Furthermore, holistic nursing facilitates consideration of the seriously defective approaches that negatively affect the patient experience in healthcare systems that struggle to achieve positive outcomes. Holism reflects the nature of human existence since people live and survive in broader social, cultural, and structural contexts that transcend their individual perspectives. Stakeholders should consider these dimensions when applying holism in nursing and healthcare. To overcome their individual biases, nurses need to expand their perspective beyond the reductionistic view of the patient and the environment to focus on the human experience and embrace the call to rethink holism about the patient experience. The rethinking of holism is imperative to capture human experience and include various person's diverse worldviews within healthcare facilities and communities.

The COVID-19 pandemic experience has provided substantial motivation for rethinking holism and pushes the boundaries of new thinking on the experiences and lessons learnt. The healthcare crisis caused by the pandemic has exposed the longstanding weaknesses and problems in many healthcare systems globally (Anderson et al., 2020; Blumenthal et al., 2020). Such weaknesses include low quality of care, rising costs and uncontrolled prices, financial barriers to access, marginalization of public health, and widespread inequities and disparities in care provision (Geyman, 2021). These elements point to the absence of a holistic approach to healthcare. The landscape for health provision across most sectors in the post-pandemic era is undergoing significant change, part of which is the outcome of efforts to strengthen the public healthcare system and make it more resilient (Sagan et al., 2021). Healthcare systems are becoming more responsive to the meaning of the global lived experiences across the spectrum of health, illness, healing, and dying. The modern approach of thinking globally and acting locally is being adopted widely as local health governance systems are embracing global health policy approaches. For example, universal health coverage and global health security now regularly appear on the agenda for higher integration in healthcare systems (Lal et al., 2021). These developments feed into the expansion of the lens of holistic thinking to achieve better inclusion and improve human experience. Enhancing holistic care requires a broader view of society, culture, economy, and the natural environment.

Defining human experience in healthcare

Health and well-being are not merely the absence of disability or illness. In the quest for health maintenance and restoration in healthcare settings, the human experience with the healthcare system is multidimensional comprising mental, physical, social, and spiritual dimensions (Oben, 2020). More precisely, the human experience in healthcare incorporates all interactions, including every encounter between patients, care partners, families, and healthcare providers and the community in which healthcare organizations and systems operate (Wolf et al., 2021). In other words, human experience encompasses the encounters of patients and their families, healthcare staff, and the communities they serve, and it weaves together the patient, workforce, and community experience (Wolf, 2020). Human experience in healthcare is not grounded in linear transactions, but rather reflects the multidimensional and relational nature of healthcare and the ebb and flow connecting both those individuals receiving and those providing care. Consequently, human experience is not simply about patients and their experience, but also encompasses the crucial and influential nature of the experience of individuals working in healthcare and recognizes and engages the communities in which healthcare operates (Wolf et al., 2021).

The notions framing patient experience have significantly influenced the conceptualization of human experience. The current definition of patient experience is the result of continuous evolution, which is at the core of understanding the term (Wolf et al., 2021). In such a way, the sum of all interactions remains crucial in reflecting that experience is related to interwoven touchpoints among and between individuals within the healthcare environment. Therefore, the concept of organizational culture becomes reinforced in healthcare settings, expanding the meanings of human experiences. The interactions where experiences happen extend beyond those between patients and caregivers to include healthcare team members, families, and communities within diverse environmental contexts (Wolf et al., 2021). In other words, conceptualizing patient perceptions means understanding that what patients, families, and care partners think about their experiences is based on their interactions and grounded in their perceptions. Therefore, an experience is influenced not only by the direct interactions, but also the context in which it occurs. In addition, the continuum of care reinforces the notion that experiences have no end and lack definite boundaries, which means that they can extend beyond healthcare settings and permeate the entire care lifecycle of an individual. Oben (2020) considers human experience key to the conceptual understanding of the patient experience. Indeed, human experience in healthcare originates from the patient experience itself, considering that patients are fundamentally human beings in an environment where they are cared for by human beings. Therefore, patient experience is a foundational element of the overall human experience in healthcare overall.

Defining patient experience

The concept of patient experience has undergone revision and expansion over the last decade, from being seen as a segment of healthcare quality to an overarching concept that reflects the integration of numerous aspects of a care encounter – from quality and safety, to cost and environment, to processes and technology and more (Wolf et al., 2021). Breen et al. (2021) define patient experience as a measure of patient-centeredness, but it comprises much more than these authors outline. A patient's experience refers to 'the sum of all interactions shaped by an organization's culture that influences patients' perceptions across the continuum of care' (Oben, 2020; Wolf et al., 2021). The definition consists of vital dimensions that frame a broader view of patient experience, not just as a measure of centeredness, but as an understanding of the impact of personal interactions and the influence of organizational and systemic culture. It is inclusive of not just one episode but reflects the multiple touchpoints one has on a care journey across the continuum of care, all of which ultimately influence patient and family perceptions.

Patient experience is found at the center of the broader human experience in healthcare. Patients desire dignified treatment with dignity being an overarching concept that consists of experience comprising social, psychological, physical, existential, and societal levels (Becqué et al., 2021). Accordingly, patient experience can comprise various aspects, such as the physiological experience of illness, customer service quality when patients interact with a healthcare facility, and individuals' lived experiences of the illness (Oben, 2020).

A positive patient experience is vital since it results in optimal patient outcomes and the restoration of good health (Wolf et al., 2021). It also plays an integral role not just as something that develops out to a broader human experience, but as a concept that is fundamentally driven by the very components of it. The experience of the health workforce has a direct impact on the experience people have on their healthcare journey. The voices of one's community have ripple effects on patient and family perceptions either before even starting a healthcare journey or how they interpret it after the experience.

It should be reinforced here that as practitioners reimagine holism, they should appreciate the role of human experience as an important aspect of the philosophy. Also, the wholeness of a system impacts how people attend work or engage in healthcare and it impacts the experience people have in workplaces. While an individual can be considered as whole by themselves, what the patient experience at the heart of human experience reminds is that an individual's holistic sense in one way may only exist to frame how they find themselves in a larger sense of systemic holism. In its essence, this systemic holism itself is the human experience in healthcare.

A starting point in rethinking holism

As a starting point in rethinking holism, it should be considered that healthcare systems consist of several key elements: individual, group, and landscape contexts of healthcare provision. These elements are dependent on one another because they are parts of one whole, which is the healthcare system. Therefore, one should consider the lived experiences of each individual, be it a patient, nurse, family member, or healthcare institution, as well as the influences of the community contexts in which healthcare organizations exist. At the same time, it is necessary to think at the level of groups within these contexts because participation in a group promotes holism and facilitates individuals sharing culture, goals, and problems. Interactions among different groups of stakeholders further shape organizational culture, which influences the human experience of each person involved and contributes to the notion of holism. Furthermore, the healthcare provision landscape extends beyond a single organization's confines. The organizational cultures of various healthcare institutions eventually shape the nature of an entire national healthcare system. These systemic efforts in unison frame global healthcare dialogues.

The elements mentioned above emphasize the need to examine the limitations of the reductionist approach to patient experience and suggest ways of transitioning to a more holistic approach. Reductionism may correct a part of a system with the naïve expectation that it will contribute to overcoming the implications of a complex phenomenon; however, unlike financial sectors, healthcare systems are more complex and cannot always be divided into small measurable components that constitute the whole – a challenge that arises from their diverse and often unpredictable interactions. Therefore, it is worth comparing reductionism to holism to understand how they differ. According to Keller (2019), reductionists hold that parts are externally (rather than internally) related to the whole. Therefore, each part is independent of the other parts, and the whole is reducible to each of its parts combined. If one knew everything there was to know about each of the parts individually, he or she would understand the whole completely. Holists take the opposite view. They hold that parts are internally related to one another. As a result, the essence of each part is partially profoundly linked to the other parts. As a result, one cannot understand the whole by exploring its parts exclusively and cannot fully explain the parts without understanding the whole.

Understanding how each part operates allows for corrective manipulation as a complete entity that enhances the wholeness of the entire system. In rethinking holism, the starting point involves considering that the whole is irreducible, and that one can correct its dysfunctional aspects by enhancing wholeness (Remde et al., 2018). In nursing, the holistic approach means providing care according to the patient's physical, psychological, spiritual, and social needs, considering their socioeconomic background and environment (Northeastern State University, 2019; Thornton, 2019). There is evidence that initial reductionist approaches integrated with holistic approaches achieve the best health outcomes. For instance, in the case of lower back pain treatment and disease prevention, holistic and reductionist approaches to care present practice dilemmas that influence treatment (Fardet & Rock, 2015; Remde et al., 2018). Consequently, holists advocate that practitioners should prioritize holism as the starting point in nursing care, regardless of the reductionistic approaches that other team members may embrace. By considering the environment and organizational culture, nurses can shift their focus from the reductionist to the holistic perspective to confirm that the patient experience pushes outward to the human experience.

Expanding one's view

Human beings exist in a system that influences their worldview in multiple ways. In a nursing context, the traditional approach to holistic care, which emphasizes the treatment of a whole person, is insufficient to address the challenges of the current environment. Thus, holism is not exclusively about the individual. Instead, it is about a system and views the individual parts as part of a more extensive system. Therefore, practitioners should not view patients simply as individuals needing care in a clinical setting. Instead, health interventions must be considered in the context that the human beings being cared for also function outside the walls of a clinical setting. People actively engage in families, among children, peer groups, communities, and even whole societies (Crawley et al., 2020). These engagements influence their sense of health and well-being and how they engage with the healthcare system. The patient requires adequate knowledge of the environments in which they live and function to understand the healthcare setting (Keller, 2019). For example, holistic care providers should consider the risk of mental health problems caused by prolonged social isolation, which became widespread during the COVID-19 pandemic (Kotwani et al., 2021). Therefore, practitioners should treat individuals physically and psychologically, including spiritual care (Heidari et al., 2020). Practitioners should also handle the shift from hospital-based to home-based care professionally to ensure that people's environment and other contextual variables are positive and health-promoting. Healthcare settings premised at home allow people to participate actively in their health promotion. At the same time, it is necessary to expand the scope of holistic thinking to include organizational cultures within hospitals and other institutions. The individual and collective experiences of healthcare teams shape organizational cultures. Organizational cultures are important because they collectively contribute to a national culture of caring, which strongly impacts the development of the entire nation and each individual that belongs in it. From a philosophical perspective, holism embraces the diversity of individuals, groups, organizations, communities, and nations (Mushi, 2020). Therefore, for healthcare providers to achieve positive results, they should integrate an awareness of all these elements and observe their complex interactions (Begun & Jiang, 2020). Holism requires healthcare providers to expand their lens and focus on human experience, which embodies thinking about patient experiences as an expression of holism. Human beings and their communities, organizations, and families influence each other. Therefore, each human being has many dimensions that stakeholders should consider when rethinking holism as a philosophy for providing holistic care.

Conclusion

Nursing practice entails interactions with patients and colleagues who hold widely varying perspectives on various issues. To effectively deliver care, nurses need to uphold a holistic viewpoint, which acknowledges the input of individual lived experiences in each interaction. While the philosophy of holism is not new, its effective application requires a wider view incorporating both group and individual involvement as part of the system that defines human experience. The appreciation of group dynamics, including families and organizations, is an important aspect of the notion of holism. Notably, it overcomes the limitations of the reductionist approach that presumes that individual components neatly amount to a whole system. Instead, the reimagined concept of holism acknowledges the unique influence of group experiences in creating an individual worldview that does not necessarily flow from distinct experiences.

References

American Holistic Nurses Association (2021). *What we do*. Retrieved from https://www.ahna.org/About- Us/What-is-Holistic-Nursing

Anderson, M., Mckee, M., & Mossialos, E. (2020). Covid-19 exposes weaknesses in European response to outbreaks. *BMJ, 368*. https://doi.org/10.1136/bmj.m1075

Becqué, Y. N., Van der Geugten, W., Van der Heide, A., Korfage, I. J., Pasman, R. W., Onwuteaka-Philipsen, B. D., Zee, M., Witkamp, E., & Goossensen, A. (2021). Dignity reflections based on experiences of end-of-life care during the first wave of the COVID-19 pandemic: A qualitative inquiry among bereaved relatives in the Netherlands (the CO-LIVE study). *Scandinavian Journal of Caring Sciences*. https://doi.org/10.1111/scs.13038

Begun, J. W., & Jiang, H. J. (2020). Health care management during Covid-19: Insights from complexity science. *NEJM Catalyst Innovations in Care Delivery, 1*(5), 1–12.

Blumenthal, D., Fowler, E. J., Abrams, M., & Collins, S. R. (2020). Covid-19—implications for the health care system. *New England Journal of Medicine, 383*(15), 1483–1488. https://doi.org/10.1056/NEJMsb2021088

Breen, W., Choi, S., Herald, K., O'Connor, S. J., Rafalski, E., & Borkowski, N. (2021). The association between an established Chief Experience Officer role and hospital patient experience scores. *Patient Experience Journal, 8*(1), 69–76. https://doi.org/10.35680/2372-0247.1508

Crawley, E., Loades, M., Feder, G., Logan, S., Redwood, S., & Macleod, J. (2020). Wider collateral damage to children in the UK because of the social distancing measures designed to reduce the impact of COVID-19 in adults. *BMJ Paediatrics Open, 4*(1), 1–4. https://doi.org/10.1136/bmjpo-2020-000701

Fardet, A., & Rock, E. (2015). From a reductionist to a holistic approach in preventive nutrition to define new and more ethical paradigms. *Healthcare, 3*(4), 1054–1063. https://doi.org/10.3390/healthcare3041054

Geyman, J. (2021). COVID-19 has revealed America's broken health care system: What can we learn? *International Journal of Health Services, 51*(2), 188–194. https://doi.org/10.1177/0020731420985640

Heidari, M., Yoosefee, S., & Heidari, A. (2020). COVID-19 pandemic and the necessity of spiritual care. *Iranian Journal of Psychiatry, 15*(3), 262–263. https://doi.org/10.18502/ijps.v15i3.3823

Keller, D. R. (2019). Reductionism, holism, and hierarchy theory. In *Ecology and Justice—Citizenship in Biotic Communities* (pp. 89–108). Springer, Cham. https://doi.org/10.1007/978-3-030-11636-1_5

Kotwani, P., Patwardhan, V., Patel, G. M., Williams, C. L., & Modi, E. (2021). A holistic care approach to combat the COVID-19 disease. *Journal of Family Medicine and Primary Care, 10*(2), 844–849. https://doi.org/10.4103/jfmpc.jfmpc_1549_20

Lal, A., Erondu, N. A., Heymann, D., Gitahi, G., & Yates, R. (2021). Fragmented health systems in COVID-19: Rectifying the misalignment between global health security and universal health coverage. *The Lancet, 397*(10268), 61–67. https://doi.org/10.1016/S0140-6736(20)32228-5

Mushi, V. (2020). The holistic way of tackling the COVID-19 pandemic: The one health approach. *Tropical Medicine and Health, 48*(1), 1–2. https://doi.org/10.1186/s41182-020-00257-0

Northeastern State University. (2019). *What is holistic nursing?* Retrieved from https://nursingonline.nsuok.edu/degrees/rn-to-bsn/what-is-holistic-nursing/

Oben, P. (2020). Understanding the patient experience: A conceptual framework. *Journal of Patient Experience, 7*(6), 906–910. https://doi.org/10.1177/2374373520951672

Remde, A., DeTurk, S., & Wojda, T. (2018). Teaching balanced patient care using principles of reductionism and holism: The example of chronic low back pain. In S. P. Stawicki et al. (Eds.), *Contemporary Topics in Graduate Medical Education.* IntechOpen. https://doi.org/10.5772/intechopen.82618

Sagan, A., Webb, E., Azzopardi-Muscat, N., De la Mata, I., McKee, M., & Figueras, J. (2021). *Health Systems Resilience during COVID-19: Lessons for Building Back Better.* World Health Organization. Retrieved from https://apps.who.int/iris/rest/bitstreams/1390564/retrieve

Schofield, J. (2021). *A Phenomenological Revision of EE Harris's Dialectical Holism.* Springer International Publishing.

Thornton, L. (2019). A brief history and overview of holistic nursing. *Integrative Medicine: A Clinician's Journal, 18*(4), 32–33.

Watson, J. (2018). *Unitary Caring Science: Philosophy and Praxis of Nursing.* University Press of Colorado.

Wolf, J. A. (2020). *Human Experience 2030: A Vision for the Future of Healthcare.* The Beryl Institute. Retrieved from https://cdn.ymaws.com/www.theberylinstitute.org/resource/resmgr/hx2030/hx2030_report_2020.pdf

Wolf, J. A., Niederhauser, V., Marshburn, D., & LaVela, S. L. (2021). Reexamining "defining patient experience": The human experience in healthcare. *Patient Experience Journal, 8*(1), 16–29. https://doi.org/10.35680/2372-0247.1594

33 Empathy and dialogue in nursing care

Fredrik Svenaeus

Introduction

Empathy is an everyday phenomenon and a basic moral capacity, and it is also the most central professional skill and ethical guiding tool of nursing care. To be empathic as a nurse means to be able to feel and see things from the point of view of the patient and act in accordance with this knowledge when caring for his good and attempting to relieve his suffering.[1] Nurses need to be dedicated but still humble when it comes to empathy: to endeavour the step into the perspective of the patient does not mean that this is possible in any total or infallible sense; only the patient feels and knows what it is like to experience this particular suffering as this particular person at this particular time. If or when empathy is complemented by a dialogue with the patient, it becomes possible to reach a more complete and confirmed understanding of his predicament (Svenaeus 2022: Chapter 5).

This emphasis on and description of the role of empathy in nursing may sound over-ambitious and idealistic to some, but it need not be, provided nurses get the appropriate time and working conditions to accomplish proper care. Some nurses are more empathically skilled than others from the beginning, but all (or perhaps rather most) nurses can learn empathy and improve their empathic performance by studying and working together with skilled colleagues. They may also profit from reading novels or watching films in which empathic acts are performed or from studying scientific or philosophical pieces on empathy, such as the present one.

It is common to distinguish between affective and cognitive empathy in nursing and health care, the former denoting a certain kind of feeling for the patient and the second consisting in a form of knowledge about his experiences and condition (Alligood 1992). It is also common to distinguish between cognitive empathy and sympathy/compassion (sometimes regarded as identical with affective empathy) (Batson 2009). As I will try to show below, such distinctions are important but they must not lead us to assume that affective empathy, cognitive empathy and sympathy are different things altogether, and we should not overlook how they are standardly fused into each other in the empathy process and the caring concerns and actions it gives rise to. Empathy is an emotional phenomenon and the thoughts and actions it fosters in nursing are developed from sympathetic feelings, experienced by the nurse in the meeting with the patient, that are developed to contain thoughts about his experiences and wishes as needing attention and care.

Accordingly, the dialogue with the patient needs to be informed by and guided by empathy to be successful in finding out what things look like from his point of view and what is most important for him in the current situation. Empathy therefore involves a curiosity about the *person* in addition to finding out more about his medical condition.

DOI: 10.4324/9781003427407-38

The psychotherapist Carl Rogers early on developed such a view on empathy as a central skill in the clinical encounter, making it possible to attain the perspective of the patient, a view which has influenced the field of caring science since a long time (Rogers 1959). But empathy is not only a source of information; it is also an *attitude* of caring sympathy for the patient aiming to help him in a professional manner. This professional attitude includes being kind and providing hope, also when things look bad from the medical point of view (Halpern 2001). Empathy is thus emotional through and through and yet a source of knowledge about the patient as well as a moral guide in the clinical encounter.

Aside from the worry that the image of empathy will provide and unrealistic ideal in health care, another common fear is that more empathy on the side of nurses will lead to burn-out and sick leaves when they invest their feelings in patients (Todaro-Franceschi 2019). This critique of empathy as a tenable ideal in nursing is related to the concern that working-life for nurses may be looked upon as a personal calling instead of as a scientific practice, similar to the profession of doctors, and thus not being respected and renumerated in an analogous way. I think all of these related worries can be dealt with by spelling out what professional empathy in nursing really means, in contrast to being emotional about patients or allowing their concerns to invade one's private life. This is what I aim to do in this chapter by presenting a blueprint for a theory of empathy in nursing: what it is, how it works and how it becomes a professional caring skill.

Empathy and phenomenology

Empathy in nursing follows a pattern that is present in all cases of empathic experiences, but which is brought under emotional control by integrating the professional role in the feeling and understanding of what the patient expresses and tells in the caring encounter. I will return to this professional aspect and to how empathy is related to interpretation in dialogue with the patient in nursing, but first I want to say a bit more about what empathy basically consists of. I will employ a phenomenological understanding of empathy that covers most of the essential aspects of the phenomenon that have been stressed by contemporary empathy theorists, including the affective, cognitive and sympathy aspects brought to attention above (Decety 2012). My chief source of inspiration will be a book written more than 100 years ago by a German and Jewish philosopher, and subsequently nun, martyr and saint of the Catholic Church: Edith Stein (MacIntyre 2007).

Stein died in Auschwitz-Birkenau 1942 at the age of 50 and *The Problem of Empathy* is her doctoral dissertation from 1916 published in a shortened version a year later (2008). After having started her doctoral studies in Göttingen for Edmund Husserl in 1914, Stein took some time off, underwent nursing training and served in the First World War in the region of Moravia during the first six months of 1915. This is rarely mentioned in presenting her thoughts, but I think the nursing experiences Stein underwent in the hospital during the war are very visible in her approach to and interest in empathy. Stein originally wanted to graduate in psychology, but the impressions made by Husserl in his lectures, and by Max Scheler, another famous phenomenologist who also taught in Göttingen, made her change her mind and turn to philosophy instead. In spite of the philosophical angle, her writings on empathy and related themes are very relevant to clinical psychologists and health care professionals, notwithstanding her rather abstract terminology, which I will do my best to unpack and systematize in what follows.

The subject of empathy for a doctoral dissertation was quite timely in 1914 as several scholars in aesthetics, psychology and philosophy had recently put the spotlight on the problem of how knowledge about the experiences of other persons is made possible in everyday life. We never access the experiences of other persons in any direct way but only via our own experiences of their condition so how can we be sure that we are right in assuming that a person is, for example, in pain when we watch and listen to her moans?

The most well-known of the empathy theorists of Stein's time was Theodor Lipps, who had started out in philosophical aesthetics and developed theories about the basic form of intersubjective experiences that were subsequently adopted in the newly established field of empirical psychology, which was developing rapidly when Stein made her contribution to empathy research (Stueber 2006: 7–9). According to Lipps, empathy rests on "inner imitations" we make of the bodily expressions of other persons when encountering them in everyday life. These inner imitations, which are associated with affective states, for instance, by inner mimicking of facial expression of feelings, are then projected onto the other person who we thereby understand to be going through certain types of emotional experiences.

Stein proceeds from the empathy theory of Lipps – and from ideas found in the phenomenological works of Scheler and Husserl – when developing her own proposal, but she also make important adjustments in order to be able to distinguish empathy from emotional contagion only and a being "swallowed up" by the feelings of the other person. Empathy, in contrast to merely being affected by and dragged into the feeling of the other person, is a way of feeling oneself *into* her experiences preserving the difference between my experience and her, as the word "Einfühlung" used by Stein and her contemporaries in the German debate makes more obvious than the English concept might do. The term "empathy" is coined as a translation of the German word and finds its way to the English language approximately at the same time as Stein is writing her dissertation (Coplan and Goldie 2011).

Stein takes empathy to be a three-step process in which the experiences of the other person (1) emerge to me as meaningful in my perception of her; I then (2) fulfil an explication of these experiences by following them through in an imaginative account guided by her, in order to (3) return to a more comprehensive understanding of the experiences of the other person (Stein 2008: 18–19). The steps (stages) that Stein discerns in the empathy process could possibly be reiterated – step three could serve as a new step one and so on – but they could also be supplemented by other ways of engaging with the other, such as talking to her or starting to do something for/to her or together with her.

However, even though Stein restricts the empathy process to the three-step model specified above – steps that do not include conversation and coordinated actions between the parties – a form of tacit communication is arguably present already in the empathy process as such, provided the target recognizes that he is being empathized with and therefore directs his expressive behaviour towards the empathizer in the process. Think of the situation in which a nurse is acknowledging and feeling herself into the experiences of a patient in sorrow and he is turning his face towards her, catching her eye and smiling sadly. This empathic feeling oneself into the experiences of the other person will be at work also in many "empathy plus" forms of human interactions, which, in addition to perception and imagination, also involve the talking, listening and acting together in the world. Which, to continue the example above, would happen when the nurse asks: "What is amiss?", and he answers, "Nothing, really, it is just…". Empathy is the starting point of understanding and sharing the experiences of other persons, which is preserved when having a dialogue with them or can be combined with receiving information in other ways about their thoughts and feelings.

A further look at the three steps of emotional empathy

In discussing and criticizing so-called simulationist accounts of the empathy process dominating contemporary philosophy of mind and cognitive science (De Vignemont and Jacob 2012), phenomenologist Dan Zahavi has pointed out that the perception of the other person as undergoing an emotional experience appears to be unmediated in nature in contrast to assumed inner mimicking of feelings on part of the empathizer (Zahavi 2011). Zahavi, in accordance with theories found in Edmund Husserl, understands empathy to be a basic *perceptual* experience of the other person in the everyday face-to-face encounter that does not include any attempts to simulate her experiences. Recently, he has also, together with Anthony Fernandez, claimed that such a concept of perceptual empathy is the most basic and important one in nursing practice (Fernandez and Zahavi 2020).

Fernandez and Zahavi are right in pointing out that nurses' empathic understanding of the patient does not in every case rely on developing the same type of feeling as he is having, but it is, nevertheless, unclear to me to which extent their phenomenological account acknowledges that empathy is an *emotional* experience. Is it, for example, possible for me to empathically understand that the other person is afraid without having *any* specific feelings about her predicament? Basic perceptual empathy, representing step one in Stein's model, is direct in the sense that the empathizer does not make any *conscious* imitations of the expressed feeling of the other person, but on the preconscious level a number of neurological processes – the most well-known one being the activity of mirror neurons – are indeed going on (Singer and Lamm 2009). Step two in Stein's model of feeling oneself into the expressed emotion of the other person also relies on an automated neurological response making the empathizer feel something similar to what he is perceiving, which is made conscious when the empathizer realizes that what he is feeling is not identical to the feeling of the other person, but precisely an empathic going along with her experiences, which is made explicit in step three of the process.

Stein's account of empathy goes beyond the perceptual level stressed by Zahavi into realms and processes of imagination typically included in simulationist accounts. Stein views empathy as a form of experience – "intentional act" – in its own right that is similar to both perception and imagination, but identical to neither (Stein 2008: 20). The idea of intentional acts (acts of consciousness) in phenomenology should not be mixed up with the idea of a person having an intention in the sense of wishing and aiming to bring something about. Intentionality in phenomenology is a much broader concept, simply indicating that the experience (act) in question has a meaning content, that is: is about something in the world.

Empathy, according to Stein, is similar to perception in presenting something – the experiencing other person – in an unmediated way, but dissimilar to perception and similar to other forms of experiences, such as imagination, in that the meaning content of the experience is not given directly to the empathizer. The terms Stein uses to get hold of this distinction is that something appears to consciousness in an "original" or "non-original" way (Stein 2008: 15). Regarding the content of an act being given in an original, as opposed to a non-original, way, the term Stein (and Husserl) often uses to stress the first form is "leibhaft gegenwärtig", or "leibhaft gegeben", that is: "given in bodily presence" (Stein 2008: 16, 31). Interestingly, in discussing the theme of the lived body ("Leib") in her book, Stein uses a third term to bridge the gap between original and non-original givenness of an experience in empathy, namely "con-originality", which is what is experienced when one living body encounters another (in contrast to encountering a non-living thing) (Stein 2008: 75). This is how Stein presents the empathy process more in detail:

> Now to empathy itself. Here, too [as in memory, expectation, or imagination, *my addition*], we are dealing with an act that is original in the sense of being a present experience but non-original as regards its content. … When it suddenly appears before me it faces me as an object (for instance, the sadness I "read" in the other's face). But when I inquire into its implied tendencies (when I try to bring the other's mood to clear givenness to myself), the experience is no longer an object for me, but has pulled me into it. I am now no longer turned towards the experience, but instead I am turned towards the object of the experience. I am at the subject of the original experience, at the subject's place, and only after having fulfilled a clarification of the experience does it appear to me as an object again.
>
> Consequently, we have in all considered cases when experiences [of other persons, *my addition*] are appearing to us three stages or modalities of accomplishment, even though in each concrete case not all of the three stages are accomplished, but we often are satisfied with stage one or stage two: 1. the emergence of the experience, 2. the fulfilling explication, and 3. the comprehensive objectification of the explicated experience.
>
> (Stein 2008: 18–19)

In the second step of Stein's model, we view the transformation of something merely perception-like into something that is also imagination-like, proceeding through the third step to something that is perception-with-imagination-like. The key to understanding this dynamics of the empathy process is, I believe, to underline the *emotional* aspects of all three steps as they typically lead into and reinforce each other (Svenaeus 2018, Szanto 2015, Vendrell Ferran 2015). Stein writes that steps two and three do not always occur in the empathic process, but I think the most fair and enlightening interpretation of her position is that other thoughts and feelings we are having and/or aspects of the situation we find ourselves in, may voluntarily or involuntarily *stop* us from proceeding from step one to steps two and three (say if we become afraid or bored). If we want to preserve the everyday meaning and use of the word empathy it appears enlightening to name cases of perceiving the expressions of other people "empathy" only when they are in some way attempting to *investigate* the experiences of other persons in their own right. It seems strange to name them cases of empathy if, instead of bringing myself to proceed with the experience of the other (step two), they are immediately followed by a turning away from the person in question, not taking any interest in her experiences as such but instead doing other things.

Rather than taking empathy to be a basic, obligatory ingredient in all everyday encounters in which we perceive and act with others, it is in my view therefore more intuitive to comprehend empathy as an attempt to understand the experiences of other persons in their own right. Such an endeavour to understand the other can, as mentioned above, move beyond perception and imagination when we engage in dialogue and coordinated actions with the other, but it will only remain an empathic endeavour if the goal of communicating and acting is to understand the other person. Such an understanding of empathy is especially enlightening in aiming to understand experiences and activities of trying to help a needful person by way of assisting and healing her, such as is the case in nursing and health care.

Professional empathy in nursing

It is a common move to stress the importance of dialogue for empathy in medical practice and health care (Halpern 2001). It is obvious that a dialogue with the patient could enhance the nurse's understanding of his experiences, but one should take care to not confuse dialogue with empathy in every case. After all, patients do not only or necessarily speak about themselves when approached in health care. Empathy rather paves the way for adequate questions and responses provided by the suffering party in the clinical encounter than consisting in oral communication itself. As Stein writes, there is a difference between approaching what the other says as a statement about things in the world and as an emotional expression found in his *voice* (Stein 2008: 99–100). The patient talks from a position and with an emotional expression that the nurse aims at understanding in the empathy process; if she directs her attention towards the object of the statement without regarding it as specifically *the patient's* words, then she is no longer empathizing: she is no longer feeling herself into the patient's world, but rather judging claims about a common world that may not have anything specifically to do with *his* experiences.

Empathy with the patient in nursing care is a feeling process that opens up the life world of the patient to be explored by way of imagination and dialogue (Gallagher 2012, Ratcliffe 2014). The starting point for empathy is not the "medical body" – that is, the body understood as a set and system of biological functions in potential disorder – but the "lived", expressive body of the patient. Stein actually makes this point in one passage in *On the Problem of Empathy*, discussing how the doctor must empathize with the patient in order to access the living realm of her illness before making the diagnosis (Stein 2008: 87–88). However, she also adds that the doctor in reality often stays with the first level of empathy (compare above) and consequently does not take into account the lived realm of illness in any substantial way. Indeed, her analogy with the gardener and his plants indicates that she takes the doctor to deal mainly with the medical body of the patient in establishing the diagnosis, most often *not* considering his lived body as a starting point for a dialogue exploring life-world issues (Stein 2008: 77, 80). This is obviously a prioritized territory for the nurse, making use of empathy in the multistep fashion we explored with Stein above: not only perceiving his pain but also projecting herself into his experiences and views by way of her feelings and imagination.

While the medical body is the object of the clinical gaze in search for medical diagnosis and possible therapeutic interventions (pharmaceutical drugs, surgery, etc.), the lived body is the anchoring point of the experienced, meaningful world of the patient. The biomedical paradigm needs to be balanced and combined with a hermeneutic, practical perspective, focusing upon the experiences and being-in-the-world of the patient, since health care professionals meets not only with a potentially diseased biological organism, but also with a person who is ill and suffering (Svenaeus 2017). Empathy is the point of entrance to this world of personally experienced illness that must be taken into account if nurses and doctors should be able to help their patients in a sufficient way. For the nurse, as well as for other health care professionals, to not acknowledge or attempt to understand the patient as a person, would not only be potentially unethical, it would also be bad medical practice given the complex relationship that exists between diseases and illness experiences in medical diagnostics and in the everyday life of patients.

The attuned nature of the empathy process, as presented above, explains the manner we are attracted to and develop an interest for the situation of the other person and are guided in this emotional process by her expressive lived body that makes us "go along" in a compassionate manner. We normally come to *care* for the other person in the empathy process and this is the reason why we want to understand her predicament, and also, possibly, want to do something about it (if the other is suffering, for instance). Even if empathy may not develop into *sympathy* (compassion) for the other person in every case, some type of *attuned interest* (concern) is always guiding the empathy process. That empathy is an emotional process therefore means that an emotionally based judgement is instantiated in the face-to-face meeting with the other person. Emotions are ways of feeling and judging states of the world to be good or bad in certain ways and empathy is an important, maybe the most important, example of this (Colombetti 2014).

As I have elaborated upon above, the most basic form of concern for the other person consists in a being *touched* by his feelings (bodily and facial expressions) in a perceptual process. This basic form of empathy takes its starting point in contagion (mirror neuron processes and other related neural circuits), but as soon as the empathizer realizes that the source of her feelings is the target and not herself, the possibilities of empathy open up (Singer and Lamm 2009). If the empathizer shies away and relieves her feelings of distress by looking after herself rather than the other person, the empathic possibilities are not realized. If, however, the concern becomes other-directed, empathy is initiated and can be developed in various ways: through continued attention on the actions and expressions of the other person and through attempts to interact with him and/or imaginatively step into his perspective.

When empathic feelings are lived through imaginatively by the empathizer, the experiences being investigated are filled with cognitive content making them meaningful. Say, for instance, that a nurse is empathizing with a patient who looks sad. In following through the sadness expressed in his face she remembers a visit he had the same morning by a relative. Could the sadness be about something that he was told, or which happened in the encounter with the daughter? Affective empathy in this process turns into cognitive empathy not because the nurse is changing her approach to the patient, but because the feelings initiating and guiding the empathy process become filled with content (Svenaeus 2018). Feelings are still the subject of what is referred to as cognitive empathy, but they are now explored as having specific contents – they are about things in the world (Goldie 2011).

The success of such continued empathic engagements depends upon the extent to which the empathizer is able to tune in to the experiences and contextual horizon of the other person by caring about his predicament in various ways. If feelings are the starting point for empathy, in health care as well as in other forms of practices, dialogue and narrative may be thought about as the main paths in bringing it forward and making it more cognitive in respect of our understanding of the other person (Gallagher 2012). The best way to understand the world of the other is no doubt a dialogic engagement with his life experiences. The imaginations of what it would be like to be in his shoes that we are able to form without engaging in dialogue are no doubt fairly restricted and certainly fallible. In the example above, the natural way to proceed for the nurse is therefore probably to ask something about the visit made by the daughter.

Consequently, empathy is not only a feeling of the other person, it is also a way of *responding* to his feelings and in this concern attempting to understand his predicament because we care for him. The interpersonal understanding we are able to develop on the basis of empathy is best thought about as a form of *hermeneutics*, as Martin Heidegger acknowledged, even though he and other phenomenological philosophers, such as Hans-Georg Gadamer, hesitated to make use of the term empathy (*Einfühlung*) because of its association with a Cartesian model of the mind (Stueber 2006: 204 ff.). We do not feel ourselves into the life of the other person by way of finding a door to his enclosed house of mind; we feel with him in sharing a world and trying to find out how *he*, particularly, fits into the picture. This is how empathy works, in health care and in other essential human encounters (Ratcliffe 2014).

In view of the proliferating tendency in philosophy and cognitive science to understand empathy and sympathy as different phenomena altogether (Prinz 2011), Stein's philosophy provides important clues in explicating how empathy is linked to concern for the other person and to ethics. Empathy is the founding ground of (caring) ethics for Stein, since it provides the starting point for getting to know the world of other persons in which the structures of human values are found that frame and determine the good life (MacIntyre 2007). The concern developed through empathy in nursing is a focus on the patient precisely as a person the nurse has the duty to understand, care for an aid in respect of her education and position. The patient is therefore not a friend in private but he is nevertheless a person whose feelings, experiences, and situation the nurse feels herself into in an empathic process by way of concern (Slote 2007). Such professional concern can lead to feelings of pain and helplessness on the part of the health care professional, and in such cases it becomes detrimental to good care. But it need not do so if nurses are offered adequate training and knowledge about the empathy process, time to meet their patients and respond to their needs in a dialogue, and opportunity to reflect upon their feelings with other professionals (Jack and Levett-Jones 2022, Taylor et al. 2020).

Conclusion

Interpersonal understanding of the patient's feelings, thoughts and predicament in health care is developed by way of empathy and in dialogue with the suffering party. Empathy and dialogue are key philosophical subjects for nurses since they name two interconnected aspects of all meetings with patients that are indispensable to good care. In this chapter, I have presented a phenomenological theory of empathy, inspired by Edith Stein, by way of examples from nursing practice which brings out the emotional aspects of the phenomenon in concordance with its cognitive features. Professional empathy has been distinguished from private-life sympathy, nevertheless insisting on the emotionally concerned aspect of coming to understand the patient's experiences and situation. The phenomenology of empathy has been linked to hermeneutics by way of pointing towards the interpretative structure of clinical dialogue, which strengthens and develops empathic understanding and makes it possible to provide good care attuned to the patient's personal needs.

Note

1 I will use the female pronoun for the nurse and the male pronoun for the patient to avoid the cumbersome "(s)he" and "her/his". Needless to say, there are quite a number of male nurses and female patients in contemporary health care.

References

Alligood, M. R. 1992. Empathy: the importance of recognising two types. *Journal of Psychosocial Nursing and Mental Health Services* 30 (3): 14–17.

Batson, C. D. 2009. These things called empathy: Eight related but distinct phenomena. In J. Colombetti, G. 2014. *The Feeling Body: Affective Science Meets the Enactive Mind*. Cambridge, MA: MIT Press.

Coplan, A. and Goldie, P. 2011. Introduction. In A. Coplan and P. Goldie (Eds.), *Empathy: Philosophical and Psychological Perspectives* (pp. ix–xlvii). Oxford: Oxford University Press.

Decety, J. (Ed.) 2012. *Empathy: From Bench to Bedside*. Cambridge, MA: MIT Press.

De Vignemont, F. and Jacob, P. 2012. What is it like to feel another's pain? *Philosophy of Science* 79 (2): 295–316.

Fernandez, A. V. and Zahavi, D. 2020. Basic empathy: Developing the concept of empathy from the ground up. *International Journal of Nursing Studies* 110: 103695.

Gallagher, S. 2012. Empathy, simulation and narrative. *Science in Context* 25 (3): 355–381.

Goldie, P. 2011. Anti-empathy. In A. Coplan and P. Goldie (Eds.), *Empathy: Philosophical and Psychological Perspectives* (pp. 302–317). Oxford: Oxford University Press.

Halpern, J. 2001. *From Detached Concern to Empathy: Humanizing Medical Practice*. New York: Oxford University Press.

Jack, K. and Levett-Jones, T. 2022. A model of empathic reflection built on the philosophy of Edith Stein. *Nurse Education in Practice* 63: 103389.

MacIntyre, A. 2007. *Edith Stein: A Philosophical Prologue*. Lanham, MD: Rowman & Littlefield.

Prinz, J. J. 2011. Is empathy necessary for morality? In A. Coplan and P. Goldie (Eds.), *Empathy: Philosophical and Psychological Perspectives* (pp. 211–229). Oxford: Oxford University Press.

Ratcliffe, M. 2014. The phenomenology of depression and the nature of empathy. *Medicine, Health Care and Philosophy* 17 (2): 269–280.

Rogers, C. 1959. *A Theory of Therapy, Personality, and Interpersonal Relationships, As Developed in the Client-Centered Framework*. New York: McGraw-Hill.

Singer, T. and Lamm, C. 2009. The social neuroscience of empathy. *Annals of the New York Society of Sciences* 1156: 81–96.

Slote, M. 2007. *The Ethics of Care and Empathy*. London: Routledge.

Stein, E. 2008. *Zum Problem der Einfühlung*. Freiburg im Breisgau: Verlag Herder.

Stueber, K. R. 2006. *Rediscovering Empathy: Agency, Folk Psychology, and the Human Sciences*. Cambridge, MA: The MIT Press.

Svenaeus, F. 2017. *Phenomenological Bioethics: Medical Technologies, Human Suffering, and the Meaning of Being Alive*. London: Routledge.

Svenaeus, F. 2018. Edith Stein's phenomenology of sensual and emotional empathy. *Phenomenology and the Cognitive Sciences* 17 (4): 741–760.

Svenaeus, F. 2022. *The Hermeneutics of Medicine and the Phenomenology of Health: Steps Towards a Philosophy of Medical Practice, Sec. Rev. Ed*. Dordrecht: Springer.

Szanto, T. 2015. Collective emotions, normativity and empathy: A Steinian account. *Human Studies* 38: 503–527.

Taylor, R. et al. 2020. Teaching empathy and resilience to undergraduate nursing students: A call to action in the context of Covid-19. *Nurse Education Today* 94: 104524.

Todaro-Franceschi, V. 2019. *Compassion Fatigue and Burnout in Nursing: Enhancing Professional Quality of Life*. New York: Springer.

Vendrell Ferran, I. 2015. Empathy, emotional sharing and feelings in Stein's early work. *Human Studies* 38: 481–502.

Zahavi, D. 2011. Empathy and direct social perception: A phenomenological proposal. *Review of Philosophy and Psychology* 2: 541–558.

Part 6

Questions for nursing

34 Navigating the edges of critical justice theory through the logic of nursing

Barbara Pesut

Introduction

Recent encounters have made me question my identity as a nurse, or more precisely my identity as a *good* nurse. In the first encounter, I was teaching a first-year research class and we were discussing evidence. A student enthusiastically put up their hand and informed the class that their people had discovered the cure for cancer. But they went on to explain to the class that it would never become mainstream because there was too much money involved in curing cancer. What could I possibly say to that claim in front of the class while guarding their dignity? As we were in a class focusing on evidence, I gently queried what evidence there was to support this treatment. They went on to explain that requiring evidence was a colonial construction (not in those exact words) that was not appropriate to their worldview.

In the second encounter, I was teaching a relational practice course. As we approached a sensitive topic, a student put up her hand and asked to be excused from class. She stated that she was feeling unsafe because of her own history. I excused her, but as this situation was one that she likely to encounter in clinical, I later met with her and probed around her strategy should this topic arise in the context of her patient care. She simply stated that this was a topic that she was incapable of dealing with and further suggested that I was being unjust by expecting her to do so.

The third encounter happened with a colleague. Over the course of a meeting, I could see him become increasingly withdrawn. He finally stated that he was very morally distressed and indicated that the language I was using was triggering him. I apologized and asked if he could help me better understand what language I should avoid. Exasperated, he stated that it was not his job to teach me what I should already know.

These encounters left me with a variety of emotions, the most significant one being moral culpability. Generally, I see myself as one who cares about people, is modestly open to new ideas, and would never intentionally cause someone to feel unsafe. Clearly, I had missed something along the way that was affecting my interactions with others in an important way. Further, these encounters left me with difficult questions. In the case of the student who had the cure for cancer, how do I reconcile the scientific and evidence-based aspects of nursing with the need to accommodate diverse worldviews? How would I feel about them providing advice to oncology patients? In the case of the student who felt unsafe, should I help students to feel safe in the classroom by avoiding certain topics when I know they will be required to confront these issues in practice? In the case of the colleague, how do I use non-triggering language when my work comes with a set of language conventions that structures the nursing and academic community?

DOI: 10.4324/9781003427407-40

I now understand that my encounters were the result of an influential theoretical movement that is shaping Canadian nursing and academia more profoundly than anything I have experienced in my 40-year career. This theoretical movement is one in which we have become increasingly conscious of the moral obligation to seek equity and inclusion for those persons who have not been represented – or poorly represented – in nursing (Morrison et al., 2021; Sanchez, 2021). In this chapter, I am going to describe this theoretical movement, which I am going to name critical justice theory (CJT).[1] I will then provide an overview of the development of this theoretical movement in nursing. Next, I will discuss four moral *edge states* of this theoretical movement that have been discussed widely in the social science literature. Drawing upon Thorne's (2016) work in Interpretive Description, I will then outline how the logic of nursing provides an anchoring point by which we might avoid falling off the edge of this important theoretical movement.

Awakenings: the rise of critical justice theory

North American institutions have been influenced by the social movement of CJT, a melding of postmodernism and social justice (Pluckrose & Lindsay, 2020). This movement has been so pervasive and influential that Pluckrose and Lindsay have given it the moniker THEORY. CJT is based on the following assumptions: (1) knowledge is socially constructed and so may take on a different nature depending upon its cultural context; (2) such knowledges are epistemologically equivalent; (3) knowledge is created by powerful factions of society and is used to oppress those less powerful; and (4) persons are defined primarily by their group identity, an identity that is constituted of oppressors and the oppressed (Pincourt & Lindsay, 2021). The moral ethos of CJT is one of freedom from oppression and harm (Pincourt & Lindsay, 2021). Examples of this moral ethos include Indigenous reconciliation and the Black Lives Matter Movement.

The underlying assumptions and moral ethos of CJT are closely related to the idea of equity, diversity, and inclusion (EDI). EDI acknowledges that many groups have been excluded, oppressed, and harmed by society. The assumptions of CJT are important in opening the intellectual landscape for their inclusion. EDI mandates are now embedded within many North American social institutions, including universities. Canadian universities have committed to EDI in teaching, policy development, research, and hiring practices. Hence, as a university-embedded profession, CJT has profoundly affected theoretical developments within nursing.

A turn towards CJT in nursing

Social justice and health equity have been important aspects of nursing theoretical thinking long before it arose as a popular social movement (Fowler, 2017; Rudner, 2021). Nursing has a long history of being concerned for vulnerable populations, and nurses were pioneers in creating systems and programmes to overcome health inequities. Traditionally, the focus of social justice and equity research was on gaining a fulsome understanding of the issues faced by those living with vulnerability and finding ways to facilitate heath equity. However, more recently such scholarship has focused on critiquing the profession itself for its contribution to inequities through its racialized and colonial history. For example, a declaration against anti-Black racism developed by the Canadian Nurses' Association (CNA) states: "Historically Canadian nursing schools, administrators, associations, and regulatory bodies have also contributed to establishing white, European-centric models of nursing and health, thereby explicitly or implicitly maintaining anti-Black racism" (Canadian Nurses Association, 2021a). A similar declaration of anti-Indigenous racism available on the same CNA website fails to name nursing's complicity, instead focusing on nursing's role as part of the solution: "To that end, as nurses, we unconditionally condemn all acts of racism and discrimination against Indigenous peoples and call for social justice to address racism and health inequity to Indigenous communities" (Canadian Nurses Association, 2021b).

A recent journal issue dedicated to racism in nursing provides further examples of nursing's self-critique. D'Antonio (2022) grapples with the colonial and racist history of Florence Nightingale and the consequent structural implications. De Sousa and Varcoe (2022) argue for the use of Black feminist thought to decentre the whiteness and femininity that has characterized nursing. Similarly, Allan (2022) reflects on whiteness, its inherent relationship to racism, and the obligation we all have to "make whiteness visible and thus, our complicity in racism" (p. 3). Thorne, in her editorial, suggests that only a small fraction of the problem is individual racist attitudes but rather our inability or reluctance to grasp our complicity in systemic racism (2022). She encourages nurses to peel back the layers of our own complicity and to measure ourselves by "how much regard you are prepared to pay to the compromised lives of those who have experienced them" (p. 1).

In summary, the turn towards CJT in nursing has been a move from advocating on behalf of those experiencing inequities towards acknowledgement of our own complicities as white people and nurses. For example, this year when filling out my fitness to practise questionnaire for the renewal of my practising registration, I had to report how often I search out and seek to ameliorate Indigenous racism. This particular theoretical turn in nursing is an intensely moral one with high stakes. Louie-Poon et al. (2022) argue that Canadian nursing has not demonstrated a moral commitment to anti-racism despite its ethical guidelines to promote social justice (p. 3). With a similar sense of urgency, Thorne quotes Moorley et al., "The world stands at a juncture of justice and Nursing must not be caught on the wrong side of history" (cited in Thorne 2022).

But as with any powerful social movements there are always risks. Halifax (2018), a medical anthropologist, social activist, and Buddhist teacher, describes the journey of altruism as one in which we stand on an edge with precipitous cliffs on both sides. Every altruistic aspiration has an extreme with the potential for harm. Numerous recent books have been published on the potential harms of a CJT approach and so I will now turn to summarizing the major arguments from this literature. It is important to note that none of these critiques take issue with the moral goodness of CJT. Rather, they focus on particular risks, or edge states as I will refer to them, that come with this theoretical approach.

Falling off the edge: unintended consequences of CJT

Recent work on CJT places the edge states of this theoretical movement within four primary categories: a fractured common life, an emphasis on emotional thinking, moralizing, and the co-opting of vulnerability. The first edge state is that of a fractured common life (Mering, 2021; Pluckrose & Lindsay, 2020). The logic embedded within CJT that persons are characterized primarily by difference makes it difficult to find ommonality across groups, and nowhere is this more apparent than in the use of language as the foundation of epistemology. This fractured common life is illustrated by an interesting story told by Mering (2021) of the evolution of the commencement service at Wellesley College, a prestigious women's college in the United States. Each year, they sing America the Beautiful as part of the commencement ceremony, which in the original included the term brotherhood. What began as brotherhood, became sisterhood, and then siblinghood; until now, it is a cacophony of self-identified relationships at this point in the singing.

What this story is meant to illustrate is that the fracturing of our common life often starts with language. We are continually reconstructing language to honour the diversity within which we find ourselves in our common life. University campuses now regularly offer workshops on how to speak the new language, and more specifically, what language to avoid (UBC, 2021). The Canadian Broadcasting Corporation recently published a list of terms to avoid including the following examples: *blackmail, blacklist, black sheep, ghetto, inner city, spooky, grandfathered in, spirit animal, tribe, first world problem, blindsided* (Hwang, 2021).

Although the respectful intent of this approach is admirable, it does come at a cost in terms of our communal life. It can be difficult to stay current with rapidly changing language convention. Civil conversation is then at risk. Individuals who care about respecting their colleagues may become silent out of fear that the intent of the language they use will be misread. Such was the case with interactions with my colleague that I described in the introduction. I was not sure how to reframe my research language so that it was non-triggering and so entered into all further conversations with some degree of trepidation. Further, CJT has a language of its own. Here are just a sample of these terms from a recent article on exposing racism in nursing: *white supremacy; epistemological ignorance, epistemological etiquette; democratic, structural, covert, and overt racism; structural violence; settler colonialism; and heteronormativity* (Louie-Poon et al., 2022). Use of this language requires both translation and interpretation. As language is so constitutive of our realities, the use of language that is inaccessible and/or elitist can be problematic to common life.

The second edge of CJT is the substitution of emotional thinking for reasoning and fact (Nadler & Shapiro, 2021; Saad, 2020). This risk arises out of a misunderstanding of what constitutes epistemological equivalency. Epistemology arises from a particular worldview. For example, an Indigenous worldview may result in a different epistemology than a Western scientific worldview. Epistemological equivalency does not suggest that we can simply mix and match these epistemologies but rather that they have an internal logic and validity in keeping with the underlying ontology. In contrast, the mix and match approach to epistemological equivalency makes it difficult to lay claim to any particular truth or way of reasoning. This is not a new concern; this point has been made for decades within nursing (Browne, 2000). However, the difficulty of establishing truth and fact has reached a new level of intensity. Nadler and Shapiro (2021) refer to this as an epistemic crisis as we enter a time when people believe ideas that do not require any substantiation, and worse, they push policy in relation to these ideas. These authors describe this as a strange epistemic stubbornness that rapidly becomes a slippery slope. Once individuals become willing to accept beliefs without sufficient evidence, this, in turn, weakens their powers of discernment and they become credulous.

To illustrate how easy it is to create a pandemic of misinformation, *The New York Times* recently profiled a story in which a young man created a popular movement based upon the absurd premise that birds were not real but rather had been replaced by spy drones in the 1950s and 1960s (Lorenz, 2022). Such conspiracy movements have become a regular part of our daily lives as we have moved through the last years of the COVID-19 pandemic. Saad (2020) refers to these as infectious ideas and argues for a rigorous return to freedom of speech and rigorous scientific methods.

Further, reasoned debate is at risk of being replaced by emotional reasoning. Lukianoff and Haidt (2018) provide a compelling reflection on the emotional reasoning that is now pre-eminent in Western Higher Education. They outline several untruths that are being taught widely to students in academic contexts including the following: students are inherently fragile, emotions should always be trusted, and "life is a battle between good people and evil people" (p. 4). They argue that the emphasis on emotional safety in the classroom is particularly nefarious for it leads to an obsession with real and imagined threats that, ironically, make it more likely that students will be fragile and hurt. Here is where the student I described in the introduction needed to leave the classroom when a topic of patient care arose that felt unsafe. These habits of emotional reasoning mimic the cognitive distortions that have long been recognized to contribute to anxiety and depression (Lukianoff & Haidt, 2018). In summary, the underlying assumptions of CJT create potential edge states where emotional reasoning and the acceptance of unsubstantiated ideas become the norm, with the unintended mental health consequences in those who adopt such ideas.

The third edge state is moralizing. I am using the term moralizing to describe moral reflections that are made in an excessively indignant or righteous way. The challenge of achieving EDI for all peoples is an honourable one and worthy of our best efforts. But taken unproblematically, the delineation of multiple identities and the subsequent stereotyping of those identities into oppressor and oppressed is fertile ground for a particular type of righteous indignation (Longstaff, 2022). Longstaff suggests that this righteous indignation develops in a typical cycle: we start from a genuine ethical wrong, we amplify that sense of wrong, we rally the sentiments of those who desire to do good, then fashion an index of commitment whereby those who want to do good are judged by their level of performance on the index. The more extreme, the more committed. This dynamic is exemplified in *cancel culture* in which individuals are thrust out of social or professional circles if their speech or behaviour, either current or past, does not conform to the current performance checklist of acceptable social behaviour. However, Dean (2022) suggests that virtue is actually destroyed in the realm of these extremes. This edge state of moralizing is even more likely in a social media climate in which outrage generates engagement which generates profit (Dean, 2022).

Sacks (2020) provides further insight into why an identity-focused morality in a social media climate is the perfect storm for indignant moralizing. He suggests that morality is not learned through abstract theorizing but rather through our day-to-day relationships. In these relational encounters, morality is about unself-help. It is about strengthening our relationships with others through openness, listening, conversations, and reciprocity. In contrast, a morality based on abstract theorizing about identity tends to un-situate the self, a self which then has an obligation to focus on what makes us different rather than on what unites us. These differences are then played out in a social media climate in which we are taught to ignore the humanity of those we are interacting with. This, in effect, teaches us to unlearn morality. Sack's (2020) point is an important one because it introduces the cost of morality. Moralizing, a form of arm chair theorizing, costs us little and so it is easy to go to excess. In contrast, it is costly to "un-self" in the day-to-day context of relationships.

Finally, there is the edge state of co-opting vulnerability. This edge is particularly risky when there is a powerful moral righteous indignation, as described above, alongside a means to power for those who adopt such indignation. Fleming (2019), in a podcast on the Philosopher's Zone, discusses how radical positions, and in particular radical *theoretical* positions, are highly saleable in our current cultural climate. An important emphasis in this theoretical radicalism is finding and championing victims. We claim status at the centre by co-opting the margins. The problem is that we must create more and more victims to establish and maintain this power. However, he suggests that this can deteriorate into a *quasi-imperialism* when such a fight becomes a means to power and status. This potential is heightened when EDI initiatives are developed within institutional meritocracies. When important goods such as research dollars, awards, promotions, and hiring practices are linked to championing those considered at risk for inequities and exclusion, there is a means to power. The performance-based meritocracy is simply replaced by an EDI meritocracy, rather than dismantled in a meaningful way that promotes authentic inclusiveness. EDI institutional initiatives are important; however, how they are implemented can make the difference between righting longstanding injustices and creating one more mechanism for a will to power.

In summary, the virtuous aspirations of CJT have edge states with important risks. The underlying assumptions and moral ethos of CJT carry particular risks related to a fractured common life, emphasis on emotional reasoning, moralizing, and the recreation of colonialism in new forms. However, falling off the edge of CJT is not inevitable. Rather, it tends to happen when legitimate ethical issues are treated in what David Brooks (2018) has referred to as *maximalist* terms. Here is where we tend to catastrophize and simplify complex issues, leaving no room for the types of subtleties, nuances, and mitigating factors that are necessary to actually resolving injustice. These edge states present particular risks when our main mechanism of advancing the agenda is through theorizing. One important way to test our theorizing is to attempt to work it out in the real world. How might these ideas hold up in practice, and in nursing practice in particular?

The logic of nursing

Understanding the logic of a discipline is necessary to understanding its primary mandate in the world. For example, the logic of science is to describe, explain, and predict (Dahnke & Dreher, 2016). Likewise, nursing has an internal logic that enables it to fulfil its primary mandate in the world, and without that logic there is no sense-making in practice. Thorne (2016), in her book Interpretive Description (ID), addresses this nursing logic in the context of nursing enquiry, citing the limitations of using social science methods for a practice discipline. When Thorne et al. (1997) initially envisioned ID, nursing qualitative research was drawing primarily upon methods developed within disciplines such as anthropology and sociology. The problem with these social science underpinnings was that there was no requirement for real-world applications. The results of such studies therefore took the form of theory that could not be readily applied at the bedside. For example, Fagerhaugh and Strauss's (1977) classic ethnography on the problem pain patient produced theory that was deeply illuminating about the social contexts on medical units but it gave little practical direction to those charged with solving those problems. With ID, Thorne developed a design logic for enquiry consistent with the epistemology of nursing, an epistemology that requires a dialectic of subjective and objective knowledge in the context of practice. Thorne (2016) suggests this design logic should meet three criteria: (1) a real-world question, (2) an understanding of what we do and do not know on the basis of all empirical evidence, and (3) an appreciation for the conceptual and contextual realm within which a target audience is positioned to receive the answer we generate. An adaptation of these questions provides an excellent foundation for considering the applicability and limitations of CJT within the logic of nursing.

But before I discuss these questions it is important to note that I am beginning from the assumption that the internal logic of nursing must be grounded in practice. While nursing research, leadership, and teaching are legitimate spheres of practice, they exist primarily to serve the nurse at the point of care. If there was no point of care practice, the other spheres of practice would cease to be relevant.

Does it have a real-world application?

To determine what might be the real-world application of CJT for point of care nurses I spent some time carefully reading the recent journal issue cited previously that focused on racism in nursing. After reading each article, I asked the question, if I was a point of care nurse what could I take away from this article to apply in my practice? I discovered that apart from heartfelt and compelling arguments against racism, there were few pragmatic applications that went beyond self-reflection. This was in part due to an underlying assumption within these articles that individual acts of racism in nursing are not the issue (Thorne, 2022). Rather, most authors are arguing for nurses' responsibility for dismantling social and structural contributors to racism, (Essex, Markowski, & Miller, 2022) while engaging in dialogue and introspection about their own contributions to maintaining those structures (Allan, 2022; De Sousa & Varcoe, 2022; Essex et al., 2022). There are examples of how nurses might go about dismantling these structures. For example, Darbyshire (2022) argues for a systematic and careful approach that entails gathering evidence, holding off on change until the needed changes are clear, and then working with individuals by providing them with specific acts they can do to promote positive change. Likewise, Essex et al. (2022) suggest nurses become involved in disruptive action at a local level, although they caution that only those who are in leadership positions can implement significant change. But at the end of the reading, I was still unclear about what my real-world action would be as a point of care nurse.

Such unclarity is inherently risky because it leaves nurses in an uncomfortable position of knowing they have a moral obligation to do something important without knowing how to fulfil that obligation. This is not a minor point. I hear stories from practice that illustrate the challenges that nurses experience trying to fulfil the moral obligations of CJT at the point of care. A nurse failed to properly triage a patient whose primary problem was gynaecological because the patient self-identified as male. A nurse was disciplined for racism after following suggestions from a cultural safety workshop, actions that the patient experienced as demeaning and stereotypical. A nurse resigned after being unable to reconcile her need for physical safety with idealized approaches to care that failed to recognize the violent behaviours of those under the influence of substances. It is not enough to encourage point of care nurses towards reflection. They need to know how to engage in the realities of practice while honouring the moral ethos of CJT.

An important contributor to this theory practice gap is the political nature of CJT. One important role of politics is about bringing diverse interests together to decide who gets what, when and how (Boswell, 2020). In the context of CJT in nursing, it is about using the political process to ensure health equity for diverse populations. However, there is another aspect of politics that is less about the distribution of resources and more about identity, culture, and the ways in which we narrate and frame problems (Boswell, 2020). This aspect of politics is ideological in that it presents "idealized, universalized, and detached expressions of actual social relations" (Martin, 2015 p. 18). It is this more ideological political approach that is particularly problematic for CJT and the logic of nursing. When we write and teach about CJT, we tend towards idealized visions, and as academics and leaders we can do so in a detached manner. We are not obligated to work out our ideas at the point of care. We need our practice-based colleagues to test and refine our ideas in real-world applications. For it is at the fulcrum of practice that we test our theoretical integrity.

Is it congruent with the epistemology of the discipline?

Nurses have long grappled with the implications of epistemological diversity in nursing. Ever since the seminal work of Barbara Carper (1978) on the ways of knowing in nursing, there has been acceptance that nursing draws upon knowledge beyond science. As Risjord (2010) has pointed out, there has been little guidance on how to prioritize these ways of knowing in practice. However, this debate was still largely about knowledge within a Western viewpoint. The rise of postmodern epistemologies, derived from diverse worldviews, provoked great debate among nursing scholars in the 1980s and early 1990s. Some nursing thinkers were in favour of diverse epistemologies; others opposed, while still others argued for a pragmatic approach depending upon the nature of knowledge. For example, Thorne and Sawatzky (2014) argued for the need to reconcile generalizable knowledge (e.g., science) with particular knowledge (e.g., patient experience) in a way that would support epistemological integrity within a practice discipline.

In the context of CJT, the acceptance of diverse epistemologies tends to go unchallenged and even becomes a moral issue. Pluckrose and Lindsay (2020) suggest that, whereas early postmodern epistemology was playful, diverse, and meant to deconstruct rather than reconstruct, that all changed about 2010. A reified postmodernism arose that began to assert the absolute truth of postmodern ideas. In other words, a radical acceptance of diverse epistemologies arose, an inevitable product of a commitment to reacting against the colonial influence of Western liberalism. Within CJT theory, this epistemological diversity is now anchored within the worldviews of diverse populations for whom we desire to create equitable space. There is therefore now a moral weight to accepting diverse epistemologies that was not there in the classic debates about ways of knowing or postmodern ideas.

An important example of this advancement has been the evolution of Indigenous knowledge within the academy. While the reconciliation of Western and Indigenous ways of knowing used to be embraced in the idea of "two-eyed seeing" (Bartlett, Marshall, & Marshall, 2012), more recent developments constitute a uniquely Indigenous methodology that has its own measures of goodness, veracity, and meaning based upon an Indigenous cosmology (Kovach, 2021). The adoption of this has required radical revisioning of what constitutes scholarly work in the academy. For example, we need to reconsider who is qualified to serve on graduate student committees, how scholarship should be evaluated, and what constitutes knowledge translation in the context of Indigenous ownership of knowledge. Such radical revisioning is described in a recent paper reflecting on decolonial futures (Stein et al., 2020). The authors use a compelling graphic to illustrate visions of reform in relation to the "house that modernity built". They describe how true reform of modern ideas requires changes in cosmology, ontology, and epistemology.

Such reform is currently being experienced at the heart of university educational decision-making. However, such a radical revision of epistemology at point of care nursing care raises many questions. Can we conceivably undergo such a transformation of our ontology and epistemology in the practice environment? Is it possible to reform and de-emphasize our understanding and use of the scientific method? And if we did, what might be the underlying epistemological structure of the discipline that would replace it or would there be multiple structures depending upon our patients? Such questions naturally lead to a reflection on how worldviews operate and whether one can indeed mix and match cosmologies and epistemologies to reflect our diverse cultures within a practice discipline?

Such questions were put to the test during the COVID-19 pandemic. This situation provided an important real-world context within which to answer these questions. In the face of competing claims, how willing were we to accept diverse epistemologies about the nature and origin of the virus, the safety and efficacy of vaccines, and the necessary public health approaches? Within British Columbia, the location from which I am writing, there was no tolerance for anything that appeared to be an anti-science stance within healthcare. Nurses who refused to be vaccinated in keeping with the best scientific evidence were no longer allowed to work within publicly funded healthcare settings. Those who actively advocated the dangers of vaccination were at risk of losing licence to practice. Despite these strong policies, nurses continued to ensure that those patients who were not vaccinated received optimal care without prejudice. These real-world scenarios tell us important things about what we will and will not tolerate in relation to epistemological pluralism. Without denying that there are other ways of looking at the world, and the veracity of the knowledge that arises from that cosmology, I suspect that the logic of Western nursing at a practice level is, and will continue to be, deeply embedded within a scientific worldview.

Conclusion

Social theory provides angles of vision in nursing that we might not otherwise see. CJT, in particular, is important because its focus on social justice and inclusiveness has historically formed the moral underpinnings of the nursing profession. But, like any worthy moral endeavour, there are risks. In the context of CJT, these risks have largely to do with idealized, universalized, and detached theorizing that fails to account for the logic of nursing as enacted through nursing's point of care practice. When such idealized approaches are given serious moral weight, there must be a concurrent practical means through which nurses can act. CJT must transcend detached expressions of social relations and provide practical strategies for nurses as moral agents. With such practical strategies, I could have better negotiated the situations I described at the beginning of this chapter. We need to have honest conversations about the benefits and challenges of CJT. It's a moral cliff with steep edges worthy of climbing.

Note

1 The terminology of CJT will be used as an umbrella term to describe a number of different theoretical approaches. I will rely upon the underlying assumptions and moral ethos to delineate which approaches might fit under this description.

References

Allan, H. T. (2022). Reflections on whiteness: Racialised identities in nursing. *Nursing Inquiry*, 29(1), e12467. https://doi.org/10.1111/nin.12467.

Bartlett, C., Marshall, M., & Marshall, A. (2012). Two-eyed seeing and other lessons learned within a co-learning journey of bringing together Indigenous and mainstream knowledges and ways of knowing. *Journal of Environmental Studies and Sciences*, 2(4), 331–340. https://doi.org/10.1007/s13412-012-0086-8.

Boswell, C. (2020). What is politics? Available from https://www.thebritishacademy.ac.uk/blog/what-is-politics/ [Accessed 30th March 2022].

Brooks, D. (2018). The problem with wokeness. *The New York Times*. Available from https://www.nytimes.com/2018/06/07/opinion/wokeness-racism-progressivism-social-justice.html [Accessed 30th March 2022].

Browne, A. J. (2000). The potential contributions of critical social theory to nursing science. *Canadian Journal of Nursing Research*, 32(2), 35–55.

Canadian Nurses Association. (2021a). Nursing declaration against anti-black racism in nursing and heatlh care. Available from https://hl-prod-ca-oc-download.s3-ca-central-1.amazonaws.com/CNA/2f975e7e-4a40-45ca-863c-5ebf0a138d5e/UploadedImages/documents/Nursing_Declaration_Anti-Black_Racism_November_8_2021_FINAL_ENG_Copy.pdf. [Accessed 30th March 2022].

Canadian Nurses Association. (2021b). Nursing declaration against anti-Indigenous racism in nursing and health care. Available from https://hl-prod-ca-oc-download.s3-ca-central-1.amazonaws.com/CNA/2f975e7e-4a40-45ca-863c-5ebf0a138d5e/UploadedImages/documents/Nursing_Declaration_Anti-Indigenous_Racism_November_8_2021_ENG_Copy.pdf. [Acessed 30th March 2022].

Carper, B. A. (1978). Fundamental patterns of knowing in nursing. *Advances in Nursing Science* 1(1), 13–24.

Dahnke, M.D., & Dreher, H.M. (2016). *Philosophy of science for nursing practice* (2nd ed.). New York: Springer.

D'Antonio, P. (2022). What do we do about Florence Nightingale? *Nursing Inquiry*, 29(1). https://doi.org/10.1111/nin.12450. 1–3.

Darbyshire, P. (2022). How to appear fully committed to doing nothing at all about structural and systemic racism: A modest proposal for health and higher education services. *Nursing Inquiry*, 29(1), 1–3. https://doi.org/10.1111/nin.12405.

De Sousa, I., & Varcoe, C. (2022). Centering Black feminist thought in nursing praxis. *Nursing Inquiry*, 29(1), 1–10. https://doi.org/10.1111/nin.12473.

Dean, T. (2022). Social media is a moral trap. Available from https://ethics.org.au/social-media-is-a-moral-trap. [Acessed 30th March 2022].

Essex, R., Markowski, M., & Miller, D. (2022). Structural injustice and dismantling racism in health and healthcare. *Nursing Inquiry*, 29(1), e12441. https://doi.org/10.1111/nin.12441.

Fagerhaugh, S. Y., & Strauss, A. L. (1977). *The politics of pain management: Staff-patient interaction*. Boston, MA: Addison Wesley Longman Publishing Company.

Fleming, C. (2019). *Politics at the extremes* Available from https://www.abc.net.au/radionational/programs/philosopherszone/politics-at-the-extremes/11466710. [Acessed 30th March 2022].

Fowler, M. D. (2017). Why the history of nursing ethics matters. *Nursing Ethics*, 24(3), 292–304. https://doi.org/10.1177/0969733016684581.

Halifax, J. (2018). *Standing at the edge: Finding freedom where fear and courage meet.* New York: Macmillan.

Hwang, P. K. S. (2021). Words and phrases you might want to think twice about using. *Canadian Broadcasting Corporation.* Available from https://www.cbc.ca/news/canada/ottawa/words-and-phrases-commonly-used-offensive-english-language-1.6252274. [Accessed 30th March 2022].

Kovach, M. (2021). *Indigenous methodologies: Characteristics, conversations, and contexts* (2nd ed.). Toronto: University of Toronto Press.

Longstaff, S. (2022). The tyranny of righteous indignation. Available from https://www.abc.net.au/religion/simon-longstaff-tyranny-of-righteous-indignation/13730108?sfmc_id=90118124&utm_id=1808993&utm_source=sfmc%E2%80%8B%E2%80%8B&utm_medium=email%E2%80%8B%E2%80%8B&utm_campaign=abc_specialist_religion_sfmc_20220131%E2%80%8B%E2%80%8B&utm_term=%E2%80%8B. [Accessed 30th March 2022].

Lorenz, T. (2022). *A movement to fight misinformation with misinformation.* New York Times Available from https://www.nytimes.com/2022/02/09/podcasts/the-daily-why-would-anybody-claim-that-birds-arent-real.html. [Accessed 30th March 2022].

Louie-Poon, S., Hilario, C., Scott, S. D., & Olson, J. (2022). Toward a moral commitment: Exposing the covert mechanisms of racism in the nursing discipline. *Nursing Inquiry, 29*(1), e12449. https://doi.org/10.1111/nin.12449.

Lukianoff, G., & Haidt, J. (2018). *The coddling of the American mind: How good intentions and bad ideas are setting up a generation for failure.* New York: Penguin Books.

Martin, J. L. (2015). What is ideology? *Sociologia problemas et Praticas, 77,* 9–31. https://doi:10.7458/SPP2015776220.

Mering, N. (2021). *Awake, not woke: A Christian response to the cult of progressive ideology.* Gastonia, NC: Tan Books.

Morrison, V., Hauch, R. R., Perez, E., Bates, M., Sepe, P., & Dans, M. (2021). Diversity, equity, and inclusion in nursing: The pathway to excellence framework alignment. *Nursing Administration Quarterly, 45*(4), 311–323. https://doi.org/10.1097/naq.0000000000000494.

Nadler, S., & Shapiro, L. (2021). *When bad thinking happens to good people: How Philosophy can save us from ourselves.* Princeton, NJ: Princeton University Press.

Pincourt, C., & Lindsay, J. (2021). *Counter wokecraft: A field manual for combatting the woke in the university and beyond.* Orlando, FL: New Discourses, LLC.

Pluckrose, H., & Lindsay, J. (2020). *Critical (Cynical) theories: How activist scholarship made everything about race, gender, and identity and why this harms everybody.* Durham, NC: Pitchstone Publishing.

Risjord, M. (2010). *Nursing knowledge: Science, practice and philosophy.* Oxford: Wiley-Blackwell.

Rudner, N. (2021). Nursing is a health equity and social justice movement. *Public Health Nursing, 38*(4), 687–691. https://doi.org/10.1111/phn.12905.

Saad, G. (2020). *The parasitic mind: How infectious ideas are killing common sense.* Washington, DC: Regnery Publishing.

Sacks, J. (2020). *Morality: Restoring the common good in divided times.* New York: Hachette Book Group.

Sanchez, M. (2021). Equity, diversity, and inclusion: Intersection with quality improvement. *Nursing Management, 52*(5), 14–21. https://doi.org/10.1097/01.Numa.0000743408.29021.85.

STEIN, S., ANDREOTTI, V., SUŠA, R., AMSLER, S., HUNT, D., AHENAKEW, C., JIMMY, E., CAJKOVA, T.., Valley, W.., Cardoso, C., Siwek, D.., Pitaguary, B.., D'Emilia, D., Pataxó, U., Calhoun, B.., & Okano, H.. (2020). Gesturing towards decolonial futures: Reflections on our learnings thus far. *Nordic Journal of Comparative and International Education, 4*(1), 43–65.

Thorne, S. (2016). *Interpretive description: Qualitative research for applied practice* (Second ed.). New York: Routledge.

Thorne, S. (2022). Moving beyond performative allyship. *Nursing Inquiry, 29*(1), e12483. https://doi.org/10.1111/nin.12483.

Thorne, S., Reimer Kirkham, S., & Mcdonald-Emes, J. (1997). Interpetive description: A noncategorical qualitative alternative for developing nursing knowledge. *Research in Nursing & Health, 20,* 169–177.

Thorne, S., & Sawatzky, R. (2014). Particularizing the general: Sustaining theoretical integrity in the context of an evidence-based practice agenda. *Advances in Nursing Science, 37*(1), 5–18.

UBC Office of Faculty Development and Educational Support. (2021). Inclusive language guide. Available from https://med-fom-fac-dev-sandbox.sites.olt.ubc.ca/files/2021/05/2021-05-19_Inclusive-Language-Guide.pdf. [Access 30th March 2022].

35 Anxiety and moral courage
The path to authentic nursing?

Dawn Freshwater

Introduction

It is well understood that nurses experience stress and burnout that can not only have a detrimental impact on their own mental and physical health, but may also lead to poorer quality of care, decreased professionalism, increased turnover and absenteeism, and a lack of overall job satisfaction associated with loss of meaning and purpose.

Anxiety, along with resilience, is commonly referred to as an influential and contributing factor in both the personal experience of stress, anxiety and burnout, and the effective management of the self through individual and social coping mechanisms. In health-related fields, some of the earliest and definitive theses on this subject stem from the work of Menzies-Lyth (1970, 1988). Menzies-Lyth did much to surface the role and function of institutionalized anxiety across and within nursing and the caring professions. In the five decades since Menzies-Lyth (1970) first published her research, there has been significant advances in the understanding of the dynamic interactions between the individual intrapersonal world of the nurse; the interpersonal relations across nursing teams, with patients and families, and with other disciplines; and the workplace environment as a social system, within broader societal systems. Advancing these ideas further, Abdollah et al. (2021) explore the relationship between anxiety, resilience and moral courage, which they, and others, contend are highly correlated with creating an appropriate moral climate in the workplace.

In this chapter, I examine the historical and social context of anxiety as it relates to nursing work, unpicking the framing of anxiety both in, and as, the social practices of nursing. In doing so, I will draw on the works of Soren Kierkegaard, who situated anxiety as structural to human existence, directly relating anxiety to the ability to 'do' and to 'be' in the world, and to find meaning through both in work. Importantly, Kierkegaard correlates this active negative with the freedom and determination to live an authentic life.

It is argued that whilst anxiety may be transmuted into specific individual coping mechanisms, it simultaneously needs to be understood as producing useful social practices within the nursing disciplines (Jackson and Everts, 2010). Anxiety thus, potentially, provides the energy and force to stimulate the qualitative leap into morally infused nursing built on good faith and authenticity.

Moral courage is proposed as one device through which nurses may better manage and understand their own anxieties, including death anxiety, and enhance resilience in themselves and their charges. It is also proposed as way of understanding and managing how anxieties are institutionally and sociologically framed. Moreover, anxiety and moral courage are framed as one route to creating more purposeful and authentic nursing practices, that are values-led and both personally and socially meaningful.

DOI: 10.4324/9781003427407-41

Background

Stress, anxiety and emotional labour in nursing

It is well known that nurses, the largest of any occupational cohort in the Health and Medical field, suffer stress and burnout related to their work, and that this can lead to detrimental mental and physical health outcomes for some professionals (Kim and Chang, 2022; WHO, 2020; Freshwater and Cahill, 2010; Yarbrough et al., 2017). In general, levels of physical and psychological ill health have been identified as being higher in healthcare workers, which at the very least, given the size of the healthcare workforce globally, is a significant drain on healthcare systems with an associated economic burden.

Increasing levels of vulnerability of nurses to stress and anxiety have been attributed to many factors, including organizational contexts, workload, constant change, inadequate resourcing and skill levels, and the long-term emotional consequences of exposure to acute and chronic suffering and dying. It is to this latter point that I would like to sharpen our understanding.

The short- and long-term impacts of exposure to suffering and dying are well documented in the nursing literature, often referred to as the burden of emotional labour; that is the effort required for 'emotional management' of the self to be achieved. This is most often framed as a way of meeting the expectations and the demands experienced within the work environment, a way perhaps of presenting a convincing professional facade (see, for example, Walsh (2007); Hochschild (1983); Nolan and Walsh (2012); Walsh et al. (2012); Walsh (2009); and Mann and Cowburn (2005) who specifically focus on mental health nursing; Freshwater and Cahill (2020) who hypothesized that in essence it is the action of emotion suppression or emotion management which has the tendency to create emotional discomfort and stress; and Kim and Chang (2022) who emphasize connections with resilience). More recently, emotional labour has been explicitly linked with the concept of moral courage, death anxiety, and empowerment (Khoshmehr et al., 2020; Mohammadi et al., 2022).

Whilst there are differing perspectives on the nature, causes and impacts, idiopathic or not, of emotional labour, the concept remains highly relevant to healthcare staff. It frequently appears in the nursing literature and in more mainstream organizational psychology writings and is often associated with anxiety, both individual and institutional. For example, Hirschorn (1988) and Menzies-Lyth (1970, 1988), using organizational theories, explicated the complex psychological interplay between anxiety and control, subjective boundaries and the execution of power in shaping the nature of work and individual identity in social systems.

Hirschorn (1988: 36) argued that the interdependency of anxiety, boundaries and aggression 'highlight the paradoxical roots of the normal psychological injuries of working'. Menzies-Lyth's (1988) early work in caring environments, illustrated via exemplars 'psychological injuries of working', in hospital settings. Menzies-Lyth's earlier works also observed that defensiveness and anxiety led to rigid individual boundaries and reduced quality of care.

Despite it being rooted in the 1970s and 1980s, Menzies-Lyth's analysis continues to be helpful in illuminating the tensions invoked by nursing work, whatever the setting, but especially those that are characterized by the necessity to attend to high levels of risk. Such settings can vary from intensive care settings, to prison healthcare and mental health settings and of course to dealing with the fallout of global health emergencies such as pandemics.

Menzies-Lyth's research exposed some of the social systems, and active negatives, that nurses constructed in order not to think about the psychological difficulties associated with their work; a way of avoiding anxiety created through being a part of the system per se, the social system being a part of the solution. Deconstructing the authentic self, emotionally and physically, in order to construct the professional nurse self, was experienced as not only personally beneficial, but institutionally and educationally encouraged.

Menzies-Lyth's essays reported the dysfunctional outcomes for staff and patients when employing institutional defences that served to routinize and depersonalize human contact. In this sense, it was a decisive work, first postulating that nurses coped with the frequent exposure to suffering and dying within a social system through supported objectification of both their patients and themselves. Later works further comprehended that experiencing both caring and 'good' and hating 'bad' feelings for the same patient, something that is difficult to tolerate for most nurses, required constant calibration for even the most conscious and emotionally mature nurse (Freshwater and Bryant, 1998). Splitting off polarized feelings helped nurses tolerate these ambivalent and conflicting feelings, (splitting is a concept well-rehearsed in psychoanalytic fields; see, for example, Klein, 1975).

The closer and more concentrated the helping relationship, the more anxiety the nurse was likely to experience. Put simply, levels of anxiety and distress were made more manageable by the nurse relating to themselves and to their patients as objects, previously elaborated by Martin Buber (1937) as the I–it (object) relationship. Keeping one's distance and ensuring professional boundaries were maintained were the order of the day. This approach was also found to be inherent in the management, administration and organization of nursing, which advocated splitting up the nurse's contact with the patient through task allocation. In this mode of functioning, each nurse was placed in a position of responsibility and power, and yet simultaneously experienced a lack of self-determination and varying degrees of disempowerment and disengagement.

Psychological impacts of the splitting process (or ritualized repression) lead to significant levels of cognitive dissonance, or in relation to emotional labour 'emotional dissonance' (Ashforth and Tomuiuk, 2000). This cognitive and emotional dissonance, in turn, generates anxiety and discomfort, and thus paradoxically perpetuates the experience of individual and institutionally produced anxiety that the nurse is attempting to defend against through splitting off.

Contemporary nursing literature shifts our thinking in foregrounding death anxiety, most notably through the incidence of COVID-19, with its high morbidity and mortality. The pandemic has caused nurses and other caregivers to experience unprecedented levels of fear and death anxiety. Mohammadi et al. (2022), for example, correlate caregivers' fear and anxiety of death strongly with their resilience and ability to provide quality care to COVID-19 patients. Resilience, they purport, is important; it is a positive adaption to adverse situations along with the ability to adapt to life-threatening situations successfully and courageously.

Anxiety, and particularly death anxiety, can have a deleterious impact on the moral courage of nurses, the corollary being that overcoming fear and anxiety assists nurses to provide safe and principled care for their patients. And, therein, to lead a more fulfilling professional life.

Before advancing the arguments around the value and integration of anxiety to authentic nursing work, and to deriving personal meaning through morally courageous work, this next section applies a philosophical lens to the concept of anxiety, seeking to deepen our awareness of anxiety itself.

Anxiety: a route through to living and ethical and moral life?

Anxiety is an important and fundamental human emotion, commonly experienced by us all on a personal level, viewed as one of the foundational development emotions along with sadness, anger, happiness, disgust. It is a perfectly normal and human emotional reaction to many of the events within our lives, carrying us through both positive and negative experiences. For some, anxiety becomes a psychological disorder, referred to as neurosis in Medical and Psychiatric circles, first described by Freud, in the 1890s as anxiety neurosis.

Freud's early work on anxiety proved definitive and has been a cornerstone for much of the past and present theories and practices of understanding and treating anxiety and anxiety related disorders. Standardized measures of the nature and severity of anxiety abound, with the intent of directing and specifying aetiology and treatment of the same. Interestingly for Freud, anxiety was a natural part of everyday life, rather than a particular affliction. Of course, much has been done to both pathologize and socialize anxiety in the decades since Freud's earlier work, alongside which our understanding of anxiety as psychosocial phenomena has advanced considerably. Although, sadly, it is most often negatively linked to fear and agitation, seen simply as an emotional response to a perceived threat. Serving little, if any other, purpose. Jackson and Evert (2010) write about this as the normative baggage of the concept of anxiety.

Similarly in nursing professions and through some of the earlier studies quoted in this chapter, it is relatively easy to take the rather superficial line of least resistance, viewing anxiety and nurses anxiousness, including death anxiety and system failure, through a psychological and pathological lens, denoting some lack of personal resilience, an inability to set and sustain sufficient emotional boundaries, and to focus purely on personal responsibilities: rather than viewing anxiety as a deeper call to authenticity. In this sense, preferring the normative baggage over other, perhaps, more authentic and essential, interpretations.

Freud's (1953–1975) works have been subjected to extensive interrogation and questions of credibility; nevertheless, the foundations of anxiety as a psychiatric and psychological phenomena and its relatedness to the body and somatization cannot be ignored.

It is, though, but one theoretical prism through which to comprehend this curious nodal concept called anxiety, a point at which multiple and varied important questions converge. Jackson and Evert (2010: 2793), for example, distinguish between personal individual anxieties (individual pathology) and anxiety that is essentially a social condition. They quote historian Bourke (2003), whom

> suggested anxiety (and other emotions) can be approached as a kind of language game, tracing the circumstances and terms in which anxieties are expressed and how they are articulated within wider social relations of power.

This provides an instructive perspective when viewed in the context of Menzies-Lyth (1970, 1988) theses of institutional containment of anxiety, specifically in relation to experiences of power and empowerment. What it doesn't do however is dig deeper into the archaeology of anxiety, to see through the neurotic foreground, to the much more intense and complex alignment with the background of living: to freedom, choice, authenticity and moral courage. To understand these connections better, I turn to the existential interpretations of anxiety as translated by the existential philosophers, such as Nietzsche (1961), Heidegger (1978) and Kierkegaard (1980). All of whom saw anxiety as a riddle whose solution would cast a flood of light.

Anxiety as the call to authenticity

Modernist philosophical treatments of anxiety, bought to bear by the writings of Nietzsche (1961), Heidegger (1978), Kierkegaard (1980) and other existential philosophers, have significantly shaped current thinking around the concept. The writings of Danish existential philosopher Soren Kierkegaard (1980) are particularly influential; Kierkegaard also did much to habilitate the concept of angst, which he linked with fear of freedom, fear of choices and fear of possibilities.

Kierkegaard straddled philosophy, psychology and theology amongst other disciplines and asked subjective questions about how people should live their lives and what they valued. He went on to inspire many, including Nietzsche (1961), Heidegger (1978) and Sartre (1943).

Kierkegaard himself, fascinated by indirect communication, explored novel ways of engaging with his audience often indirectly (opting to use pseudonyms to write about many ideas, including values, faith, freedom, fear and importantly, in the context of this chapter, alienation and anxiety). One of his definitive writings, 'The concept of Anxiety' (1980), is specifically devoted to describing and defining anxiety as it relates to the human condition. Kierkegaard conceived of anxiety as both terrifying and simultaneously compelling.

Jackson and Evert (2010: 2795) explain this compulsion as such:

> In the state of anxiety, humans come to realize their own position within the world and to distinguish themselves from their surrounding environment.

This provides an interesting lens through which to conceptualize and contextualize the anxiety experienced (consciously or unconsciously) by nurses in their everyday practices, in the work setting and in relationship to their patients. For some commentators it is clear that distinguishing oneself from one's environment is not the same as keeping a professional distance through splitting off and objectification.

Multiple scholars have attempted to break down Kierkegaard's writings on anxiety into simply digestible, sometimes rather formulaic, ideas, all linked to the ways in which people can lead their lives. Most agree that as individuals we pass through stages of realization (or consciousness) of our position in the world, and that anxiety is a fundamental precursor to action (progress) or paralises (stasis) in this regard.

In summary, being in the first aesthetic stage of realization individuals have little or no concept or awareness of the existence of a higher purpose; instead we are focused on what Freud and other psychoanalytic theorists might have termed the pleasure principle. Freud (1953–1975), and others, would advance that this lack of consciousness around higher purpose, and self-awareness, is a neurotic defence against anxiety of an existential nature, or existential angst.

The second ethical stage of realization is the realm in which individuals begin to take responsibility for themselves, their choices and their actions, and the impacts of the same on the other. Psychoanalytic thinkers link this to the move away from the inevitable narcissistic development of the self in early childhood, to a more mature recognition and appreciation of self and other relations. Moving through these stages of development is seen as fundamental to the creation of mature healthy personal relationships and the 'moral absolute' (Jacobs and Freshwater, 2023). This then is a stage of realization, during which there is a move beyond the individual self to appreciate not only the self and other, but also the self and other in the sense of a higher purpose.

Jackson and Evert (2010: 2795) describe these two stages as such:

> individuals pass through different stages, from ignorance and purposeless seizing of this or that opportunity, through becoming a thoughtful and responsible individual, to the realization that everything is grounded in nothingness, opening up the possibility of true faith....

The final stage of realization emphasizes the relationship with the transcendent; in the case of Kierkegaard's text 'Fear and Trembling' (1946), the transcendent is God. Where the ethical stage is based on reason, the third stage of realization, as Jackson and Evert (2010) note, is underpinned by faith. Choosing God (or faith as many authors prefer), Kierkegaard argues, means transcending the ethical, and submitting to a higher power.

Paradoxically then, Kierkegaard and others contend that what a faithful, ethical and authentic life demands is *more* anxiety, as opposed to less. Moreover, they contend that anxiety is the emotion most tightly aligned with the burden of mortality and meaning, and the ability to live an authentic and moral life: a life perhaps of good faith.

For Kierkegaard, the ground between the ethical stage of realization and one of living through faith in the higher purpose is ambiguous and requires what he calls the qualitative leap. The qualitative leap describes the movement that closes the gap between these two stages. A gap that, according to Kierkegaard, is one in which the anxiety between possibility and actuality resides. Kierkegaard suggests that if possibility and actuality are marked as points along a linear path, there lies between them an ambiguous realm.

Kierkegaard argues that anxiety, also translated in *The Concept of Anxiety* (1980) as dread, shrinks the ambiguous space between possibility and actuality, bringing the two ends closer towards one another, enabling the individual's transition between them. Moreover, the ambiguous space which anxiety shrinks is itself anxiety.

Here, possibility describes a sort of abstraction in which the ultimate end is concretization; let me substitute this suggesting that it also describes a commitment to ethical, moral and authentic practice. This commitment is the concretization of the pursuit of progression based not only on moral courage, but also faith and trust in a higher purpose. A practice not driven by endless doing as a way to cope with anxieties and dissonances, rather one that is based as much on being in the world, as it is on doing.

In essence, the actualization of possibilities comes to us via anxiety, forcing, as it does, the qualitative leap. More straightforwardly, Kierkegaard proposes that the anxious person is anxious about the reality of endless possibilities, colliding with one another, culminating in an assault on their very existence. To quote Boss (2020):

> ...Dasein exists as a whole assembly of possibilities for being in the world and that in any given moment it may "carry out" only one of these while each of the others remain simply "uncarried out".

Kierkegaard (1980) also writes that whoever is educated (by possibility) remains with anxiety; he does not permit himself to be deceived by its countless falsifications and accurately remembers the past. This is to say that the person who understands the possibility manifest in anxiety knows not to deny anxiety. Rather, it is a personal goal to 'accurately remember the past', which describes moments of anxiety and the path onto which one is led upon seizing possibility. Importantly, welcoming anxiety is akin to welcoming the path to freedom, authenticity and a moral life (Kierkegaard, 1964). Understanding this in the context of contemporary nursing practice, education and research is not a mere philosophical reverie; importantly, it is crucial to the very being of the profession as it struggles and strives to continue to be taken seriously and in good faith.

And so, to clarify, according to Kierkegaard, the ultimate learning is to have learned to be anxious in the right way. The abstract notion of the ultimate is rendered concrete if anxiety is regarded as the tool with which individuals navigate through space and time. Assuming anxiety is the tool Dasein uses in order to project one's self forward, and each movement brings the individual closer towards the goal of authentic existence, then using anxiety to one's advantage is in fact the most important knowledge Dasein can and should acquire (Boss, 2020).

By learning anxiety, it is possible to avoid the *misfortunes* of being without anxiety, or to succumbing to anxiety as neurosis. This is an interesting shift in Kierkegaards writing, as it is almost as if he is stating that to be educated properly, one needs to live with and understand anxiety from the inside out, and that anxiety is a masterful teacher, he notes that:

> If at the beginning of his education he misunderstands the anxiety… then he is lost. On the other hand, whoever is educated (by possibility) remains with anxiety…

Simply put, Kierkegaard emphasizes the importance of learning to be anxious in the right way.

This leaves us with some fundamental questions about how we teach nurses to learn anxiety, how we engage with anxiety provoking systems and experiences, how we translate that learning into moral courage for authentic practice, and as importantly, how do we enable those in our charge also to learn from anxiety. This is an especially a thorny question for mental health nurses.

Discussion

Anxiety as the route to authentic nursing?

How then are we to think about nurses, nursing, nursing practice, nurse education and indeed nursing research when seen through such perspicacity.

Knowing, as we do, that the nursing profession not only stimulates individual anxiety, but also produces social anxiety through habituative and institutionalized regimes, that ironically are meant to lend themselves to coping.

Knowing as we do, that nursing values and care statements are embroidered in multiple mission and purpose parchments, and yet the gap between espoused theories and theories in action continue to be a key factor in the well-being, retention and recruitment of nursing staff.

Knowing, as we do, that nurses are often understood to be stuck in the aesthetic stage of realization, seen as self-serving and not always consciously focused on caring for the other and the best outcome for that person, even when it is not the most comfortable outcome for the caregiver; rather deriving ego strength and pleasure from caring, for the purpose of suring up the insecure ego (self) and the unconscious desire to be needed. Thereby avoiding anxiety of one's own mortality and choices.

Knowing, as we do, that the nursing curriculum and its approach to learning and teaching is not necessarily focused on creating personal ethical and morally challenging learning experiences for nurses to reflect deeply on. To privilege graduate attributes such as deliberative action; conscious purposeful practice; intentional decision-making.

Nurses need anxiety. Nurses need to have the right sort of anxiety and to be aware that to avoid anxiety is to flee from freedom, from a life and a profession, full of possibilities.

Nurses need to learn that anxiety is necessary for the absolute progression of possibilities of practice to translate into actuality; to live their espoused theories and to work and live meaningfully and authentic working lives through moral courage: a life full of hope when faced with suffering and dying.

As alluded to earlier, moral courage is variably defined as a virtue or value that assists nursing in doing the right thing; that is making correct decisions when faced with ethical dilemmas. Moral courage is also related to personal values (Kleemola et al., 2020; Numminen et al., 2017). Whilst some writers emphasize the role that moral courage plays in helping caregivers adhere to the principles and values of professional ethics in caring for the patient, others see morality as an indispensable part of human life, a practical philosophy looking for right and wrong and determining good and bad in a collection of behaviours under certain conditions (Murray, 2010; Kleemola et al., 2020).

Nurses face moral and ethical problems daily. Identification of ethical problems necessitates a moral sensitivity and an awareness of ethical principles. Nonetheless, Khoshmehr et al. (2020) argue that possessing moral sensitivity and knowledge is not sufficient enough to deal with moral and ethical dilemmas. Nurses also have to possess moral courage in order to:

> perform on the basis of what is considered ethically right provided personal values and criteria correspond to the accepted healthcare values.

When a nurse struggles to act according to the correct ethical performance, moral courage helps them to apply their best effort to achieve their ultimate goal, regardless of the consequences. In doing so, they consider moral principles and perform a correct act that is not easy to do: I refer to this as right action.

Studies demonstrate that moral courage is related to concepts concerning assessment of ethics under certain conditions such as sensitivity to justice, perception of control over one's emotions and performance such as emotional self-regulation and self-efficacy (Abdollah et al., 2021; Kleemola et al., 2020; Khoshmehr et al., 2020). We might think about this as doing the right thing even when you are not being watched. Observing and feeling the anxiety and fear that comes with doing the right thing and taking the qualitative leap.

Right action is not always comfortable, requiring courage in the face of potential alienation from peers and colleagues. Negative consequences that can be created through moral courage include stress, anxiety, fear of being scolded and rejection by colleagues and seclusion. However, moral courage is also a motivating force that assists nurses to overcome many fearful barriers, enabling them to care for and protect the patient effectively.

I have argued here for a revitalization of morally infused nursing that is values-led and which embraces anxiety and death anxiety as fundamental to the delivery of faithful care and the emergence of the authentic self. And perhaps for the future survival of our profession. This demands of nurses and nursing that we create an environment within which the stages of realization, according to Kierkegaard are not only fostered, but actively cultivated.

As Kierkegaard framed it, to escape from 'the dizziness of freedom' from the realization of boundless possibilities, is to live a stagnant life, devoid of hope. The right sort of anxiety has the potential to lead to empowerment, the power to create new possibilities, to opportunity pursue those possibilities even with the inherent (real or perceived) risks, to explore the edges of our knowing and imagination, and in that sense to determine the limits of our capabilities. Anxiety is deeply connected to the lived experience of freedom. Without this, the loss and shameful lack of support and mis-reading of nursing, nurse education and nursing practice remains.

If, as Menzies-Lyth (1970, 1988) and others insisted, empowerment is a key solution to the reduction of nursing burnout and stress, and a potential window to strength in moral courage, then surely our only option is to run towards, anxiety rather than flee from it, in the process to discover moral courage.

References

Abdollah, R., Iranpour, S., and Ajri-Khameslou, M. (2021) Relationship between resilience and professional moral courage amongst nurses. *Journal of Medical Ethics and History of Medicine*, 14: 3.

Ashforth, B., and Tomuiuk, M. (2000) Emotional labour and authenticity: Views from service agents. In Fineman, S. (ed.) *Emotion in Organizations*, 2nd Ed. London: Sage.

Boss, M. (2020) Recent considerations in daisenanalysis. *The Humanistic Psychologist*, 28 (1–3): 210–230.

Bourke, J. (2003) Fear and anxiety: Writing about emotion in modern history. *History Workshop Journal*, 55: 113–133.

Buber, Martin (1937) *I and Thou*. Translated by Ronald Gregor Smith. Edinburgh: T. & T. Clark.

Freshwater, D., and Cahill, J.L. (2010) Care and compromise: Developing a conceptual framework for work-related stress. *Journal of Research in Nursing*, 15 (2): 173–183.

Freud, S. (1953–1975) Inhibitions, symptoms, and anxiety. In Strachey, J. (Trans) *An Autobiographical Study: Inhibitions, Symptoms, and Anxiety: The Question of Lay Analysis and Other Works*. Vol. 20. London: Hogarth Press.

Freshwater, D. and Robertson, C. (2002) *Needs and Emotions. Core Concepts in Psychotherapy*. Buckinghamshire: Open University Press

Freshwater, D., and Bryant, S. (1998) Exploring mutuality within the nurse-patient relationship. *British Journal of Nursing*, 7 (4): 204–206.

Heidegger, M. (1978) *Being and Time*. Oxford: Blackwell.

Hirschorn, L. (1988) *The Workplace Within: Psychodynamics of Organizational Life*. Cambridge: MIT Press.

Hochschild, A. (1983) *The Managed Heart*. California: University of California Press.

Jackson, P. and Everts, J. (2010) Anxiety as social practice. *Environment and Planning*, 42: 2791–2806.

Jacobs, M. and Freshwater, D. (2023) *The Presenting Past* (5th Edition). Open University Press Oxford

Khodaveisi, M., Oshvandi, K., and Bashirian, S. (2021) Moral courage, moral sensitivity and safe nursing care in nurses caring of patients with COVID-19. *Nursing Open*, 8 (6): 3538–3546. https://doi.org/10.1002/nop2.903.

Khoshmehr, Z., Barkhordari-Sharifabad, M., Nasiriani, K., and Fallahzadeh, H. (2020) Moral courage and psychological empowerment among nurses. *BMC Nursing*, 19: 43.

Kierkegaard, S. (1946) *Fear and Trembling*. Oxford: Oxford University Press.

Kierkegaard, S. (1964) *Repetition: An Essay in Experimental Psychology*. London: Harper.

Kierkegaard, S. (1980) *The Concept of Anxiety*. Princeton, NJ: Princeton University Press.

Kim, E.Y. and Chang, S.O. (2022) Exploring nurse perceptions and experiences of resilience: A meta-synthesis study. *BMC Nursing*, 21: 26.

Kleemola, E., Leino-Kilpi, H., and Numminen, O. (2020) Care situations demanding moral courage: Content analysis of nurses' experiences. *Nursing Ethics*, 27 (3): 714–25.

Klein, M. (1975) *The Writings of Melanie Klein Vol 3*. London: Hogarth.

Mann, S., and Cowburn, J. (2005) Emotional labour and stress within mental health nursing. *Journal of Psychiatric and Mental Health Nursing*, 12 (2): 154–162.

Menzies-Lyth, I. (1970) *The Functioning of Social Systems as a Defence Against Anxiety*. London: Centre for Applied Social Research.

Menzies-Lyth, I. (1988) *Containing Anxiety in Institutions: Selected Essays (Vol 1)*. London: UK Free Association Press.

Mohammadi, F., Masoumi, Z., Oshvandi, K., Khazaei, S. and Bijani, M. (2022) Death anxiety, moral courage, resilience in nursing students who care for COVID-19 patients: A cross-sectional study. *BMC Nursing*, 21: 150.

Murray, J.S. (2010) Moral courage in healthcare: Acting ethically even in the presence of risk. *Online Journal of Issues in Nursing* 15 (3), https://ojin.nursingworld.org/MainMenuCategories/EthicsStandards/Resources/Courage- and-Distress/Moral-Courage-and-Risk.html.

Nietzsche, F. (1961) *Thus Spoke Zarathustra. A Book for Everyone and No One*. Translated by R.J. Hollingdale. London: Penguin.

Nolan, G. and Walsh, E. (2012) Caring in prison: The intersubjective web of professional relationships. *Journal of Forensic Nursing*, 8 (4): 163–169.

Numminen, O., Repo, H., and Leino-Kilpi, H. (2017) Moral courage in nursing: A concept analysis. *Nursing Ethics*, 24 (8): 878–891. DOI: 10.1177/0969733016634155.

Sartre, J.-P., (1943) *Being and Nothingness*. London: Routledge.

Walsh, E. (2007) An exploration of the emotional labour of prison nurses. PhD Thesis. Bournemouth University: Bournemouth.

Walsh, E. (2009) The emotional labour of nurses working in Her Majesty's (HM) prison service. *Journal of Forensic Nursing*, 5 (3): 143–152.

Walsh, E., Freshwater, D.M. and Fisher, P. (2012) Caring for prisoners: Towards mindful practice. *Journal of Research in Nursing*, 18 (2): DOI: 10.1177/1744987112466086.

World Health Organization (2020) State of the World's Nursing Report-2020. https://who.int/publications/i/item/9789240003279. Accessed 20/01/2023.

Yarbrough, S., Martin, P., Alfred, D., and McNeill, C. (2017) Professional values, job satisfaction, career development, and intent to stay. *Nursing Ethics*, 24 (6): 675–85.

36 Freedom of speech as a philosophy in nursing

Roger Watson

Introduction

I became acutely aware of the issue of freedom of speech, especially as it relates to my profession of nursing, through personal experience. In early 2020, COVID-19 appeared and changed the world forever. I had been in Wuhan at the start of what the World Health Organization later declared a pandemic but had been completely unaware that there was a novel coronavirus spreading across China and further afield. The mainstream media was reporting widespread deaths in Wuhan and even showing reports of people collapsing in the streets and dead bodies being found on the pavements. I had just been there, had used crowded trains, given lectures in crowded hospitals and walked extensively in the city of Wuhan and my experience directly contradicted what was being reported. But I made a mistake by telling people.

Clearly, I managed to leave China prior to the draconian travel restrictions and only on return to the United Kingdom was I aware of the novel coronavirus. Concerned, I asked my Chinese colleagues—and kept asking them throughout 2020—if any of them had caught COVID-19 or knew anyone who had died. In both cases, the answer was negative. Studying the figures for infections, infection fatality rate and age profile of deaths from Wuhan, it was clear that the virus was contagious but that it had a fatality rate like influenza and was also fatal for the same group of people, the very old and the medically compromised. While not doubting that there was a novel and possibly dangerous virus spreading, I was aghast at the measures that were being proposed early in 2020 and subsequently introduced.

However, it is not my purpose here to justify my views further or to weigh up their veracity against the established facts regarding COVID-19 and the efficacy of the non-pharmacological methods that were introduced. I began expressing my view that, perhaps, we were getting things out of proportion regarding COVID-19 and linked these articles to my social media accounts. I expected, and most certainly received, opposition in brief in Twitter, at length on Facebook and by email. I fully expected and welcomed this. What I did not expect was to be shunned (Watson, 2021) and called out by some very good colleagues who were very personally critical of me but who would neither engage in debate nor offer alternative views and figures. Finally, I was shocked by a tweet from the Chief Executive of our local city council which said: "Aren't you the Professor of Nursing @uniofXXXX and should you not be supporting our @XXXXXX our Public Health Officer?" The tweet itself was shocking as it implied that as a nurse, I should not have the freedom to express an opinion contrary to the line that was being taken regarding COVID, the 'Covid narrative'. What was worse was the Twitter 'pile on' which

DOI: 10.4324/9781003427407-42

called on my university to dismiss me and some very threatening tweets. The tweets subsided and I had to answer to my employees for my actions and the fact that I had spoken locally and anti-lockdown rallies. I had had the good sense to say, on record, that I was not representing my university, and a supportive email from Toby Young of the Free Speech Union copied to the university stemmed any further action. Literally overnight, I had gone from being naïve about the issue of freedom of speech to being acutely aware, however mildly in my case, of the potential consequences when it is not respected. Others have not been as lucky.

Whistleblowing and freedom of speech

I had the privilege many years ago, at the height of the publicity surrounding him, to meet the late Graham Pink. In the late 1980s and early 1990s, Pink had complained copiously about the poor standard of care being provided for older patients in his hospital, providing some concrete examples of what he was observing. Lack of action by the hospital led him to write to his local Member of Parliament and these letters were subsequently published by *The Guardian* newspaper (Brindle, 2013). Pink was dismissed from his job on the basis that he was undermining confidence in the hospital. He subsequently took his health authority to an industrial tribunal, won his case and was awarded damages. Eventually, the concept of whistleblowing became enshrined in law in the Public Interest Disclosure Act 1998 and others have used the freedom it enshrined to criticise, for example, the National Health Service with impunity if such criticism was found to have substance. This is exemplified by the complaints made by nurses (and the public) about the poor level of care and abuse of patients in Mid-Staffordshire which resulted in the Francis Report (2013).

Nursing and freedom of speech

Nursing has roots in both religious orders and military structures, organisations that are not traditionally associated with freedom of speech. Despite raising the educational level of nursing in recent decades, nurses continue to work within a medical and nursing hierarchy where freedom of speech may also not be a foremost consideration.

However, freedom of speech is important at several levels such as the need to have open and appreciative debate about nursing issues at an academic level, the ability to speak out in clinical practice—whistleblowing—when poor care appears to be institutionalised and even in rapidly developing clinical situations where patient safety may be compromised.

This chapter will initially examine freedom of speech as a philosophy underpinning academic debate. I will then explore some current issues where the exercise of freedom of speech has been curtailed by social media mobbing and even by termination of employment. The limits of freedom of speech will be explored, and some current measures and movement intended to preserve it. Finally, ways of ensuring the inculcation of freedom of speech with nursing students will be discussed.

Freedom of speech

Freedom of speech, properly understood, is an important concept and in society generally, there is evidence that this is being eroded (Doyle, 2021). Freedom of speech has largely been something taken for granted, until relatively recently. Properly understood, it has meant the freedom to express an opinion, even if that opinion offends, with impunity. However, in expressing an offensive view, it is assumed that there is some reason (i.e. in the application of reason) underlying it and that the view can be challenged fairly and robustly. The true spirit of expressing a well-formed and deeply held view is that of reserving the right to be wrong and being open to challenge and even to the possibility of having one's mind changed.

However, like all things, freedom of speech exists on a spectrum and that spectrum stretches from freedom of speech absolutism at one end to approval of freedom of speech only if it accords with one's own views at the other end. Exemplified, this ranges from—at the absolutist end of the spectrum—to the right to shout 'fire' in a crowded theatre simply for the fun of watching people panic and evacuate (Doyle, 2021) to, at the more restrictive end of the spectrum, only being in favour of freedom of speech when you operate it, without affording others the right to do the same.

Clearly, both ends of the spectrum represent extremes in freedom of speech and, as such, are likely, when exercised, to lead to folly. The folly of saying whatever one feels like, simply for effect, is on the one hand unlikely to win you a large circle of friends and is likely to have been socialised out of you at a relatively early age. On the other hand, freedom of speech absolutism can endanger lives, lead to civil unrest and weaken the fabric of society. It seems, where freedom of speech is concerned, that there must be some constraints.

But at the other end of the spectrum, where freedom of speech is severely constrained, then there is likely to be great harm to society and great harm to individuals. Constraints to freedom of speech are evident in totalitarian regimes such as the one exemplified in George Orwell's (1949) dystopian novel *Nineteen Eighty-Four*. Orwell's world of Oceania was fictional, but we can witness in several modern regimes how the curtailment of freedom of speech is used to control the media and thus the narrative about current events and thus the population. Violations of these curtailments can lead to severe punishment. 'This could not happen here', we say; yet, it has, and it is exemplified by what has become known as 'cancel culture' (Williams, 2022) to which media stars, academics and students have succumbed often with the loss of career, job and mental health.

Cancel culture

Cancel culture is not operated by the state but by powerful groups of individuals who put pressure on institutions such as universities to expel students or dismiss staff who express views that they deem unpalatable. The issues that lead to cancellation are cases *par excellence* of freedom of speech. They are not efforts to incite civil unrest, promote violence or even deliberately to offend. In fact, in expressing some of the issues that have led to cancellation the person expressing the view meant no more than to share their sincerely held view. These can range from countering an argument by restatement of the blindingly obvious to asking a question about something that is not fully understood. The freedom of speech issue arises in the eye of the beholder; in other words, the person objecting to the view obviously does not agree with it but also, has taken offence. The response and clarion call of the freedom of speech adherents is 'nobody has the right not to be offended' (Doyle, 2021) which seems like a less eloquent version of Orwell's "If liberty means anything at all, it means the *right* to tell people things they do *not* want to hear" (Orwell, 1972).

The origins of freedom speech

While it is impossible to pinpoint the precise origins of freedom speech, there is certainly no record of it having existed, for example, in ancient China or ancient Egypt. Indeed, from what we know about the structures and beliefs of these societies, it is unlikely that freedom of speech existed in any form that we would recognise today. The earliest recorded codification of freedom of speech seems to be in ancient Greece—for those who were considered to be citizens—where there were two understanding of the term *isegoria and parrhesia*. Respectively, these can be defined as follows (Bejan, 2017): "*isegoria* described the equal right of citizens to participate in public debate in the democratic assembly; *parrhesia*, the license to say what one pleased, how and when one pleased, and to whom". In other words, one description governed the right to freedom of speech while the other governed the content of that speech. That said, freedom of speech was not without its penalties in ancient Greece as Aristotle discovered. Accused of impiety and corrupting the youth with his methods, he defended his views, literally, to the death. He was executed in 399 BC.

The fortunes of freedom of speech have varied over the centuries and across different cultures and empires. In biblical times, up to an including *The New Testament*, whether taken allegorically or historically, freedom of speech was frowned on if it did not accord, for example, with scriptural teaching and the pivotal event in Christianity—the execution of Jesus—could be considered an issue of freedom of speech. The Romans, who ruled Palestine at the time of the execution of Jesus, while freedom of speech was not explicitly prohibited, did not have any laws specifically encoding freedom of speech. It has certainly been a continuing feature of most major religions through The Reformation and up to and including the present day, that freedom of speech, where it contradicts the essential tenets of the religion, is frowned upon, often with fatal consequences. Where Christianity has largely conceded in terms of, for example, blasphemy laws, militant Islam has taken over with some notable and bloody incidents which were the direct consequence of freedom of speech legally exercised within the countries, such as France and the United Kingdom where such incidents have taken place (Doyle, 2021).

Notable philosophers have given expression to freedom of speech. Voltaire notably and nobly is alleged to have said: "I disapprove of what you say, but I will defend to the death your right to say it". He never, in fact, said that; it was a fabrication in a biography written 300 years after his death (The Quotations Page, 2018). Nevertheless, it was supposed to be a summary of Voltaire's commitment to the defence of freedom of speech. More notably, freedom of speech was advocated and promoted by the philosopher John Stuart Mill (1860) who, in his book *On Liberty*, stated that even wrong opinions, including false ones, should be freely permitted as it was only by open discussion and debate that the truth could be reached. He also reserved the right to be wrong and to have his own opinions changed if they were shown to be wrong.

Many international bodies such as the United Nations and European Union provide for the protection of freedom of speech and, as a result, many of the countries—but by no means all—associated with these bodies provide protection for freedom of speech in their laws and even, where they have one, in their constitutions. That said, the United Nations includes countries such as Mainland China and the Russian Federation where freedom of speech is notably curtailed. Perhaps most prominent among

Western countries to enshrine freedom of speech in its constitution and, thereby, in law is the United States of America. The famous First Amendment of the Constitution of the United States of America enshrines freedom of speech. Specifically, the First Amendment says:

> Congress shall make no law respecting an establishment of religion, or prohibiting the free exercise thereof; or abridging the freedom of speech, or of the press; or the right of the people peaceably to assemble, and to petition the Government for a redress of grievances.

Initially aimed at ensuring the separation of church and state, the scope of the amendment has been expanded by testing in courts of law beyond, for example, freedom of the press and freedom of assembly to such things as pornography.

The recent history of freedom of speech

Freedom of speech has come into sharp focus in very recent years, with some notable incidents which I will use to exemplify the kinds of issues that can arise, lead to problems and also have consequences for the individuals. For the purposes of the argument, I will present three very different cases, none related specifically to nursing but which will serve to illustrate a range of issues related to freedom of speech.

Politics

In 2018, the Spectator columnist Toby Young was appointed by then Prime Minister Theresa May to the new higher education regulatory body Office for Students which was formed after the dissolution of the Higher Education Funding Council for England. Toby Young had appropriate experience being a Fulbright Commissioner and having set up the first free school in London and being employed by the charity which he established to help others to set up further free schools and to oversee the work of existing free schools. Free schools were established with government funding but were free from local government control and were not religiously affiliated. The free schools he established, which did not select on educational achievement proved to be very successful and quickly developed waiting lists. Young was already quite a controversial character and being conservative in his politics was not universally popular. People— referred to by Young as 'offence archaeologists'—quickly got to work attempting to discredit him by searching his back catalogue of articles and trawling through his social media (Murray, 2018). As Young says 'it didn't take them long' to find some controversial articles and some regrettable tweets. The remainder of the story is a matter of public record (Phipps, Rawlinson & Mason, 2018). Suffice to say, for comments made and articles written some many years before, which had no bearing on Young's ability to work with the Office for Students and for which he apologised, he was not appointed. Furthermore, he had to resign as a Fulbright Commissioner, give up an honorary fellowship at a university and ultimately to resign from the charity which he established, which he ran and which paid his salary. It is worth noting that nothing Young had said was illegal, aimed at any individuals or in any way connected with the role to which he had been appointed.

Health

British doctor and general practitioner Professor Carl Henegan, director of the University of Oxford's Centre for Evidence-Based Medicine, was a prolific commentator on the COVID-19 pandemic of 2020–2021 which persisted in some areas of the world well into 2022. Professor Henegan was considered a calm voice of reason throughout the pandemic and made regular television and radio appearances and wrote regularly in several media outlets. However, unlike many of his colleagues, he was not prone to hyperbole regarding the likely outcome of the pandemic in terms of deaths, he never catastrophised the situation and he politely and effectively questioned the established narrative around the pandemic that was being promoted by the government advisory group SAGE and especially the sensationalist headlines that were being promulgated by most newspapers and the remainder of the mainstream media. Despite his considerable expertise as an epidemiologist and his demonstrable ability to evaluate evidence he was rapidly shunned by the mainstream media, making very few appearances on, for example, the BBC, ITV or Sky News. Instead, he was interviewed on channels such as talkRADIO and the then emerging GB News channels which took a more independent line. He defended his fellow Oxford epidemiologist Professor Sunetra Gupta (Dodsworth, 2021), one of the founders of the Great Barrington Declaration which urged protection of the vulnerable while avoiding economic lockdown and he defended oncologist Professor Karol Sikora (also a victim of cancel culture) who warned about a looming cancer crisis due to lockdown (Sikora, 2022) and who likewise had to depend on outlets such as talkRADIO and UnHerd's Lockdown TV for interviews where he warned about the detrimental effect of closing the NHS on oncology services. Essentially, the message from Carl Henegan, often reinforced by Karol Sikora was that we must get back to normal as soon as possible before the NHS and the economy were in crisis and people suffered undue mental health and other problems. Once the pandemic was, essentially, over and restrictions had been lifted, the analysis began and it emerged that, perhaps, the number of deaths from COVID-19 (as opposed to with or at the time of COVID) had been inflated and *The Mail* published an article to that effect. That COVID-19 deaths had been inflated was the view of Carl Henegan and, as he agreed with the figures in *The Mail* article, he retweeted the article on his Twitter feed. Twitter suspended him for 24 hours and made him delete the tweet as a condition of lifting the suspension (Powell, 2022).

Education

In 2021 at the height of the pandemic restrictions, students were prevented from attending lectures on university campuses and were confined to residences or to their homes from where they received lessons online. During an online seminar for final-year law students at Abertay University in Scotland, the participants in the modules titled 'Gender, feminism and the law' and 'Human Rights' were discussing the issues of gender and transgender issues, surrogacy and contraception. Following the seminar, one student, Lisa Keogh, was summoned by the university to a formal investigation into an allegation that she had made 'inappropriate' comments (Williams, 2022). During the discussion during which students had been invited to comment on whether 'women have vaginas' and 'not all men are rapists', Lisa had offered the view, which she has never denied, and which reflected her beliefs, which was that only women had vaginas. She also shared that she thought biological men should be excluded from contact sports with women as, due to their greater strength there was a physical risk to women. These comments had offended a member of the discussion group, which Lisa believed to be an open discussion where she had freedom to express her views and that member had reported her to her university.

Lisa was a mature student, a single mother and, with her final examinations approaching, she was on the verge of fulfilling her dream of becoming a solicitor. However, life was made very hard for her as she was told that the investigation, which was no longer into 'comments' but into inappropriate behaviour, would proceed and that if she was found to be in breach of university procedures then her studies would be terminated, and she would be expelled from the university. Supported by the Free Speech Union and through crowdfunding for legal support Lisa fought the case and won. She was found not to be in breach of the university regulations and proceeded to and passed her final examinations. However, she felt that considerable damage had been done and that she may be unemployable because of the allegations and the investigation. Lisa was deeply distressed by the investigation and, while she was found to be innocent and not punished, she considered that the process was the punishment and is taking legal action against the university for the damage it has done to her.

Reflection

The three cases presented above illustrate the consequences for people whose freedom of speech is violated. The three cases, while representing different levels of freedom of speech violation due to the extent to which the initial offending comments were made are all very different in content. The incident of Toby Young illustrates that the right to make offensive comments, however much in jest, can be used against you to the extent that you lose your job and other prestigious positions which you had earned. The underlying issue here was, undoubtedly one of disagreement with Young's well known political views. The second incident illustrates how freedom of speech can be violated when views expressed contradict a current narrative; in this case, the COVID-19 narrative even if the views were expressed in the form of a retweet by a recognised expert in the field. In neither of these above cases was there any access to appeal; Young was never appointed to the Office for Students and did not return to his job. Carl Henegan, while there were no further consequences, was forced to delete an innocuous tweet. In the third case, the subject was the victim of current views and activism associated with the transgender movement where the concept of binary sexuality or biological determination of sex and gender is denied. Her innocent, heartfelt views which were based on commonly accepted views of sex and gender held by most people were considered offensive and an investigation was initiated without care for the well-being of the individual at the end of the allegation. What they all have in common is that an individual's right to make comments with which others disagree was eroded and escalated from individual offence to organisational action.

Caring professionals who get cancelled

It is not only public figures and unfortunate students who get cancelled. Nurses and other caring professionals have been the subject of cancel culture too. There is at least one incidence of a nursing student being expelled from her programme for expressing her views, based on her Christian belief, that marriage could only be between a man and a woman. Similarly, at the University of Sheffield, social worker student Felix Ngole was expelled in 2016 from his programme for expressing opposition, based on his devout Christian belief, that homosexuality was a sin, and that marriage could only take place between a man and a woman. It should be noted that he expressed these views as part of a debate on Facebook over the issue of a Christian registrar in the United States of America refusing to register same sex marriages. Mr Ngole had not put these comments up with the intention of offending, but they came to the attention of LGBT activists who demanded of the university that he be expelled. He was duly expelled but in 2019 his case was heard at the Court of Appeal and Sheffield was asked to reconsider it.

In Ngole's case, the university considered that his comments may be incompatible with his role as a social worker, but why? His view was legitimate and one that would be expected from some devout Christians. He did not express any hatred of gay people or even of people who were in same sex marriages; he expressed a view about what he considered constituted a valid marriage in the Christian sense. It I could be considered illogical to extrapolate and say that made his unfit to be a social worker, even one coming into contact with gay people or people in same sex marriages.

As the Editor-in-Chief of *Journal of Advanced Nursing*, I came under pressure over a freedom of speech issue for publishing an editorial by Niall McCrae and Jonathan Portes, both of King's College London (McCrae & Portes, 2019). The editorial was based on a small survey of nurses and their beliefs regarding Brexit. The study was not suitable for publishing as an original article, but I considered that it had sufficient currency, originality and interest for publication as an editorial which might stimulate discussion. This was certainly achieved in the form of a complaint about me to the publisher Wiley for publishing the editorial by someone who had not declared their involvement in a pro-Brexit organisation (McCrae was a member of pro-Brexit Bruges Group), how the editorial was biased and political and clearly promoting one view and asking how it could be published when it was not peer reviewed. I permitted the authors to write a counter editorial—to which I responded—and, while we did consider that, in future, we should indicate two aspects of all editorials: (1) that they were not reviewed in the normal manner and published at the discretion of the Editor-in-Chief; and (2) a declaration of interests (as with other articles) statement where necessary, what the offended authors has not realised that in the two authors, both sides of the Brexit debate were represented. Jonathan Portes is a committed Remainer and was regularly interviewed on the BBC Radio 4 *Today* programme to that effect. In fact, the editorial represented the precise opposite to what the complainants had claimed, and it was also an exemplar of freedom of speech and how two people with opposing views could work together regardless of those views. Once this fact was conveyed to them, there was no further correspondence on the matter.

Is there a problem regarding freedom of speech in nursing?

In my experience, there is. For example, I hold and have expressed the view that paying bursaries to nursing students is not appropriate. This is not the place to rehearse my reasons which are a matter of public record (Watson, 2018). Of course, in stating these views, I understand that people will oppose me and, indeed, I have lost the argument in the sense that bursaries were reinstated after a short spell when they were withheld. I also realise that, for many, it is an emotive issue and that there are a great many legitimate arguments in favour of paying bursaries to nursing students. However, even as someone in the public eye on the issue and prominent within my profession, nothing prepared me for the reaction on two occasions. I was booed off stage at a staff development conference on one occasion with absolutely no opportunity to explain my position, the only time in my career when that happened.

But even worse was the reaction to my article in *The Conversation* which continues to elicit hundreds of responses the vast majority disagreeing with me. On face value, this is perfectly acceptable but I was unprepared for the frank hatred that was displayed in some of the comments, the Twitter pile-on and letters to the Vice-Chancellor of my university demanding my resignation. I also received direct emails from people expressing their disgust at me. To all my detractors I suggested they write a constructive response to my article for *The Conversation* and, latterly, I offered them space in the editorial pages of *Journal of Advanced Nursing* where they could make their case about nursing bursaries or about my opposition to them. The offer is extant at my current journal *Nurse Education in Practice*. Nobody has taken up the offer.

Is there a place for freedom of speech in the nursing curriculum?

The nursing curriculum is already packed, and I would be reluctant to add more to it, especially something that, to the general public who already hold a negative view about university educated nurses may question. Moreover, nursing may not be alone in requiring some understanding of freedom of speech as other groups of students, for example, those whose political views do not accord with the majority of students, say that they are reluctant to express those views.

There are two sides to the freedom of speech issue, and one is being educated to realise that this is a right that we have, albeit that it needs to be exercised responsibly; the other side is learning to allow others the right to freedom of speech and not to shut them down, shout them down or cause opprobrium to be heaped upon them.

Perhaps, rather than having a curricular strand dedicated to freedom of speech—akin to having sessions on 'critical thinking' which should be an underlying principle to university education—opportunities, for example, debates, need to be created where students can exercise freedom of speech, both the transmission and reception of controversial ideas in an atmosphere where the 'bottom line' is freedom of speech.

Conclusion

Nursing and many individual nurses have made considerable progress in recent decades in achieving places at the 'high tables' of policy and decision making, for example, in government committees, research councils and charities alongside their medical and other peers. In these forums, they need to be able freely to express controversial ideas which may counter the established narrative without fear and to accept controversial ideas which may counter their beliefs without taking offence. This will work to ensure that their voice is heard, their views are challenged and changed where necessary and should lead to better outcomes from the bodies in which nurses are involved.

Those of us who advocate freedom of speech and purport to practise it should both expect and accept it from others. '*Audi alteram partem*' (listen to the other side).

Declaration

The author is a member of the Free Speech Union.

References

Bejan, T.M. (2017) The two clashing meanings of 'free speech'. *The Atlantic*, 2 December. https://www.theatlantic.com/politics/archive/2017/12/two-concepts-of-freedom-of-speech/546791/; accessed 13 July 2022.

Brindle, D. (2013) Why whistleblowers' voices must continue to be heard. *The Guardian*, 27 November. https://www.theguardian.com/society/2013/nov/27/whistleblower-voices-heard-nhs-elderly-care-graham-pink; accessed 15 July 2022.

Dodsworth, L. (2021) *A state of fear*. Pinter & Martin, London.

Doyle, A. (2021) *Free speech and why it matters*. Constable, London.

Francis, R. (2013) *Report of the Mid Staffordshire NHS Foundation Trust Public Inquiry*. TSO, London.

McCrae, H., Portes, J. (2019) Attitudes to Brexit: A survey of nursing and midwifery students. *Journal of Advanced Nursing* 75(1):1–9. doi: 10.1111/jan.13706. Epub 2018 Jul 8.

Mill, J.S. (1860) *On liberty*. John W. Parker & Son, London

Murray, D. (2018) *The madness of crowds*. Bloomsbury Continuum, London.

Orwell, G. (1949) *Nineteen eighty-four*. Secker & Warburg, London.

Orwell, G. (1972) *TLS: The Times Literary Supplement* 15 September p.1039 (https://quoteinvestigator.com/2020/07/06/hear-liberty/; accessed 19 July 2022).

Phipps, C., Rawlinson, K., Mason, R. (2018) Toby young resigns from the office for students after backlash. *The Guardian*, 9 January (https://www.theguardian.com/media/2018/jan/09/toby-young-resigns-office-for-students; accessed 19 July 2022).

Powell, M. (2022) Twitter bans Oxford academic who shared this Mail on Sunday article - but allows anti-vax rants amid fears over new 'online safety' powers letting tech giants censor legitimate journalism. *MailOnline*, 26 March (https://www.dailymail.co.uk/news/article-10655577/Twitter-bans-Oxford-academic-shared-MoS-article-allows-anti-vax-rants.html; accessed 20 July 2022).

Sikora, K. (2022) Britain's looming cancer crisis. *spiked*, 7 April (https://www.spiked-online.com/2022/04/07/britains-looming-cancer-crisis/; accessed 20 July).

The Quotations Page. (2018) (http://www.quotationspage.com/quote/331.html; accessed 19 July 2022)

Watson, R. (2018) Nurses don't need bursaries – here are four reasons why. *The Conversation*, 17 April (https://theconversation.com/nurses-dont-need-bursaries-here-are-four-reasons-why-94938; accessed 19 July 2022).

Watson, R. (2021) Ostracised, for the sin of speaking my mind over Covid. *The Conservative Woman*, 2 April (https://www.conservativewoman.co.uk/ostracised-for-the-sin-of-speaking-my-mind-over-covid/; accessed 20 July 2022).

Williams, J. (2022) *How woke won*. Spiked, London.

37 Using philosophical inquiry to dismantle dominant thinking in nursing about race and racism

Annette J. Browne, Colleen Varcoe, Lydia Wytenbroek, Ismalia De Sousa, and Chloe Crosschild

Introduction and overall purpose

The purpose of this chapter is to leverage philosophical inquiry as an entry point for discussing and critiquing dominant thinking in nursing about issues of race and racism. In Part I, we provide an analysis of the deeply ingrained structures and mechanisms underlying thinking about race and racism in nursing, and demonstrate the value of drawing on subaltern[1] perspectives and angles of inquiry to illuminate and unseat structural influences on thinking about race and racism. In Part II, we highlight how Chicana and Black feminist theorizing, and Indigenous knowledges can create new possibilities for nursing philosophizing, theory and knowledge.

Writing is an act of scholarly resistance and our relationships shape our learning and co-production of knowledge. We are each involved in academic nursing research and education in Canada: Annette J. Browne is a white woman whose research program is in health and healthcare inequities, with a focus on working in partnership with Indigenous and non-Indigenous peoples to mitigate the negative effects of racism and intersecting forms of discrimination. Colleen Varcoe is a cisgender woman of Indigenous and English immigrant ancestry who works to mitigate structural and interpersonal violence and their impacts. Lydia Wytenbroek is a white woman, nurse and historian, with interests in the histories of nursing and healthcare as they intersect with gender, race and place analyses. Ismalia De Sousa is a Black European ciswoman, nurse and doctoral candidate whose nursing philosophy is informed by lived experience theorizing and Black and Chicana feminisms. Chloe Crosschild is a cisgender Blackfoot[2] woman from the Kainai Nation, nurse and doctoral student whose nursing philosophy is informed by Siksikaitsitapi (Blackfoot ways of knowing).

Part I: Explicating the deep structures influencing thinking in nursing about racism

In this chapter, we deliberately use "Western" to signal the dominant, taken-for-granted genre of Western-White[3]-Eurocentric philosophical thinking in nursing, not to imply that all nursing is Western but to prompt attention to excluded and previously disqualified knowledges in nursing such as Indigenous and Black ontologies and epistemologies. As we emphasize below, Western professional nursing arose from Christian and colonial contexts and is consequently aligned with those dynamics and their underlying ideologies. Race-based thinking, essential to European colonialism and slavery, has persisted in nursing, buttressed by liberal individualism, the ideology underlying capitalism.

DOI: 10.4324/9781003427407-43

The influence of colonialism, the legacy of chattel slavery and influences on thinking in nursing about race and racism

"The West" is an invented category, not a geographical reality, and was produced and deployed to facilitate white European imperialistic conquest. As Edward Said (1978, 1993) problematized, the scholarly production of "the West" and "the East" presents these entities as monolithic, static and oppositional. This process of discursive othering constructed "the West" as "superior" in contrast to "the East" as "inferior", and served to justify white European and American geopolitical domination, colonial occupation and exploitation. Understanding how "the West" was constructed offers a way to think about the evolution of "Western" nursing and its disciplinary orientation toward race and racism.

The concept of race was invented as a means of classifying human beings for the purpose of legitimizing the power of white people over Black and Brown people. Racial classification schemes were established during European colonialism and functioned as a tool of the empire to justify colonial expansion, state formation and the establishment of hierarchies that determined access to power in the form of material, social, cultural or natural resources.

As Rana Hogarth (2017) notes, physicians and scientists in the 18th and 19th centuries had a key role in "medicalizing" Blackness or constructing Blackness as a medically significant marker of difference. Physicians deployed science in the invention of race and racial hierarchies to reinforce and reproduce white privilege and power. The ideas of British and American race scientists were well-received in Canada, but used for specific ends. Canadian physicians argued that race science supported the assimilation of Indigenous peoples and the appropriation of material resources (land, natural resources). The ideological currents that underpin(ned) anti-Blackness are(were) extended to Indigenous bodies and knowledges. Nursing was infused with these prevailing forms of thinking.

At the end of the 19th century, white women sought to create and construct nursing as a "socially acceptable and respectable" profession for white women. In North America, women who were Indigenous, Black or People of Colour (IBPOC)[4] were either segregated in separate nursing schools (United States) or barred from entering nursing schools until the mid-20th century (Canada). Although IBPOC nurses were active in their communities and contributed to the development of nursing knowledge, anti-Black and anti-Indigenous sentiments founded on racist ideologies functioned to largely exclude non-white/non-dominant knowledges.

Although nurses trained in the Nightingale model[5] influenced reforms in nursing globally, the veneration of Nightingale as the "founder" of nursing[6] has (a) obscured the contributions of IBPOC nurses, (b) reinforced white, Anglocentric views of what it means to be a nurse and (c) perpetuated the dominance of Western-White-Eurocentric thinking that continues to dominate nursing. Imbricated within these legacies are the Christian roots of nursing's orientation toward charity for others (often racialized people). For example, in Canada, the French Catholic nursing tradition is often upheld as a heroic account of a vast nurse-run hospital system, with no mention of the negative impact Catholic missionaries had on Indigenous peoples. Professional nursing expanded globally in tandem with colonialism and imperialism. Consequently, whiteness has dominated nursing theorizing and philosophizing, and has shaped the definitions of professional nursing with little attention to the role of nurses in the inherently racist and materialist aims of colonial projects.

We highlight these contexts to draw attention to exclusions in nursing – that is, the exclusion of knowledges of IBPOC people, scholars and philosophical perspectives – and an overall lack of critical questioning about prevailing schools of thought. IBPOC folks who enter nursing schools typically encounter pedagogical systems that continue to denigrate and exclude subjugated knowledges.[7,8] In order to "make it", IBPOC nurses often have had to adapt and conform, or create their own covert politics of dissent within white colonial structures and institutions. Ongoing anti-Black and anti-Indigenous sentiments continue to exclude diversity of thought and philosophizing in nursing, further entrenching dominant thinking. The dynamics sustaining the dominance of Western-White-Eurocentric philosophical perspectives in nursing align with other well-argued critiques of nursing philosophical perspectives: nursing's alignment with scientific racism and uncritical engagement with race-based thinking, and nursing's uptake of liberal individualism.

Nursing's uncritical engagement with race-based thinking

The persistence of misinformed categorical conceptualizations of race as a biological entity in nursing research, education and philosophical thinking directly reflects the colonial context in which nursing's disciplinary knowledge has evolved. Despite repeated arguments dispelling myths about the biological basis of race-based categories, the idea that race is a biological category endures. As Gilroy (2000) has argued, the pervasiveness of "raciological thinking" is persistent, even among researchers and scholars who are attempting to orient themselves toward decolonial, intersectional theoretical and philosophical perspectives (p. 30). Despite widely accepted evidence to the contrary (e.g., Krieger, 2020; Roberts, 2021), race continues to be understood, taken up and presented in nursing research, textbooks and pedagogy as a biological reality, and as a legitimate category of difference. The often-unquestioned uptake in categorical uses of race as a stand-in for genetic differences, socioeconomic status and other social determinants of health continues to detract from examining the broader, complex, social and structural factors that lead to unfair and unjust social, economic, legal, political policies and systems that sustain racialized inequities.

These critiques of race-based thinking do not diminish the importance of continually recognizing the harms of racism (Koshy, 2021). As Gilroy (2000) reminds, the

> disruption of race-thinking presents an important opportunity. There is here a chance to break away from the dangerous and destructive patterns that were established when the rational absurdity of 'race' was elevated into an essential concept and endowed with a unique power to both determine history and explain its selective unfolding
>
> (p. 14)

Supporting such disruption in nursing requires fundamental shifts in philosophical thinking at a disciplinary level.

Philosophical inquiry requires that we critically reflect on knowledge claims, epistemological assumptions and predominant and often taken-for-granted patterns of thinking (Rehg & SmithBattle, 2015). For example, the genealogy of race-based thinking in nursing and science ought to be foregrounded in nursing analyses to scrutinize the philosophical motivations underpinning calls for more race-based evidence as prerequisite for anti-racism actions. Philosophical inquiry can enable us to tread cautiously, embrace a degree of tentativeness and avoid dogmatic philosophical positions; we are prompted to recognize that it is not as straightforward as saying, "dispense with race-based analyses". On the contrary, as Gilroy (2000) writes, for many, the "ideas of racial particularity… provide sources of pride" and "for many racialized populations, 'race' and the hard-won, oppositional identities it supports are not to be lightly or prematurely given up"…and may be "precious forms of solidarity and community" (pp. 12–13). Further, as noted below, scholars such as Krieger have deployed race-based data to demonstrate inequities (Krieger, 2012; Shavers et al., 2012).

While the axiom "no data, no problem" has been used strategically, both scientifically and politically, to make the impacts of racism visible (e.g., Krieger, 2012), there is now an extensive body evidence documenting the harms of racial categorizing, racism and intersecting forms of discrimination. This leads us to question whether calls for more "evidence to inform actions" can be interpreted as delay tactics or to deflect engagement with more radical actions. In the UK, the Workforce Race Equality Standard (WRES) serves as an example of how continuous data collection does little to redress inequities. Since 2016, the WRES has collected data on healthcare providers to document progress in addressing racial inequities in the National Health Service. In 2022, the WRES report identified that white applicants were more likely to be chosen from a shortlist of candidates than Black and Minority Ethnic (BME) applicants, and were more likely to be offered non-mandatory training and professional development (Wilkinson-Brice, 2022). BME staff continued to occupy fewer senior leadership positions and were more likely to experience harassment, bullying or abuse from staff, and discrimination at work. The overall lack of improvement since 2016 reflects a broader issue: a lack of change in the dominant institutional cultures and structures that maintain health and social inequities. Thus, the analytic leverage of philosophical inquiry lies in its potential to raise questions about the presumed assumption that more data are needed to support actions or changes at the structural level. It is worthwhile asking, for example, why is extant knowledge of health and social inequities not held out as a sufficient and credible body of evidence for implementing action? To whose benefit is it to continue to call for more race-based evidence as a requirement for action? How might current calls for evidence-based justifications as prerequisite for structural changes be exacerbating inequities? And, how does race-based data, typically collected at the individual level, reify individualism and obscure racialized collective patterns of inequity?

How liberal individualism continues to influence understandings of racism in nursing

Since the early 1990s, nursing scholars have drawn attention to the influence of liberal political ideology on nursing science, focusing on the impact of individualism, egalitarianism and a preference for politically neutral knowledge development (e.g., Browne, 2001; Doane & Varcoe, 2021; O'Neill, 1992). Currently, neoliberalism is increasingly co-constituted with race-based thinking to further entrench, for example, common sense populisms regarding the value of ethnonationalism, protectionism and xenophobia, creating a context for the normalization of racism and other forms of discrimination in everyday life, including new narratives of white victimhood and meritocratic-individualism (MacLeavy, 2019). The political backdrop of neoliberalism intersects with populist rhetoric about the ideals of corporate equity, diversity and inclusion (EDI) to dilute the critical social justice underpinnings of health equity aims. We see these "inclusionary" practices intersecting with deepening disinterest in analyses of how racism, power and privilege operate to shape health and healthcare – despite popularized calls within health sector for "more" EDI. With regard to implications for nursing, EDI discourses can give way to new forms of depoliticization, referring not to the removal of politics, but to the denial of politics as shaping social dynamics. Depoliticization also smooths the way for avoiding analyses of new variations of liberal-sounding, meritocratic discourses that further reinforce beliefs in systems as essentially egalitarian. In Canada, for example, liberal individualism combines with policy-entrenched multiculturalism to contribute to "democratic racism" and a climate which promotes rhetoric about Canada as a just society, while egregious forms of racism are tolerated, with "culture" frequently used as a euphemism for "race" (Henry et al., 2010, p. 15). Consequently, racialized others are held accountable for their life circumstances and health, simultaneously obscuring racialized patterns of inequity. For instance, lack of perinatal care and poor perinatal outcomes are often blamed on women and their "cultures" rather than understood as differential access due to rurality, poverty, avoidance of racism and so on.

Against this backdrop, "it is impossible to deny that we are living through a profound transformation in the way the idea of "race" [and racism] is understood and acted upon" (Gilroy, 2000, p. 12). While the anti-racist movements of 2020 may have heralded the start of new era of permissiveness in nursing with regard to critiques of racism, the pervasiveness of liberal individualistic understandings of racism continue to dominate, contributing to "a more individualistic anti-racist culture, which is keen on checking privilege and affirming the validity of other people's experiences, but has trouble creating durable institutions or political programmes" (Koshy, 2021). At a philosophical level, this reinforces the position that "because I am confident that personally I am not a racist, my behavior need not be called into question, and therefore I am under no obligation" to explore new perspectives that might unseat my assumptions, for example, that society (and healthcare) is essentially egalitarian, despite evidence to the contrary; that racism is ultimately the problem of a "few bad apples"; or that the problem of structural-level racism should be solved at the individual level in nursing by focusing on "training" to remediate individual behaviors. Thus, the notion of democratic racism continues to have currency as a philosophical frame of reference for explaining how racism can continue to exert its harmful effects at a systemic level while at the same time, nursing disciplinary doctrines such as Codes of Ethics and mission statements espouse liberal democratic principles of equality, tolerance, fairness, and the existence of an equal playing field, epitomized in the phrase, "we treat everyone equally", or "we are steadfastly colour blind" (Henry et al., 2010; Hilario et al., 2017). As Thorne (2022) recently emphasized, this kind of liberal individualistic stance and orientation can be depicted as the "reigning ideological buttress of a corresponding and distinct form of structural white supremacy" (Mueller, 2017, p. 220).

Despite the now often mandated requirements for addressing for EDI in health system strategic plans, these tend to be enacted at a rhetorical level in the absence of broad structural change, often reflecting "non-performative" diversity policies – in the sense that they pledge commitment to discursive EDI, but do not necessarily commit resources to enact concrete actions to transform institutional cultures (Ahenakew and Naepi, 2015). Thus, tokenism, rhetoric and surface level actions often function to protect deep structures, aligned with current politically correct discourses, and assuage guilt. As Gilroy writes in today's context, this can mean little more than "keeping unjust societies as they are, except with a few 'black and brown bodies' in the corporate boardrooms" (cited in Koshy, 2021). We argue that nursing has yet to fully grapple with the magnitude of these philosophical legacies. In the following section, we discuss approaches for transcending these structures underlying dominant thinking in nursing.

Part II: Leveraging philosophical inquiry to unseat the structures that influence our thinking in nursing

We have argued in the section above that philosophical and theoretical shifts are needed not only to tackle white dominance (Thorne, 2022) and inadequate anti-racist competence (Bell, 2021), but to develop strategic responses to "the discourses of individualism, multiculturalism, color blindness, political correctness and denial" that are often deployed by our profession to "reinforce the belief in an essentially fair and just society while avoiding the need to acknowledge the persistence of racist discourses and ideologies" (Hilario et al., 2017, p. 1). Next, we discuss three philosophical lenses useful in informing and unseating dominant thinking in nursing with regard to race and racism. We offer insights from what might be considered subjugated knowledges in the spirit of pushing back against any semblance of "intellectual complacency" (Koshy, 2021) in our disciplinary thinking and philosophizing in nursing about racism.

Chicana feminist thinking

Chicana feminist thought can be useful in eliminating the epistemic erasure and politics of exclusion rooted in and continuously asserted by Western-White-Eurocentric colonialism and coloniality. By centering this kind of thinking in nursing philosophy, the intention is not to "include them" (as an inclusionary othering practice), but to offer a new praxis of being. It is a (re)new(ed) philosophy about being and seeing the other that can support nursing in grappling with the influence of colonialism, chattel slavery and related discourses, mainly with regard to race-based thinking and individualism.

Chicana feminists' Borderlands theory and a "nos/otras" epistemology[9] directly critique notions of othering that gave rise to discourses deployed in service of historical and ongoing colonial expansionism and slavery. Centered on the lived experiences of Chicanas and using the U.S.-Mexican border as a metaphor, Chicana feminist Anzaldúa, a "border woman", lays the foundational ground for an ontological view of relationality. This view of relationality can be useful in unseating nursing's individualistic disciplinary orientation. For example, in Western ways of thinking, a border is a lugar (space) of division between us and them/the other, between the safe and unsafe, the "normal" and los atravesados (Anzaldúa, 2012). This way of being and seeing the other as different from oneself is constructed to reinforce a social hierarchy, excluding particular bodies and erasing ontologies and epistemologies that are not "like us" in order to "protect ourselves from them". In contrast, Anzaldúa (2012) sees the border as a place of transition between countries, cultures, languages and social systems. This "ethic of interconnectivity" that characterizes the border is what Anzaldúa reminded us of when telling "todas somos nos/otras" (Anzaldúa, 2002, p. 3), "who and what we are depends on those surrounding us, a mix of our interactions with our alrededores/ environments, with new and old narratives" (Anzaldúa, 2015, p. 69).

The interconnection between nos and nosotras, between us and our environments, offers a way to theorize about identity, as contextual and constructed by individual lives, experiences and intergenerational learning, ourselves and our environments. Identity is also boundaryless, fluid and ever-evolving, in opposition to binary constructions of identity (e.g. women/men, femininity/masculinity). In the discourse on race within nursing, this conceptualization of identity reminds us that the focus is not solely on a critique of the problematic and wrongful acceptance of race as a biological reality. The problem is also tethered to its use as an exclusionary categorization of difference, by which peoples' identities are constructed thus diminishing individual lived and living experiences and the environment. Such exclusionary categorizations reify, protect and maintain power differentials, the us versus them, under the guise of defining identity.

Recognizing the interconnectivity among nosotras will also allow the creation of bridges. Bridging is leaving the safety of our existing knowledges (Anzaldúa, 2002); it is a back-and-forth process of questioning our existing ontologies and epistemologies while simultaneously creating relationships with those who might be on the opposite shore. Bridging is not a form of inclusionary othering – there is no inclusion or othering because nosotras is an epistemology against division and separation – it is pro-coalition, an antithesis to othering and a praxis of being in relation with all of us.

Black feminist thought

While Chicana feminism deconstructs the ontologies and epistemologies of othering, individualism and exclusion that are built in the scaffolding of the settler-colonial project, intersectionality through the lens of Black feminism can help expand understandings of categories of difference reconstructed by discourses centered on systems of power (Collins, 2019). Black feminism is a standpoint rooted in the lived experiences of African-American women that arose as a disruption to the hegemonic canon of white middle-class liberal feminism, and has extended throughout the African diaspora (Barriteau, 2009; Collective, 1982; Collins, 2000, 2022). For nursing, Black feminist thought prompts engagement in philosophical inquiries that consider the dominance of white privilege, discrimination, racism and the other various intersectional systems of power.

Intersectionality as the paradigm that underpins Black feminist thought favors a structural analysis of health inequities experienced by made-marginalized individuals by offering an analytic viewpoint for nursing praxis that considers the web of systems of power (i.e. racism, sexism, cis-heteronormativity, ableism, classism and so forth), the trappings of coloniality and their influence on individuals and their collective experiences (De Sousa & Varcoe, 2022). By drawing attention to systems of power, away from the problematics of the categorizations of identity (and difference) and individualism, intersectionality underlies a structural analysis that can move nursing to rekindle its interest and action toward the actual problems that drive health inequities (Anderson, 2002, 2004a, 2004b). Anderson (2004a), drawing on theoretical underpinnings from Collin's (2000) scholarship on postcolonial feminism, raises questions at a philosophical level that we see as crucial to continually ask, such as: to what extent are we, as members of a privileged group ("the centre") constructing a marginalized and racialized other?; how is this reinforcing positions of power at the center?; what resistances and tensions arise as privilege is contested?; and, what are the ways in which we in nursing might be reinforcing the very power structures we seek to dismantle, by undermining resistances at "the margins"? In the process, we are inspired to revisit the analyses that Anderson (2004a) urges: "how might we move forward as we work towards a liberatory discourse?" by exposing "how privilege is retained by some and denied to others", and "by making situated experience the starting point of analysis, instead of the 'categories' in which we are positioned" (p. 14).

Indigenous knowledges

Indigenous knowledges are invaluable in expanding dominant philosophical thinking in nursing and the health sciences (Ahenakew, 2016, 2019; Crosschild et al., 2021), pushing beyond the prevailing knowledges that structure thinking in nursing about racism. Indigenous scholars highlight the pervasiveness of cognitive imperialism as a form of cognitive manipulation used to repudiate the value of other knowledge bases, and as directly linked to the settler architecture used to justify ongoing Indigenous dispossession and oppression (Battiste, 2005). These perspectives have ramifications for nursing's engagement with issues of racism, and the colonial and postcolonial enterprise focused on the accumulation and protection of material wealth and privilege (Coulthard, 2014). Colonial dispossessions of Indigenous peoples are inextricably connected to the advancement of White-Western-Eurocentric rationalization and discourses of Indigenous "savagery" and "deficiency", all salient features of cognitive imperialism and conquest. Specifically, White-Western-Eurocentric ideas, such as individualism, science, capitalism and Christianity, were driving forces that placed Indigenous peoples into a society predicated on their dispossession and desired elimination (Wolfe, 2006). This imperialist world-making project is concerned with the material restructuring of the world wherein White-Western-Eurocentric ways of being and knowing have been ascribed as universal common sense (Smith, 2012). According to Maori scholar Linda Tuhiwai Smith (2012), material conquest was tethered to the notion of "progress" as the signifier to assert "a sense of innate superiority and an overabundance of desire to bring progress into the lives of indigenous peoples" (p. 114).

Nursing as a discipline and the prevailing genres of philosophical thinking that shape our discipline are often overlooked as contributing to settler-colonial agendas, including actions or inaction related to systemic racism and the impacts on health (Burnett, 2007; Henry et al., 2018). At the core of the discipline, nursing philosophy values and privileges White-Western-Eurocentric philosophical paradigms that continue to exert power through the subordination of Indigenous knowledges by depicting them as inferior, primitive or as non-knowledges altogether (Battiste, 2011).

Indigenous knowledges and philosophies are articulated through notions of energy, offering nursing the potential to disrupt both the process of othering, which is essential to racism, and individualism, which obscures the structural and material conditions shaping health. In this understanding of Blackfoot paradigms, Little Bear (2000) explains Indigenous knowledges and philosophies as articulated through ontologies of human/non-human relationality:

> The idea of all things being in constant motion or flux leads to a holistic and cyclical view of the world. If everything is constantly moving and changing, then one has to look at the whole to begin to see patterns.
>
> (p. 78)

While Indigenous knowledges can make visible and mitigate colonial knowledge systems, care must be taken in doing so. Indigenous knowledges have been appropriated and misappropriated to advance colonial aims of conquest (Kelm, 1998). For instance, Maslow's Hierarchy of Needs was appropriated from the Blackfoot beliefs and value systems (Feigenbaum & Smith, 2019). Briefly, Maslow's theory suggests that humans can achieve their individual potential through levels of motivating factors beginning with fulfilling the most basic of needs (food, clothing, shelter), advancing to safety, security, love and intimacy, and self-esteem. Maslow spent time on the Blackfoot reserve with friends who were conducting anthropological research. Blackfoot value systems inherently shaped his model and "Theory of Human Behavior" (Maslow, 1943), which is widely used in alignment with liberal individualism and the promotion of capitalist consumerism.

One of the many problems with appropriating Indigenous knowledges is that the intended teachings or messages that do not fit within the parameters of White-Western-Eurocentric rationalization are often missed entirely. For example, Maslow's White-Western-Eurocentric lens and valuing of individualism dismissed Indigenous philosophy and the valuing of holism inherent in Blackfoot philosophy. Blackfoot philosophies, specifically the Blackfoot value of relationality between human and non-human kin, push the concept of self-actualization past the individual and toward the collective, including the natural environment. From a Blackfoot perspective, the purpose of achieving self-actualization is not to benefit self, but to benefit the collective.

Such approaches could offer nursing an enhanced perspective on race and racism by expanding these concepts past individuals to collectives, collectives that comprise human and non-human kin, explicitly thinking about the relationships nurses and nursing have with places (geographical locations, facilities, etc.), spaces (environments, history, etc.) and structures (institutions, language, etc.). The intention is not to bifurcate values of individualism and collectivism, but to consider how Blackfoot philosophy offers understanding of the world outside of singularity, objectivity, conquest, and individualism. Racism can then be understood as a structural issue that is deeply entrenched in the culture of nursing – in our history, norms, traditions, and organization – and functions to uphold privileges of whiteness and resources (Crosschild & Varcoe, 2021).

Utilizing philosophies that push the bounds of nursing knowledge is essential to the growth of the discipline. Nursing can move toward deeper structural analyses by drawing on diverse philosophies, such as the examples we offer above, and asking thought provoking questions. What knowledges are used in nursing that we take for granted or deem as common sense? How might we challenge ourselves to reach a position of self-actualization that also is accountable to the collective? Moreover, how might we push the discipline to expand its philosophical underpinnings to recognize various intersectional forms of power including racism?

Closing comments

In nursing, and society at large, we often overlook how racism is intertwined with political-economic realities and real material resources. In Western societies, we tolerate or even applaud consumerism and wealth accumulation; however, we do so at the expense of ignoring the ongoing appropriation of Indigenous lands and resources, and contemporary forms of slave labor of racialized others. Without discounting the harms of oppression, we call for alternate angles of inquiry, not necessarily "about" oppression, but about upholding dominance, whiteness and privilege, particularly (in the case of this chapter) in relation to philosophizing in nursing. This requires grappling with philosophical questions regarding how society and dominant forms of knowledge structure our thinking about the existential problem of racism, and how these structures and knowledges exert their influence within systems of power. These are philosophical issues that require re-thinking. As Harding (2015) enjoins, "finding or creating even just a little distance from prevailing assumptions and interests can be sufficient to enable critical perspectives to illuminate issues in new ways" (p. 10). Hence, we urge nurses to undertake philosophical inquiry with constant attention to the pernicious effects of approaches steeped in race-based thinking. Chicana feminism, Black feminism and Indigenous knowledges are examples of philosophical approaches that can support nursing to mitigate the impact of its colonial and race-based roots toward evolving our knowledge-base in support of equity, collective wellbeing and population health.

Notes

1 "Subaltern" is used to draw attention to knowledges subjugated within the dynamics of race-class-gender and colonial conquest (Spivak, 1988).
2 The Blackfoot are a North American Indigenous tribe that crosses the Canadian and American border in southern Alberta and northern Montana. The Blackfoot Confederacy is composed of four Nations: Kainai, Piikani, Amskapi Piikani and Siksika.
3 "Whiteness" is not used to mean "the identity of white people", but to conceptualize the historical legacy of colonialism, chattel slavery and imperialism, the foundation for and justification of white privilege and form of structural privilege (Rasmussen et al., 2001). Except for "Western-White-Eurocentric", "white" and "whiteness" will not be capitalized to decenter whiteness as the standard and norm (Backhouse, 1999).
4 This acronym reflects populations and terminology used in Canada. In jurisdictions such as the UK, other terms are used, e.g., Black, Asian and Minority Ethnic (BAME).
5 Nursing in the Nightingale tradition involved a personal and professional pledge to a particular Christian, colonial ontological and epistemological orientation (McCallum, 2014). In North America, the Nightingale pledge was used until recently, and its use continues in various contexts, e.g., in Portugal and Ecuador.
6 Nursing has a longer history than typically acknowledged. In Japan, the career of Iwako Uryu (born in 1829) paralleled Nightingale's. Long before white European settlers colonized North America and established hospitals and nursing schools, Indigenous peoples had extensive healing traditions and health practices with formalized social structures for care.
7 "Subjugated knowledges" as articulated by Foucault (1980) include forms of "erudite" knowledges and "disqualified" knowledges (Bacchi, 2022).
8 The colonization of nursing is extensive, structuring educational curricula, professional debates, and tenure and scholarly trajectories for nurse researchers globally.
9 In offering an interpretation of the literary works of Anzaldúa, we do not seek to ignore other Chicano/a/x authors or Chicana feminisms writ large.

References

Ahenakew, C. (2016). Grafting Indigenous ways of knowing onto non-Indigenous ways of being: The (underestimated) challenges of a decolonial imagination. *International Review of Qualitative Research*, 9(3), 323–340.

Ahenakew, C. (2019). *Toward scarring our collective soul wounds*. Guelph: Musagetes. https://decolonialfutures.net/towardsscarring/

Ahenakew, C., & Naepi, S. (2015). The difficult task of turning walls into tables. In A. Macfarlane, M. Webber, & S. Macfarlane (Eds.), *Sociocultural theory: Implications for curricular across the sector* (pp. 181–194). Christchurch: University of Canterbury Press.

Anderson, J. M. (2002). Toward a postcolonial feminist methodology in nursing: Exploring the convergence of postcolonial and black feminist scholarship. *The International Journal of Research Methodology in Nursing and Health Care*, 9(3), 7–27. http://web.ebscohost.com/ehost/detail?vid=15&hid=8&sid=61ee7910-b7b6-4c5b-b273-1dbc493b63e8%40sessionmgr7

Anderson, J. M. (2004a). The conundrums of binary categories: Critical inquiry through the lens of postcolonial feminist humanism. *Canadian Journal of Nursing Research*, 36(4), 11–16.

http://web.ebscohost.com/ehost/detail?vid=25&hid=8&sid=61ee7910-b7b6-4c5b-b273-1dbc493b63e8%40sessionmgr7

Anderson, J. M. (2004b). Lessons from a postcolonial-feminist perspective: Suffering and a path to healing. *Nursing Inquiry, 11*(4), 238–246. https://doi.org/10.1111/j.1440-1800.2004.00231.x

Anzaldúa, G. (2002). (Un)natural bridges, (un)safe spaces. In G. K. Anzaldua (Ed.), *This bridge we call home: Radical visions for transformation* (pp. 1–5). New York: Taylor & Francis Group. https://doi.org/10.4324/9780203952962

Anzaldúa, G. (2012). *Borderlands: The new mestiza = la frontera* (4th ed.). San Francisco, CA: Aunt Lute Books.

Anzaldúa, G. (2015). *Light in the dark - Luz en lo oscuro: Rewriting identity, spirituality, reality* (A. Keating, Ed.). Durham, NC: Duke University Press.

Bacchi, C. (2022). *"Situated knowledges" OR "subjugated knowledges"*. Retrieved from https://carolbacchi.com/2018/09/03/situated-knowledges-or-subjugated-knowledges/

Backhouse, C., & Osgoode Society for Canadian Legal, H. (1999). *Colour-coded: a legal history of racism in Canada, 1900–1950*. Published for the Osgoode Society for Canadian Legal History by University of Toronto Press, Toronto.

Barriteau, V. E. (2009). The relevance of Black feminist scholarship: A Caribbean perspective. In S. M. James, F. S. Foster, & B. Guy-Sheftall (Eds.), *Still brave: The evolution of Black women's studies* (pp. 413–434). New York: The Feminist Press.

Battiste, M. (2005). Indigenous knowledge: Foundations for First Nations. *World Indigenous Nations Higher Education Consortium (WINHEC) Journal, 1*(1), 1–12.

Battiste, M. (2011). Cognitive imperialism and decolonizing research. In C. Reilly, V. Russell, L.K. Chehayl, & M. M. McDermott (Eds.), *Surveying borders, boundaries, and contested spaces in curriculum and pedagogy* (pp. xv–xxviii). Charlotte, NC: Information Age Publishing.

Bell, B. (2021). White dominance in nursing education: A target for anti-racist efforts. *Nursing Inquiry, 28*(1), e12379–n/a. https://doi.org/10.1111/nin.12379

Browne, A. J. (2001). The influence of liberal political ideology on nursing science. *Nursing Inquiry, 8*(2), 118–129. https://doi.org/10.1046/j.1440-1800.2001.00095.x

Burnett, K. (2007). *Building the system: Churches, missionary organizations, the Federal state, and health care in southern Alberta Treaty 7 communities, 1890–1930. Journal of Canadian Studies, 41*(3), 18–41. https://doi.org/10.3138/jcs.41.3.18.

Collective, T. C. R. (1982). A Black feminist statement. In G. T. S. Hull, P. Bell-Scott, & B. Smith (Eds.), *All the women are white, all the blacks are men, but some of us are brave: Black women's studies* (pp. 13–22). The Feminist Press. The Combahee River Collective.

Collins, P. H. (2000). *Black feminist thought: Knowledge, consciousness, and the politics of empowerment* (2nd ed.). New York: Routledge.

Collins, P.H. (2019). *Intersectionality as critical social theory*. Durham, NC: Duke University Press.

Collins, P. H. (2022). *Black feminist thought, 30th anniversary edition. Knowledge, consciousness, and the politics of empowerment*. New York: Routledge.

Coulthard, G. S. (2014). *Red skin, white masks: Rejecting the colonial politics of recognition*. Minneapolis: University of Minnesota Press. https://doi.org/https://doi.org/10.5749/minnesota/9780816679645.001.0001

Crosschild, C., Huynh, N., De Sousa, I., Bawafaa, E., & Brown, H. (2021). Where is critical analysis of power and positionality in knowledge translation? *Health Research Policy and Systems, 19*(1), 92–92. https://doi.org/10.1186/s12961-021-00726-w

Crosschild, C., & Varcoe, C. (2021). Commentary: Piinaat'stikaanookiinan: A call to action for nursing leaders to decolonize nursing. *Nursing Leadership (Toronto, Ont.), 34*(4), 144–150. https://doi.org/10.12927/cjnl.2021.26677

De Sousa, I., & Varcoe, C. (2022). Centering Black feminist thought in nursing praxis. *Nursing Inquiry, 29*(1). https://doi.org/10.1111/nin.12473

Doane, G. H., & Varcoe, C. (2021). *How to nurse: Relational inquiry in action* (2nd ed.). Philadelphia, PA: Wolters Kluwer.

Feigenbaum, K. D., & Smith, R. A. (2019). Historical narratives: Abraham Maslow and Blackfoot interpretations. *The Humanistic Psychologist*, 48(3), 232–243. https://doi.org/10.1037/hum0000145

Foucault, M. 1980. Two lectures. In C. Gordon (Ed.), *Michel Foucault power/knowledge: Selected interviews and other writings 1972–1977 by Michel Foucault*. New York: Pantheon Books.

Gilroy, P. (2000). *Against race: Imagining political culture beyond the color line*. Cambridge, MA: The Belknap Press of Harvard University Press.

Harding, S. G. e., U. (2015). *Objectivity and diversity: Another logic of scientific research*. Chicago, IL: The University of Chicago Press. https://press.uchicago.edu/ucp/books/book/chicago/O/bo19804521.html

Henry, F., Rees, T., & Tator, C. (2010). *The colour of democracy: Racism in Canadian society* (4th ed.). Toronto, ON: Thomas Nelson.

Henry, R., LaVallee, A., Van Styvendale, N., & Innes, R. A. (Eds.). (2018). *Global indigenous health: Reconciling the past, engaging the present, animating the future*. Tucson: The University of Arizona Press. https://doi.org/https://doi.org/10.2307/j.ctv513dtj.

Hilario, C. T., Browne, A. J., & McFadden, A. (2017). The influence of democratic racism in nursing inquiry. *Nursing Inquiry*, 25(1), e12213, Article e12213. https://doi.org/10.1111/nin.12213

Hogarth, R. (2017). *Medicalizing blackness: Making racial difference in the Atlantic world, 1780–1840*. Chapel Hill: University of North Carolina Press.

Kelm, M.-E. (1998). *Colonizing bodies: Aboriginal health and healing in British Columbia 1900–1950*. Vancouver: UBC Press. https://go.exlibris.link/8lB7jwg5

Koshy, Y. (2021). The last humanist: How Paul Gilroy became the most vital guide to our age of crisis. https://www.theguardian.com/news/2021/aug/05/paul-gilroy-britain-scholar-race-humanism-vital-guide-age-of-crisis

Krieger, N. (2012). Methods for scientific study of discrimination and health: An ecosocial approach. *American Journal of Public Health*, 102(5), 936–945. https://doi.org/10.2105/AJPH.2011.300544

Krieger, N. (2020). Measures of racism, sexism, heterosexism, and gender binarism for health equity research: From structural injustice to embodied harm—an ecosocial analysis. *Annual Review of Public Health*, 41(1). https://doi.org/10.1146/annurev-publhealth-040119-094017

Little Bear, L. (2000). Jagged worldviews colliding. In M. Battiste (Ed.), *Reclaiming Indigenous voice and vision* (pp. 77–85). Vancouver: UBC Press.

McCallum, M. J. L. (2014). *Indigenous women, work and history 1940–1980*. Winnipeg: University of Manitoba Press.

MacLeavy, J. (2019). Neoliberalism and the new political crisis in the West. *Ephemera*, 19(3), 627–640. http://www.ephemerajournal.org/contribution/neoliberalism-and-new-political-crisis-west

Maslow, A. H. (1943). A theory of human behavior. *Psychological Review*, 50, 370–396.

Mueller, J. C. (2017). Producing colorblindness: Everyday mechanisms of white ignorance. *Social problems (Berkeley, Calif.)*, 64(2), 219–332. https://doi.org/10.1093/socpro/spw061

O'Neill, S. (1992). The drive for professionalism in nursing: A reflection of classism and racism. In J. L. Thompson, D. Allen, & L. Rodrigues-Fisher (Eds.), *Critique, resistance, and action: Working papers in the politics of nursing: Papers from the second national conference on critical and feminist perspectives in nursing*, Toledo, OH.

Rasmussen, B. B., Klinenberg, E., Nexica, I. J., & Wray, M. (2001). *The making and unmaking of whiteness*. Durham, NC: Duke University Press.

Rehg, E., & SmithBattle, L. (2015). On to the 'rough ground': Introducing doctoral students to philosophical perspectives on knowledge. *Nursing Philosophy*, 16(2), 98–109. https://doi.org/10.1111/nup.12077

Roberts, D. E. (2021). Abolish race correction. *The Lancet (British edition)*, 397(10268), 17–18. https://doi.org/10.1016/S0140-6736(20)32716-1

Said, E. W. (1978). *Orientalism*. London: Routledge & Kegan Paul Ltd.

Said, E. W. (1993). *Culture and imperialism*. New York: Knopf.

Shavers, V. L., Klein, W. M. P., & Fagan, P. (2012). Research on race/ethnicity and health care discrimination: Where we are and where we need to go. *American Journal of Public Health*, 102(5), 930–932. https://doi.org/10.2105/AJPH.2012.300708

Smith, L. T. (2012). *Decolonizing methodologies: research and indigenous peoples* (2nd ed.). London: Zed Books.

Spivak, G. C. (1988). Can the subaltern speak? In C. Nelson & L. Grossberg (Eds.), *Marxism and the interpretation of culture* (pp. 271–313). Urbana, IL: Macmillan Education.

Thorne, S. (2022). Moving beyond performative allyship. *Nursing Inquiry*, 29(1), e12483.

Wilkinson-Brice, E. E., A. (2022). *NHS Workforce Race Equality Standard*. https://www.england.nhs.uk/wp-content/uploads/2022/04/Workforce-Race-Equality-Standard-report-2021-.pdf

Wolfe, P. (2006). Settler colonialism and the elimination of the native. *Journal of Genocide Research*, 8(4), 387–409.

38 Perpetuating the whiteness of nursing
Enculturation and nurse education

Debra Jackson

Introduction

As a service discipline and an area of research and scientific endeavour, nursing stands on a platform of equity of health care for all people and recognition of the essential humanity and dignity of all people. These espoused values can be clearly seen in the numerous professional proclamations, declarations and mission statements that are used to describe, represent and govern nursing. Such statements appear in multiple nurse education documents such as curricula documents and subject outlines, and also frequently appear on web sites of schools and nursing organisations and influential and authoritative bodies. Furthermore, despite declared platforms of equity and inclusion, and the frequent statements that assert the commitment to social justice, oppression and privilege, based on colour and race, continue to dominate nursing. However, there is compelling evidence of white dominance in nurse education.

Many years ago, when I was a student of nursing, I can remember hearing talk of *the whiteness of nursing*, and (a much younger me) can remember being confused by this. On hearing this term, I would look around at my peers and colleagues many who were from First Nations communities, all regions of the world, and all cultural and socio-economic backgrounds, and think, well, perhaps in some places this may be the case, but not here. It took me many more years, to work out that 'white' is so much more than a category of skin colour (Puzin 2003), and that this phrase, *the whiteness of nursing*, refers to the seen and the unseen, the acknowledged and the unacknowledged discourses that shape nursing. Whiteness forms the means through which power is distributed and held in nursing, and the ways that people of all cultural backgrounds become enculturated into Western nursing.

In this chapter, I will consider enculturation as it relates to nurse education, and in particular, focus on the dominant orthodoxies and discourses in nursing, and how in adopting and accepting these, nursing students may become blinded to alternate ways of thinking and seeing the world. I argue that nurse educational programmes promulgate *the whiteness of nursing*, through *enculturation of whiteness*. Enculturation into white normativity is reproduced and regularised through the teaching strategies and artefacts that are used, and this enculturation affects the ways that nursing students are able to understand, speak, relate to and meet (or not) the needs of diverse communities within and without of nursing.

Becoming a nurse

Students of nursing enter into a range of educational programmes that are designed to provide graduates with the knowledge and skills to effectively practice as a nurse. Through their programmes of study, students are socialised and enculturated into

DOI: 10.4324/9781003427407-44

nursing. Over time, they are exposed to the knowledge, attitudes and ideas that will shape their thoughts about being a nurse, the values they hold as a nurse, and the ways they enact nursing. This process is part of socialisation and enculturation into nursing. Socialisation and enculturation are used as synonyms in many instances. *Enculturation* (also inculturation) is the term to describe the process in which the behaviours and values associated with the culture or group are gradually acquired. Generally, enculturation is not overtly or deliberately taught; rather, enculturation occurs as a result of cultural knowledge being acquired through prolonged and direct observation of others within the culture. *Socialisation* into nursing refers to the process of acquiring the norms, values and roles associated with nursing and how to respond and interact in ways that are acceptable and understood within the context of being a nurse. Many learning activities in nurse education are provided with a view to aiding student socialisation into nursing.

Much nurse education takes place on university campuses and in other, similar institutions of higher education. These settings have been described as bastions of 'privileged whiteness and white supremacy' (Bell 2020: 9) that are privileged and elite settings dominated by white ways of being, doing and thinking, and in which other forms of knowing, such as culturally informed knowledge(s), are subjugated, marginalised and devalued. In addition to on-campus learning, a considerable amount of undergraduate learning also occurs in health care settings and services. Writing from an Australian Aboriginal perspective, Nielsen, Stuart and Gorman (2014) assert that white cultural norms and expectations permeate the Australian health care system. Furthermore, during clinical practice learning, students may not have the opportunity to work alongside Black, Indigenous or persons of colour as colleagues, because of underrepresentation of some populations within nursing (Nielsen, Stuart & Gorman 2014).

Through the educational activities held in on-campus and clinical sites, students are not only exposed to opportunities to develop the knowledge and skills needed to be a nurse, they are actively absorbing the culture of nursing. Through their teaching and learning activities and through exposure to nurses' work and observation of how nurses are in the world, students are able to learn what is expected of nurses, how nurses can and should respond to particular situations, what it means to be a 'good' nurse, and what 'acceptable' behaviour in nurses looks like. Over time, students come to internalise these (and other) ideas and patterns of behaviour.

The nature of nurse education

In reflecting on nurse education and on how it is framed and constructed, it is important to take a moment to consider both liberal and vocational educational ideologies. *Liberal education* refers to a broad, general education and preparation for leadership, based on the development of intellectual abilities, whereas *vocational education* has more of a narrow focus on the development and acquisition of professional skills for purposes of employment. Paterson (2015: 11) describes liberal education as having a concern with 'what kind of person it [education] would shape – not just facts or ideas they would learn'. The importance of students of nursing having a 'solid base in liberal education' (AACN 2008) has been recognised by influential and authoritative bodies as being essential to the continued development of the discipline and such an education has even been described as the 'cornerstone for the practice and education of nurses' (AACN 2008). The American Association of Colleges of Nursing (2008) identified nine essential graduate outcomes for baccalaureate nurses and the first of these was for a liberal education as a 'distinguishing cornerstone for the study and practice of professional nursing' (AACN 2008: 11), and called for integration of liberal and nursing education (AACN 2008: 12).

Achieving liberal education for nurses has proven to be easier said than done. Nursing is first and foremost a practice discipline and so when designing educational programmes for nursing, providers are required to have a familiarity with the requirements for nurse registration in their jurisdictions, and design and deliver learning activities to ensure that graduates can meet the requirements of registration authorities. Ideally, students are exposed to concepts that also foster critical thinking, understanding of human experience, cultural and spiritual knowledge, the ability to find, critically analyse and interpret information, as well as a spirit of scholarly enquiry and openness to ideas.

In reality however, nursing has had a difficult relationship with what might be called the more liberal aspects of nurse education. Carr (2009) wrote of the tensions between liberal and vocational approaches to education, and this he terms the liberal-vocational dichotomy. This dichotomy is clearly evident when considering nurse education. There is a large discourse on the 'theory-practice gap' (Allmark 1995), and in 1986 in a very influential work, Dunlop posed the question 'is a science of caring possible', in which distinctions between a science for caring and a science of caring were drawn. Walker (1997) described the process of 'enfleshment' through the 'training' of nurses, and how through this process, nurses came to understand that being a 'good' nurse meant being busy, nice, obedient and docile (Walker 1997). Writing more recently Walker (2009) examined the undergraduate nursing curriculum in Australia to reveal continued tensions between 'book' learning and clinical learning. Tensions between 'thinking' and 'doing' nursing (Walker 1997) (also known as the theory-practice gap) dominated the development of nursing curricula and the application of pedagogy in nurse education.

Despite the move from an apprenticeship style model of learning in many parts of the world, nurse education remains subject to the external oversight of various regulatory bodies who are charged with the responsibility for monitoring, approving and reviewing the development and implementation of nursing curricula. This means groups external to the educational provider are able to exercise ultimate control over what is taught to students of nursing, how it is taught and by whom. Even though nursing regulatory bodies often have strong mission statements attesting to their commitment to diversity, equity and inclusion, many of these regulatory bodies are primarily concerned with provision of a docile workforce ready to 'hit the ground running' (Wilson et al. 2020) to (mostly) hospital or other in-patient settings, and so there is often a focus on the rapid acquisition of clinical skills or competencies, frequently at the expense of socio-political content. The ideologies of those who have the power to shape and control the development and delivery of curricula in nursing may therefore be at odds with the more liberal aspirations of university-based educators, meaning that attempts to add more of a liberal flavour to nurse education may be stifled by regulatory bodies who tend to be more focussed on the acquisition of vocation knowledge and skills. This focus on the acquisition of (psychomotor) skills over a more liberal approach to education is in line with the strongly vocational educational roots of nursing.

Furthermore, an audit of the persons who comprise membership of the regulatory bodies with oversight of the nursing curriculum generally reveals homogeneous groups of people who collectively, in no way embody the diversity and inclusion statements of the organisations they represent. In addition, mechanisms for authentic engagement by influential and authoritative nursing bodies (including regulatory bodies) generally do not reveal robust and transparent procedures for genuine engagement and involvement with minority communities.

Whiteness in nursing curricula

At this point, it is useful to consider the formal, informal and hidden aspects of curricula (Hafferty and Franks 1994). These aspects have been framed as being multidimensional and interrelated (Raso et al. 2019). The formal curriculum refers to the intended and stated outcomes of the curriculum as represented in official documents and statements of intent (such as graduate attribute statements); the informal curriculum refers to the learning that occurs beyond the traditional teaching and learning setting, The hidden curricula refer to the unintended and unstated values that are passed on through learning activities and the ways these act to shape and reinforce social and professional norms, values and behaviours, and have been linked to the development of professional identity (Raso et al. 2019).

Most nursing curricula feature preambles, or other introductory statements, many of which include declarations attesting to the host institutions' strong commitment to diversity, equity, inclusion, social justice, respect for and recognition of the importance of cultural values in health care and other similar sentiments. They generally go on to state that these beliefs both reflect the beliefs of the organisation and inform the development and delivery of curricula. However, recent evidence suggests this is not the case, and that such sentiments and ideologies are not making through to the classroom. Reporting a United Kingdom-based study on nurse education in relation to pressure injuries, Oozageer Gunowa et al. (2021) found that classroom teaching activities were:

> predominately framed through a white lens with white normativity being strongly reinforced... through two main themes: (i) dominance of whiteness in the teaching and learning of pressure injuries in undergraduate nurse education and (ii) the impact and implications for student nurses of whiteness as the norm in pressure injury teaching
>
> (Oozageer Gunowa et al. 2021: 4511)

There is compelling evidence that within nursing curricula, cultural issues are presented in ways that reinforce whiteness as normative, and through the lens of cultural diversity, students of nursing are schooled that health beliefs and practices of cultural minority groups must be identified and reframed within a white and colonialist model of health care (Puzin 2003, Oozageer Gunowa et al. 2021). This is evident both in classroom teaching settings and through analysis of curricula documents (Oozageer Gunowa et al. 2020, 2021). Where health-related racial disparities exist, these are often presented to students as being rooted in biology rather than being a result of race-based oppression (Bell 2020). Bell (2020) has positioned this (mis)representation of race as 'a major ongoing flaw in nursing education... which reproduces scientific racism in the form of deficit thinking' (p.4). She goes on to cite numerous examples of scientific literature in which racial disparities are noted and presented as biologically significant, with a failure to acknowledge or address the racist oppression that contributes to these health outcomes. When considering whiteness in relation to nurse education, Puzin commented:

> Whiteness is depicted not as a preordained biological property, but as a socially constructed category of race, wherein non-white people are racially designated, while whites escape such designation and occupy positions which allow them to carry on as if what they say is neutral, rather than historically and ideologically situated.
>
> (Puzin 2003: 193).

Deficit discourses

Health education, including nurse education, is shaped, informed and under-pinned by deficit discourses. The term *deficit discourses* refers to narratives that characterise people in terms of failure, negativity and deficiency (Smallwood et al. 2022), and apportions blame and responsibility to people for their own predicaments without considering the socio-economic factors that create social inequity (Fogarty et al. 2018). Deficit discourses are pervasive and become unquestioningly accepted, and so because of this can be ingrained into the thinking and attitudes of university staff. Active measures are required to shift these ingrained deficit views (O'Shea et al. 2016, Curtis et al. 2021).

Much of what is considered scientific or scholarly writing in relation to Black, Indigenous and minority ethnic communities is deficit-focussed and contributes to a racially based, discriminatory and marginalising narrative (Bell 2020). This deficit narrative is evident in many articles and papers in the literature, and reinforces deficit-focussed ways of seeing people, particularly people from minority backgrounds (Smallwood et al. 2022). This deficit-focussed standpoint then becomes part of the broader discourses that reinforce enculturation of whiteness and white cultural dominance in nurse education. For the purposes of this current discussion, it is important to recognise the discourses of colonisation and how they are presented to students of nursing through their learning, and how this contributes to continued deficit ways of framing minority people, communities and populations.

Denial and silence around racism

Racism is known to be harmful to people and has been linked to multiple health and social issues. Many health services and systems feature entrenched systemic racism (Davidson et al. 2012), and so (unsurprisingly) there is a long history of disparity and inequity in health services along racial lines. The outcomes of this inequity can be seen in the copious data that reveals people belonging to racial and ethnic minorities suffer greater levels of sickness, disability and death than white populations, and that this occurs across the spectrum of health conditions, including hypertension, cardiovascular disease, diabetes, renal disease and childbirth outcomes, as well as life expectancy and barriers to accessing health care (Leech et al. 2019, Williamson et al. 2021, CDC 2022, Yan Li et al. 2022). For these reasons alone – its harmful effects on people and communities, and the role of nursing in upholding racist systems, racism should be prominent in nursing curricula. However, it has been noted that talk of racism in nursing is largely taboo (Barbee 1993, Thorne 2017).

When we think of racism, many people think of overt racism, of racism that is easy to recognise – of white supremacist groups or of people who openly and actively dislike and or seek to harm persons of particular racial backgrounds. However, in reality and much more often, racism can be far more complex and nuanced; and in nursing has been described as 'subtle and mundane' (Mapedzahama et al. 2012); more in keeping with the concept of 'everyday racism' which is easily overlooked and dismissed. Though subtle and mundane, it is none-the-less- powerful, and Allen (2022) argues that not only is racism present in nursing, nursing is complicit in upholding racist health systems and services. Racism is evident interpersonally and structurally in nursing and has been so since the beginning of modern nursing and nurse education. Reflecting on the history of nurse education, Barbee (1993: 347) has articulated how Black nurses have been marginalised within nursing, and how the racially bound experiences and concerns of minority nurses are 'trivialized, marginalised and denied' by white nurses.

Many authors have noted the absence of acknowledgement of racism in nursing curricula, position statements, policies, and other guiding documents. In 1993, when considering racism in nursing, Barbee stated: 'In nursing, the denial of racism is enacted in several ways. Both historically and currently, problems of racism are avoided by simply not using the term' (Barbee 1993: 350), and went on to identify an orthodoxy that being a nurse transcended racism (despite considerable evidence to the contrary), meaning that racism need not be specifically addressed. Furthermore, enculturating student nurses into being 'nice' and conflict avoidant has been linked to racist practices and behaviours in nursing (Barbee 1993, Jackson 2022), through acting to silence those who would speak out against such practices and behaviours (Jackson 2022). However, there is increasing discomfort at this silence and invisibility in some areas of nursing. Writing in 2017, Sally Thorne observed, 'Over the years, there has been a growing cadre of nurses trying to raise the alarm with respect to the problem of nursing silence around racism' (Thorne, 2017).

The failure to address or even acknowledge racism in the discourses that both shape and reflect nursing effectively amounts to a denial of racism (Mapedzahama et al. 2012, similarly: Hilario et al. 2018, Burnett et al. 2020). However, this denial very much depends on any individuals' standpoint. Writing in 1993, Barbee asserted:

> Black, Latina, Asian, and Native American nurses are acutely and chronically aware of racism in the profession and in health care generally. They spend much time and energy combating racism in the profession, while Euro-American nurses spend as much time and energy denying that racism exists.
>
> (Barbee 1993: 347)

Adopting a colour-blind perspective occurs when white people assert that they don't notice the colour of a minoritised person (Hilario et al. 2018). Such positioning permits the view that all people are treated the same, and that recognition and acknowledgement of race are irrelevant and unnecessary, further contributing to the invisibility and silence around racism. Refusal to acknowledge skin colour fosters continued denial of racism creating cultures that actively silence and suppress those who would speak up about racism (Barbee 1993), and means discussion and acknowledgement of difference are only able to be framed as being without colour' (Hilario et al. 2018).

Furthermore, the lack of acknowledgement of racism also arises because racism is often invisible to those who do not experience it. The lack of racial awareness is highlighted by Martin-McDonald and McCarthy (2008) in their discussion on whiteness, who assert that the hegemony of whiteness is upheld and reinforced through powerful social, legal and economic systems and traditions. These authors refer to the dominance and privilege of whiteness and provide insights into the lack of awareness of hegemonic whiteness, stating that, 'whiteness is invisible to those of us who are white… our whiteness is always present, visible and better known to those who are not white' (Martin-McDonald & McCarthy 2008, p. 129).

Similarly, the white dominance of nursing has been generally uncritically accepted and not recognised, problematised or addressed. In 2003, Puzin argued the pervasiveness of whiteness, not only in practice, but within nurse education. Writing more recently, Allen (2022) reflects on the structural domination of whiteness in nursing, and on the lack of attention to whiteness in nursing. These later works all lend support to Puzin's (2003) earlier assertions that whiteness is strongly upheld, and that this is the case, even where there is a non-white nursing workforce. For further focussed consideration on race and racism, see Chapter 32 (Varcoe and Browne).

Whiteness of the nursing academic workforce

There is a raft of literature attesting to the white dominance of the nursing academic workforce (see, for example, Scammell & Olumide 2012, Allan 2017, Bell 2020), particularly at senior levels (Kaur-Aujla et al. 2021). The vast majority of the continuing or tenured nursing academic workforce is white and female. There has been increasing recognition in some parts of the world of the need for nursing to be more inclusive and to take steps to improve awareness of the needs of diverse communities and the participation of people from minority groups in nursing, including academic nursing. Resulting actions have seen a focus on recruitment of some minority groups in some countries. However, despite these well-intentioned (but largely ineffective efforts), there has only been very little focus on the nature of nursing knowledge, how it is imparted and by whom in the process of nurse education.

Allan (2017) raises issues about discriminatory procedures and systems within nurse education that mitigate against persons of colour and their ability to progress their careers. While many institutions have stated commitment to increasing diversity in faculty positions, such efforts are 'notoriously unsuccessful' (Bell 2020: 4). Applicants for faculty jobs have reported being interviewed by all-white interview panels, and a sense they were being interviewed only to fill quotas, rather than being seen as talented people with strong skillsets to bring to their roles (Loyd 2015). Loyd (2015) also reported minority applicants applying for positions in all-white faculties, and seeing white applicants successfully appointed while they themselves were unsuccessful, despite having had more experience. There was also a sense that minority persons were hired into less secure roles, some with very short contracts and less benefits than other faculty positions (Loyd 2015).

After appointment, minority faculty report many issues of concern, including unsupportive and even hostile work environments, invalidation, discrimination, racism, marginalisation and being 'the only' person of colour within the department or faculty, with all of the stress and expectation that can bring (Beard & Julion 2016, Loyd 2015). Similarly, Barbee (1993) has described Black women being marginalised in nursing in multiple ways, and the additional burden of being positioned as an 'ambassador' for their race. More focussed attention is paid to race and racism elsewhere in this text (see Chapter 31, Varcoe and Browne), but what is important in relation to this discussion is that in having largely white faculty, we again enculturate students into the whiteness of nursing in and through their learning activities.

Exclusionary practices in the construction and transmission of knowledge

Given the overwhelming dominance of particular ways of seeing and understanding the world – largely through a monocultural, white, colonial lens – it is hardly surprising that much nurse education is shaped by this world view. There are many tensions and a large literature around what counts as knowledge, and there is much talk of evidence-based practice (EBP). However, these discussions often assume the evidence is out there, that it exists, and it is simply a matter of finding and evaluating the evidence and embedding it into practice. Yet, in reality, much of what passes as nursing knowledge is drawn from white, settler perspectives. Thus, the dominant and racialised discourses and processes that influence the generation of knowledge not only shape (what passes for) knowledge, but also impedes our ability to adequately interrogate health disparities (Hilario et al. 2018). These factors coalesce so that the perspectives that dominate, shape and regulate nurse education overwhelmingly represent the needs, concerns and experiences of particular dominant groups, and do not adequately prepare graduates to meet the needs of people who do not belong to these dominant groups. There is also the issue of marginalisation of minority ethnic people, particularly Black and First Nations nursing in the literature. Reflecting on her experience of writing her influential and important paper about racism in nursing, Barbee stated:

> From the outset, I experienced several difficulties in writing this article. The first, and perhaps most basic, obstacle was deciding how to write about a problem that, at least according to the nursing literature, does not exist. The traditional approach of reviewing the current, relevant literature created a dialectic. As a Black nurse with 30 years of experience in the profession as a nursing student, hospital staff nurse, graduate nursing student, and nursing school faculty member, I am convinced that racism is deep seated and pernicious in nursing. On the other hand, the literature contradicts my experiences.
>
> (Barbee 1993: 347)

Barbee's experience was of writing on a topic (racism) about which the nursing literature said (at that time) did not exist. Even today, and despite the productivity of many Black, First Nations and minority scholars, the bulk of nursing text and literature is still dominated by white voices and white perspectives. This situation contributes to both overt and covert (and combined) racism in texts, and continues to reinforce (largely) unquestioning acceptance of racial stereotypes and biological determinism.

Opportunities to publish and have access to research funds to address contemporary issues in health care involves dealing with many gatekeepers who are in the position to control and filter access to information and essential resources. These gatekeepers have enormous influence over what research will be funded or unfunded, what papers will be published or remain unpublished and whose voices will be heard and whose will remain hidden. Through these mechanisms, these powerful gatekeepers get to decide what information will be presented as knowledge, and therefore become available to nursing students. It is important to acknowledge that while most authors and researchers of all ethnicities are subjected to various gatekeeping processes, the difference for white scholars and scientists is that the gatekeeping processes tend to be dominated by white interests, concerns and perspectives.

Citation bias also acts to maintain white domination of nursing knowledge. Ioannidis et al. (2020) produced data on 100,000 international scientists drawing on indices to calculate career long citation impact (to 2019), and single-year metrics for 2019. These authors calculated impact to both include and omit self-citations. This large and broad data set of was subjected to a secondary analysis with a focus on nursing in Australia and New Zealand to find out more about a number of factors, including gender, level of appointment and cultural diversity of these leading researchers in the field (Jackson et al. 2021). From the more than 35,000 authors in the larger data set (Ioannidis et al. 2020), 147 scientists with nursing as their subfield discipline were identified from a total of 38 Australian and New Zealand institutions. Findings of this secondary analysis showed that within that data set, no First Nations nurse scientists were included, despite there being several well-known and very well-published First Nations nursing scientists in both Australia and New Zealand. This lack of inclusion of First Nations researchers raised the question of systemic citation bias against work authored by First Nations nurse scientists (Jackson et al. 2021). In addition to transmitting knowledge, citations play an important role in demonstrating impact and so failure to cite First Nations scientists and scholars likely contributes to discrimination faced by First Nations faculty, particularly around issues such as promotion and tenure. Thus white domination of the nursing academy continues, and is a powerful force in the enculturation into nursing that occurs through nurse education programmes.

Concluding thoughts

Even today, nurse education is dominated by white perspectives at all levels – from the regulatory overseers of curricula, to the overwhelmingly white teaching workforce and the contexts that nurse education takes place in – largely white, colonised institutional settings such as universities, colleges, hospitals and other health environments. When developing and implementing activities that will contribute to the enculturation of students into nursing, we must carefully reflect on what behaviours and values we are imparting, consciously or unconsciously. We must interrogate (formal, informal and hidden) curricula to challenge and disrupt the strong and entrenched discourses in nursing that deny racism.

As nurse educationalists we have an important role to play in challenging the discourses that perpetuate racism and the white domination of nursing. We must recognise, acknowledge and mitigate the many ways that whiteness is centred and reinforced and understand how this underpins the enculturation processes for students of nursing. While ever nurse educationalists continue to create and disseminate narratives of biological essentialism, and uncritically and unquestioningly accept biological explanations of racially based health inequities and disparities, not only do we fail to address racism, we continue to promulgate the enculturation of whiteness that occurs in and through nurse educational programmes. All who are involved in nurse education have an essential responsibility to act to interrupt and challenge the factors that reinforce student acquisition of race(ist) ideologies and world views during their enculturation into nursing.

References

AACN. (2008). *The Essentials of Baccalaureate Education for Professional Nursing Practice.* American Association of Colleges of Nursing. https://www.aacnnursing.org/portals/42/publications/baccessentials08.pdf (accessed 02/06/22).

Allan, H. (2017). Editorial: Ethnocentrism and racism in nursing: Reflections on the Brexit vote. *Journal of Clinical Nursing*, 26, 1149–1151. https://doi.org/10.1111/jocn.13627

Allan, H. (2022). Reflections on whiteness: Racialized identities in nursing. *Nursing Inquiry*, DOI: 10.1111/nin.12467

Allmark, P. (1995). A classical view of the theory-practice gap in nursing. *Journal of Advanced Nursing*, 22, 18–23. https://doi.org/10.1046/j.1365-2648.1995.22010018.x

Barbee, E. (1993). Racism in U.S. nursing. *Medical Anthropology Quarterly*, 7(4), 346– 362.

Beard, K., & Julion, W. (2016). Does race still matter in nursing? The narratives of African-American nursing faculty members. *Nursing Outlook*, 64(6), 583–596. https://doi.org/10.1016/j.outlook.2016.06.005

Bell, B. (2020). White dominance in nursing education: A target for anti-racist efforts. *Nursing Inquiry*, 28, e12379. https://doi.org/10.1111/nin.12379

Burnett, A. et al. (2020). Dismantling racism in education: In 2020, the year of the nurse and midwife, it's time. *Nurse Education Today*.

Carr, D. (2009). Revisiting the liberal and vocational dimensions of university education. *British Journal of Educational Studies*, 57(1), 1–17, DOI: 10.1111/j.1467–8527.2009.00425.x

CDC (2022). *Impact of racism on our nation's health*, Centers for Disease Control and Prevention, https://www.cdc.gov/healthequity/racism-disparities/impact-of-racism.html (accessed 18/6/22).

Curtis, S., Mozley, H., Langford, C., et al. (2021). Challenging the deficit discourse in medical schools through reverse mentoring—using discourse analysis to explore staff perceptions of under-represented medical students. *BMJ Open*, 11, e054890. https://doi.org/10.1136/bmjopen-2021–054890

Davidson, P.M., MacIsaac, A., Cameron, J., Jeremy, R., Mahar, L., Anderson, I. (2012). Problems, solutions and actions: addressing barriers in acute hospital care for indigenous Australians and New Zealanders. *Heart, Lung and Circulation*, 21(10): 639–43. doi: 10.1016/j.hlc.2012.07.005.

Dunlop, M.J. (1986). Is a science of caring possible? *Journal of Advanced Nursing*, 11, 661–670. https://doi.org/10.1111/j.1365-2648.1986.tb03383.x

Fogarty, W., Bulloch, H., McDonnell, S., & Davies, M. (2018). *Deficit Discourse and Indigenous Health: How Narrative Framings of Aboriginal and Torres Strait Islander People Are Reproduced in Policy*, The Lowitja Institute, Canberra. https://www.lowitja.org.au/content/Document/PDF/deficit-discourse-summary-report.pdf (accessed 10/06/22).

Hafferty, F.W., & Franks, R. (1994). The hidden curriculum, ethics teaching, and the structure of medical education. *Academic Medicine*, 69(11), 861–871.

Hilario, C.T., Browne, A.J., & McFadden, A. (2018). The influence of democratic racism in nursing inquiry. *Nursing Inquiry*, 25, e12213. https://doi.org/10.1111/nin.12213

Ioannidis, J.P., Boyack, K.W., & Baas, J. (2020). Updated science-wide author databases of standardized citation indicators. *PLoS Biology*, 18(10), e3000918. https://doi.org/10.1371/journal.pbio.3000918

Jackson, D. (2022). When niceness becomes toxic, or, how niceness effectively silences nurses and maintains the status quo in nursing, *Journal of Advanced Nursing*, https://onlinelibrary.wiley.com/doi/10.1111/jan.15407

Jackson, D., Usher, K., Durkin, J., & Wynne, R. (2021). What can we learn from citation metrics? Measuring nurse researchers in Australia and New Zealand. *Journal of Advanced Nursing*, 78, e33–e35. https://doi.org/10.1111/jan.15035

Kaur-Aujla, H., Dunkley, N., & Ewens, A. (2021). Embedding race equality in nursing programmes: Hearing the student voice. *Nurse Education Today*, 102, 104933. https://doi.org/10.1016/j.nedt.2021.104932

Leech, T., Irby-Shasanmi, A., & Mitchell, A.L. (2019). "Are you accepting new patients?" A pilot field experiment on telephone-based gatekeeping and Black patients' access to pediatric care. *Health Services Research*, 54(Suppl. 1), 234–242. https://doi.org/10.1111/1475-6773.13089

Loyd, V. (2015). Illuminating the experiences of african-american nursing faculty seeking employment in higher education in nursing. *Dissertations*, 140. https://irl.umsl.edu/dissertation/140

Mapedzahama, V., Rudge, T., West, S., & Perron, A. (2012). Black nurse in white space? Rethinking the in/visibility of race within the Australian nursing workplace. *Nursing Inquiry*, 19, 153–164. https://doi.org/10.1111/j.1440-1800.2011.00556.x

Martin-McDonald, K., & McCarthy, A. (2008). 'Marking' the white terrain in Indigenous health research: Literature review. *Journal of Advanced Nursing*, 61(2), 126–133. https://doi.org/10.1111/j.1365-2648.2007.04438.x

Nielsen, A.M., Stuart, L.A., & Gorman, D. (2014). Confronting the cultural challenge of the whiteness of nursing: Aboriginal registered nurses' perspectives. *Contemporary Nurse*, 48(2), 190–196. https://doi.org/10.1080/10376178.2014.11081940

Oozageer Gunowa, N., Brooke, J., Hutchinson, M., & Jackson, D. (2020). Embedding skin tone diversity into undergraduate nurse education: Through the lens of pressure injury. *Journal of Clinical Nursing*, 29, 4358–4367. https://doi.org/10.1111/jocn.15474

Oozageer Gunowa, N., Hutchinson, M., Brooke, J., Aveyard, H., & Jackson, D. (2021). Pressure injuries and skin tone diversity in undergraduate nurse education: Qualitative perspectives from a mixed methods study. *Journal of Advanced Nursing*, 77, 4511–4524. https://doi.org/10.1111/jan.14965

O'Shea, S., Lysaght, P., Roberts, J., & Harwood, V. (2016). Shifting the blame in higher education – social inclusion and deficit discourses. *Higher Education Research & Development*, 35(2), 322–336. https://doi.org/10.1080/07294360.2015.1087388

Paterson, L. (2015). *Social Radicalism and Liberal Education*. Luton, Bedfordshire: Andrews UK Ltd. ProQuest Ebook Central. https://ebookcentral-proquest-com.ezproxy.library.sydney.edu.au/lib/usyd/detail.action?docID=4393933 (accessed 23/11/22).

Puzin, E. (2003). The unbearable whiteness of being (in nursing). *Nursing Inquiry*, 10(3):193–200.

Raso, A., Marchetti, A., D'Angelo, D., Albanesi, B., Garrino, L., Dimonte, V., Piredda, M., & De Marinis, M.G. (2019). The hidden curriculum in nursing education: A scoping study. *Medical Education in Review*, 53, 989–1002. https://doi-org.ezproxy.library.sydney.edu.au/10.1111/medu.13911

Scammell, J., & Olumide, G. (2012). Racism and the mentor-student relationship: Nurse education through a white lens. *Nurse Education Today*, 32(5), 545–550. https://doi.org/10.1016/j.nedt.2011.06.012

Smallwood, R., Usher, K., Woods, C., Sampson, N., & Jackson, D. (2022). De-problematising Aboriginal young peoples' health and well-being through their voice: An Indigenous scoping review. *Journal of Clinical Nursing*, 32, 2086–2101. https://doi.org/10.1111/jocn.16308

Thorne, S. (2017). Isn't it high time we talked openly about racism? *Nursing Inquiry*, 24, e12219. https://doi.org/10.1111/nin.12219

Walker, K. (1997). Dangerous liaisons: Thinking, doing, nursing, *Collegian*, 4(2), 4–14.

Walker, K. (2009). Curriculum in crisis, pedagogy in disrepair: A provocation, *Contemporary Nurse*, 32, 1–2, 19–29. https://doi.org/10.5172/conu.32.1–2.19

Williamson, H.J., Armin, J.S., Stakely, E., Masimi, B., Joseph, D.H., Meyers, J., & Baldwin, J.A. (2021). *Annals of International Occupational Therapy*, 4(3). https://doi.org/10.3928/24761222-20201202-02

Wilson, N.J., Hunt, L., Lewis, P., & Whitehead, L. (2020). *Nursing in Australia: Nurse Education, Divisions, and Professional Standards*. Melbourne, Routledge.

Yan Li, A.S., Lang, Q., Cho, J., Nguyen, V.S., & Nandakumar, S. (2022). Cultural and structural humility and addressing systems of care disparities in mental health services for black, indigenous, and people of color youth. *Child and Adolescent Psychiatric Clinics of North America*, 31(2), 251–259.

39 What can queers teach us about nursing ethics?

Maurice Nagington

Introduction

This chapter will explore what queerness and its specific sub-cultural history can teach healthcare professionals about an ethics of care that extends beyond how to treat LGBT+ people, and instead teaches us about how our ethics of care can be critiqued from a queer perspective. The ethics of how healthcare professionals and LGBT+ people relate to one another has a long history of discussion. In more recent times, particularly in Western Europe, there has been an aim to reduce prejudice and develop more compassionate, stigma-free, and culturally appropriate approaches to care that affirm LGBT+ people's identities. In more distant times from roughly the 1960s through to the 1980s, LGBT+ people who experienced prejudices commensurate with wider society were often able to find understanding straight allies or LGBT+ healthcare professionals to meet their needs in ways that were ethically sound and free from prejudice (this was particularly true in more cosmopolitan areas). Where this was not possible, sexuality may have been hidden from professionals, sometimes causing difficulties, sometimes not. One of the major catalyses for change between these two very different approaches to LGBT+ people was the AIDS pandemic which left gay men and trans* people radically more vulnerable and reliant on healthcare services. The needs for care became so great, and so urgent, that in the face of needing hospital admissions for AIDS-related illnesses, choice of service provider and withholding information about one's sexuality could no longer function as an adequate insulator against prejudice. As such, in the 1990s, literature began to address how nurses, who were often seen as providing some of the most intimate care as well as advocacy, had to examine and rid themselves of these prejudices in order to provide adequate care (Mackereth, 1995). In addition, novel ethical quandaries began to be raised in the literature about how to limit the spread of a highly stigmatised disease, whilst adhering to other ethical principles such as confidentiality that pertained not only to the disclosure of a pathology, but also at times meant maintaining confidentiality about the sexuality of ones' patients (Lichtenstein, 2000; Mackereth & Harrison, 1995). Alongside all of this, decision making for patients who lacked capacity was often complicated by having to mediate between homophobic families and families of choice that were rooted in the LGBT+ community consisting of lifelong partners and friends (Kadushin, 1999).

In a post-AIDS era, again particularly in Western Europe, discussions about the ethics of care for LGBT+ people have tended towards discussions such as how to use correct pronouns. Yet across the recent history of LGBT+ people's interactions with healthcare professionals, one common theme remains: that nurses must change the way they care for LGBT+ people. The discourse remains structured so as to isolate the changes that

DOI: 10.4324/9781003427407-45

occur so that they only pertain to LGBT+ people, thus limiting broader critique of care structures than can benefit everyone. This chapter argues that rather than limiting our thinking to the ethical treatment of LGBT+ people with regard to the specific issues that they face, we should instead think about what a queer critique of care may mean more widely for our approach to the ethics of care. In order to do this, I take inspiration at least in part from Ward's (2020) argument that queer people can act as critical allies to the prevailing normative culture with regard to engaging in ethical relationships. This chapter uses this inspiring inversion to argue that no longer should we think about the ethical problems that LGBT+ may face, but instead ask what LGBT+ people's radically different sub-cultural history and experiences of care structures can teach about the ethics of care. I term this a "queer ethics of care".

I will explore what a "queer ethics of care" may mean from multiple angles, each taking inspiration from the care practices and theories forged within an LGBT+ sub-culture that has been deeply affected by, and forced to respond creatively to, the deep-seated prejudices and the devastating effects of the AIDS pandemic. In order to introduce this, an outline of relevant areas of queer theory is outlined, highlighting their unique relevance for developing a novel approach to care ethics. I then consider four key aspects of a queer ethics of care. First, how care practices developed by the LGBT+ community recognise and value shared vulnerability. Following on from this, the boundaries that are maintained in professional nursing codes of conduct are critiqued for being unhelpful in producing ethical care practices, and an alternative promiscuous care approach is suggested. Third, critiques of power that emerge from queer theory will be explored for their potential to transform care into an ethico-political act. Fourth, the potential points of failure that LGBT+ themselves discovered during this process of forming novel approaches to care are outlined in order to help nurses avoid them. Finally, mpox (formerly known as monkeypox) is reflected on with regard to how a queer approach to ethics critiques the various responses to it.

Queer theory as an approach to care ethics

Queer theory is a broad and often highly contested field. It is also not uncommon for people to claim that it has little to no application to the real world, with many critiques of it increasingly tending towards homophobic and transphobic ideologies that try to re-affirm heterosexuality and cis-gender (a term to denote people who are not trans-gender) identities as natural or even morally superior. Such critiques however miss the primary point of queer theory which aims to deconstruct the very claim that there is such a thing as a natural expression of gender or sexuality, and instead argues that both are merely coalescences of the prevailing power structures within which contemporary subjectivity is formed. It is this critique of how power attempts to make itself appear natural and normal that forms a central departure point for how queer theory allows critiques of areas outside of gender and sexuality. Indeed, whilst seeming at first to be the territory of high-brow theorists, queer theory has spurred on and has had an iterative relationship with social justice activism. As Halperin quips, those protesting to improve care for AIDS people had a metaphorical copy of Foucault's *The History of Sexuality* in their back pockets (Halperin, 1997). Queer theory therefore has a very intimate relationship with political action, and interventions from queer theorists such as Judith Butler have turned the insights gained from experiencing oppression into more general commentaries about the ethics of how to live (Butler, 2009). Just as queer theory critiqued the so-called bases for gender and sexuality, imploring us to find more capacious ways to experience bodies and pleasures free from an identity politics that traps us in oppositional ways of understanding the self and the other, queer theory has now developed a strand of moral and ethical frameworks that argues for broadening our response to the ethical call of how to live alongside those who we may not feel connected with. Butler argues that this stems from recognising the vulnerability we share to things that can harm and extinguish life and that we are all therefore interwoven in producing one another's living (Butler, 2015). This insight itself is deeply rooted in the heightened sense of precarity and vulnerability that many LGBT+ people have experienced secondary to state and/ or societal homophobic violence and/or indifference to the threats (such as HIV) that disproportionately affected (and in some communities continue to affect) the LGBT+ community. This iterative development of experience and theory results in a set of ethical frameworks that form the core of a queer ethics of care.

Professional boundaries

In almost all nursing codes of conduct, there are ideological positions that require distance which is maintained between the cared for (the patient) and carer (the professional). For example, both the UK's Nursing and Midwifery Council (2010) and International Council of Nurses (2021) codes of conduct contain very similar statements imploring nurses to set professional boundaries between themselves and their patients. In these two codes, there is little in the way of nuancing how or why boundaries are set. The American Nurses Association (2015) goes some way to developing the concept of boundaries, but only in so much as to say that nurse-patient relationships should contain different boundaries to those between friends or colleagues, at the same time muddying their thesis by saying that nurse-patient relationships are "inherently personal". At this point, it is necessary to highlight that I am not suggesting that boundaries are not helpful in preventing abuse; indeed, the Canadian Nurses Association (2017) points out that the boundaries between nurses and patients are often symbolic of power differentials that may not always be beneficial to transgress. Yet, the CNA draws a distinction between "boundary crossings" which can be helpful in developing therapeutic relationships, and "boundary violations" which are acts of abuse. This more liberal and nuanced approach to transgressing boundaries allows "brief excursions" beyond the boundaries, but only the CNA makes explicit some of the boundaries that must not be crossed such as romantic and sexual ones. To be clear, in what comes next, I am not advocating for all nurses to begin sexual relationships with their patients; there remain significant ethical reasons not to do this considering the unequal power dynamics inherent in the nurse-patient relationship. However, what I am suggesting is that there remains something to be learned about the ethics of how LGBT+ people have constructed and transgressed the normative boundaries of care work.

Constructing boundaries

In the early days of the AIDS pandemic in the UK, Dickinson et al. (2022) note how boundaries between the carers and the cared for were often policed far beyond the necessities for infection control, highlighting that staff would often go nowhere near patients with an AIDS diagnosis. Much of the excessive boundary policing could at best be seen as naivety to the transmission risks of AIDS, or more latterly wilful ignorance that was "underscored by fear and ignorance [which] meant patients were often poorly treated" (Dickinson et al., 2022, 7). One could argue that death has always prompted the production of boundaries between the living and the soon-to-be-dead which is a necessary condition of living; reinforcing one's ego from the ever pressing fear of death and disease is a necessary condition of making the experience of finitude bearable (Becker, 1973). Yet in the case of AIDS, whilst some people amplified this process of boundary making, others responded to the vulnerability by sharing it and producing a closeness. Dickinson et al. note that gradually many LGBT+ healthcare professionals and allies chose to work with AIDS patients, and that this often produced a closeness via a shared sense of identity. However, a mutual sense of identity is not a necessary condition of producing a more mutual sense of caring for one another. As demonstrated by responses to AIDS in Northern Thailand in the 1990s (where homophobia was essentially non-existent), communities would offer care, education, and mutual support regardless of the gender or sexuality of the patient (Borthwick, 1999). One can therefore read the prejudice in Western contexts as being a reworking of antecedent aversions to homosexuality where earlier aversions are "dredged up, re-worked and re-distributed" (Kagan, 2018, 131) to maintain the so-called natural boundaries around the charmed circle of heterosexual and monogamous relationships. Anything outside of these boundaries is met with revulsion in order to shore up the identities which remain within the charmed circle (Rubin, 1984). As such, culturally mediated boundaries came to impinge on the provision of care by reproducing boundaries within the informal support networks of families and friends, with fathers being particularly prone to enacting the worst forms of prejudice and abandonment of their gay sons (Kadushin, 1996, 1999). Yet whilst such boundary making activities were incredibly harmful for those who were the wrong side of them and in need of care, the homophobic boundaries became a source of political resistance to the antipathy of AIDS (Borthwick, 1999) and resulted in new ways of working that broke down, and continue to offer a critique of, the boundaries enacted in healthcare practice.

Transgressing boundaries

One of the most comprehensive examples of how the boundaries produced by fear were transformed into caring practices is expressed by the charity *Gay Men's Health Crisis*. GMHC was founded in 1981 in New York, USA; the aim was to provide emotional, nutritional, and legal support alongside a diverse array of activities encompassing everything from relaxing and shopping through to hands on care of the dying (Katoff & Dunne, 1988). Care partners were allocated to those needing care and they were organised into clusters of around 12 people that ensured back-up care was always available. These groupings also functioned as mutual support for the carers. Additionally, the distinction between carers and cared for was often porous, with 25% of those needing care returning to be volunteers providing care and support for others. Other models of mutual care demonstrate that the opposite was equally true, that those who began as carers would often turn to the very same services as they developed AIDS themselves, and that this often resulted in people becoming politicised to bring about change to broader care structures (Kayal, 1991). This produces new ethico-political philosophies because of how the AIDS crisis compressed and inverted the ideological distinction between carer and cared for, sometimes repeatedly switching between the two, until distinctions became meaningless which had radical effects on the care network relationships that formed zduring the AIDS crisis. First, whilst an AIDS diagnosis may have often produced a distance towards natal family and the caring professions, this intermingling of the cared and cared for highlighted the value of reciprocity in interpersonal relationships that prevented people constantly feeling like a dependent victim, on the contrary structuring caring relationships around mutualism helped promote self-esteem (Hays et al., 1990). Such intermingling of carer and cared for mean that care was provided on the basis of need (Kayal, 1991), not whether people fulfilled particular characteristics such as nationality, sexuality, or insurance status. Brier (2007) highlights that this approach resulted in "a community of practice... [where] everyone was an insider" (p. 240). As such, no one becomes subjected to the power dynamics of a pathologising gaze, nor is anyone operating it. Instead, there is a continual and mutual gazing that looks for opportunities for mutual care regardless of status. These interminglings provide an ethical argument for differently constructing caring relationships that may at first appear anathema to nursing ethics. However, as I will demonstrate, they offer valuable insights into why and how nurses must come to work with a queer ethics of care that is characterised not by the care of the individual, but as reframing care as a social endeavour that is always and already looking to exceed the boundaries placed on it.

Promiscuity

The Care Collective (2020) draw on many of the theoretical underpinnings above. In doing so, they identify that one of the key ethical problems with contemporary forms of care lies in how a need for care has become pathologised. This pathologisation operates in two ways: first, it disavows the shared reality of human frailty and constructs those needing care as pejoratively dependent. Second, pathologisation simultaneously demands that those dependent on care must self-regulate to reduce (and preferably eliminate) the care that they receive from others. Where this cannot be eliminated they identify that society is organised via a look-after-our-own logic, mostly pertaining to natal families taking on caring responsibilities, but also eliminating the right to care for migrants and others who are on the margins of societies. Such models of organising care always result in care occurring within a system of (supposed) limited resources where care for one person always means care for another is removed or lessened in some unarticulated way. Competition for care and metrics to justify and distribute it become the underpinning moral philosophy. Drawing on the moral philosophies of care developed during the AIDS crisis, The Care Collective argue for "promiscuous care". This draws inspiration from how promiscuity amongst gay men was constructed by Douglas Crimp (1987) as not the cause of the AIDS crisis, but as a source of an all-encompassing philosophy rooted in experimental approaches to intimacy which could result in new ways for gay men to care for another. Expanding this philosophy, The Care Collective argue care must become promiscuous, without boundaries, where there is no distinction between "our own" and those we consider to be "others". What this logic teaches us is that the contemporary boundaries produced in healthcare between the self and other, nurse and patient, carer and cared for are most often in place to regulate the production of care and enable profit extraction and/or produce efficiencies via a marketised logic. It also demonstrates that many of the most valuable aspects of engaging in care are a sense of mutuality, connectedness, and patience, which marketised logics have no vocabulary for, nor any way to capture and measure.

Day's (2021) work is particularly helpful in thinking about how queer legacies of care help conceptualise boundaries in alternative ways. Her work (done in collaboration with Holly Hey) centres around David's House, an HIV hospice in Toledo Ohio that opened its doors in 1990 and stopped being an independent HIV hospice in 2003. It was set up in an old Catholic rectory and relied heavily on community fund-raising events held in the local LGBT+ spaces of Toledo. Toledo is not a wealthy place; instead, as Day describes, it is a part of the USA that has seen a severe decline in its economy with little in the way of assistance from the state to stem the parallel declines in social and healthcare provision. David's house offered a model for mutual care and assistance when many were arguing that money needed to be invested in more traditional medical care facilities. Many of the residents also doubled up as care workers, not in a paid capacity, but in a way that ensured care was available to all. Day argues that the porosity of bodies to HIV infection that in other more medicalised facilities resulted in a harsh policing of boundaries was instead reconceptualised as a porosity to providing mutual care, regardless of one's status, that became reflected in an attunement "to the wide variety of needs of the HIV community" (Day, 2021, 1536). The openness that this went on to form produced a coalition between those who were marginalised. However, the radical boundary challenging model of care that typified David's house became a victim of its own success when it was encouraged to expand to become an agency bidding for government contracts to run services. Plans for an extension to David's house to provide housing became altered to provide offices for paid staff, and eventually David's house was taken over by larger and larger umbrella organisations. No longer was David's house an organisation "for, and supported by, unruly queers" (2021, 1537); instead, it had become co-opted into the very marketised systems of care that it had aimed to resist and provide radically different care to.

In summary, whilst a queer ethics of care recognises the need for state support in providing funds, training, and infrastructure to care, it must remain critical to the almost pervasive underlying ideologies within which states function that aim to maximise efficiency and/or profit. When this ideology permeates, patients become tasks that are measured and efficiently completed (Nagington et al., 2013) with little no power over how they can redirect their care (Nagington et al., 2015). This results in them being unable to engage with and critique and alter care structures and instead transforms them into increasingly passive recipients whilst claiming that they are in fact active consumers. A queer ethics of care must always be attentive to these unequal power dynamics and ensure that there is a consistent critique of the prevailing political structures within which ethical care is (not) produced.

Care as an ethico-political act

Between various decriminalisations and legalisations of homosexuality in a post-World War II liberal democracies, but before the AIDS crisis, gay men and lesbians had begun to live relatively separate lives both socially and politically (Summerskill, 2012). This changed as the AIDS crisis began to envelop the gay male community, lesbians offered practical support such as organising blood donation drives and hands on care, and as time progressed also started highlighting the feminist arguments around how practical elements of care raise political arguments (Brier, 2007). A queer ethics of care inherits this legacy and is therefore not just concerned with the care of individuals, but also to challenge the structures of society so that people are better able to care for one another. To put it another way, a queer ethics of care highlights that caring is not just an act, but is an ethico-political act, one that recognises to draw from one of the major rhetorical phrases of second-wave feminism, "the personal is political". The hours of caring for one another, doing the so-called dirty work, for the so-called dirty people, who had contracted a so-called dirty disease, were not just something to contain within oneself. No longer was the body, its diseases, and displeasures something to keep as a private affair; instead, under the influence of this strand of politics, and supported by their lesbian friends, gay men began the ethically complex task of transforming their personal experiences into political acts. Simple examples exist such as the work of Bobbie Campbell who rather than sitting patiently and quietly in an outpatient department waiting to see a doctor to be diagnosed and treated, instead began publicly declaring his status as an AIDS patient suffering from Kaposi's Sarcoma (a very visible form of cancer that leaves bruise-like lesions on the skin) (Wright, 2013). Campbell, against the wishes of his doctors began hanging around in outpatient departments creating a community with other patients who were suffering through similar experiences, these people then began to join together, publicly sharing their experiences. It must be noted that at the time to be an "out" AIDS patient was to expose oneself to significant shame and stigma. However, rather than allowing this to silence themselves, Campbell and others ensured that such small acts gradually built to larger communities of people coming together on the streets campaigning for (and achieving) improved care for people living with AIDS. Transforming the personal into the political in this way brings with it a sense of collective power that can transform the prevailing structures to produce more caring outcomes.

Failure

A queer ethics of care does however sometimes fail, and it is important to highlight these failures in order to learn from them. Organisations like the *Gay Men's Health Collective*, whilst often radical in their (re)structuring of healthcare and mutualism, still failed at times to engage in a continually queer approach to ethics that has been outlined above. For example, as the HIV/AIDS pandemic came to be recognised as affecting a wider demographic than just gay men, there was a desire expressed amongst many gay men to maintain a narcissistic form of community where "changing demographics and heterosexualisation of AIDS and the volunteer corps" (Kayal, 1991, 299) was spoken about in worried tones as potentially leaving people disinclined to volunteer. In this context, racial inequalities were also being noted as being poorly addressed with a similar inability to recognise the multiple and intersecting oppression that BAME people faced (and still do face) in relation to HIV/AIDS. This demonstrates that to "queer" something is not a one-time act, and that the ethics that stems from queer theory is never a static achievement. To queer something is in fact best thought of as a continuous present verb (Sullivan, 2003) one that is always examining power relationships and the boundaries that they create. A queer approach to ethics therefore aims to always recognise that there is a continual need to bring more people into more equal forms of relationships that can be the basis for enhancing our ability to care for one another; and, that rather than constructing boundaries to protect ourselves and society from imagined threats, or constructing boundaries to disavow threats as somehow not relevant to "us" because they only pertain to "them", we instead respond to those on the other side of boundaries in ways that always holds out the possibility of transgression as an ethical act to caring.

Mpox

At the time of writing, possibly the most current and pressing application of a queer ethics of care that has the potential to teach us about what taking a queer approach could mean for nursing ethics is the ongoing outbreak of mpox (formerly known as monkeypox). Mpox is a virus in the same group of orthopox viruses such as smallpox. Two strains exist, one with very low mortality rate at around 1%, and one with a significantly higher at around 10% (World Health Organization, 2022a). Both produce uncomfortable and at times highly painful lesions across the body which can scar, clinical recommendations state that people isolate for 21 days to prevent spread. Additionally, mpox can infect other mammals, meaning that there is potential for human-animal transmissions that could lead to the infection becoming endemic across multiple species, all but eliminating the possibility of stopping the virus becoming endemic. Smallpox vaccines are highly effective at preventing outbreaks. Mpox, is already endemic to areas in Western Africa and was first identified in 1970. Various countries have seen small outbreaks totalling tens of patients all of whom had identifiable first-person contact that could be managed with contact tracing and isolation, but since early 2022 there has seen widespread community transmission occurring in the Americas, Europe, and Australia (World Health Organization, 2022b). Whilst surveillance and data remain nascent, outside of Western Africa, the overwhelming majority of cases have been occurring between gay men, with the majority being linked to sexual transmission (Allan-Blitz & Klausner, 2022). With regard to inside Western Africa, the mechanism of transmission is less well agreed upon, but for several years sexual transmission has been documented as an important route, even if the sexuality of those involved lacks reliable data (Yinka-Ogunleye et al., 2019).

A queer ethics of care can help critique the responses that have been seen with regard to mpox. Much discussion has been devoted to whether mpox should be considered an STI or not (Iglesias et al., 2022); some suggest that constructing it as such is vital to help with targeted campaigns that engage communities most at risk so that vaccines can ultimately be provided to those most in need (Mack, 2022), and stopping mpox from becoming endemic in countries outside of Western Africa. Some even go so far as suggesting that doing so can help reassure those who are not at significant risk, such as children in school where close contact is thought to only pose a small risk. Yet, this places gay men in a particular subjective position which they are all too familiar with, where a sense of threat is projected onto them leaving them as the outsider that harbours a disease that must be contained, with some even expressing "optimism" that it is only "spreading within a defined community" i.e. gay men (Branswell, 2022); as if rapid spread amongst gay men were an acceptable form of collateral damage because "they" are not "us". Additionally, identification of mpox as an STI also places its treatment onto one specific part of healthcare systems: sexual health services, which have been defunded for years in the UK (Local Government Association, 2022). As a result of this, the responsibility for containing mpox is then thrust upon gay men who, despite having homophobic tropes from the HIV/AIDS era being recycled to refer to them "gross and irresponsible" (Dreher, 2022) for spreading mpox, still subject themselves to a public health that requires them to stand in line waiting for a vaccine for up to 6 hours, to the point where some people pass out secondary to heat stroke (Vesty, 2022). In such situations gay men shoulder huge responsibility and burden with little sense of solidarity from society or political institutions. In the case of mpox (unlike COVID-19), little to no Central Government resources have been mobilised in the UK beyond procuring the minimum necessary vaccine doses. There were few centralised campaigns or administrative systems, and there was little to no support to help raise awareness in communities that were slow to take up the vaccine. Instead all this work was done by charities and sexual health clinics that drew time and resources away from other important work. Any sense of mutual care and support remains entirely within the LGBT+ community who, echoing the days of the AIDS pandemic, self-organised to get drugs into bodies. A queer ethics of care would recognise that defunding one area of healthcare effects everyone and that producing an ethical approach to care is about recognising the synergistic and non-linear relationships that we have with one another, and that these relationships cannot be disavowed just because "they" are not "us".

A queer ethics of care also challenges us to think who "us" is in a way that is always looking to bring more people into more equal relationships with one another. As noted above, mpox has remained largely ignored by the very countries who are now rapidly trying to vaccinate their populations, despite one of these countries (the USA) stockpiling 100 million doses of a suitable vaccine which was never offered to West African countries to help contain the pandemic. Instead, vaccines were hoarded out of the fear of a bioweapon attack by an imagined potential future other, and not offered in solidarity to those with real and current needs. Instead, the vaccine expired and was binned in 2014 (Ferrannini, 2022). A queer ethics of care recognises that boundaries need to be critiqued and transgressed, and that attempting to calculate the risks and benefits of one's actions can never be the basis for an ethical form of care. Rather the basis for ethical action is engaging in acts of solidarity with those in need because we recognise our shared vulnerability, not because we want to protect ourselves from "them". In doing so, ideas of sexuality, nationality, insurance status, ethnicity or any other characteristics are no longer boundaries between "us" and "them" but instead offer us ways to recognise power imbalances that can be responded to through acts of solidarity that aim to reduce the difference between "us" and "them" producing a mutually supportive "we".

Conclusion

A queer ethics of care therefore draws from the sub-cultural experiences of LGBT+ people, which has led theorists and activists alike to synergistically develop an ethical framework that is rooted in the increased precarity that comes from being subjected to homophobia, sexism, and diseases like HIV and mpox that amplify and replay this precarity. Emerging from this a queer ethics of care can be described as a resolutely mutual way to think about ethics that turns the experience of precarity into an affirmation of our shared vulnerability and interdependency. This recognition of shared vulnerability also encourages a critique of how and why boundaries are constructed and places an ethical call on those in positions of power to always be attentive to the inequalities that exist and emerge. Most importantly, because power is always operating and always needs critiquing it highlights that ethical practice is always and already at risk of experiencing failure, yet that failure only really exists when one fails to be attentive to the constancy of needing to queer practices.

References

Allan-Blitz, L., & Klausner, J. D. (2022) *Is Monkeypox a sexually transmitted infection?* Retrieved 25/8/22 from https://medium.com/@drklausner_3821/is-monkey-pox-a-sexually-transmitted-infection-19dd2f533d03

American Nurses Association. (2015) *Code of ethics with interpretative statements*. Maryland: American Nurses Association.

Becker, E. (1973) *The denial of death*. New York: Free Press.

Borthwick, P. (1999) HIV/AIDS projects with and for gay men in northern Thailand. *Journal of Gay & Lesbian Social Services*, 9(2–3): 61–79.

Branswell, H. (2022) *With monkeypox spreading globally, many experts believe the virus can't be contained*. Retrieved 25/08/22 from https://www.statnews.com/2022/07/19/monkeypox-spread-many-experts-believe-the-virus-cant-be-contained/

Brier, J. (2007) Locating lesbian and feminist responses to AIDS 1982–1984. *Women's Studies Quarterly*, 35(1/2): 234–246.

Butler, J. (2009) *Frames of war: When is life grievable?* London: Verso.

Butler, J. (2015) *Notes toward a performative theory of assembly*. Harvard: Harvard University Press.

Canadian Nurses Association. (2017) *Code of ethics for registered nurses*. Ottawa: Canadian Nurses Association.

Crimp, D. (1987) How to have promiscuity in an epidemic. *Aids: Cultural Analysis/Cultural Activism*, 43: 237–271.

Day, A. (2021) Care, crisis, coalition: Imagining antiprophylactic citizenship through AIDS hospice activism. *Culture, Health & Sexuality*, 23(11): 1532–1544.

Dickinson, T., Appasamy, N., Pritchard, L. P., & Savidge, L. (2022) Nursing a plague: Nurses' perspectives on their work during the United Kingdom HIV/AIDS crisis, 1981–96. In Weston, J. and Elizabeth, H.J. (eds.) *Histories of HIV/AIDS in Western Europe* (pp. 109–138) Manchester: Manchester University Press.

Dreher, R. (2022) *Why did Sebastian Köhn get monkeypox?* Retrieved 25/8/22 from https://www.theamericanconservative.com/why-did-sebastian-kohn-get-monkeypox/

Ferrannini, J. (2022) *Why 100 million vaccines the US already has aren't being used for monkeypox* Retrieved 25/8/22 from https://thehill.com/homenews/wire/3584521-why-100-million-vaccines-the-us-already-has-arent-being-used-for-monkeypox/

Halperin, D. M. (1997) *Saint Foucault: Towards a gay hagiography*. Oxford: Oxford Paperbacks

Hays, R., Chauncey, S., & Tobey, L. (1990) The social support networks of gay men with AIDS. *Journal of Community Psychology*, 18: 374–385.

Iglesias, J. G., Nagington, M., Pickersgill, M., Brady, M., Dewsnap, C., Highleyman, L., de Novales, F. J. M., Nutland, W., Thrasher, S., & Umar, E. (2022) Is monkeypox an STI? The societal aspects and healthcare implications of a key question. *Wellcome Open Research* https://doi.org/10.12688/wellcomeopenres.18436.1

International Council of Nurses. (2021) *Code of ethics*. Geneva: International Council of Nurses.

Kadushin, G. (1996) Gay men with AIDS and their families of origin: An analysis of social support. *Health & Social Work*, 21(2): 141–149.

Kadushin, G. (1999) Barriers to social support and support received from their families of origin among gay men with HIV/AIDS. *Health & Social Work*, 24(3): 198–209.

Kagan, D. (2018) *Positive images: Gay men and HIV/AIDS in the culture of 'Post-Crisis'*. I.B. Tauris.

Katoff, L., & Dunne, R. (1988) Supporting people with AIDS: The Gay Men's Health Crisis model. *Journal of Palliative Care*, 4(4): 88–95.

Kayal, P. (1991) Gay AIDS voluntarism as political activity. *Nonprofit and Voluntary Sector Quarterly*, 20(3): 289–312.

Lichtenstein, B. (2000) Secret encounters: Black men, bisexuality, and AIDS in Alabama. *Medical Anthropology Quarterly*, 14(3): 374–393.

Local Government Association (2022) *Councils warn of pressure on sexual health services due to rising number of Monkeypox cases.* Retrieved 25/8/22 from https://www.local.gov.uk/about/news/councils-warn-pressure-sexual-health-services-due-rising-number-monkeypox-cases

Mack, D. (2022) *Let's speak clearly: Monkeypox is mostly being transmitted via sex.* Retrieved 25/08/22 from https://www.buzzfeednews.com/article/davidmack/monkeypox-sex

Mackereth, P., & Harrison, T. (1995) HIV/AIDS. Maintaining confidentiality when tracing contacts. *Nursing Times*, 91(2): 25–26.

Mackereth, P. A. (1995) HIV and homophobia: Nurses as advocates. *Journal of Advanced Nursing*, 22(4): 670–676.

Nagington, M., Luker, K., & Walshe, C. (2013) 'Busyness' and the preclusion of quality palliative district nursing care. *Nursing Ethics*, 20(8): 893–903.

Nagington, M., Walshe, C., & Luker, K. (2015) Quality care as ethical care: A post-structural analysis of palliative and supportive district nursing care *Nursing Inquiry*, 23(1): 12–23.

Nursing and Midwifery Council (2010) *The code: Standards of conduct, performance and ethics for nurses and midwives.* London: NMC.

Rubin, G. (1984) Thinking sex: Notes for a radical theory of the politics of sexuality. In Vance, C. (ed.) *Pleasure and danger.* New York: River Oram Press.

Sullivan, N. (2003) *A critical introduction to queer theory.* New York: NYU Press.

Summerskill, C. (2012) *Gateway to heaven: 50 years of Lesbian and Gay oral history.* London: Tollington Press.

The Care Collective (2020) *The care manifesto: The politics of interdependence.* London: Verso Books.

Vesty, H. (2022) *Person 'collapses' in queue for monkeypox jab as hundreds wait 'hours in direct sun'.* Retrieved 25/8/22 from https://www.manchestereveningnews.co.uk/news/greater-manchester-news/person-collapses-queue-monkeypox-jab-24754608

Ward, J. (2020) *The tragedy of heterosexuality.* New York: New York University Press.

World Health Organization (2022a) *Monkeypox.* Retrieved 25/8/22 from https://www.who.int/news-room/fact-sheets/detail/monkeypox

World Health Organization (2022b) *Multi-country monkeypox outbreak: Situation update.* Retrieved 25/08/22 from https://www.who.int/emergencies/disease-outbreak-news/item/2022-DON393

Wright, J. (2013) "Only Your Calamity": The beginnings of activism by and for people with AIDS. *American Journal of Public Health*, 103(10): 1788–1798.

Yinka-Ogunleye, A., Aruna, O., Dalhat, M., Ogoina, D., McCollum, A., Disu, Y., Mamadu, I., Akinpelu, A., Ahmad, A., & Burga, J. (2019) Outbreak of human monkeypox in Nigeria in 2017–18: A clinical and epidemiological report. *The Lancet Infectious Diseases*, 19(8): 872–879.

40 No as an act of care

A glossary for kinship, care praxis, and nursing's radical imagination

Jessica Dillard-Wright, Favorite Iradukunda, Ruth De Souza, and Claire Valderama-Wallace

Radical imagination and the transformations that ensue are fundamentally collaborative, connected, and conscious. In an effort to first imagine and then cocreate a more just, equitable present/future for nursing and those with whom we care in the spirit of radical imagination, this chapter examines nursing care as praxis and the shifts that occur in embracing kinship as a reciprocal model for nursing. In so doing, we challenge embedded power structures within the healthcare-industrial complex – and thus nursing – as we currently know it. Using feminist, queer, anticolonial, anti-imperialist, and abolitionist insights, we imagine a present/future for nursing liberated from the capitalist political economy entrenched in a boundless society of control. This speculative vision is urgent, encompassing, and material, bursting open the boundaries of nursing as we consider with whom we align and how we build toward a future on a deteriorating planet.

> Ruth DeSouza (RDS): It helps us think about what we don't want, because it's also "no" as generative. No - it's not closing something. It opens up something. So what are we opening up if we say no?

> Favorite Iradukunda (FI): When we say no, people assume it is the easy way out. The pain and the processing that goes into the decision to say no, decisions to challenge the system - none of it is wrong - we are working toward the same goal, often, but those who choose to say no are regarded by those who resist within as abandoning ship.

As we began our collaborative efforts in first imagining and then writing these words on kinship, care praxis, and radical imagination, we found that much of our time together inspired connection, experimentation, and creativity, seeking to expand our circles of kinship in an effort to broaden the reach of care through engaged intertexuality (The Care Collective, 2020). Ideas weaving from one topic to the next, resonating and ringing, urgent and emergent across geopolitical and academically institutionalized borders. Snippets sliding in symbiosis. This led us in the direction of "tiny texts," a first-person writing technique that allows us to tackle many ideas in a discrete but connected fashion (Thomson, 2019). Tiny texts complement the polyvocality of our ongoing conversations: concordant with historian Elsa Barkley-Brown's (1991, 1992) theorization of histories, our words connected and collided and converged and conflicted, reflecting layered ideas, multiple rhythms, and an improvisational quality of historical being, doing, knowing, worldbuilding. Our collective work here is also inspired by Eve Tuck and C. Ree's (2013) "A Glossary of Haunting," formulated without expository context, an entire story punctuated with key terms, explaining, distancing, connecting all at once. Haunting resonated for us

DOI: 10.4324/9781003427407-46

as nurses invested in nursing: haunting as poignant, evocative. Haunting as persistently and disturbingly present in our minds. Thinking of the etymology of haunting, its origins in Old French *hanter*, of Germanic origin; distantly related to home ("Haunt, v.," n.d.). To what terms do we return? What terms stay with us?

As we framed out our vision for this chapter, community was/has been/is central, creating a context of caring collaboration rooted in community as much as scholarship. Our meetings began with check-ins, a time of pausing and visiting. On visiting, educator and theorist Eve Tuck again, with collaborators Haliehana Stepetinb, Rebecca Beaulne-Stuebinga, and Jo Billows (2022) wrote, "As a practice of being in relation across space and time, visiting enacts futurity and remembrance in the present" (p. 1), prioritizing relation and an ethos of caring, pointing to an embodied practice of philosophy. While also serving a social function, the act of visiting takes on philosophical importance that gets at something historical – as the past meets the present, we are at a confluence where we might redirect the unfolding of the future, if we choose (Benjamin, 2018; Dillard-Wright, 2022; Kaba, 2021).

As members of various communities with rich linguistic traditions and scholars attuned to the power of language, our use of the word "we" is an expression of collective learning, seeing, writing, and invoking as authors. We also use "I" on occasion because, as we write in English, we find ourselves limited to "we" or "I." English does not conceptualize relationships in a nuanced fashion. Linguistically, English "we" does not distinguish speaker/audience dynamics the way other languages do. This is a product of empire: English has not always been – and *never* has been – the only language of knowledge production (Gobbo & Russo, 2020). The primacy of English as *the* language of science, of knowledge, of nursing naturalizes intellectual arrogance perched atop an array of violent colonial assumptions around power, authority, and knowledge. We wish to make no such assumptions, readily acknowledging the limitations and pitfalls while living, writing, working, achieving, caring in English language-dominated spaces. In further service to this refusal, we make use of words and definitions that are untranslated *and* untranslatable. This is both political and ontological (see, for example, Benjamin, 2016).

This preamble is designed to orient you, the reader, to visit our polyvocal, multirhythmic tiny texts. We have organized this work in two overlapping ways: the first a glossary and the second a conversation, imbricated and interconnected. The glossary and conversation cross over insofar as the words gleaned for the glossary come from our collective conversations. The words that form the glossary were plucked from our visits with one another, bouncing off conversations and lines of flight they inspired (Deleuze & Guattari, 2007). In doing so, we transgress embedded power structures that shape nursing as we currently know it. Using feminist, queer, anticolonial, and abolitionist insights, we imagine a present/future for nursing liberated from the carceral capitalist political economy entrenched in a boundless society of control. This speculative vision is urgent, encompassing, and material, bursting open the boundaries of nursing as we consider with whom we align and how we build a future on a deteriorating planet. We begin with accountability.

Accountability, what is it? Accountability, to whom?

Is accountability an act of caring or a burden? The interpretation depends on who has the power and privileges to demand – or politely request, as power differentials may require – accountability. What if we considered accountability as an act of caring?

A friendly reminder that we are relational beings. As a way to cede/share power, could accountability be understood as a gift?

> FI: Accountability is also an act of care and it's not always welcomed. But really I think talking about how we got here and the conversation we had at the very beginning– how interconnected we are even being across very, very different time zones and continents, and I like how we connected with our roots, talking about what we eat, what we have from home. Just having those multiple identities. In a way I felt cared for by being accountable to you all.

I am accountable to you, you are accountable to me! We are accountable to families, friends, communities/villages, societies, lands, water, flora, fauna, planet, past, present, and future. To space and the great beyond. We are accountable to those with less power, those who have been wronged by the lack of accountability. We imagine a circle of care that includes everyone and centers, that elevates and amplifies the ignored or those exploited by systems that depend on their labor. Recognizing also that this foregrounding benefits us all. We know that the most exploited among us are not merely patients, clients, constituents, stakeholders – they [you] are valued kin. Maybe accountability is also a privilege. Someone cares about what you are doing and how you are doing it. Accountability as a verb, part of a process of repair.

Audience

As authors, we are accountable in some ways to you as an audience and ask, how are you today? What do you hope to derive from reading this chapter? How is everyone today? How often do you, readers, think about the ways in which you are writing to a particular sort of audience? Chapters such as this speak from a place of **AUTHORITY** and will be gathered together in important works such as this handbook. Rather than something definitive, however, the concepts, constructs, and constellations we speak to in this particular chapter are negotiated, dialectic, processual, relational, dialogic. We believe – we know, we see, we experience, we find, we make – meaning is made in intertextuality. That we are in relation.

This text is also for those among us – nurses, careworkers, care receivers, students, descendants of care workers – who do not always see ourselves in the accepted and dominant stories (past, present, and future) of nursing. It is for the folks who still mask in spite of the overwhelming failure of institutions and structures and other people to extend the same courtesy. We imagine an audience in raucous, lively community, of which we are a part, and with whom we wish to move, think, work. We also imagine talking back to an audience who might more readily adhere to and identify with institutional and structural power within healthcare and nursing.

Bodily autonomy/bodily entropy

Questions of bodily entropy and bodily autonomy pulsed through our shared and solo experiences. Calendars, time changes, family, illness, caregiving, care receiving, self-care, celebrations, sorrow, frustrations, joys. For a discipline that is theoretically and *practically* about bodies, nursing pays scant attention to bodies, particularly in academic spaces.

Care

Care when "quantified" and packaged as commodity fluctuates, its value increases or decreases based on whatever agenda it is attached to. But what is the real value of care? Can it be quantified? What is the harm in not quantifying it? According to whose metrics? To what ends? Does the commodification of care lead to the commodification of those who provide it? To those who receive it? When caring is a community practice, everyone has more time, strengths, and inspiration to care. We begin to view care as a joyful expression of love, of resistance, of survival, of thriving – rather than a burden to be shouldered by a few, provided by only the skilled, housed in designated spaces, contained within institutions.

Caring in diaspora

Global connectedness is a matter of family and collective, not an academic exercise of awareness nor reconnaissance for trivia. The policies and practices of separation, erasure, and displacement enact and internalize loss. The pandemic reveals global dependence on labor exportation, care work as commodity, and the care vacuum behind while simultaneously carrying a disproportionate exposure burden (Nazareno et al., 2021). The daily grind of capitalism and imperialism reduces wholeness and healing to an individualized extracurricular activity rather than a prerequisite for sustained collective empowerment. About this, poet and Nap Bishop Tricia Hersey (2022) writes, "our collective rest will not be easy. All of culture is collaborating for us not to rest," a sobering commentary on the challenge of resisting neoliberalism, trying to flourish.

Communities

Positioned often as separate from healthcare/acute care/nursing/hospital and definitely from academia, communities become the object of nursing care. They are reduced to objects of intellectual curiosity and an undertheorized space for what's devalued. Places where knowledge is extracted, a resource to be mined, instead of places where people negotiate how to live well with illness or disability. Community health is marginalized and destituted, while politicians invest in profitable infrastructures like hospitals as a demonstration of care instead of in the constellations and networks that already nourish and support well-being and care. The reality is that health, well-being, and liberation does not and cannot happen in these acute care and institutional settings, underscoring the colonial hubris of healthcare institutions.

Complexity/wholeness

Multiple dimensions, realities, interpretations can exist at the same time. We should always question our urge to simplify complexity, to be certain, and sure, upholding one dimension or interpretation as unique or superior.

Deadlines are violent and rooted in impulses of white supremacy. Literally. The etymology of "deadline" is immediately carceral, initially referring to the perimeter around a Confederate prison camp (O'Conner & Kellerman, 2009). Demarcating no man's land, the deadline marked the boundary across which no person would pass, hazarding death themselves as guards were charged with shooting transgressors. "Deadline" did not become common parlance regarding paperwork until sometime in the early 20th century (O'Conner & Kellerman, 2009). Challenging urgency, we instead wish to consider the ways in which accountability, community, and care are more suitable relations for nursing and nursing education and nursing community.

See also: promotion and tenure dossier evaluations, chapter drafts, course evaluations, meeting agendas, grades, enforced lingua franca; impatience, urgency.

Divided self

Who and what shows up in any given space: nurse, mom, sister, comrade, friend, parent, spouse, partner, writer, artist, academic, baker, knitter, chauffeur, scheduler, keeper of things, knower of things. All at once, pulled in every direction.

Doing it all?

Mythology of unrealized and unrealizable expectations. The specter of exploitation cloaked in martyrdom, but perhaps also not trusting that the collective will show up.

Ethics

Nursing can be about building the worlds we wish to see, concordant with liberation, moved to transform that which does not fit into this vision, following the insurrectionist ethics proposed by philosopher Leonard Harris (Harris, 2020; Mcbride, 2017). This is a question of the ethics we choose to embrace and enact, both ontological and axiological (Braidotti, 2020; de la Bellacasa, 2011; Puig de la Bellacasa, 2017; Thorne, 2014). In this way, care is always in some form or fashion about ethics – not in a facile "it is or it is not ethical" – but rather, the care we do/are/give enacts what we value, hopefully in relation with those for and with whom we care.

Food as care, as community

"Kumain na ba kayo?" Have you (all) eaten yet? This is how my mom would greet me when I was away at college – and how she greets me on the phone now to gauge how my kids are doing. To offer food without question, to make each other's favorite dishes, to bring back favorites not yet commodified into trendiness in the US. This connects with feelings of home and comfort, as well as hospitality. The word "hospitality" is etymologically related to hospital, and yet there is much to be desired when it comes to the food hospitals provide to the folks in respite there. What might shift if we moved toward thinking about the nourishment provided in hospital settings as actively part of care? If we allowed families and communities to bring food and culture as part of care and healing (DeSouza, 2021)? If we thought about hospitals as sites for and of community? If the site of care was where the care receiver needed it to be rather than organized around the demands of all forms of institutionalized care. If nursing institutions took heed of the calls to action put forth by communities around the world, how might our very ideas of food and the supply chain – and our relationship to land – shift?

Gatekeeping

Violent practices to extract, co-opt, and own notions, knowledge, resources, based on pillars of elitism, racism, ableism, ageism, and heteronormativity. Narratives of impostor syndrome and indicators of attrition are just a few of the manifestations of gatekeeping, with the lens focused on individuals, guided by deficit thinking and framing. Futures shaped by silencing and erasure, facilitated by mechanisms of professionalization.

Gaze

Foucault (1994) calls our attention to the ways in which clinical gazes enact power relations (Greenhalgh, 2001). This maneuver individualizes, narrows, normalizes a circumscribed perspective for carers that focuses on constructed care interactions, divorcing the person and their care from wider contexts, even as those very contexts structure reality. Cultural safety as a process and outcome of care reverses the clinical gaze and instead attempts to re-calibrate power differentials by elevating the voice of the recipient of care (DeSouza, 2022).

> RDS: That's the thing about the reductionist medical gaze. Individualising the body, the person, and not considering the context. So how do we widen or reverse the gaze?

Generations

Eurocentric epistemological and ontological views of time are codified into institutional practices. These, combined with the primacy of individualism, focus the actions and mindsets on the here and now – on me, rather than the relationships connecting the past, the present, and our future. Generations also show up in intergenerational conflict – a generational blame-game, if you will. All too familiar in nursing where people are expected to pay their dues, tow the line… …or else. Sometimes referred to as "eating our young," this adversity is a shorthand for the specific sort of gendered violence of bullying in nursing (Rudge, 2011). And while it is often leveled at new – and ostensibly younger – nurses, it can also be understood as a veiled tactic to discount, discourage, diminish, discriminate, distort, deny, dishonor nurses that do not, cannot, will not conform to nursing's hegemonic norms. This is often shrouded in calls to respect nursing's heritage, nursing's legacy, nursing's history – as if this is an uncomplicated and straightforward thing.

Grief

When care and caring relations endure, they can be subtle, overwhelming, disquieting, and freeing. A living mirror with lessons to consider. Neoliberal institutions compel us to give our all in service to our communities, but the grinding pace prevents us from truly connecting to our grief, to each other. How does interrupted grief seep into our relations, our work, our hopes?
    See also: Unraveling.

Hope

To what degree do we situate ourselves within matrices of change, what Sara King (2022) might call tapestries – within the deep conviction that how things are not have they will or must be? Hope not as a transient feeling but a stance, a disposition, a practice toward engaging in action that ushers in collective strength and liberatory changes. This characterization of hope can be located in the work of prison abolitionist and movement-maker Mariame Kaba's (2021) work and is a central feature of Rosi Bradoitti's feminist new materialism. Hope as a practice can be generative but it can also be a signal of dreams and justice deferred, denied, a colonial reality explored by Chelsea Watego (2021) in a compilation of essays entitled *Another Day in the Colony*. In some frames, hope provides buoyancy necessary to keep on going. In others, hope is an indicator of things all fucked up.

Imagination

Imagine everything we could do with knowledge-power-wisdom if we embraced the connectedness that binds us together instead of resisting it, seeing the constellations instead of focusing on the individual stars (Kaba, 2021).

Kapwa

Recognizing shared identity of an inner self shared with others. Being in kapwa with each other is not merely a rooted sense of collective identity but how this manifests in our relationships with each other.

Kinship

The idea of kin, in my professional experience, boils down to the legal concept of "next of kin," a hierarchy invoked when healthcare decisions must be made and/or conflicts managed. Structured around white supremacist, cisheteronormative, patriarchal institutions, and expectations of family (Benjamin, 2018), this vision of kinship is narrow and problematic, predicated on individualism and imagined norms. (See, for example, de Vries et al., 2022. Queer folks are presented as a "special case" for advanced care planning, noting family estrangement, poverty, and precarity.) In these structures, kinship is reduced to legalities designed to protect (fictive, imagined) bloodlines, whatever those are (Butler, 2002). Kinship need not be so narrow. Sociologist of Technology Ruha Benjamin (2018) imagined "meta-kinship," a relation that "exceeds biological relatedness" (p. 49), unbound by space, time, species, blood relation, institutions, or even death. Kin might, but does not have to, include blood relations. Kin is the family we choose, who we show up for, who shows up for us. Pandemics and climate change mean that we also need to consider interdependence and how we widen these circles of care beyond the idealized nuclear family.

Lived experience

Lived experience is an embodied, vast, complex, and nuanced way of knowing and being in the world. This kind of knowing and being is – in our lived experiences as nurses and lived experiences from our various perspectives and embodied realities and lived experiences we learn about from those we love and care for – not understood as epistemically rigorous or ontologically valid in spite of its materiality and standpoint. What does nursing look like when folks' lived experiences, material realities, and radical imaginings guide care?

Experience, however, is not the be-all, end-all. It does not stand outside space and time. Speaking to realities of the historical record, feminist theorist and historian Joan Scott (1991) articulated the trouble with historical records when it comes to experience. Experiences, filtered through the perspective of historians, become evidence for difference which essentializes differences, failing to attend to the constructed quality of lived experience.

Movements

At the heart of movements is change, active struggle for just and liberatory futures – alternatives to dominant systems and ideologies which exist today. Nursing as a field is determined to establish and cement relevance against medical hegemony, status, and disciplinary autonomy through professionalization which inhibits the emergent, the unsettled, the unknown. Serving the people in the pursuit of justice, particularly in the carceral order of nursing things, despite the Code of Ethics, is an extracurricular endeavor for nursing. But it does not have to be. Justice can be, following neuroscientist and activist Sara King (2022), loving awareness in action that is deeply inclusive. The idea that, if you have a body, you deserve well-being. This is congruent with feminist philosophers Berenice Fisher and Joan Tronto's (1990) vision for care, which is any "*species* activity that includes everything that we do to maintain, continue, and repair our world so that *we* can live in it as well as possible. That world includes *our bodies, our selves, and our environment, all of which we seek to interweave in a complex, life-sustaining web*" (p. 40, emphasis added). This is not a solitary endeavor. Instead, it requires us to move. Together.

No

Drawing on Eve Tuck and Wayne Yang (2014a, b) and Ruha Benjamin (2016) and others' work on refusal, we want to enjoin the generativity of no. "No" which makes other yeses possible. No conserves, no protects. No allows for other possibilities to become. No means self-care.

> "You don't owe anybody anything" but wait - that is not true. What about accountability? In my experience most people who don't value/appreciate our "NO" are not necessarily concerned with accountability.

Nurse

This whole conversation is about problematizing what it means to be a nurse, to do nursing.

Precarity

Manufactured discomfort under the pressures of late stage capitalism, where many labor for the benefit of a scant and ever-narrowing few, precarity is now-normal, ever-present, always-expanding (Dionne, 2021). The threat – and eventual convergence – of disaster in neoliberal economies is the logic of precarity, following Naomi Klein's (2007) work in *Shock Doctrine*. Corporations – including hospitals, nursing homes, clinics – engineer near-precarity for their workers through just-in-time supply and lean staffing, leaving no flex for problems that bubble up, nevermind cataclysms that might occur. When these problems and cataclysms do unfold, systems bear up to ride out extreme precarity, folks coming together to accomplish a common goal, assured that, one day, things will return to normal. That day never comes and the new bare bones that worked in crisis times become normalized, till the next time, when the last drops of marrow are sucked from the dry bones (Klein, 2007).

Radical

While radical is not a word often associated with professionalized practices of care like nursing (Dillard-Wright, 2022), radical simple means "grasping at the root." This is a concept that, we find, suits nursing as a practice of caring well. Getting to the bottom of what people need, planting seeds that allow us to grow, nourishing folks in as many ways as we can. Nursing can be, should be radical.

Relational, not transactional

Commitment to program implementation allows peoples in complex ecosystems to be reduced to benchmark indicators, gatekeeping, and adherence. What might be relational becomes transactional.

Settler colonialism

Our relationships to each other, the lands from which we and our ancestors come, and to the Indigenous peoples on whose land we live are inextricably situated within settler colonialism as an ongoing system of displacement, dispossession, extraction, and exploitation. Connected to what Patrick Wolfe (2006) called an "organizing grammar of race" (p. 387), settler colonialism structures realities in a present and ongoing confrontation. Not a past gone by. A structure (Kauanui, 2016).

Talking shit as a precursor to care

The hard stuff cannot be addressed without being in relation first, and being able to talk about the small stuff. Can we learn banter and small talk, the micro communication skills that build a foundation of trust and care? This trust is built brick by brick, conversation by conversation even around routine tasks. Talking to/with people and their families is crucial work, particularly as nurses are witness to the best and worst experiences a person, family, or community will undergo.

Time, questions of

Time, running out of

Time to think

Oftentime, sometimes, many times, out of time, in time, over time... What if we had more time?

424 Jessica Dillard-Wright et al.

Triage

If you are reading this, you are probably a nurse? Maybe a nurse, anyway. If you are a nurse, you are almost certainly familiar with triage as a way to decide who gets what and when. We employ it here in our collective writing as we try to write in dialogue according to our shared values. Maybe just like care has to be triaged in a resource-bound commodified sense, we also have to triage our kinship-based care, ensuring folks get what they need while also ensuring we get what we need. And part of what we need is a healthy community where our comrades and kin thrive.

See also: Care as Commodity, Care as Community, Care as Collective, Care, of Self.

Ubumuntu

The essence of what makes us human, relational, relatable, imperfect and in need for one another – the making of our shared humanity. It is embedded in how we care for others and how they respond to our care. In the context in which this word is used it is not assumed that every human "umuntu" always chooses to share their humanity "ubumuntu" for the common good so part of collective accountability is to remind individuals to be "human."

Unraveling

A process that allows for emergency, return, reclamation – not supported by the daily conditions of capitalism – pausing the pausing of one's self.

Whose [standards of] care?

As we have written this chapter, we have continually wrestled with care according to whose standards, to what ends, and how. Part of our collaborative process has been rooted in care for one another, but it remains unclear whether or how this would be recognized as nursing or care in other contexts.

Yes but

A colonially acceptable way to stop, shutdown, gatekeep, reject, energy vampire, or otherwise defang a potentially exciting, sometimes provocative idea, plan, or process. A no-as-barrier disguised as something else.

Zapatista Movement

As we come to the end of the alphabet, we think of social movements like CASSANDRA Radical Feminist Nurses Network, the People's Power Movement in the Philippines, Queer EcoJustice Project, the Young Lords, and the Zapatista Movement. No one of us has lived experience with or in the Zapatista movement, it is important to note. The Zapatista Movement coalesced at the turn of the 21st century, a collective of Mayan people organized for sovereignty, international solidarity, and resisting neoliberalism (Rethinking Schools Editors, 1999; Zapatista Army of National Liberation, 2005). What if we were guided by and collectively held to principles in action predicated on community accountability and solidarity rather than the static Code of Ethics that many don't see, don't read, don't have access to, didn't help to write, feel unmoved by? What might nursing care look like if we prioritized obeying in order to lead, proposing rather than imposing, modeling alternative modes of power, building consensus rather than overwhelming dissent, build rather than destroy, for many and not one, as the Zapatista Movement teaches (Oikonomakis, 2015)? Or in centering values of culture, consciousness, community, and collaboration, the priorities that drive the Queer EcoJustice Project (n.d.)? Or the Peace and Power process outlined by Charlene Eldridge Wheeler and Peggy Chinn (1984) in their feminist organizing which held up consensus and process over majority rule? While we cannot and do not embody all of these lived experiences, we are inspired by the community, accountability, solidarity, power-sharing, and care that guide these groups in their relations, finding alternatives that could transform nursing care relations, were we to embrace these principles. We leave you with this provocation in closing as both the final word and an invitation.

References

Benjamin, R. (2016). Informed Refusal: Toward a Justice-based Bioethics. *Science, Technology, & Human Values*, 41(6), 967–990. https://doi.org/10.1177/0162243916656059

Benjamin, R. (2018). Black AfterLives Matter: Cultivating Kinfulness as Reproductive Justice. In A. Clarke & D. Haraway (Eds.), *Making Kin Not Population* (pp. 41–66). Prickly Paradigm Press.

Braidotti, R. (2020). "We" Are In This Together, But We Are Not One and the Same. *Journal of Bioethical Inquiry*, 17(4), 465–469. https://doi.org/10.1007/s11673-020-10017-8

Brown, E. B. (1991). Polyrhythms and Improvisation: Lessons for Women's History. *History Workshop*, 31, 85–90.

Brown, E. B. (1992). "What Has Happened Here:" The Politics of Difference in Women's History and Feminist Politics. *Feminist Studies*, 18(2), 295–312. https://doi.org/10.2307/3178230

Butler, J. (2002). Is Kinship Always Already Heterosexual? *Differences: A Journal of Feminist Cultural Studies*, 13(1), 14–44.

de la Bellacasa, M. P. (2011). Matters of Care in Technoscience: Assembling Neglected Things. *Social Studies of Science*, 41(1), 85–106. https://doi.org/10.1177/0306312710380301

de Vries, B., Gutman, G., Soheilipour, S., Gahagan, J., Humble, Á., Mock, S., & Chamberland, L. (2022). Advance Care Planning Among Older LGBT Canadians: Heteronormative Influences. *Sexualities*, 25(1–2), 79–98. https://doi.org/10.1177/1363460719896968

Deleuze, G., & Guattari, F. (2007). *A Thousand Plateaus: Capitalism and Schizophrenia* (B. Massumi, Trans.). University of Minnesota Press.

DeSouza, R. (2021). Going Without: Migrant Mothers, Food, and the Postnatal Ward. In T. M. Cassidy & A. O. El-Tom (Eds.), *Moving Meals and Migrating Mothers: Culinary Cultures, Diasporic Dishes and Familial Foodways* (pp. 171–180). Demeter Press. https://doi.org/10.2307/j.ctv1tgwzz4

DeSouza, R. (2022). Using Arts-Based Participatory Methods to Teach Cultural Safety. In J. Dillard-Wright, J. Hopkins Walsh, & B. B. Brown (Eds.), *Nursing a Radical Imagination: Moving from Theory and History to Action and Alternate Futures* (pp. 152–165). Routledge. https://doi.org/10.4324/9781003245957-13

Dillard-Wright, J. (2022). A Radical imagination for Nursing: Generative Insurrection, Creative Resistance. *Nursing Philosophy*, 23(1), e12371. https://doi.org/10.1111/nup.12371

Dionne, E. (2021). Resisting Neoliberalism: A Feminist New Materialist Ethics of Care to Respond to Precarious World(s). In M. Hamington & M. Flowers (Eds.), *Care Ethics in the Age of Precarity* (pp. 229–259). University of Minnesota Press.

Fisher, B., & Tronto, J. (1990). Toward a Feminist Theory of Caring. In E. Abel & M. Nelson (Eds.), *Circles of Care Work and Identity in Women's Lives* (pp. 35–62). SUNY Press.

Foucault, M. (1994). *The Birth of the Clinic: An Archeology of Medical Perception* (S. Smith, Trans.). Vintage Books.

Gobbo, F., & Russo, F. (2020). Epistemic Diversity and the Question of Lingua Franca in Science and Philosophy. *Foundations of Science*, 25(1), 185–207. https://doi.org/10.1007/s10699-019-09631-6

Greenhalgh, S. (2001). *Under the Medical Gaze: Facts and Fictions of Chronic Pain*. University of California Press.

Harris, L. (2020). *A Philosophy of Struggle: The Leonard Harris Reader* (L. A. M. III, Ed.). Bloomsbury Academic.

Haunt, V. (n.d.). In *OED Online*. Oxford University Press. Retrieved December 1, 2022, from http://www.oed.com/view/Entry/84641

Hersey, T. (2022). *Rest Is Resistance: A Manifesto*. Little, Brown Spark.

Kaba, M. (2021). *We Do This Till We Free Us: Abolitionist Organizing and Transforming Justice*. Haymarket Books.

Kauanui, J. K. (2016). "A structure, not an event": Settler Colonialism and Enduring Indigeneity. *Lateral*, 5(1). https://doi.org/10.25158/L5.1.7

King, S. (2022). The "Science of Social Justice": An Interdisciplinary Theoretical Framework Grounded in Neuroscience, Education, and Anthropology towards Healing Intergenerational Trauma. *The Journal of Contemplative Inquiry*, 9(1), Article 1.

Klein, N. (2007). *The Shock Doctrine: The Rise of Disaster Capitalism*. Macmillan.

Mcbride, L. A. (2017). Insurrectionist Ethics and Racism. In N. Zack (Ed.), *The Oxford Handbook of Philosophy and Race* (pp. 225–234).). Oxford University Press. https://doi.org/10.1093/oxfordhb/9780190236953.013.52

Nazareno, J., Yoshioka, E., Adia, A. C., Restar, A., Operario, D., & Choy, C. C. (2021). From Imperialism to Inpatient Care: Work Differences of Filipino and White Registered Nurses in the United States and Implications for COVID-19 through an Intersectional Lens. *Gender, Work, and Organization*, 28(4), 1426–1446. https://doi.org/10.1111/gwao.12657

O'Conner, P. T., & Kellerman, S. (2009). *Origins of the Specious: Myths and Misconceptions of the English Language*. Random House.

Oikonomakis, L. (2015, Winter). Why We Still Love the Zapatistas. *ROAR Magazine*, Winter(0). https://roarmag.org/magazine/why-we-still-love-the-zapatistas/

Puig de la Bellacasa, M. (2017). *Matters of Care: Speculative Ethics in More than Human Worlds* (3rd ed.). Univ of Minnesota Press.

Queer EcoJustice Project. (n.d.). *About*. Queer EcoJustice Project. https://www.queerecoproject.org/about

Rethinking Schools Editors. (1999). Introduction: Zapatista Movement. *Rethinking Schools*, 14(1), 14–16.

Rudge, T. (2011). The 'well-run' System and its Antimonies. *Nursing Philosophy*, 12(3), 167–176. https://doi.org/10.1111/j.1466-769X.2011.00495.x

Scott, J. W. (1991). The Evidence of Experience. *Critical Inquiry*, 17(4), 773–797.

Thomson, P. (2019, February 11). Tiny Texts – Small Is Powerful. *Patter*. https://patthomson.net/2019/02/11/tiny-texts-if-not-beautiful%e2%80%8b-small-is-pretty-darn%e2%80%8b-useful/

Thorne, S. (2014). Nursing as Social Justice: A Case for Emancipatory Disciplinary Theorizing. In P. Kagan, M. Smith, & P. L. Chinn (Eds.), *Philosophies and Practices of Emancipatory Nursing* (pp. 70–90). Routledge.

Tuck, E., & Ree, C. (2013). A Glossary of Haunting. In S. Holman Jones, T. Adams, & C. Ellis (Eds.), *Handbook of Autoethnography* (pp. 639–658). Left Coast Press.

Tuck, E., Stepetin, H., Beaulne-Stuebing, R., & Billows, J. (2022). Visiting as an Indigenous Feminist Practice. *Gender and Education, 35*(2), 144–155 https://doi.org/10.1080/09540253 .2022.2078796

Tuck, E., & Yang, K. W. (2014a). R-words: Refusing Research. Humanizing research: Decolonizing qualitative inquiry with youth and communities, 223, 248.

Tuck, E., & Yang, K. W. (2014b). Unbecoming Claims: Pedagogies of Refusal in Qualitative Research. *Qualitative Inquiry*, 20(6), 811–818. https://doi.org/10.1177/1077800414530265

Watego, C. (2021). *Another Day in the Colony*. University of Queensland Press.

Wheeler, C., & Chinn, P. (1984). *Peace and Power: A Handbook of Feminist Process*. Margaret-daughters, Inc.

Wolfe, P. (2006). Settler Colonialism and the Elimination of the Native. *Journal of Genocide Research*, 8(4), 387–409. https://doi.org/10.1080/14623520601056240

Zapatista Army of National Liberation. (2005, June). Sixth Declaration of the Selva Lacandona. *Enlace Zapatista*. https://enlacezapatista.ezln.org.mx/sdsl-en/

Part 7
Scholarship, research, technology

41 Phenomenology and nursing

Dan Zahavi

Phenomenology is one of the influential movements in 20th-century philosophy.[1] It has over the years made major contributions to many areas of philosophy and offered incisive analyses of topics such as subjectivity, intentionality, perception, corporeality, temporality, and sociality, and is also known for its persistent criticism of various forms of reductionism, objectivism, and scientism. One of its central claims has been that if we want to understand the world we live in, we need to consider the role played by embodied, perceiving, thinking, and feeling agents (Zahavi 2019).

When hearing about phenomenology, people might think of Edmund Husserl's theory of the lifeworld, Martin Heidegger's analysis of anxiety, or Jean-Paul Sartre's description of the gaze. All three authors had a penchant for writing weighty tomes with daunting titles such as *Logical Investigations*, *Being and Time*, and *Being and Nothingness* and it might initially be hard to imagine how they could possibly contain ideas of relevance for the discipline of nursing. Since its inception, however, phenomenology has been seen by many as offering a refreshingly new way to philosophize, one that didn't get bogged down in dry abstractions and empty speculations, but which connected with everyday experience in a way not normally found in philosophy. As Husserl famously wrote:

> We can by no means be satisfied with 'mere words' [...]. We must return to 'the matters themselves'.
>
> (Husserl 2001: 168)

> The true method does not follow our prejudices and models, but rather the nature of the case to be investigated.
>
> (Husserl 1965: 102)

Already quite early, such insistence on the importance of carefully attending to the phenomena in their full concreteness and of avoiding what Spiegelberg calls the "premature strait-jacketing of the phenomena by preconceived theories" (Spiegelberg 1972: 308) started to have an influence on empirical science and the world beyond academic philosophy. Already prior to World War I, disciplines such as psychiatry and experimental psychology took inspiration from Husserl's ideas, and not long after, sociology and anthropology also started engaging with the work of the phenomenological philosophers. It took a bit longer for nursing science to catch up. Patricia Benner's 1984 book *From Novice to Expert*, which is a phenomenological study of how nurses develop embodied expertise, was a watershed (Benner 1984). Benner's account of nursing practice drew

DOI: 10.4324/9781003427407-49

heavily on Hubert Dreyfus' account of expertise and skill acquisition, which, in turn, was inspired by the work of Heidegger and Merleau-Ponty. Following the success of Benner's work, nursing researchers increasingly turned to phenomenology, and for the last 35 years journals such as *Nursing Inquiry, Qualitative Health Research, Nursing Philosophy, International Journal of Nursing Studies, Nurse Researcher,* and *Journal of Research in Nursing* have published numerous articles detailing how nurses might use phenomenology in their research and clinical practice.

On closer consideration, it is perhaps not that surprising that many nurses have turned to phenomenology when seeking to develop their own methodology and theoretical foundation. Phenomenology has a particular interest in subjective experience, in meaning, and in the lifeworld. This is an interest that phenomenologists share with nurses, who typically strive to take the experiential claims and concerns of their patients seriously. By being interested in patient experience, by striving to understand people's experiences of health, illness, and care, the discipline of nursing might ultimately have more affinities with the social sciences and its qualitative methods than with medicine and its reliance on the quantitative methods of the natural sciences. Indeed, if the aim is to provide proper care for, say, stroke patients, or patients with diabetes or Alzheimer's disease, it is important to have some understanding of what it is subjectively like to live with such conditions just as it is important to understand the meaning the patients attach to the events that disrupt their lives. Importantly, this focus on patient experience isn't simply about monitoring (and increasing) patient satisfaction. It is about obtaining information that will allow for more adequate health care. Some of the concerns that are part of nursing practice consequently seem to fit rather naturally with the phenomenological approach. Indeed, one reason why nursing science became interested in phenomenology was precisely because the latter was seen as a resource that could bridge the gap between research and practice. It could not only shape the way nursing research was conducted, but also inform clinical practice. It might in short help ensure that the academic field of nursing research actually led to an improvement of nursing practice.

Even if nurses had good reasons for turning to phenomenology, their engagement with that philosophical tradition hasn't been uncomplicated. Phenomenology is a heterogeneous movement. Should one take inspiration from Husserl or Heidegger? Merleau-Ponty or Levinas? Schutz or Sartre? Even more importantly, how deeply rooted in phenomenological philosophy must the nursing practice and research be in order to qualify as phenomenological? Must it, for instance, accept various theoretical core commitments found in phenomenological philosophy or would it be sufficient for it to simply consider the first-person perspective of the patient?

Only a minority of nursing researchers have gone directly to the classical sources themselves. The majority have chosen a different strategy, and instead sought guidance from leading proponents of phenomenology as a qualitative research method. In recent years, the work of Jonathan Smith, Max van Manen, and Amedeo Giorgi have been particularly widely used and referenced by nursing researchers. But, unfortunately, all three authors differ rather markedly in their methodological recommendations and in their view of how narrowly or broadly one should define what counts as phenomenological.

Smith, for instance, has argued that his own approach, which is called *Interpretative Phenomenological Analysis* (IPA), is phenomenological because it seeks to "explore the participant's view of the world and to adopt, as far as is possible, an 'insider's perspective' of the phenomenon under study" (Smith 1996: 264). But is it sufficient to simply consider the perspective of the informant in order to make the approach phenomenological? Is this sufficient to make the approach distinct from other approaches in qualitative research? Van Manen has deemed this to be a far too shallow and superficial use of phenomenology and argued that Smith's approach is "hopelessly misrepresentative of phenomenology in any acceptable sense" (van Manen 2018: 1962). For van Manen himself, the "basic method of phenomenological analysis consists of the epoché and the reduction" (2017b: 820). In one of his books meant to introduce phenomenology in a non-technical manner to researchers who are not themselves professional philosophers, van Manen goes further and distinguishes what he calls the heuristic, hermeneutic, experiential, methodological, eidetic, ontological, ethical, radical, and originary reduction as important elements of the phenomenological method (van Manen 2014: 222). But is it reasonable to propose that health care professionals interested in using phenomenology in their research or practice should master this complicated apparatus? This is certainly not the view of Giorgi, but he as well has argued that any qualitative research which is to qualify as phenomenological must employ part of Husserl's method, in particular the epoché and reduction, and thereby withhold "existential assent of the phenomena" (Giorgi 2012: 4).

What is this epoché and reduction? In a Husserlian context, both notions are explicitly connected to very specific philosophical aims and pursuits. To quickly recap Husserl's line of argumentation. In our everyday pre-philosophical life, we all take it for granted that the world is simply there. But if we really wish to engage with the fundamental epistemological and metaphysical questions in a radical and unprejudiced manner, we must subject this basic trust in the absolute and mind-independent existence of the world to a critical examination. To do so, we must first perform an epoché vis-à-vis "the being or non-being of the world" (Husserl 1960: 36), i.e., we must first suspend or bracket any assumptions we might have regarding its mode of being. Rather than taking worldly reality as the unquestioned point of departure, we should instead attend to the phenomena and examine how worldly objects are given to us. Doing so will bring us to the realization that reality is always revealed and examined from some experiential perspective or another, and we will thereby come to appreciate the importance of our own contributing subjectivity. When Husserl speaks of the reduction, what he has in mind is precisely the systematic analysis of the relation between experiencing subjectivity and objective world; an analysis that will eventually lead us to the insight that consciousness, reason, truth, and being are essentially interlinked (Husserl 1982: 340). These are important philosophical ideas. It is much less obvious that they are also ideas that everybody seeking to apply phenomenology outside of philosophy must constantly bear in mind (Zahavi 2021). Indeed, is it reasonable to insist that nurses, who want to use phenomenology to better understand the changed life-circumstances of diabetes patients must first learn to suspend various deep-seated metaphysical assumptions about the mind-independent status of the world and "resist from positing as existing whatever object or state of affairs is present" (Giorgi 2012: 4)?

Given the lack of agreement between Smith, van Manen, and Giorgi (Giorgi 2012; van Manen 2017a; Smith 2018; Zahavi 2020), it is perhaps not overly surprising that nursing research's turn to phenomenology has met resistance from some quarters. One persistent critic has been John Paley who has not only accused nurses of mostly misinterpreting the philosophical ideas they claim to rely on, but who has also argued that the approaches of Smith, van Manen, and Giorgi lack methodological rigor and are permeated by personal idiosyncrasies (Paley 2017: 28, 147). Paley's recommendation has not been that nurses should turn to the primary sources and become more familiar with the philosophy they are basing their research on, but rather that they should abandon their attempts to ground their research on phenomenological philosophy altogether (Paley 1997: 192). This message has started to resonate through nursing studies to such a degree that some have even started to ask the question, "Is there nursing phenomenology after Paley?" (Petrovskaya 2014).

I don't think the turn to phenomenology was a mistake. Phenomenology contains important resources of relevance for nursing, but it is urgent to strike the right balance between a too superficial and a too orthodox engagement with its philosophical ideas.

As we have just seen, a standard assumption has been that if nursing research (and practice) is to engage with phenomenology, it has to adopt its method, it has to perform the epoché and reduction. I have already expressed reservations about this assumption. Nurses are, of course, welcome to explore both of these quite technical concepts, but the question is whether their use is mandatory for any clinical research or practice that wants to call itself phenomenological. This is what I am disputing. Rather than primarily focusing on the question of whether nurses are using phenomenology in a manner that accords as much as possible with Husserl's (or Heidegger's or Levinas', etc.) philosophical method, a far more productive focus would be on whether the phenomenological concepts or analyses drawn upon allow for new insights or better therapeutic interventions (Zahavi & Martiny 2019).

Perhaps this proposal will be resisted. The very idea that one should draw on pre-existing phenomenological concepts or analyses might appear problematic. After all, is the phenomenological approach not precisely characterized by a jettisoning of prior theories and theoretical commitments? Is the phenomenological attitude not ultimately about obtaining a "sense of wonder and openness to the world" that will allow one to "meet the phenomenon in as fresh a way as possible" (Finlay 2008: 2, 12)? One place where such ideas have surfaced in the nursing literature is in interview guides. Although extensive clinical observations can certainly provide important insights, nursing researchers and practitioners will typically also have to interview the patients. But how are these interviews to be conducted? According to one approach, nurses must be very careful in not asking any guiding questions. If the aim is to understand how particular events and life episodes are experienced by the individuals in question, the interviewees must be allowed to express themselves about their own experience without being unduly influenced or constrained by the interviewer's research agenda. This is why, Wood, for instance, in an article published in *Rehabilitation Nursing* suggests that "in true phenomenological research only one question is usually asked to elicit data" (Wood 1991: 196). Typically, the opening question will be quite broad and non-directive, and simply be a question that encourages the interviewee to start describing his or her experiences. This approach is, however, confronted with multiple problems. One of them is the following: What if the participants who are being interviewed and who are requested to provide rich descriptions of, say, what it is like to live with depression or chronic obstructive pulmonary disease, are only able to offer very coarse and superficial descriptions? But why assume that the interviewee is from the outset able to offer detailed descriptions and that the task of the interviewer is simply to register everything that is being said? Why not instead view the interview as a collaborative process, where the task of the interviewer is to help the interviewee obtain new insights of his or her own. To adopt a hands-off approach, where one simply asks the patient to describe his or her experiences and then sits back and listens, is clearly not the right way. Moreover, although one should, of course, be prepared to revise one's theoretical assumptions in the face of what the patient is saying, a methodological prerequisite for doing the interview is by no means that one initially strips one's own mind of preconceived ideas. On the contrary, it is all about conducting the interview in light of quite specific ideas and notions, notions taken from phenomenological theory. To conduct a phenomenological interview is consequently not simply a question of being open-minded and interested in first-person experience. It is very much also about adopting and employing a comprehensive theoretical framework that will allow one to ask the right questions in order to determine how different dimensions of human existence are affected in pathology, illness, or difficult life-circumstances.

Let me exemplify. As pointed out by Dahlberg, if we wish to offer proper care, we shouldn't focus on the symptoms in isolation, but need to understand how the illness in question affects the more general life-situation of the patient (Dahlberg et al. 2009). We need to understand how it affects the patient's being-in-the-world, e.g., his or her intentional, temporal, spatial, and social sense-making. But this is precisely where a health care professional can profit from phenomenological investigations of intentionality, embodiment, temporality, empathy, spatiality, etc. Consider a classical phenomenological distinction such as that between the time of the clock and lived time. Consider how the experience of time can change as a result of a diagnosis. Consider how it might affect short- and long-term planning; consider how it might change one's experience of the openness of the future. Consider how an hour in pain, or an hour waiting for treatment, might feel much longer than an hour spent watching an exciting movie, even though the hour still contains the same number of minutes. Or consider other phenomenological distinctions such as that between geometric space and lived space, between empathic and imaginative interpersonal understanding,[2] or between the body as object and the body as subject.

Perhaps this still sound too abstract, so let me try to offer a slightly more detailed example and pick a notion with immediate relevance for nursing, namely *embodiment*.[3] How do phenomenologists approach the body? Supposedly by attending to the way it appears. But how is the body given? Is it primarily given as a perceptual object in space? That it can be given in such a way is evident from any anatomy lesson, but phenomenology has long insisted on the need for recognizing the difference between the body that is perceptually given as an object among many, and the body as it is subjectively lived through. While the body as object captures how the body is apprehended from an observer's point of view, where the observer might be a scientist, a physician, or even the embodied subject herself, the notion of a subjective body captures the way the body is lived through from an embodied first-person perspective.

The distinction between the body as subject and the body as object is a phenomenological distinction. It is a distinction between two ways in which we can experience and understand the same body and is not a distinction between two different bodies. A further claim made by many phenomenologists is that the lived body precedes the perceived body. In the first instance, I am not conscious of my body as an intentional object. I do not perceive it; *I am it*. Indeed, rather than simply being an object that I perceive in space, the body is precisely what allows me to perceive spatial objects in the first place. Moreover, we do not observe the world from a distance, but are placed right in its middle, and as Husserl remarks, the world reveals itself to us according to our bodily ways of inhabiting it:

It is thus that all things of the surrounding world possess an orientation to the Body [...]. The 'far' is far from me, from my Body; the 'to the right' refers back to the right side of my Body, e.g., to my right hand. [...] I have all things over and against me; they are all 'there' – with the exception of one and only one, namely the Body, which is always 'here'.

(Husserl 1989: 166)

The fact that the world is given to us as a world of affordances, i.e., as situations of meaning and circumstances for action, as allowing or preventing specific bodily activities, the fact that the body is operative in every perception and every action, the fact that it constitutes our point of view and our point of departure is, however, not something we normally attend to. In normal life, our bodily capacities are taken for granted. When riding our bike or brushing our teeth, we seldomly attend to our bodily skills. They remain in the background as something we can count on. But of course, this can quickly change, because of pain, exhaustion, illness, or disability. What was previously taken for granted is suddenly problematized. As Carel writes:

Cases of illness make apparent not only the bodily feeling of confidence, familiarity, and continuity that is disturbed, but also a host of assumptions that hang on it. For example, one's future plans depend on bodily capacities and thus are limited by ill health. One's temporal sense is radically changed by a poor prognosis. One's values and sense of what is important in life are frequently modified in light of illness; bodily limitations impact on one's existence generally.

(Carel 2013: 184)

This is also why we cannot simply view illness as something inhabiting a less than perfect physiological machine. To understand illness, we need to understand how it affects the patient's being-the-world. Consider, for example, how a person who finds himself bound to a wheelchair doesn't simply undergo a change in embodied self-experience. He finds the environment changed as well. What used to be an easily accessible storeroom in the basement might now appear as an inaccessible and unusable part of the house. Even if the distance to the top shelf of the cupboard remains the same when measured in centimeters, it is now out of reach. In some cases, illness can also be identity transforming. A diabetic long-distance runner who loses her left foot due to gangrene might have to struggle with the task of redefining who she is, since the goals and activities that she used to consider identity defining are no longer available. Or consider somebody with locked-in syndrome, who is conscious and cognitively unimpaired, but paralyzed and unable to communicate verbally. In such circumstances, the body might well be experienced as an antagonist rather than as (part of) who I am.

These brief remarks only touch the surface of a phenomenological analysis of the body, but should make it evident, I hope, why such an analysis might be relevant to nurses, might aid them in understanding how illness or disability can affect the life of the patient (Leder 1990; Toombs 1992; Svenaeus 2000). A familiarity with phenomenological theorizing about the body can, however, not only help health care professionals better tailor their care to individual patients; by using these phenomenological ideas in clinical practice, by being oriented toward and concerned with the life situation of concrete patients, by attending to specific aspects or dimensions that the phenomenological philosophers might have overlooked, the nurses can also contribute to theory development, and help refine the phenomenological analyses and distinctions. In the cognitive science literature, this situation has been labeled a relationship of *mutual enlightenment* (Gallagher 1997), since it isn't merely a question of importing and applying readymade ideas from philosophy to a given domain; rather in the best of cases, it is a two-way exchange, where both sides can profit from the interaction.

The relevance of phenomenology for nursing is not restricted to these kinds of analyses, however. Phenomenology also offers insights of a more systemic nature. One interesting application of these can be found in an older study by Ashworth and colleagues (1992). The idea that patients should be actively involved in rather than simply passive recipients of health care decisions is widespread and has in particular been considered decisive for increased patient compliance. But what is the right way to involve the patient and what are the obstacles to such involvement? In order to address these questions, the authors turned to the phenomenological sociologist Alfred Schutz and his work on social interaction. They briefly presented some of his core ideas, and in particular highlighted Schutz's discussion of the social distribution of knowledge. The authors then immediately proceeded to show how these ideas might be used in everyday clinical practice. Participation is always contextual; it is participation in a shared cultural practice that often relies on a number of taken-for-granted assumptions. One obvious challenge to proper patient participation is that the patients are encouraged and invited to participate in a medical setting involving specific tasks, procedures, aims, roles and statuses that they are often quite unfamiliar with, and where they and the health care professionals are not at all on equal footing. While the nurses are trained experts who are thoroughly familiar with all the standards routines connected to admission, history taking, ward rounds, discharge etc., many of these procedures will be quite bewildering to the patients, who will attempt to make sense of them on the basis of their own past experiences. The mismatch between the nurse's and patient's stock of knowledge can easily lead to miscommunication and misunderstanding. Indeed, the very attempt by the nurses to actively involve the patients in their own health care decision, might even come as a surprise to the patients and be interpreted as evidence of the nurses' lack of care and concern. If the nurses are to succeed in involving the patients in genuinely patient-centered care, it is consequently crucial that the nurses are aware of and recognize the patients' varied life experiences.

Let me in conclusion outline three challenges that current nursing research and practice are confronted with when it comes to a successful engagement with phenomenology.

The first challenge is that of being *too superficial*. Occasionally, a study is being presented as phenomenological simply because it contains careful first-person descriptions of experience. But is it really appropriate to qualify a study or an approach as phenomenological simply because it considers the perspective of the informant, is qualitative and non-reductive, and seeks to provide rich experiential descriptions? Would such an approach really differ from other approaches in qualitative research, would such a study allow for insights that one could not have obtained otherwise? Is there not far more to phenomenology than simply being open-minded and interested in first-person experience?

A possible remedy against the superficiality charge is to engage with the classical texts and seek inspiration from them. Indeed, it seems reasonable to expect any researcher or practitioner who claims to be using a phenomenological method, procedure, or approach to have some familiarity with phenomenological theory. This immediately confronts us with the next challenge, however, which is that of being *too philosophical*, i.e., operating with too many technical philosophical concepts or methodological requirements whose clinical relevance remains unclear. It is essential that phenomenology is being used in a transparent way, i.e., in such a way that it is clear which elements are being used and what role they are supposed to play. A certain pragmatism is consequently appropriate. One should only employ concepts and methodological tools that are pertinent for the task at hand, and which can make a valuable difference, i.e., which can allow for new insights or better therapeutic interventions. The pursuit of purity or orthodoxy is a red herring. It is not coincidental that many of the leading figures that initially used ideas from phenomenology in psychology, psychiatry, or sociology adopted a quite heterodox approach to phenomenology. In the conclusion to his impressive survey *Phenomenology in Psychology and Psychiatry*, for instance, Spiegelberg explicitly warns against "an orthodox return to Husserl" (Spiegelberg 1972: 366) and argues that one has to free oneself from some of the technicalities of Husserl's philosophy if a true two-way exchange between psychology and phenomenology is to be possible.

This finally brings me to the third charge, which is that of remaining *too insular*. Over the years, phenomenology has found use in a variety of disciplines. Somewhat surprisingly, however, insights from one successful disciplinary application have rarely been taken up by other disciplines. While there are ongoing debates regarding the relevance of phenomenology in, for instance, nursing research, sociology, anthropology, psychology, psychiatry, and embodied cognitive science each of these disciplines have only to a quite limited extent engaged with and profited from ongoing discussions in the other disciplines. This is a missed opportunity. The way forward is to collaborate across the disciplines and to draw on and learn from exemplary approaches and best practice models. Were qualitative researchers, nursing scholars, anthropologists, psychologists, psychiatrists, and philosophers to collaborate in the development of an applied phenomenology everybody would profit?

As should be clear from what I have written, my take on how phenomenology is best to be used in a non-philosophical context is very much a pragmatic one. To qualify as good phenomenological research, the phenomenological tools being employed must show their pertinence, must make a valuable difference. We should assess the value of the procedure on the basis of the results it delivers, and not on the basis of its orthodoxy or purity.

Notes

1 An earlier and much shorter version of the present text was originally published in the online magazine *Aeon* under the title "A sage on the ward."
2 For some discussions of how nurses might benefit from phenomenological discussions of empathy, see Fernandez and Zahavi 2020, 2021.
3 The following example is adapted from Zahavi 2020.

References

Ashworth, P. D., Longmate, M. A., & Morrison, P. (1992). Patient participation: Its meaning and significance in the context of caring. *Journal of Advanced Nursing* 17: 1430–1439.
Benner, P. (1984). *From Novice to Expert: Excellence and Power in Clinical Nursing Practice.* Menlo Park, CA: Addison-Wesley Publishing Company.
Carel, H. (2013). Bodily doubt. *Journal of Consciousness Studies* 20/7–8: 178–197.
Dahlberg, K., Todres, L., & Galvin, K. (2009). Lifeworld-led healthcare is more than patient-led care: An existential view of well-being. *Medicine, Health Care and Philosophy* 12: 265–271.
Fernandez, A. V., & Zahavi, D. (2020). Basic empathy: Developing the concept of empathy from the ground up. *International Journal of Nursing Studies* 110: 103695.
Fernandez, A. V., & Zahavi, D. (2021). Can we train basic empathy? A phenomenological proposal. *Nurse Education Today* 98: 104720.

Finlay, L. (2008). A dance between the reduction and reflexivity: Explicating the "phenomenological psychological attitude". *Journal of Phenomenological Psychology* 39: 1–32.

Gallagher, S. (1997). Mutual enlightenment: Recent phenomenology in cognitive science. *Journal of Consciousness Studies* 4(3): 195–214.

Giorgi, A. (2012). The descriptive phenomenological psychological method. *Journal of Phenomenological Psychology* 43: 3–12.

Husserl, E. (1960). *Cartesian Meditations: An Introduction to Phenomenology*, trans. D. Cairns. The Hague: Martinus Nijhoff.

Husserl, E. (1965). Philosophy as rigorous science, trans. Q. Lauer. In Q. Lauer (ed.), *Phenomenology and the Crisis of Philosophy* (pp. 71–147). New York: Harper & Row.

Husserl, E. (1982). *Ideas Pertaining to a Pure Phenomenology and to a Phenomenological Philosophy. First Book. General Introduction to a Pure Phenomenology*, trans. F. Kersten. The Hague: Martinus Nijhoff.

Husserl, E. (1989). *Ideas Pertaining to a Pure Phenomenology and to a Phenomenological Philosophy. Second Book. Studies in the Phenomenology of Constitution*, trans. R. Rojcewicz and A. Schuwer. Dordrecht: Kluwer Academic Publishers.

Husserl, E. (2001). *Logical Investigations I-II*, trans. J. N. Findlay. London: Routledge.

Leder, D. (1990). *The Absent Body*. Chicago, IL: University of Chicago Press.

Paley, J. (1997). Husserl, phenomenology and nursing. *Journal of Advanced Nursing* 26: 187–193.

Paley, J. (2017). *Phenomenology as Qualitative Research: A Critical Analysis of Meaning Attribution*. London: Routledge.

Petrovskaya, O. (2014). Nursing phenomenology after Paley. *Nursing Philosophy* 15: 60–71.

Smith, J. A. (1996). Beyond the divide between cognition and discourse: Using interpretative phenomenological analysis in health psychology. *Psychology & Health* 11(2): 261–271.

Smith, J. A. (2018). 'Yes it is phenomenological': A reply to Max Van Manen's critique of interpretative phenomenological analysis. *Qualitative Health Research* 28/12: 1955–1958.

Spiegelberg, H. (1972). *Phenomenology in Psychology and Psychiatry: A Historical Introduction*. Evanston, IL: Northwestern University Press.

Svenaeus, F. (2000). *The Hermeneutics of Medicine and the Phenomenology of Health: Steps Towards a Philosophy of Medical Practice*. Dordrecht: Kluwer.

Toombs, S. K. (1992). *The Meaning of Illness: A Phenomenological Account of the Different Perspectives of Physician and Patient*. Dordrecht: Kluwer.

van Manen, M. (2014). *Phenomenology of Practice: Meaning-giving methods in phenomenological research and writing*. Walnut Creek, CA: Left Coast Press.

van Manen, M. (2017a). But is it phenomenology? *Qualitative Health Research* 27/6: 775–779.

van Manen, M. (2017b). Phenomenology in its original sense. *Qualitative Health Research* 27: 810–825.

van Manen, M. (2018). Rebuttal rejoinder: Present IPA for what it is—Interpretative psychological analysis. *Qualitative Health Research* 28: 1959–1968.

Wood, F. G. (1991). The meaning of caregiving. *Rehabilitation Nursing* 16/4: 195–198.

Zahavi, D. (2019). *Phenomenology: The Basics*. London: Routledge.

Zahavi, D (2020). The practice of phenomenology: The case of Max van Manen. *Nursing Philosophy* 21: 12276.

Zahavi, D. (2021). Applied phenomenology: Why it is safe to ignore the epoché. *Continental Philosophy Review* 54/2: 259–273.

Zahavi, D., & Martiny, K. M. M. (2019). Phenomenology in nursing studies: New perspectives. *International Journal of Nursing Studies* 93: 155–162.

42 Is there anyone here who has a genuine medical problem? Health, illness and Aristotle

Peter Allmark

Introduction

The issue of how we should "pin down", that is define, specify, describe or model health and related concepts, such as illness and disease, has come to be seen as a central question in healthcare philosophy.[1] Philosophy has developed many ways to analyse concepts. In this handbook, for example, John Paley sets out four types of conceptual or concept analysis. I will use a combination of two: first, ordinary language (OL) philosophy and, second, what Paley terms conceptual analysis, or the method of cases. First, though, why might it matter to pin down health terms?

Why pinning down health terms might matter

"Is there anyone here who has a genuine medical problem?"[2]

The above quote is taken from a scene in the UK TV comedy drama, Doc Martin, in which the eponymous GP rails against his waiting room full of what he views as time wasters and hypochondriacs. It takes us to the first reason that pinning down health terms might matter, that is, to settle disputes concerning whether certain phenomena truly constitute health issues. Foremost here is the dispute about whether mental illness is a true illness or, say, a way in which society controls behaviour it disapproves of (Szasz, 1998). There are also disputes about whether myalgic encephalitis (ME), long COVID, chronic pain and mild-to-moderate depression are genuine illnesses. There has also been a discussion about whether teenage pregnancy, smoking and obesity should be seen as health problems dealt with by public health bodies or whether they are, at most, social problems and bad habits. Related to this, the UK government has recently been discussing which activities constitute healthcare and which social care, in order to decide budgetary responsibilities.

A second reason concerns moral and legal responsibilities for action. If, for example, mental health is simply a myth, then presumably the defence of not being guilty on grounds of diminished responsibility would be impossible to maintain. If ME is not a genuine illness, then doctors will not write sick notes for employees who wish to take time off for it.

There is also a concern about the scientific basis of healthcare. Ian Kennedy (1983) took Szasz's argument on from mental health, applying it to all health terms. He argued that illness and disease are not facts but judgements on facts. At the time, there was a furious response from medics who viewed this as a threat to the view of medicine as objective and scientific.

DOI: 10.4324/9781003427407-49

One final reason that pinning down health terms might matter concerns issues of measurement and justice. We might wish to measure the health status of individuals or groups within society; alongside this, we might have concerns about health inequalities. But both measurement and action for justice would presumably require that we know what is meant by health and how to measure it; it would also require us to say why health inequality is a matter of justice.

Attempts to pin down health terms

This gives us some initial reasons why we might desire to pin down health terms; let us turn next to some attempts at doing so. Haverkamp et al. (2018) provide a helpful overview of five accounts of health. They compare these accounts across various features. One is that of naturalism versus normativism. Naturalistic accounts of health view it as a natural state, a descriptive term that can be discerned from biological facts; normative accounts say that any statement concerning health involves some form of value judgement or evaluation. This distinction between naturalist and normative accounts also tends to be reflected in a distinction between reductionist and holist accounts. Reductionist accounts view health as the product of a summation of healthy parts, while holist accounts view it as something that emerges from but is more than the sum of such parts. There are also distinctions to be made concerning (amongst others) the relationship between health and well-being and the relationship between health and disease.

Haverkamp et al. (2018) suggest that all five accounts capture something correct about the concept of health. But rather than develop yet another account which tries to capture all of these correct features, they suggest a pluralist approach. They argue that health practices differ in their purposes and character. This plurality requires a complementary variety of health concepts. They give three examples. The first is biomedical research, which is well served by relatively objective and naturalistic accounts of health against which to test treatment. The second is care of the chronically ill, where, they say, the health concepts should primarily be subjectivist. The third is health inequality: this requires an account of health that is measurable but which answers to the needs and desires of the different populations to be compared. They also suggest that the account of health may need to focus on the wider environment rather than simply the healthy or unhealthy individual.

Using this pluralist approach, rather than seeking the correct meanings for health terms, we look at how health terms are used in particular contexts. This approach can be given philosophical heft: we can say that health terms are used in a wide variety of ways and have a variety of meanings which ultimately bear some family resemblance. This notion of family resemblance is inspired by Wittgenstein, who used the term to cover conceptual terms such as games and numbers; others have suggested terms such as art. The idea is that such terms do not have a shared single feature, core or essence but instead share sets of features, none of which are possessed by all examples. The term, disease, shows this clearly. While there are many diseases, it does not follow that there is a set of necessary or sufficient conditions by which we can clearly or definitely categorise something as disease-in-general. Instead, diseases share a family resemblance.

Earlier, we set out some puzzles and problems relating to health terms as a way of showing why we might want to pin them down. I mentioned the UK government dispute about which practices count as healthcare or as social care. On the pluralist account, this is not a problem to be resolved by getting clear about our definitions; rather, it is to be decided by thinking through the best way to organise budgets and bureaucracy. We might decide that healthcare should include care of the disabled, the old and frail, the sad and lonely; in doing so, we will be expanding our meaning of the term health. Alternatively, we might shrink the term health down to mean only those things that are currently treated by medical or surgical interventions.

Puzzles

Are there puzzles that the pluralist account does not satisfactorily resolve? It is clear that the pluralist account is, despite its cover-all nature, normative rather than naturalist. While it allows the use of a naturalist account in some circumstances, it nonetheless requires that practitioners make judgements about what to include under the umbrella of health terms and healthcare. And this, in turn, leaves some of the problems faced by other normative accounts. Chief amongst these is the question of which values should be used to decide health issues. Is it simply fiat by which, for example, practitioners come to define some behaviour as mental illness or to allow the defence of insanity in court? Why is being unhoused not included as a health issue while teenage pregnancy is? On the basis of whose values should inequalities in health be a concern from the viewpoint of justice?

To begin my attempt to develop an account that is better able to deal with such problems, the next section of the chapter will analyse health terms using the OL approach mentioned earlier. It will then use the insights from this to develop an account of health terms that maintains the strengths of the pluralist account while providing a basis to tackle the puzzles set out.

Ordinary language and health terminology

OL philosophy is based in the idea that everyday language, for the most part, works well in enabling people to express and communicate. OL philosophers say that we should not leave behind or forget the way language is ordinarily used when using language in a philosophical context. Hence in his *Sense and Sensibilia*, JL Austin, who is closely associated with OL philosophy, criticises philosophers influenced by logical positivism, particularly AJ Ayer, for their account of knowledge and perception which is entirely detached from ordinary speech (Austin, 1962). This is not to say that ordinary speech is a benchmark for correct usage but rather that close attention needs to be paid to it in philosophical analysis. If we want to know what is meant by conceptual words such as health, illness and disease, we should look to how those words are used.

In one paper, JL Austin bemoans the lack of time and space to look at how words are actually used by real commentators on real incidents or by narrators of fictional incidents (Austin, 1956). Austin tells us that, therefore, he can only use imaginary cases. Such cases are limited by the individual philosopher's own imagination and experience. This problem can now be overcome thanks to the development and continuing growth of corpuses, databases of huge numbers of examples of actual use of language. For this chapter, I looked at two: the British National Corpus (BNC), which collates examples of British usage of English, and the Corpus of Contemporary American English (COCA), which collates American English.

Both BNC and COCA give an indication of the frequency of terms. They also categorise use of words into different sources, such as academic, newspaper, magazine, fiction and spoken sources, particularly television and radio. Health is a high-frequency term in both corpuses. This means it turns up often in the sources collated. It is most commonly seen in academic sources but also appears frequently in newspapers and magazines; it is least common in fiction. Illness and disease are also high-frequency terms although less common than health which is at least twice as common as the other two terms. There was (at least) one reference to a political movement as a disease (fascism). In addition, we might have a vehicle health check, a sick building, an unhealthy economy and many more.

It might seem surprising that health is more commonly used than illness and disease, given that the latter terms seem less abstract. Nonetheless, all the terms are high-frequency and the examples show decisiveness in their use – I saw no cases where the terms were applied with any doubt as to their use or meaning. We might say, therefore, that the terms are normal and firmly established.

There is also some univocity in meaning. All health terms apply to something internal to the entity that has them; hence, bad if it's diseased or ill, good if it's healthy or in good health. Illness and disease are unambiguously bad for the entity that has them. They might not necessarily be bad from our viewpoint, for example, where disease is deliberately introduced to counter threat from an invasive plant species. Health, by contrast, is neutral – an entity can be in good or bad health. Often, the term, health, implies good health but this implication is usually clear in the context. From this basis in OL, let us now develop the account of health terms.

Method of cases

If someone is wealthy then they have wealth, if stealthy, stealth; the relationship is direct. By contrast, if someone is healthy, they do not merely have health, they have good health. Health is something that can be attributed to all people, only some of whom would be called healthy. Thus, health is like an attribute such as height or weight; we require more information before we can say anything meaningful about the individual: "he has (a state of) health" is no more useful a statement than "he has height and weight".

In addition, it is useful to distinguish two ways in which health terms are used; let us call these sense 1 and sense 2.

- Sense 1 is the state of health of the entity, as when we speak of a healthy animal or plant.
- Sense 2 is the capacity of an entity to affect the health of someone or something else, as when we speak of an unhealthy diet.

Health is almost always a sense 1 term, as are the terms ill and diseased; by contrast, disease and illness, being the entities that can affect the health of other entities, are generally sense 2 terms. Hence, when we ask what types of entity can be said to be healthy or not, we need to be clear that we speak only in sense 1 terms. As noted, a diet can be healthy (sense 2) but it cannot be in good health (sense 1). What, then, are the entities to which we attribute health terms in sense 1?

The clue lies in the idea that an entity's health or illness is something internal. A vehicle fails its health check if it has faulty spark plugs causing it to be unable to move; it does not fail if it is locked in a garage and the key is lost, even though it is also unable to move. Similarly, an animal with plentiful food but an inability to digest it is ill; this is something internal to it. An animal with an ability to digest but no food available is not ill (although it will soon become so); this is something external to it. The ability to have internal problems signifies that the entity is a whole that is made up of interconnected parts. A pebble has no such interconnected parts and health terms in sense 1 cannot be attributed to it; a car, by contrast, does.

Described in this way, the entities to which health terms, sense 1, apply can be called systems: these are entities made up of component parts that work together to produce some outcome. In particular, they are end-based or teleological systems, that is, they are organised towards some outcome or outcomes. A weather system, for example, may produce certain outcomes but is not organised towards that outcome; as such, we would not describe as unhealthy (sense 1) a weather system that breaks down, such as a potential storm that fails to eventuate. We might, however, say that a car which is unable to start because it lacks working spark plugs is unhealthy (sense 1) or, more likely, that it has failed its health check. I propose, therefore, that health terms in sense 1 are applied to systems, particularly, end-based or teleological systems.

One objection here is that the attribution of health terms to manufactured end-based systems is uneven. In many cases, it would be more idiomatic to talk simply in terms of whether it is working or not. Those inanimate systems we talk of in health terms tend to be those we anthropomorphise, such as cars to which we might give a name and might describe, say, as being poorly. There is something in this criticism, although there are other artefacts to which it doesn't apply so easily, such as when we have a PC health check. The key point, however, is the univocity noted earlier; we readily and easily apply health terms to these end-based systems and not to other human creations, such as objects of art or music or diets.

More substantial objections might arise with the idea that organisms are end-based, however. In responding, I will take it is unproblematic that organisms are systems and that they contain subsystems, that is, systems within them that have a specific purpose in themselves (as the eye has the purpose of enabling sight) but which, in turn, serve the needs of the organism overall. But in what sense can we say that organisms themselves have a purpose or end, in the light of which we deem them to be healthy or not? Let us leave aside the possibility that organisms are created for a purpose by a creator and stick with the view that organisms have evolved by chance processes of interaction between the environment and genetic drift. In this picture, there are at least two ways in which organisms may be described as end-based systems, one narrow and one broad.

A typical narrow account would be based in evolutionary science, saying that the end or purpose of an organism is to survive and reproduce; more narrowly still, it might be said the purpose is to replicate its own DNA. A broad account might typically draw on Aristotelian philosophy. This would describe the end or purpose (Greek, *telos*) of an organism as being found in the way it flourishes; another way of describing this is to say the organism's *telos* is seen in the activity of the best examples of its kind. This will include reproduction and survival – but this is found in all organisms; it doesn't mark out the difference in *telos* between one organism type and another. That is to be found, rather, in the characteristic way in which the organism survives and flourishes.

To illustrate the difference between narrow and broad accounts, imagine a species of big cat that is native to cold, forest areas but which no longer survives in such areas. Instead, the surviving cats are maintained in protected zones, such as zoos, where they are fed, have the services of a veterinary service and breed successfully. On the narrow account, the cat is achieving its end and is, therefore, healthy; on the broader account, it is not because it is not flourishing *qua* that species of cat.

The narrow account seems best to fit with OL usage of health terms. Any individual cat in the protected zone would be thought healthy if it is able to survive and reproduce without undue difficulty from internal sources, that is, diseases or illnesses. The broad account is too demanding: animals can be healthy without flourishing *qua* that type of animal. This opens a gap between flourishing and health. The cats in their controlled environment are healthy; but we might doubt they are flourishing. The cats are healthy because they *could* flourish– but the environment is such that they are not doing so. In this case, good health seems to be the wherewithal, the lack of internal physical or mental barriers, to flourish.

EBSAH – the ends-based systems account of health terms

Let us term the account we have developed an ends-based system account of health terms (EBSAH). An end-based system's health is a measure of its ability to achieve its ends, given the right external circumstances. In some cases, the gap between health and achieving ends is narrow; a healthy plant in the right environment will flourish; in the wrong environment, it will not flourish but it will also cease to be healthy. However, the health to flourishing gap widens in higher animals. A person can be in good health but, say, imprisoned, friendless and generally unhappy, and, as such, does not seem to be flourishing.

In examining EBSAH, we can start by asking whether it provides a naturalist or normative account of health terms. The EBSAH links health terms to systems, particularly natural entities and the ways they flourish. In plants, as we've seen, there is little or no gap between good health and flourishing; here, a naturalist account of health terms seems plausible. In other words, the good health of a plant can be described entirely in fairly objective, natural terms.

In higher animals and humans, it is more problematic. Flourishing in these cases is not identical with good health. It also involves evaluation. We saw with the cats which, despite their ability to live disease-free and without great suffering or want, might not be described as flourishing. Could we perhaps say, therefore, that the description of health in these cases is naturalistic, as it is with the plants, but the description of flourishing is evaluative? This would be a naturalist interpretation of the EBSAH. Roughly it would state that evaluation is necessary to describe human flourishing but that once this is done, a description of the internal wherewithal humans need to achieve human flourishing can be done without evaluation. Take the following syllogism:

1 Humans need the capacity for social contact and recreation,
2 Parkinson's Disease inhibits this,
3 Therefore, PD is an illness or disease,

AND

4 PD is an internal feature of some human beings that can be described in non-evaluative terms,
5 Therefore, at least some diseases (and other health terms) are naturalist, non-evaluative terms.

An evaluative judgement of what is needed for human flourishing is set out in premiss 1. But premiss 2 simply states a naturalistic fact; it says that if humans need the capacity for social contact and recreation then PD inhibits that capacity. In addition, PD itself can be described in biochemical terms that involve no value judgements. This could work in a similar way for mental illness if, for example, we replace the term PD with "bipolar disorder".

This has implications for some of the puzzles. We noted earlier that Szasz and the anti-psychiatry movement declare that mental illness is a myth; it is not a fact about human beings but rather a judgement about the ways in which some of us behave. Kennedy took this further and noted that all declarations of something to be an illness involve a value judgement. This led us to speculate that the arguments here were about what we mean by terms such as health and illness. If the EBSAH is correct, however, the arguments are actually about what we mean by human flourishing; the disagreements lie there. Whether, say, bipolar disorder is genuinely an illness or not depends on the view taken of human flourishing. Those who say it is illness declare such behaviour to be significantly out of line with flourishing, whereas those who say it is not believe it to be part of the different ways in which individuals flourish. It is this difference that lies at the heart of the debate between Szasz and those who say mental illness is real precisely because it inhibits flourishing (Megone, 2000).

Let us now set the EBSAH against the pluralist account of health with which we ended the third section – Attempts to pin down health terms.

EBSAH and the pluralist account of health

The pluralist account of health terms belongs to a recent trend. There have been a number of articles that have suggested it is an error to attempt a monistic theory of health terms; several of these invoke Wittgenstein and the idea of family resemblance (Haverkamp, Bovenkerk and Verweij, 2018; Nordby, 2019; van der Linden and Schermer, 2022). The EBSAH may seem compatible with this pluralist tradition but this is only insofar as it is incomplete; it tells us that health terms arise from the ends which a system, such as a vehicle, animal or human, has. But the specification of these ends is normative, as is particularly clear in the case of human beings. Once the EBSAH is paired with an account of ends, its ceases to look like a pluralist account of health terms. In other words, once the end is specified, the states of health and illness are objective and non-pluralist.

For example, Aristotle's *Nicomachean Ethics* is devoted to setting out what human flourishing consists in, concluding that it is an active life of virtue plus a number of external goods. Good health is one of those external goods, important to but not identical with a flourishing human life. By contrast, a libertarian account might state that human flourishing consists in having the liberty through which each individual is able to find their own way to a flourishing life, something that will vary from one to another. In such an account, health, disease and illness will also vary from one individual to another. Thus, where an Aristotelian account would view schizophrenia and hearing voices as a barrier to flourishing, a libertarian account might say that, for some individuals, the so-called symptoms are actually just part of their way of flourishing.

For our purposes here, we do not need to favour one or other account of human ends. What we have established, though, is that the EBSAH is not pluralist once the ends of the system have been specified. However, the EBSAH is wide-ranging, covering the health of all animate systems and some inanimate. In addition, it covers subsystems. This allows it to retain the idea that health terms are context dependent both to the system and to the subsystem they are applied to. This is why health terms have such a wide range of application because there are many end-based systems and subsystems.

In addition, therefore, unlike the pluralist accounts, the EBSAH explains the univocity of the terms and the ease with which they are applied in everyday speech. We are surrounded by end-based systems and easily apply health terms to their ability to achieve ends or not. We do not generally apply health terms beyond such systems except in sense 2 usage. In explaining univocity, the EBSAH also fills out the family resemblance of health terms. For example, despite the wide range of phenomena to which a term like disease applies, once we have divided sense 1 and 2 usage, all the sense 1 diseases share their likeness in applying to a system or subsystem and the barrier they (that is, diseases) create to the system working or functioning properly.

Finally, unlike the pluralist accounts, EBSAH is a naturalist rather than normative account of health terms. The specification of the ends is normative, as with the Aristotelian and libertarian examples above. But once this specification is made, the judgement of whether or not different internal conditions are illnesses or not is factual, not evaluative.

Returning to the puzzles

We have already seen how the EBSAH tackles some of the puzzles left by the pluralist approach. It explains univocity and family resemblance, for example. Of itself, however, the EBSAH is no better able than the pluralist account to tackle the problems of what constitutes a true illness, whether mental illness exists, whether teenage pregnancy is a health problem or whether we should be concerned by health inequality as a matter of justice. Tackling these questions requires providing detail of the system ends, which, in the case of human beings, is a philosophical, ethical undertaking.

As is probably clear, my preferred filling-out of the EBSAH is Aristotelian. This approach provides reasons to believe that mental illness is true illness. Indeed, *pace* Kennedy (1983), the wide range of health conditions are correctly diagnosed by health scientists and carers even though an evaluation of human ends is involved. In addition, an Aristotelian EBSAH can link up to a well-established theory of human welfare or well-being, the Capability Approach (CA).

The CA says that in order for an individual to live well (or flourish) they need the ability to do and to be various things. These "beings and doings" are human capabilities. Originating in economics, CA provides an alternative to the idea that economic welfare (measured in, say, Gross National Product) is an adequate measure of human welfare. Nussbaum provides a provisional list of core capabilities that a person needs in order to flourish (Nussbaum, 2011). These include bodily health but also bodily integrity (approximately, freedom to move freely without assault), the capability to use senses, imagination and thought, to express emotions, to affiliate with others, to enjoy recreation, and to plan and have some control over your life. The list need not detain us: for our purposes, the point is that being in good health is only one of the capabilities: without the others, good health alone does not result in a flourishing individual.

The CA provides a basis from which it is possible to argue why health inequality is a matter of justice. Roughly, if the goal of humans is to flourish then the purpose of principles of justice is to ensure that, insofar as it is possible, people have the means to do so. Those means are the core capabilities, one of which is health that is good enough to open up a reasonable set of life possibilities for people. If there is health inequality, there is injustice because some people (avoidably) are inhibited from flourishing.

Conclusion

The OL analysis shows that health terms are commonly and easily applied across a wide range. Such ease is hard to account for in a pluralist account which would appear to require people to switch definitions from one context to another. The EBSAH provides an alternative which captures the univocity behind the broad range. It also provides a naturalist rather than normative account of health terms. It does this by separating health terms from the account of flourishing on which they are based. In discussion of health issues, including what constitutes a true illness, why health inequality is an issue of justice, and so on, our focus should be on the philosophical discussion of flourishing, not on the relatively straightforward issue of accounts of health and disease.

Acknowledgement

Thank you to John Paley who made helpful comments on an earlier draft that led to important changes to this version.

Notes

1 I shall use the term "pin down" to capture the broad range of defining, describing and modelling health and related terms. Similarly, I shall use the phrase "health terms" to mean "health and related terms such as illness and disease".
2 https://tvtropes.org/pmwiki/pmwiki.php/Series/DocMartin

References

Austin, J. (1956) 'A Plea for Excuses?', *Proceedings of the Aristotelian Society*, 57, pp. 1–30.
Austin, J. (1962) *Sense and Sensibilia*. Edited by G. Warnock. Oxford: Oxford University Press.
Haverkamp, B., Bovenkerk, B. and Verweij, M. F. (2018) 'A Practice-Oriented Review of Health Concepts', *The Journal of Medicine and Philosophy*, 43(4), pp. 381–401.
Kennedy, I. (1983) *The Unmasking of Medicine*. London: Granada.
Megone, C. (2000) 'Mental Illness, Human Function, and Values', *Philosophy, Psychology and Psychiatry*, 7(1), pp. 45–65.
Nordby, H. (2019) 'Who Are the Rightful Owners of the Concepts Disease, Illness and Sickness? A Pluralistic Analysis of Basic Health Concepts', *Open Journal of Philosophy*, 09(4), pp. 470–492.
Nussbaum, M. (2011) *Creating Capabilities: The Human Development Approach*. Cambridge, MA: Belknap/Harvard University Press.
Szasz, T. (1998) *The Myth of Mental Illness: Foundations of a Theory of Personal Conduct*. Revised. New York: Harper & Row.
van der Linden, R. and Schermer, M. (2022) 'Health and Disease as Practical Concepts: Exploring Function in Context-Specific Definitions', *Medicine, Health Care and Philosophy*, 25, pp. 131–140.

43 Concept analysis

John Paley

Introduction

Concept analysis, as it is understood in the nursing literature, originates with Walker and Avant (1983). There are scattered references to 'concept analysis' and nursing during the 1970s, usually in the context of specific empirical studies, but very few of them are in nursing journals, and there is nothing which closely resembles the genre that has become established since the publication of *Strategies for Theory Construction in Nursing*.

Walker and Avant's account of concept analysis is rooted in an interpretation of the aims and methods of analytic philosophy as it was practised in the 1950s and 1960s. Their primary source is Wilson (1963), a book written by a UK high school teacher for his students. I will say a bit more about this later, but the important point now is that concept analysis, as Walker and Avant described it, was based on a reading of post-war Anglophone philosophy.

Since then, analytic philosophy has moved on. The approach described by Wilson is still recognisable in 2023 (although there is a continuing debate about its aims and methods). However, there is much greater diversity. For example, there has been a revival of metaphysics and metametaphysics after Quine; the development of pragmatics after Grice, and intensive discussion of the relation between pragmatics and semantics; a renewed interest in Wittgenstein and Carnap; the arrival of theories of direct reference with Kripke; the emergence of inferentialism and modern forms of expressivism, especially after Brandom; a focus on the ontology of concepts after Fodor; innovations in experimental philosophy; signs of a partial convergence with linguistics; a turn to conceptual revision instead of concept description.

If concept analysis in nursing is to be derived from a reading of philosophy, there are more possibilities now than there were in 1963 or 1983. Here, I'll briefly describe four. I start with *conceptual analysis*, the expression used by philosophers to describe what they do (or what some of them do). I then consider *concept analysis*, the nursing term, suggesting that, while it is based loosely on conceptual analysis, it adopts very different methods. Next, I discuss one version of *ordinary language philosophy*, drawing on Wittgenstein and linguistics. Finally, I consider a form of *revisionism*: 'conceptual amelioration'. All of these options are derived from distinctive understandings of what philosophy tries to achieve and how it tries to achieve it.

Method of cases (conceptual analysis)

The origins of conceptual analysis can be traced back to the emergence of analytic philosophy early in the 20th century. In contemporary philosophy, there are a number of

DOI: 10.4324/9781003427407-50

different threads, not all of which pull in the same direction. I won't try to disentangle these threads here. Instead, I will focus on a procedure which analytic philosophers often employ. This is the 'practice of theorizing on the basis of the "application" of terms to "cases"' (Baz 2017: 1), sometimes called 'the method of cases'.

The method of cases is a contemporary version of the procedure Wilson writes about. As an example, suppose you want to know what *knowledge* is, or what the structure of the concept of 'knowledge' is. The idea is to propose an analysis of the concept such that (i) the analysis identifies conditions which are individually necessary and jointly sufficient for the application of the term/concept 'knowledge'; (ii) the analysis does not include the word 'know' or its cognates. Consider a schematic sentence such as the following:

(k)   *S* knows that *p*

An analysis can now be proposed which specifies the necessary and sufficient conditions for the truth of this statement. For much of the 20th century, the starting-point analysis looked like this:

'*S* knows that *p*' is true if and only if:
(a)   *S* believes that *p*
(b)   *S* is justified in believing that *p*
(c)   *p* is true

This analysis was typically summarised as the claim that 'knowledge is justified true belief' (the 'JTB analysis'). It is often referred to as the 'traditional' view, though it is not clear that many philosophers ever held it. What *is* clear is that few, if any, contemporary epistemologists think it is adequate.

A pivotal moment occurred when a paper called 'Is justified true belief knowledge?' (Gettier 1963) was published. In this paper, Gettier outlined two 'cases'. Both are vignettes describing situations in which conditions (a), (b), and (c) all hold, and yet we would *not* be inclined to say that statement (k) is true. In other words, somebody has a belief, the belief is true, and the person is justified in believing as she does – and yet she cannot be said to *know*. The widely accepted conclusion is that the JTB analysis does not work. It does not succeed in specifying a *sufficient* condition for the truth of (k) – this is what Gettier's vignettes are taken to show – even if all three of its components are *necessary*. So the hunt is on for a further condition which will make the set jointly sufficient as well as individually necessary.

The logic of conceptual analysis is as follows:

A.1   An analysis of the target concept is proposed.
B.1   The analysis is tested against cases, whether real or invented.
C.1   If there are cases in which the conditions implied by the analysis hold but the target concept does not apply, the analysis is taken to be wrong.
A.2   A new, or amended, analysis is proposed.
B.2   The new analysis is tested against further cases.

… and this process can continue over numerous iterations. Very roughly, then, the logic is *hypothesis testing*. Any proposed analysis is a hypothesis, which is then tested against the 'evidence' (cases). If the hypothesis is disconfirmed by this evidence, it is amended or (sometimes) abandoned. It is true that the initial hypothesis may be prompted by a review of the literature; to that extent, there may be (but is not necessarily) an 'inductive' phase. However, the central point is that the hypothesis, whatever its origins, is *tested* against something that counts as evidence. This is why much contemporary philosophy consists of suggesting *counter-examples* to somebody else's analysis. The counter-examples are used to test the proposed analysis, with the writer suggesting that they disconfirm it.

Concept analysis (nursing)

Most readers of this chapter will not need a tutorial on Walker and Avant's method of concept analysis. So I will jump straight into a comparison of the Walker and Avant approach and the procedure described in the previous section. They have things in common, but there are also significant disparities. However, this isn't a *they-got-it-wrong* argument; it's a *notice the similarities (S) and differences (D)* suggestion.

S (1)   Walker and Avant assume that concepts are (relatively) stable *structures*. They are mental items or abstract objects. Being structures, they have 'components' that can be identified; and they can be used as 'building blocks' for more complex structures such as theories. Concepts can change (or 'evolve'), but they are durable enough to permit analysis. The analysis takes the form of 'decomposition'. Walker and Avant say that a concept can be broken into 'simpler elements', and that the analyst can 'get inside' the concept, and 'see how it works'. The analogy with physical objects is clear; but that is also a feature of the philosophical literature on concepts, whether they are taken to be mental 'particulars' (Fodor 1998) or abstract entities (Peacocke 1992).

D (1)   In the two disciplines, concepts are not identified in the same way, and the 'components' are not of the same type. In philosophy, an indicative sentence typically represents the target concept: '*S* knows that *p*', say, rather than 'knowledge'. Similarly, the 'components' have indicative form, as in sentences (a), (b), and (c) above. In nursing, by contrast, concepts are identified by a noun, or a noun phrase, or a noun clause. The components are a mixed bag: nouns, adjectives, participles, indicatives. The concept is a grammatical subject, and its defining attributes are the predicates attached to it.

S (2)   However, the 'breaking into simpler elements', the 'decomposition', is roughly parallel. In both cases, components are listed and each represents a necessary condition. In one case, the 'components' are, like (a), (b), and (c), indicative sentences which are necessary conditions for the truth of the target indicative sentence (k). In the other, the components are features which must be present if the concept (represented as a noun or noun phrase) is to be applied. It is the same basic idea, realised in a somewhat different form.

D (2)   However, the logic of concept analysis is not hypothesis testing. The proposed analysis is not *tested*. Cases are not used as 'evidence' capable of disconfirming the analysis/hypothesis. There are no attempts to find, or invent, cases which might be counter-examples (this is the key move in conceptual analysis). Occasionally, authors will point out that an analysis seems inadequate in some way (Hupcey *et al.* 1996; Bergdahl & Berterö 2016), but this is rarely because they have devised Gettier-style cases. In concept analysis, testing-by-cases is not part of the method.

D (3) The role of cases is almost a touchstone for the difference between the two forms of analysis. In conceptual analysis, as I have suggested, they are 'evidence', potential counter-examples. Their role is to test a hypothesis, to determine whether the sentences which comprise the analysis really do amount to a set of necessary and sufficient conditions for the truth of the target sentence. In concept analysis, by contrast, cases are *illustrations*. They are appended to the analysis, they are not an essential part of it. 'Here are the defining attributes of the concept, derived from my analysis; and here are some concrete illustrations: a case in which the concept can be applied, a case in which it can't...', and so on. This is not a form of testing.

D (4) The logic of concept analysis is *inductive*. The defining attributes are derived from data: usually, the literature dealing with the topic, but sometimes also dictionaries, fiction, and interview data. Walker and Avant's account is extremely clear: review the literature to determine what is said about the concept in question, and identify

> the characteristics of the concept that appear over and over again. This list of characteristics, called defining characteristics or defining attributes... help you and others name the occurrence of a specific phenomenon as differentiated from another similar or related one.
>
> (Walker & Avant 2005: 68)

Note that the characteristics most frequently referred to *are* the defining attributes of the concept. Frequency is a very simple – arguably simplistic – criterion for defining attributes; and several variations have been proposed. But, on this account, the logic of concept analysis is undeniably inductive.

The assumption that the defining attributes can be derived, *somehow*, from the literature (perhaps with the addition of empirical data) has remained intact, despite various modifications of Walker and Avant's method. The procedure is obviously different from the hypothesis testing logic of conceptual analysis, and the examples described by Wilson. The hypothesis testing method tries to get something *right*; and the conclusion may be at odds with the rest of the literature. The inductive method sets out to *synthesise* what has already been written.

Ordinary language philosophy and linguistics

The writers often bracketed as 'ordinary language philosophy' (OLP) – the later Wittgenstein, Austin, Ryle, Strawson, and others – did not see themselves as a school of thought sharing a method. However, there are similarities. A useful initial account is this: OLP is the idea that many traditional philosophical problems arise, not from a mistaken answer to a legitimate and intelligible question, but rather from 'the question itself, and the assumption that, as raised in the philosophical context... it makes clear sense and has a correct answer' (Baz 2017: 5). Here, I will focus on what I personally take from Wittgenstein (1963), and what I think can usefully be done with his understanding of language. And note: language. This is not an approach which has much to say about concepts. In fact, I suggest that there are no such things (Paley 2021).

OLP, on my understanding, does not formulate a hypothesis about the 'structure' of a concept, and test it with cases, in the way conceptual analysis does. Nor does it use inductive inference to infer 'defining attributes' from the literature, as concept analysis does. Its aim is not to identify necessary and sufficient conditions for the truth of a target indicative sentence, or for the application of a concept-as-abstract-noun. It does not try to define the structure of a concept *at all*. Instead, it assembles what Wittgenstein calls 'reminders' of how we employ the relevant words ordinarily.

This may sound a rather trivial exercise. It isn't. The reminders are necessary because, when we start theorising about the *concept of X*, we lose sight of how the word 'X' is actually used. We inadvertently restrict our awareness of its use to an extremely narrow range. A careful examination of the pattern of usage generally shows that it is *much* more complex than we had assumed, and that the word's function varies with morphology, syntax, and linguistic context. Hence the need for reminders. The goal of the investigation is not to produce a conclusion, but to provide an understanding of this complexity, and so motivate greater caution when theorising about ('analysing') the concept.

For example, accounts of hope in the nursing literature usually take the form of a sentence beginning 'Hope is…'. 'Hope is a theological virtue' (Lebacqz 1985); 'Hope is a multidimensional dynamic life force' (Dufault & Martocchio 1985); 'Hope is an inner power directed toward enrichment of being' (Herth 1990). It is variously described as an emotion, a cognitive process, a disposition, an instinct, a basic need. What most of these characterisations have in common is this: they imply that hope is a state of the person. It is construed as an 'inner' something: a mental state, process, power, or mechanism.

However, when we examine actual usage of the word 'hope', we find a far more complex pattern. This is illustrated at length in Paley (2021). But here I'll just take one example: negative sentences in which 'hope' occurs. Consider the following:

(1)   Will Lee win? Not a hope!
(2)   There's not a hope in hell that Nadia will keep her mouth shut.
(3)   It's a system that most scientists say has no hope of working.
(4)   With the hiring freeze, there's no hope of hiring a trained toxicologist.
(5)   The position paper cannot hope to answer all the specifics.

In all these examples, there is no reference to anyone's state of mind, or to any mental process or power. In (1), it is *not* being claimed that Lee does not want to win, or that he does not think he can. In fact, (1) might be true even if Lee 'hopes' to win. Similarly, (2) could be true even if some of the people being addressed 'hope' that Nadia *will* keep her mouth shut. In both cases, it is possible to substitute 'chance' for 'hope' without a change of meaning. The same applies to (3) and (4). Of course, we can't substitute 'chance' in (5). But the same sense is involved: there is no chance of the position paper including every detail, or answering every question. The message is the same in each case. 'This isn't going to happen'. No states of mind are referred to. Systems and position papers don't *have* states of mind.

The definitions of hope miss this aspect of use altogether. Nor is this a footling matter, easily dismissed as marginal. When patients with potentially fatal conditions ask 'Is there any hope?', they are not asking whether *they* have a certain state of mind – presumably they would know – or whether the health care professional has that state of mind. They are asking whether there is any *chance* of them being cured, or any chance of them surviving for longer than the prognosis suggests.

This is just negations. It turns out that the word 'hope' has different functions in a range of grammatical constructions: as a count noun, or mass noun; singular or plural uses; first-person and third-person uses of the verb; with or without ellipsis; and more. If we overlook this complex pattern, the result is that our theories of hope are lop-sided. We imagine that we have provided an analysis of *hope* when, in fact, our accounts are based on a narrowly selective range of uses of the *word* 'hope'.

Conceptual amelioration

Do we have to be satisfied with a list of a certain concept's defining attributes (concept analysis); or a list of the necessary and sufficient conditions for the truth of a target sentence (conceptual analysis); or an account of the pattern of usage associated with a particular word (OLP)? In each case, there is an assumption that the aim of an analysis is to get at the truth: to identify the correct attributes, to pinpoint the necessary and sufficient conditions, to depict the pattern of usage. In effect, it is a question of accurate portrayal. But is that the end of the line? Suppose that the analysed concept or pattern of usage seems deficient in some way? Is there nothing else that can be done?

Philosophy has seen a surge of interest in such questions during the last 20 years, and there is now an extensive literature on 'conceptual engineering' and 'conceptual amelioration'. Although this is a recent development, the basic idea goes back much further. Carnap (1945) introduced the expression 'explication' to refer to a form of 'repair' undertaken on concepts which are regarded as defective. The kinds of defectiveness he had in mind were lack of clarity, ambiguity, and inexactness. An 'explication' involved the engineering of a more precise concept, and the substitution of the precise concept for the imprecise one.

However, there is more than one way in which a concept can be defective – being inexact or imprecise is just one kind of failing among others – and conceptual engineering has become popular again. Some contributions deal with narrowly philosophical themes; others discuss moral, social and political issues. Some propose new expressions; others redefine old ones. Some suggest that a re-engineered concept repairs a fault, and that a new concept fills the gap; others argue that an ameliorated concept is more useful than its predecessor: that it will serve our purposes better, and will have positive social outcomes.

Here is a moral/social/political example. Haslanger (2012) argues that we should change the meaning of the words 'woman' and 'man' by adopting different definitions. For example:

S is a woman if and only if:
  i   S is regularly and for the most part observed or imagined to have certain bodily features presumed to be evidence of a female's biological role in reproduction.
  ii   that S has these features marks S within the dominant ideology of S's society as someone who ought to occupy certain kinds of social position that are in fact subordinate (and so motivates and justifies S's occupying such a position!); and
  iii   the fact that S satisfies (i) and (ii) plays a role in S's systematic subordination, i.e., along some dimension, S's social position is oppressive, and S's satisfying (i) and (ii)plays a role in that dimension of subordination.

So according to this definition, anybody described as a woman is necessarily subordinate. Haslanger's definition of 'man' is correlative, the difference being that 'subordinate' and 'oppressive' are replaced by 'privileged', while 'subordination' is replaced by 'privilege'. By definition, there cannot be a man who is not privileged, nor can there be a woman who is not subordinate. (For an enhanced ameliorative analysis along these lines, ensuring the inclusion of trans women, see Jenkins 2016.)

Haslanger's reasons for re-engineering the words 'man' and 'woman' in this way are broadly political. The changed meanings are designed to have desirable social and political outcomes. The ultimate goal, when briefly stated, is the elimination of women (defined as above). 'I believe it is part of the project of feminism to bring about a day when there are no more women (though, of course, we should not aim to do away with females!)' (Haslanger 2000: 46). She does acknowledge the difficulty of advancing this project, but thinks her definitions will serve the goal of understanding racial and sexual oppression, and helping to achieve sexual and racial equality.

Conceptual engineering, then, is not just playing around with words or an exercise in wish fulfilment. It is a serious attempt to change things.

Knowledge

To illustrate compactly some of the principal differences between concept analysis, conceptual analysis, OLP, and conceptual engineering, I'm going to sketch how the same concept might be tackled by each approach. The concept I've chosen is 'know'/'knowing'/'knowledge'.

Method of cases

As we saw in 'Method of Cases (Conceptual Analysis)', the Gettier cases were taken to show that the JTB analysis of 'S knows that p' was incomplete: arguably, the three conditions were individually necessary but not jointly sufficient. Consequently, there has been a series of attempts to identify a fourth condition to add to the original set. Given that, in Gettier narratives, S arrives at the true conclusion by luck, one proposal is to add an 'anti-luck' condition to the other three. For example, Unger (1968) suggested:

'S knows that p' is true if and only if:
(a) S believes that p
(b) S is justified in believing that p
(c) p is true
(d) S's belief is not true merely by luck.

An alternative strategy is to abandon the search for a fourth condition, and to replace the 'justification condition' with a different requirement at (b). For example, one possibility – there are many others – is the 'causal condition', associated with Goldman (1967):

(a) S believes that p
(b) S's belief that p is caused by the fact that p
(c) p is true

Each successive proposal is tested against further evidence – that is, new cases – but no agreement has yet been reached about the correct analysis. Indeed, some philosophers now argue that the main lesson of the post-Gettier debate is that knowledge is not susceptible to analysis at all, and *cannot* be defined.

Concept analysis

There is, as it happens, a concept analysis study of 'knowing in nursing' (Bonis 2009), so I will use that as a convenient example. 'Knowing in nursing' represents Bonis's target concept. Although 'knowing' is the present participle of the verb, it can of course be used as a noun (a gerund); and this is how Bonis uses it in the article. Her search terms, in addition to 'knowing', were 'personal' and 'experience'. She explains this narrowing down from the more general idea of knowledge by referring to the ontological foundations of nursing.

The search terms were entered into CINAHL and PubMed, and 134 papers were ultimately selected, 97 being from the nursing literature. According to Bonis (1330):

> Each paper was read in its entirety to gain an understanding of the manner in which the concept of knowing was used, as well as the characteristics of the concept. Tentative themes evolved to categorize the use of the concept of knowing.

In effect, she uses the 134 papers as her data, and subjects them to a qualitative-style thematic analysis.

Bonis identifies six attributes of the concept. Each is a sentence which describes knowing in nursing:

i   It is a type of knowledge.
ii It lies in personal experience.
iii It is personal knowledge.
iv It is shaped through personal perspective.
v   It is a dynamic and changing process.
vi It evolves as a person lives and interacts in the world.

Here there is no 'if and only if', and no hypothesis testing. The attributes are inductively derived from the literature-as-data, and described in very general terms. So they represent (at best) a set of necessary conditions; and, crucially, it's not clear why the same conditions do not also apply to 'knowing' in other disciplines. In other words, however necessary this set of attributes may be, it is clearly not sufficient. It is consistent, not merely with 'knowing in nursing', but also with 'knowing in physiotherapy', 'knowing in medicine', or 'knowing in teaching' (and, I imagine, many more).

Assembling reminders

There are innumerable ways to begin an OLP analysis of 'know', so I will content myself with a quick sketch of just one. Consider the idea that there are 'multiple ways of knowing'. This is usually presented as an ontological or epistemological truth, but I think it is what Wittgenstein (1964) calls a 'grammatical remark'. It is an observation about how the word 'know' is ordinarily used, but it is often presented as if it is metaphysically profound.

In nursing, the literature on 'ways of knowing' was prompted by Carper (1978). Understanding the four patterns of knowing, Carper says, 'involves critical attention to what it means to know', but she makes no attempt to link this idea to nursing epistemology or ontology. However, later authors were quick to make this connection. Here is an example: 'The diverse patterns of knowing constitute the ontological and epistemological foundations of the discipline of nursing' (Fawcett *et al.* 2001: 117). This is a view which recent authors have rarely challenged. However, I think that to interpret Carper in this way is to read her through subsequent contributions to the literature. Perhaps we need a reading of Carper more in keeping with the Wittgensteinian view.

Suppose someone says: 'There are multiple ways of playing'. This may be puzzling until it is pointed out that we talk of playing dumb, havoc, golf, the fool, Metallica, hard to get, a hunch, the oboe, along, truant, hell, fast and loose, and dozens more. 'There are multiple ways of playing' is a slightly fanciful way of saying that. Similarly, I would argue, with 'There are multiple ways of knowing'. It is a slightly fanciful way of saying: '"Know" can be used in countless different ways'. Here's just a brief selection. They are all possible continuations of 'Do you know....?'

... where I put my phone?	... how to get this open?	... why you're here?
... if that's an orchid?	... how wicked that is?	... about Charles and Fiona?
... what the consequences will be?	... 'Over the Rainbow'?	... the solution to 15 down?
... the atomic number of gold?	... what the right dose is?	... anything about this?
... what 'metonymy' means?	... Amie Thomasson?	... how much I'm hurting?
... your multiplication tables?	... that you're acting weird?	... what her real worry is?

Now imagine, for each of these, the reply: 'Yes...', and the kind of explanation that would follow. 'Yes, I can see it in your back pocket'. 'Yes, I'm nervous'. 'Yes, I'm a chemist'. 'Yes, I have met her several times'. 'Yes, I've read the systematic review'. And so on. This isn't about four 'patterns of knowing'. It is not about any particular number. These situations are so varied, and the criteria for the legitimate use of 'know' so context-dependent, that there is no way of counting how many 'patterns' there are. I think 'There are multiple ways of knowing' is just a way of expressing that. It is a grammatical remark about the uses of 'know'. However, many writers want to inflate it, and turn it into something with ontological and epistemological ramifications.

Conceptual engineering

The idea that knowledge might well be a candidate for some kind of conceptual engineering has been around for a while (although the expression has only been used recently). For example, Papineau (2019) has described knowledge as 'a stone-age concept'. That sounds rather extreme, but in some languages, as Papineau points out, *every* assertion is marked with an 'evidential' tag indicating its provenance. 'For example, the Eastern Pomo language from California has verbal suffixes indicating whether the source of your information is direct visual observation, other sensory perception, hearsay, or inference'. In principle, we could do that to English. Instead of having the concept of 'knowledge', or using the word 'know', we could tag every assertion we make with an indication of what evidence it's based on. That would be an ambitious and immensely difficult piece of re-engineering, but it's not inconceivable.

Interestingly, Carper can be read as providing a basis for such a project in nursing. Her four patterns are empirics, aesthetics, personal knowledge, and moral knowledge. Rather than putting all of these under the heading 'nursing knowledge' or 'patterns of knowing', we could treat them in the way suggested by the Eastern Pomo language, and tag every claim made by a nurse with an *'evidential'*: assertions based on scientific findings (SF), assertions based on 'esthetic' experience (EE), assertions based on personal encounters with individuals (PI), and assertions based on judgements of moral value (MV). This would not be a 'claiming-to-know' on the basis of SF, EE, PI, or MV. Instead, the point would be to abandon the concept of 'knowing' altogether, and use 'tagging' syntax as a way of signalling the provenance of any claim (allowing others to decide for themselves what significance any particular assertion had).

I am not claiming that this was Carper's intention. It clearly wasn't: she wanted all four 'patterns' to be recognised as *knowledge*. However, it is a way of reconceptualising her work, and one that resists the ontological and epistemological weight usually placed on it. That in itself would be no bad thing. It's not going to happen, obviously, but what I am attempting to do is to suggest a different way of thinking about 'patterns of knowing', dragging the expression away from ontology and epistemology, towards linguistics.

Concluding remark

I think that a debate on the methods that can be employed in concept analysis (or something occupying the same slot) is overdue. My ambition here is to prompt a discussion about the range of options. It is *much* wider than those recognised in the current literature. To stick with just one conception of 'concept analysis', and a 60-year-old one at that, is to impose what seems an unnecessary restriction.

References

Baz, A. (2017) *The Crisis of Method in Contemporary Analytic Philosophy*. Oxford University Press, Oxford.

Bergdahl, E. & Berterö (2016) Concept analysis and the building blocks of theory: Misconceptions regarding theory development. *Journal of Advanced Nursing*, 72(10), 2558–2566.

Bonis, S.A. (2009) Knowing in nursing: A concept analysis. *Journal of Advanced Nursing*, 65(6), 1328–1341.

Carnap, R. (1945) The two concepts of probability: The problem of probability. *Philosophy and Phenomenological Research*, 5(4), 513–532.

Carper, B.A. (1978) Fundamental patterns of knowing in nursing. *Advances in Nursing Science*, 1(1), 13–23.

Dufault, K., & Martocchio, B. C. (1985). Hope: Its spheres and dimensions. Nursing Clinics of North America, 20(2), 379–391.

Fawcett, J., Watson, J., Neuman, B., Walker, P.H. & Fitzpatrick, J.J. (2001) On nursing theories and evidence. *Journal of Nursing Scholarship*, 33(2), 115–119.

Fodor, J. (1998) *Concepts: Where Cognitive Science Went Wrong*. Oxford University Press, New York.

Gettier, E.L. (1963) Is justified true belief knowledge? *Analysis*, 23(6), 121–123.

Goldman, A.I. (1967) A causal theory of knowing. *The Journal of Philosophy*, 64(12), 357–372.

Haslanger, S. (2000) Gender and race: (What) are they? (what) do we want them to be? *Nous*, 33(1), 31–55.

Haslanger, S. (2012) *Resisting Reality: Social Construction and Social Critique*. Oxford University Press, Oxford.

Herth, K. (1990). Fostering hope in terminally ill people. Journal of Advanced Nursing, 15, 1250–1259.

Hupcey, J.E., Morse, J.M., Lenz, E.R. & Tasón, M.C. (1996) Wilsonian methods of concept analysis: a critique. *Scholarly Inquiry for Nursing Practice*, 10(3), 185–210. PMID: 9009818

Jenkins, K. (2016) Amelioration and inclusion: Gender identity and the concept of woman. *Ethics,* 126, 394–421.

Lebacqz, K. (1985). The virtuous patient. In E. E. Shelp (Ed.), Virtue and Medicine (pp. 275–288). Berlin: Springer.

Paley, J. (2021) *Concept Analysis in Nursing: A New Approach.* Routledge, Abingdon, UK.

Papineau, D. (2019) Knowledge is crude. *Aeon Essays,* June, https://aeon.co/essays/kmowledge-is-a-stone-age-concept-were-better-off-without-it.

Peacocke, C. (1992) *A Study of Concepts.* MIT Press, Cambridge, MA.

Unger, P. (1968) An analysis of factual knowledge. *The Journal of Philosophy,* 65(6), 157–170.

Walker, L.O. & Avant, K.C. (1983) *Strategies for Theory Construction in Nursing.* Appleton-Century-Crofts, Norwalk, CT.

Walker, L.O. & Avant, K.C. (2005) *Strategies for Theory Construction in Nursing: Fourth Edition.* Prentice Hall, Upper Saddle River, NJ.

Wilson, J. (1963) *Thinking with Concepts.* Cambridge University Press, Cambridge.

Wittgenstein, L. (1963) *Philosophical Investigations.* Basil Blackwell, Oxford.

Wittgenstein, L. (1964) *Preliminary Studies for the "Philosophical Investigations". Generally known as The Blue and Brown Books.* Basil Blackwell, Oxford.

44 Epistemic injustice and vulnerability

Havi Carel

Epistemic injustice and vulnerability

The demands of patiency

Illness is a profound and central experience of human existence, despite being pushed to the margins in many contemporary contexts, within a culture which largely favours health, youth, and freedom to reflection on illness, affliction, and death. However, this reluctance does not reflect the realities of life. Despite much denial, we are all 'dependent, rational animals' to use Alasdair MacIntyre's (1999) eloquent phrase, and we are also all patients, now or in the future. In addition, most of us begin and end our lives within a medical setting – a hospital, clinic, or hospice. We are born into complete helplessness and dependence on others, and we die in complete helplessness and dependence on others. To mask this fact is to deny a deep and universal truth about human life (Carel 2021).

What this fact of life, so to speak, reveals to us is our profound vulnerability – physical, emotional, mental – and our deep dependence on others at all times, but especially during periods of illness and incapacitation. I use the term 'illness' to denote serious, life-changing, or life-threatening conditions that are irreversible, often chronic, and sometimes lead to premature death. I am not referring to mild, reversible, or self-limiting illnesses, such as mild flu, a twisted ankle, or a winter cold. I focus on the kind of illness that requires hospitalisation, at least for some of the time, and that also requires the ill person to change how she has lived and restrict her activities because of the illness, as well as casting a dark shadow on her future.

There are features of this kind of illness that make it particularly hard to bear and makes those who are ill vulnerable much beyond the vulnerability we all share in virtue of being contingent, limited, and finite (for a full discussion of shared vulnerability, see Carel 2021). First, being ill is physically extremely taxing. If one has been previously healthy, the experience of pain, fatigue, nausea, dizziness, weakness, and other ways of feeling unwell can be profoundly destabilising. And if it is already familiar, the dread that one will never feel better, and the drag of everyday routines being impossibly exhausting, can make one feel defeated, depleted, and hopeless. The physical symptoms become amplified and eventually are all consuming as the illness progresses and crescendos at the end of life.

Second, being ill requires us to accept others' help and care whether we want to or not, and whether we know or like them (and vice versa) or not. Being unable to get out of bed, needing the care of others for basic daily care and nourishment, and requiring intensive medical treatment are difficult for those who were previously independent and self-sufficient. It is not easy to ask for help, especially with self-care that used to be a

DOI: 10.4324/9781003427407-51

trivial part of one's autonomy, and there is a great deal of anxiety involved in knowing that one is – literally and tragically – at the mercy of others.

Third, being ill is emotionally, morally, and existentially demanding. There are a multitude of pressures: a range of difficult emotions, such as fear, dread, anxiety, worry, and stress; the impossibility of contemplating one's own death; sorrow and regret about precious things lost and opportunities foregone; the desire to negotiate, to attempt to carry on as before, to deny the illness in ways incompatible with our body's dictates; being torn away from one's familiar life fabric; frustration and anger about being ill; the moral demands of facing one's nearing death: these are all pressing aspects of serious illness. In addition, there is sometimes an urgent need to sort out financial affairs, plans, and other practicalities, as well as a feeling that time is running out and that conversations need to be had that both acknowledge, and see beyond, the current state of illness.

The profound sense of helplessness arising from physical incapacitation can be intensely amplified by worries and rumination. These are, of course, contradicting requirements, because sorting out the practicalities of one's life (housing, car, will, debts) is often incompatible with the need for quiet rest and reflective contemplation, that are already hard to come by in a hospital setting. The continuing tide of emotions and our responses to disease progression and unwelcome news of a poor prognosis require emotional, moral, and existential resources that can become altogether depleted. There is often a tacit call upon those who are very ill to be courageous, to accept their deterioration, to continue to strive, which are extremely demanding moral requirements. Finally, there is an existential and spiritual need to make sense of fast paced events, to find peace with one's ailing body and bad luck, to create a self-narrative that can offer meaning and solace, to reconnect meaningfully with oneself – these can be hard to address on a busy hospital ward, and with a lack of accepted rituals.

These challenges of illness cumulatively amount to what Ian Kidd and I dubbed 'the predicament of patients' (Kidd and Carel 2021). That predicament is marked by vulnerability and dependence on others, which take a toll on the ill person in so many ways. The ineradicable reality is that being a patient is hard, confusing, and demanding in a host of ways, which are difficult to anticipate and prepare for.

One pivotal hardship I focus on in this chapter is epistemic: that is, related to one's agency and status as a *knower*, as someone whose has epistemic agency, who can offer thoughts and ideas, explain their point of view, say what their preferences are, and express their wishes and views. When one becomes a patient, the knowledge, opinions, and preferences that provide the substance of one's distinctive individuality can get lost within the busy medical setting. As a result of this and other reasons, such as being overly focused on objective medical facts to the exclusion of the patient voice, these opinions and preferences are not always sought, taken into account, or acted upon. The result may be an epistemic injustice suffered by the ill person, who epistemic offerings (view, opinions, preferences) may be unjustly ignored or marginalised.

Even when a patient does offer her views, they can be rejected, ignored, or tuned out by the medical objective, scientific, and practical stance, which is often opaque to the patient and marked by time pressure, high workloads, and the unrelenting demands of complex multiple tasks. Information is often lost in the busy work environment and patient vigilance is always required to guard against that. In addition, this stance has little or no personal acquaintance with the patient herself. Shiftwork and the impersonal nature of medical settings also mean that strangers are thrust together at a time of great distress, and the sharp contrast between the existential crisis of patient and family and the routine work of the health care professional (HCP) can deepen both the gulf between them and the sense that the patient's stance is unheeded.

In other settings – GP surgery, outpatient clinics, and other types of ongoing care for chronic illness – this gulf can be narrowed through the creation of a shared understanding and a shared history. But in acute settings and given the large number of HCPs involved in the care of any one patient, HCPs can be oblivious to the impact of words, gestures and of course, decisions, on the individual sitting in that hospital bed. The mismatch between the reality of the hectic shift of the HCP (nurse, physician, care assistant, radiographer, and so on) and the continued turmoil of the patient, whose life has been put on hold or pushed out of orbit, often mean that a 'decisive gap', as S.K. Toombs calls it, in attitudes, worldview, and existential stance marks any communicative exchanges between patient and those who are caring for her (Toombs 1987).

Important, intimate decisions involving the ill person, her body, and her life, are made without sufficient interpretive tools to handle the differing views, perspectives, and tangible gaps in understanding between the patient's point of view and that of HCP. Amid the desire for certainty, care, and cure, there is also a powerful desire – a need, even – to be heard, to be able to communicate the reality of one's circumstances and help others to understand (Kidd and Carel 2018). This is not merely a psychological need to be heard, although this is certainly important. It is the critical need for patients to be able to put forth views and preferences for these to be an integral part of any decision-making process about their care.

The need to be seen, heard, and understood is a pervasive theme of pathographic literature devoted to describing the lived experience of illness. Abby Norman's *Ask Me About My Uterus* is subtitled *A Quest to Make Doctors Believe in Women's Pain* (Norman 2018). She reflects on the experiences of women whose testimonies about diseased bodies were ignored, citing the example of American comedian Gilda Radner who died of ovarian cancer after her appeals to her doctors were ignored:

> What resonated with me about her story [...] was the deep knowing of her own body as a woman that is seeming unworthy of anyone's consideration or respect. I find that deeply unnerving: that I might be dying, and no-one would believe me, but that feeling of inescapable truth wouldn't leave me no matter how much other people denied it.
>
> (Norman 2018, p. 56)

Such pathographies emphasise the many practical and epistemic constraints built into contemporary health care systems: the knowledge and trust gaps, the charged power dynamics between the medically trained and the rest, and the complicated relationships between the many actors – HCPs, managers, patients, families, and sometimes lawyers, social workers, and more. There are financial and political forces beyond the control of those acting within the immediate scene. There are the intellectual and moral failings of individual people, which can ramify when they interact with so many others (Carel and Kidd 2021). There are deeply entrenched structures of pathophobic assumptions and practices deeply baked into our social systems and cultural imagination.[1] Finally, there is the simple yet all-consuming state of being ill, in pain, suffering. A recent Patients Association report states that the top three terms patients used to describe being ill are 'frustrating', 'frightened', and 'vulnerable' (Being a patient: First report of the Patients Association's patient experience programme, 2020).[2]

Becoming ill means, among other things, coming to occupy a new and difficult epistemic position. Susan Sontag said that to become ill is 'to take up one's residence in the kingdom of the ill'. She added that this kingdom has its own 'landscape' – its own stereotypes, prejudices, obstacles, and dangers (Sontag 1978, p. 3). We can use that metaphor to think about the newly imposed epistemic challenges of those who have become ill. One suddenly arrives at a strange, hostile new territory complete with new and disturbing features – unfamiliar medical terms, rules that are not explained in advance, a new daily schedule the patient needs to fit into, being wheeled around to tests and investigations without knowing why. There are medical terms to learn, services to find, and new people to reluctantly involve in one's intimacies. There are decisions to be made, treatment options to consider, and practicalities to sort out. There are profound and bewildering changes to all aspects of one's life, that require mental energy, attention, emotional resources, and a lot of talking, thinking, and communicating. Becoming ill carries many intrinsic difficulties as well as bringing with it a life sentence of hard epistemic labour (Carel 2018; Kidd and Carel 2018).

To be ill is to inhabit a changed world with new challenges, needs, and risks that are tied into a complicated interpersonal world (Carel 2018). Coping with epistemic challenges is a significant burden and main aspect of one's illness experience. The term 'epistemic injustice' has been instrumental in giving clear articulation to how these distinctly epistemic challenges manifest in the domain of health care, and what particular epistemic obstacles and risks come into play within the health care setting. I now turn to this concept.

Epistemic injustice in health care

The concept of *epistemic injustice* was coined by the philosopher Miranda Fricker. Her original articulation of the concept was the landmark monograph, *Epistemic Injustice: Power and the Ethics of Knowing* (Fricker 2007). Fricker describes her work as sitting at the intersection of ethics and epistemology, and the concept of epistemic injustice as capturing an injustice done to someone in their capacity as a knower, an epistemic agent: as someone making contributions to knowledge by offering their opinions, interpretations, and knowledge. The two main kinds of epistemic injustice Fricker describes in the book are *testimonial injustice*, where negative prejudice causes a hearer to deflate the credibility assigned to a speaker, and *hermeneutical injustice*, where a collective gap in hermeneutical resources prevents understanding some or all of the social experiences of certain groups (Fricker 2007, Chapters 1 and 7). Fricker subsequently refined and elaborated her ideas in later publications, although the original framework remains central to epistemic injustice studies (Fricker 2017).

Testimonial injustice occurs when negative stereotyping leads a hearer to prejudicially deflate the credibility assigned to a speaker. The effects include reduced testimonial authority, frustration of practical and social agency, and erosion of the epistemic confidence of the speaker, which can ultimately lead them to cease trying to communicate altogether. Though originally analysed in its agential forms, as an injustice carried out by an individual agent, subsequent work has recognised structural forms of testimonial injustice, which are perpetrated by an institution or broad social structures, since acts of credibility deflation can be embedded in social structures, alongside the corrupted perceptions and judgements of individuals.

A variety of negative prejudices and stereotypes can inform testimonial injustice, including the gendered and racialised cases discussed in Fricker's original account. Moreover, further forms of intersectional epistemic injustices are now recognised, many articulated using the conceptual resources of a variety of social justice movements (see Parts II and III of Kidd, Medina, and Pohlhaus, Jr., 2017). Within this context, Kidd and I argued (Carel and Kidd 2014; Kidd and Carel 2016) that ill persons are *especially* vulnerable to testimonial injustice because appraisals of their credibility can be corrupted by pathophobic prejudices and stereotypes.

How is the credibility of ill persons eroded? First, there is pre-emptive derogation of the epistemic credibility and capacities of ill persons owing to pathophobic stereotyping – a prior view of ill persons as being confused, incapable, or incompetent, that distorts an evaluation of their actual epistemic performance. Second, hearers can presuppose that an ill person will be dominated by their illness, such that they cannot be perceived as impartial or objective. As a result of these negative stereotypes, ill persons often report the downgrading of their testimonies: this downgrading is unjust because it is based on stereotype and prejudice which occlude the credibility judgements the hearers make about the ill person.

It is important to note that these testimonial injustices are generated by *pathophobic* prejudices and stereotypes, and so track ill persons through the social world. The tenacity of these prejudices ensures their effects reach beyond the clinical setting to affect other areas of life, such as education, housing and employment. This is documented by patient activists, researchers, and patient authors, who feel compelled to adopt a 'stance of silence', when their 'actual stories' are denied the credibility needed for uptake (Hinshaw 2008, pp. 8–9).

Turning to hermeneutical injustice, this occurs when the capacity of a person or group to make intelligible certain of their bodily, existential, and social experiences to themselves or to others is unjustly constrained or undermined. The effort to make sense of our social experiences requires an array of hermeneutical practices and resources – appropriate language, metaphors, and images, shared and recognised within a community, through which we can make sense of the structure, significance, and complexities of lived experience. Often, creating and actively updating this understanding come naturally, especially to the members of hermeneutically privileged groups whose social experiences are supported by a rich interpretative structure that renders them intelligible. But this is not the case for the hermeneutically marginalised, those who cannot create or share the sense of their social experiences in comparably lucid ways (Fricker 2007, Chapter 7).

Such failures to achieve intelligibility affects both hearers and speakers, but members of these groups are differentially disadvantaged: the more privileged group tends to suffer less, epistemically and practically, and may even have an interest in *not* understanding the experiences of the underprivileged in some cases, for example, dismissive attitudes towards complaints about gender or race based mistreatment. The injustice lies in the harmfulness, unfairness, and discrimination constitutive of these hermeneutical situations in which certain illness experiences have no socially accepted way of being expressed and understood.

Unsurprisingly, therefore, forms of hermeneutical injustice can be heterogeneous, depending, for instance, on whether they arise from an absence of appropriate hermeneutical resources or from prejudices against certain communicative or expressive styles. The injustice may be that people are prevented from making sense of their experiences, or of sharing that sense with others. Moreover, forms of hermeneutical injustice may be sustained by structural or interpersonal dynamics, which, if sufficiently oppressive, can precipitate the destruction of hermeneutical agency (Medina 2017).

Kidd and I further argued that ill persons are *especially* vulnerable to hermeneutical injustice (Carel and Kidd 2014; Kidd and Carel 2016, 2018, 2021,). Ill persons suffer hermeneutical marginalisation that is specific to certain features of illness – the difficulty of talking about one's illness, its traumatic nature, the deep fear and anxiety that accompany illness, and the common tendency to shy away from discussing illness and death can all hamper expressive attempts. Illness itself intrinsically constrains hermeneutical agency, imposing difficult new demands, while disrupting one's capacities to make intelligible and share one's experiences.

Even among HCPs, there continues to be a reluctance to discuss death, existential suffering, and subjective symptoms, such as mental distress, and 'contested illnesses', such as chronic fatigue syndrome (CFS/ME). Such active silences are evident in documented cases of epistemic injustice in the case of CFS/ME, increased vulnerability to stigma in the case of mental disorder, and discomfort about discussing assisted dying (Quill 2000; Blease, Carel, and Geraghty 2017; Crichton, Carel, and Kidd 2017). There can also be situations where HCPs may want to discuss such issues when patients do not. What ought to be shared hermeneutical agency becomes unidirectional, as either practitioners or patients are unable to reciprocally respond to the other. Indeed, although most analyses of failed communication in end-of-life contexts focus on HCPs, recent research indicates that patients, their families, and HCPs often 'collude to avoid mentioning death or dying, even when the patient's suffering is severe and prognosis is poor' (Quill 2000).

Unintelligibility, confusion, and other forms of hermeneutical frustration are abiding themes of patient testimonies and core to phenomenological accounts of illness (Carel 2016, 2018). As formerly stable structures of meaning destabilise, the world ceases to be 'a space of salient possibilities', reliably reflective of one's goals and purposes. It is no longer 'a safe context that offers opportunities for activity but [becomes] something one is at the mercy of' (Ratcliffe 2008, pp. 113–115; see also Carel 2018, 2016). Understood outside the strictures of clinical medicine, illness is experienced as a 'breakdown of meaning', a harsh disclosure of the truth that 'meaning and intelligibility depend on consistent patterns of embodiment' that no longer – and may never again – obtain (Carel 2016, pp. 14–15).

Meaning and intelligibility are difficult to achieve, given the variety of obstacles encountered by ill persons in their efforts to make and share meaningful accounts of their experiences. Although some of these are harmful, it is important to note that not all are due to unjust attitudes or structures. Many of these difficulties reflect two distinctive features of chronic illness – its *inarticulacy* and *ineffability*. The inarticulacy arises from the difficulties of communicating alterations in the structures of one's lived experience, of 'finding the right words'. Since one's sense of the ordinary meanings of things becomes disrupted, as one's relationship to previous habits and lived environment are affected by illness, one's existing hermeneutical resources and competences cease to be effortlessly effective, while developing new ones appears as another set of demands imposed by illness. As S. K. Toombs explains:

> [T]he bookcase outside my bedroom was once intended by my body as a "repository for books"; then as "that which is to be grasped for support on the way to the bathroom", and is now intended as "an obstacle to get around with my wheelchair".
>
> (Toombs 1995, p. 16)

In the same way that the meaning of the word 'bookcase' has changed with her increasing limitations, other words and concepts may no longer be part of the shared meaning that underpins the intelligibility of everyday human life. That may form part of a process of hermeneutical marginalisation, where meanings become increasingly unshared and may even be experienced as entirely idiosyncratic. Such idiosyncrasy is a powerful hermeneutical obstacle, and if coupled with others' culpable failures to attend to or accept those idiosyncratic meanings, may mark some types of hermeneutical injustice.

A further difficulty is the *ineffability* of certain dimensions of the experience of illness, their resistance to any articulable understanding shareable with others. Sometimes, one can't find the words, but, at other times, there really are no words to cogently convey to others the dynamics and character of one's new, altered way of being. It may be that certain life experiences are so unique, dramatic, or traumatic, that they are accompanied by a sense of ineffability. The radically and irreducibly subjective character of certain experiences arguably generates fundamental obstacles to the possibility of collective hermeneutical agency.

In addition, there is a range of exclusionary practices, inherent in social and health care systems, that run the risk of excluding ill persons from the sites and practices in which social meanings are created and legitimated. The exclusion may be physical, epistemic, social, or some combination of these. Such exclusion prevents ill persons from participating in shared creation of medical definitions, such as diagnostic criteria, or in consensus conferences. Another example is the exclusion of patients from certain places of deliberation and decision, such as hospital committees or policy discussions.

Attempts by ill persons at participation in hermeneutical practice may also be thwarted by expressive restrictions. Corresponding to what Medina (2017) calls the 'performative' forms of hermeneutical injustice, these take the form of restrictions on the types of expressive styles accepted as legitimate. Typically, in the case of illness, legitimacy is confined to the norms, language, and terminology of biomedicine which may promote an impersonal expressive style. Such a style is stripped of the existential particularity, affective depth, and contextual richness of lived experience. It has the additional function of reducing the amount of discomfort HCPs experience by offering an objective and emotionally neutral alternative to highly personal and emotive discussions. As detailed above, many health care interactions are between people who are strangers to each other, and whose interests and perspectives are vastly different. This creates a fertile ground for shutting down expressive attempts that diverge from the standards accepted in health care discourse.

The expressive styles judged by ill persons to be adequate for the task of conveying their existential and social experiences may be quite different – anecdotal, episodic, autobiographical, rich in affective and existentially complex description and full of difficult emotions such as anger and grief. Within modern health care systems these styles and the content they are especially apt to convey are typically excluded as irrelevant or ineffective for the epistemic needs of clinical practice (for more on expressive styles, see Burley 2011; Kidd 2017).

Unjust epistemic situations can be challenged in various ways. These include patient activism, academic research, and improved uptake of the perspectives of patients, through the cultivation of approaches such as a phenomenological approach, patient-centred care, and inclusive research design. Reflecting on the testimonies of physicians who become patients, Klitzman says that often 'only the experience of becoming seriously ill finally compels them to change their thinking, and see themselves and their work more broadly, and from a different vantage point (Klitzman 2008, p. 12). Further initiatives from health care research funders and academic communities as well as patient partnerships, include public-patient involvement, including experts by experience in design of services, and a focus on patient well-being. However, a more systematic study of epistemic injustice in its unique operation within health care is still needed. More research on epistemic injustice is being continuously published, and I briefly outline some trends in this area.

Following the emergence of epistemic injustice studies, and the publication of work specifically on epistemic injustice in health care (inaugurated by Carel and Kidd 2014), scholars went on to identify other kinds of epistemic injustice. Examples include what Kristie Dotson (2011) called *testimonial smothering*: a pre-emptive self-censoring of the content and expression of testimonies by speakers. Christopher Hookway (2010) identified another pair of pre-emptive epistemic injustices. *Informational prejudices* involve prejudices about what kinds of people will possess the sense of relevance necessary to being a worthwhile informant, while *participatory prejudice* prevents one from recognising someone as a potential participant in a shared epistemic activity. Other scholars have described kinds of *contributory injustice* and *discursive injustice;* doubtless others exist (Kukla 2014; Tate 2019). David Coady (2017) argues that Fricker's account presents the wrongs of epistemic injustice in *discriminative* terms – we unfairly and harmfully discriminate against certain epistemic agents (women, disabled persons, and so on). Coady proposes an alternative *distributive* account according to which the wrongs of epistemic injustice concern misdistribution of epistemic goods, such as credibility and intelligibility, in a social environment. Dotson has argued that the real wrong of many epistemic injustices is that they are specific expressions of a wider phenomenon of *epistemic violence*, a concept introduced by Spivak (1988). If the violent character of epistemic injustices is occluded, we may risk understating their full nature and significance (Dotson 2011, pp. 237–242). Emmalon Davis (2018) suggests a further epistemic harm, which she dubs *epistemic appropriation*, in which marginalised knowers are harmed through the dissemination and intercommunal uptake of their epistemic resources, in ways that detach those resources from the knowers who created them. Moreover, such resources are utilised in dominant discourses in ways that disproportionately benefit the powerful.

The upshot of these developments since the publication of Fricker's *Epistemic Injustice* has been a substantial enrichment of our resources for conceptualising the nature, causes, wrongs, and effects of many kinds of epistemic injustice. These enriched resources are also being taken up by academics interested to put those concepts to work, often in the service of ameliorative and practical work in specific domains (see Sherman and Goguen 2019). We should beware a tendency to rely on under-articulated accounts of epistemic injustice. This can include a neglect of relevant distinctions. Not all uses of the concept require us to include all of its associated theoretical detail but in many cases the concept can only really do its work if sufficient detail and theoretical precision is used.

Conclusion

To end this survey of epistemic injustice within the context of health care, I'd like to consider how epistemic injustice might arise between HCPs, rather than between HCPs and patients. There is epistemic asymmetry between different HCPs within institutions of contemporary health care services. There are complex relationships and hierarchies between the different actors present at each health care scene: junior vs senior, medically educated vs other forms of training, core vs 'complementary', and so on. It is crucial to note that epistemic injustice – and other kinds of epistemic asymmetries – are intrinsic to such complex social situations and may therefore be present in staff and team meetings, multidisciplinary discussions, and in informal situations in which decisions are made.

In this chapter, I focused primarily on the epistemic injustice patients are more vulnerable to because some HCPs enjoy epistemic privilege owing to their training, expertise, and third-person psychology, and there is also an implicit privileging of certain styles of articulating and evidencing testimonies in ways that marginalise ill persons. But this does not cancel out the possibility of epistemic injustice occurring between other actors and groups within the complex health care system and settings. Indeed, what happens within institutions affects not only the 'service users' of that institution but also its actors and agents, who may lose trust in the institution and become alienated from it due to epistemic failings on the institutions level (for a discussion of this, see Carel and Kidd 2021).

In closing, I suggest that a phenomenological approach may be part of an effort to ameliorate epistemic injustice. This approach prioritises first person experience, provides a rich and robust framework within to study and understand that experience, and has the potential to powerfully advocate for the patient's voice. A phenomenological approach can be used to give patients tools with which to order and articulate their experiences, as well as to effectively share them with others, thus improving their self-advocacy and epistemic confidence (Carel 2012). In this sense, the theoretical development of both epistemic injustice studies and patient experience research are powerful political tools, aligned in their quest to improve patient care and experience and support those who are ill.

Notes

1 The term 'pathophobic' was coined by Ian James Kidd to describe negative attitudes (stigma, negative stereotypes, etc.) towards illness or ill persons. See Kidd 2019.
2 https://www.patients-association.org.uk/Handlers/Download.ashx?IDMF=16708179-90d6-41dd-a360-2c53b7e9ebe7

References

Being a patient; First report of the Patients Association's patient experience programme. The Patients Association. (July 2020). https://www.patients-association.org.uk/Handlers/Download.ashx?IDMF=16708179-90d6-41dd-a360-2c53b7e9ebe7 [accessed on 29 January 2023].

Blease, Charlotte, Havi Carel, and Keith Geraghty. (2017). Epistemic Injustice in Healthcare Encounters: Evidence from Chronic Fatigue Syndrome. *Journal of Medical Ethics* 43: 549–557.

Burley, Mikel. (2011). Emotion and Anecdote in Philosophical Argument: The Case of Havi Carel's Illness. *Metaphilosophy* 42: 33–48.

Carel, Havi. (2012). Phenomenology as a Resource for Patients. *Journal of Medicine and Philosophy* 37(2): 96–113.

Carel, Havi. (2016). *Phenomenology of Illness*. Oxford: Oxford University Press.

Carel, Havi. (2018). *Illness: The Cry of the Flesh*. 3rd ed. London: Routledge.

Carel, Havi. (2021). 'Creatures of a Day': Contingency, Mortality, and Human Limits. *Royal Institute of Philosophy Supplements* 90: 193–214.

Carel, Havi, and Ian James Kidd. (2014). Epistemic Injustice in Healthcare: A Philosophical Analysis. *Medicine, Healthcare and Philosophy* 17(4): 529–540.

Carel, Havi, and Ian James Kidd. (2021). Institutional Opacity, Epistemic Vulnerability, and Institutional Testimonial Justice. *International Journal of Philosophical Studies* 29(4): 473–496.

Coady, David. (2017). Epistemic Injustice as Distributive Injustice. In I. J. Kidd, J. Medina & G. Pohlhaus (eds.),

Crichton, Paul, Havi Carel, and Ian James Kidd. (2017). Epistemic Injustice in Psychiatry. *British Journal of Psychiatry Bulletin* 41: 65–70.

Davis, Emmalon. (2018). Epistemic Appropriation. *Ethics* 128(4): 702–727.

Dotson, Kristie. (2011). Tracking Epistemic Violence, Tracking Practices of Silencing. *Hypatia* 26(2): 236–257.

Fricker, Miranda. (2007). *Epistemic Injustice: Power and the Ethics of Knowing*. Oxford: Oxford University Press.

Fricker, Miranda. (2017). Evolving Concepts of Epistemic Injustice. In I. J. Kidd, J. Medina &G. Pohlhaus (eds.), *The Routledge Handbook to Epistemic Injustice* (pp. 53–60). London: Routledge.

Hinshaw, Stephen P. (2008). *Breaking the Silence: Mental Health Professionals Disclose their Personal and Family Experiences of Mental Illness*. Oxford: Oxford University Press.

Hookway, Christopher. (2010). Some Varieties of Epistemic Injustice: Reflections on Fricker. *Episteme* 7(2): 151–163.

Kidd, Ian James. (2017). Exemplars, Ethics, and Illness Narratives. *Theoretical Medicine and Bioethics* 38(4): 323–334.

Kidd, Ian James. (2019). Pathophobia, Illness, and Vices. *International Journal of Philosophical Studies* 27(2): 286–306.

Kidd, Ian James, and Havi Carel. (2016). Epistemic Injustice and Illness. *Journal of Applied Philosophy* 3(2): 172–190.

Kidd, Ian James, and Havi Carel. (2018). Pathocentric Epistemic Injustice and Conceptions of Health. In Benjamin R. Sherman & Stacey Goguen (eds.), *Overcoming Epistemic Injustice: Social and Psychological Perspectives* (pp. 153–168). New York: Rowman and Littlefield.

Kidd, Ian James, and Havi Carel. (2021). The Predicament of Patients. In *Royal Institute of Philosophy Supplements*: *How Do We Know? The Social Dimension of Knowledge* (vol. 89, pp. 65–84). Cambridge U Press, Cambridge and the editor is Julian Baggini.

Kidd, Ian James, José Medina, and Gaile Pohlhaus, Jr. (eds.) (2017). *The Routledge Handbook to Epistemic Injustice*, co-edited with. New York: Routledge.

Klitzman, Robert. (2008). *When Doctors Become Patients*. Oxford: Oxford University Press.

Kukla, Rebecca. (2014). Performative Force, Convention, and Discursive Injustice. *Hypatia* 29(2): 440–457.

Macintyre, Alasdair. (1999). *Dependent Rational Animals: Why Human Beings Need the Virtues by*. Chicago: Open Court Press.

Medina, José. (2017). Varieties of Hermeneutical Injustice. In Kidd, Medina & Pohlhaus, Jr. (eds.), *The Routledge Handbook to Epistemic Injustice* (pp. 41–52). New York: Routledge.

Norman, Abby. (2018). *Ask Me About My Uterus: A Quest to Make Doctors Believe in Women's Pain*. New York: Nation Books.

Quill, Timothy E. (2000). Initiating End-of-Life Discussions with Seriously Ill Patients: Addressing the "Elephant in the Room". *Journal of the American Medical Association* 284(19): 2502–2507.

Ratcliffe, Matthew. (2008). *Feelings of Being: Phenomenology, Psychiatry, and the Sense of Reality*. Oxford: Oxford University Press.

Sherman, B. R., and Goguen, S. (2019). *Overcoming Epistemic Injustice: Social and Psychological Perspectives*. London: Rowman and Littlefield.

Sontag, Susan. (1978). *Illness as Metaphor*. New York: Farrar, Straus and Giroux.

Spivak, Gayatri Chakravorty. (1988). Can the Subaltern Speak? In C. Nelson & L. Grossberg (eds.), *Marxism and the Interpretation of Culture* (pp. 271–313). Champaign, IL: Macmillan.

Tate, A. J. M. (2019). Contributory Injustice in Psychiatry. *Journal of Medical Ethics* 45: 97–100.

Toombs, S. K. (1987). The Meaning of Illness: A Phenomenological Approach to the Patient–Physician Relationship. *Journal of Medicine and Philosophy* 12: 219–240.

Toombs, S. K. (1995). The Lived Experience of Disability. *Human Studies* 18: 9–23.

45 A process philosophy perspective on the relationality of nursing and leadership

Miriam Bender

Introduction: the paradox of leadership in/and nursing

Nursing appears to have a foundational commitment to leadership, and yet paradoxically the existing literature demonstrates that in nursing there does not seem to be any well-defined conceptualization of nursing leadership. In a landmark report written by the Institute of Medicine (IOM) in 2011, called *The Future of Nursing: Leading Change, Advancing Health,* leadership was considered a fundamental nursing competency that is "needed to practice [nursing]" and that "strong [nursing] leadership is critical if the vision of a transformed health care system is to be realized" (p. 7). To accomplish this, the report called for leadership competencies to be "embedded throughout nursing education" and that "all nurses - from students, to bedside and community nurses, to chief nursing officers and members of nursing organizations, to researchers - must take responsibility for their personal and professional growth by developing leadership competencies" (IOM, 2011, p. 8). Yet, it is important to note that leadership was never actually defined in the report, beyond its mention as a set of "skills" or "competencies" and "the need for them" (IOM, 2011, p. 270). The report did put forth a set of research priorities for "transforming nursing leadership" that began with the identification of "personal and professional characteristics most critical to [nursing] leadership... [and] leaders" (IOM, 2011, p. 277). This knowledge was then to be used to provide nurses with leadership competence which they should then use to lead change and advance health.

This report spurred a flurry of efforts to generate leadership 'knowledge' for use by nursing schools across the United States and beyond (see, for example, a recent bibliometric analysis by Kantek, Yesilbas & Ozen, 2022). A December 2022 Google search for 'nursing leadership textbooks' identified a whopping 83 textbooks that could be used to help in this effort, with titles such as *Nursing Management, Lead like a Nurse, The Nuts And Bolts Of Nursing Leadership, Transformational Leadership In Nursing,* etc. The American Association of Colleges of Nursing (AACN), the "national voice for academic nursing" here in the United States, considers leadership an "essential" required competence for all levels of nursing education, meaning that nursing schools must teach leadership to their students in order to be accredited by the AACN (only students graduating from accredited nursing schools can sit for their state RN licensure exam).

The AACN defines "basic nursing leadership" as "an awareness of complex systems, and the impact of power, politics, policy, and regulatory guidelines on these systems" (AACN, 2021, p. 13) and provides a list of leadership curricular content to achieve this awareness that includes leadership theory, leadership styles, and leadership skills. However, it does not delineate these theories, styles, and skills. In fact, a recently developed

DOI: 10.4324/9781003427407-52

AACN "toolkit" to prepare nurses to serve as leaders reports on the massive "prolif-eration" of leadership theories, styles (they note at least 28), and attributes, and ac-knowledges that amidst all this leadership "knowledge," it remains "difficult for nursing educators to define and develop the desired skills needed for improving our healthcare delivery" (AACN, 2021, no pagination). They hope that their toolbox can be of some assistance, but the message is clear that there is no well delineated conceptualization of leadership that nurses can teach or take on unproblematically.

This lack of conceptual clarity is also the major finding of a recently published com-prehensive systematic review of "the essentials of nursing leadership" (Cummings et al., 2020). The study found no less than 58 different instruments measuring nursing leader-ship and identified an eye-popping 105 "factors" contributing to nursing leadership. These myriad factors included years of individual nursing experience, individual levels of education, and individualized traits such as emotional intelligence and conscientiousness. In terms of leadership development programs/curriculum, the authors found no com-monality in content nor duration. Overall, the systematic review found that "leadership practices by nurses remain poorly characterized" (2020, p. 8) and the authors conclude that "robust theory and research" on nursing leadership is needed.

In summary, while nursing leadership is considered essential for nursing practice, and has been conceptualized as a set of skills or competencies that each individual nurse should be educated to enact, it seems there are as many definitions of leadership as there are papers, books, and policy documents reporting on it.

Problematizing leadership as individual competency

How can we understand this paradox of a universal commitment to leadership as fun-damental to nursing practice but which appears to be undefinable in and of itself? In the systematic literature review described above, the authors were clear that "leadership practices are intricately intertwined with the context in which they occur and do not sim-ply depend on the characteristics of individuals" (Cummings et al., 2020, p. 10).

What this implies is that a conceptualization of leadership that focuses on the indi-vidual may not be the right orientation. A focus on the individual has led to inquiry into traits, characteristics, and competencies that individuals as leaders should have or enact in order to effectively lead. This is reflected in the majority of nursing leadership research which focuses on attributes such as 'years of practice' and 'conscientiousness' (Cum-mings et al., 2020). In terms of educational competencies, the focus is also individualized. For example, the recently published American Organization for Nursing Leadership's framework for leadership has every one of their competencies explicitly described as something enacted by the individual, such as "influences and persuades others… encour-ages new ideas… implements and maintains optimal, culturally competent healthcare" (Hughes, Meadows & Begley, 2022, p. 630).

This focus on the individual in terms of leadership theorizing is slowly beginning to change, however. For example, in Northouse's 9th edition of his book *Leadership: Theory and Practice* (2021), he acknowledges that "after decades of dissonance, leader-ship scholars agree on one thing: They can't come up with a common definition of leader-ship" (p. 5). Northouse then plots the trajectory of leadership scholarship from a focus on individual traits and individual behaviors toward something that happens in groups and ends up defining leadership as "a process whereby an individual influences a group of individuals to achieve a common goal" (2021, p. 6).

This is an important shift. If leadership is something that manifests in groups, then it is an interactional event and not an individual competency. The question then becomes how can we orient to leadership as an interactional event and what do we find when that occurs? While understanding what traits or skills or competencies individuals may need to enact leadership is undoubtedly important, it is also clear, as the literature has plainly shown, that these individual elements don't manifest in practice unmediated. Learning to be 'conscientious' may be important to a nurse as a first step toward leading, but the unanswered question is how can conscientiousness manifest in practice and how does that manifestation accomplish 'leadership?' If leadership is an interactional event, then elements such as context and group dynamics, including their heterogeneity, become just as important to understand, if not more so, than individual elements.

Problematizing nursing's traditional focus on the individual

The existing focus on individual traits or competencies in leadership scholarship and education is presupposed by an orientation that separates the individual from their environment; that considers the nurse as an autonomous individual in control of their knowledge and agency and who uses this agency to affect change in their environments. This 'individualistic' orientation is assumed in much nursing discourse (see Petrovskaya, 2023 for a highly insightful analysis).

We have already considered the problems of leadership when it is conceptualized as individual traits, characteristics, or competencies. Another important example is the highly influential scholarship on nurse staffing and patient outcomes. In this extensive body of research, which was a key driver in bringing staff nurse-patient ratio laws to California (AB 95, established in 1999), the nurse is conceived as individual body count and the work was to demonstrate that an insufficient number of individual nurses in hospitals was associated with greater harms to patients (see, for instance, Aiken et al., 2002; Needleman et al., 2002, 2006, 2011).

Another important example is the influential body of scholarship on nursing practice environments. The assumption driving this research is that nurses are unable to fully implement their competencies (including leadership) because of barriers within the contexts of their practice. The research has worked to demonstrate that "healthy work environments" are those where nurses can practice to their highest level of competence (see, for instance, Blake et al., 2013; Lake, 2002, 2007).

The issue with these important programs of research is that the focus on the individual nurse has not produced the intended consequences for nursing or healthcare. In terms of the California staff nurse ratio law, which did indeed manage to increase the number of registered nurses working in hospitals (Donaldson et al., 2005), numerous studies have failed to show any improvements in patient care quality and safety outcomes after the law was put into effect (Aiken et al., 2010; McHugh et al., 2012; Needleman, 2015; Spetz et al., 2013). In terms of the workforce scholarship, the very fact that the context of nursing was operationalized as completely independent from the nurse creates the alarming scenario where nurses are rendered powerless *in principle* to shape the contexts of their care. In this body of research, nursing leadership becomes in effect a meaningless concept (for a more detailed analysis, see Bender & Feldman, 2015).

There are many other examples that could be brought forth, but space prohibits. Yet, the three examples of nurse leadership, nurse ratios, and nurse work environments make clear that a primary orientation in well-funded nursing research and well-intended nursing policy is toward the nurse as distinct entity autonomous from their contexts of practice. This cleavage is conceptual in nature and has resulted in the outcomes described: a lack of understanding about what nursing leadership consists of; a body of evidence demonstrating that more nurses do not automatically result in better quality patient care; and a definition of nursing contexts that renders invisible, thus meaningless, the actual contributions of nursing in producing beneficial environments of care.

This is all to say that nursing is much more complex than the actions of specially educated individuals, and that there is an active interdependency between nurses, nursing, patients, and environments that generate quality patient outcomes. And if so the question then becomes, how can we orient to nursing in ways that do not reproduce autonomous individuals separated from their practices and their contexts?

Thinking process

One potentially fruitful way of orienting is through a process lens. A process-oriented understanding of phenomena foregrounds how, not what. It does not assume that the world is already filled with people and things that are well-defined or well-definable, such as nurses with leadership competencies. Instead, a process orientation focuses on what's happening, on how phenomenon happens, for example, how nursing leadership happens. This directs attention away from things, and people, and toward doings, actions, performances, and engagements. By focusing on the doings, the idea is that what is involved becomes 'what matters' and this is identified through the inquiry itself, and can't be pre-decided ahead of time.

What does this mean? Basically, it has to do with the idea that 'things' never exist on their own but are always dependent on other 'things.' In a fascinating paper by Annamarie Mol and Jessica Mesman (1996), they do the work of unpacking the seemingly unproblematic term 'food.' Their setting was a neonatal intensive care unit. What they found was that 'food' had many definitions that depended on what was happening. Here is an excerpt:

> What is it [food]? There isn't one word for it. there are many. The bottle contains *food* for the baby. it contains the *infusion* dripping into a vein, and a *sugar suspension*. Or part of the *120 calories for every kilo a day*. And then again the bottle's content is a fluid with a particular composition... But it is also *nutrition*. It is classified as *intake*. And it is definitely *everything that this small patient is going to get for the next 24 hours*. So there are many words for the content of a single bottle. They relate to different concerns and their value doesn't need to stay the same... [all this] helps to show that a discussion about food is also a discussion about the [many] way[s] Matthew's [a neonate] life is ordered... [that] there are many orders... different orderings co-exist.
>
> (Mol & Mesman, 1996, pp. 430–434, italics original)

This idea of ordering is powerful, making visible the fact that 'food' consists of multiple processes of ordering that interweave and intersect at the site of a neonate's incubator, including doctors making calculations and pharmacists making solutions and nurses documenting solution intake, not to mention the solution's infusion into Matthew through an enteric tube or bottle, depending on many other things, not least of which are the decisions about whether doctor's orders or baby's sleep requirements will be met during a particular feeding time. All these orderings result in what we hope becomes Matthew-growing-stronger so he can get out of the intensive care unit.

Considering 'food' through this lens of multiplicity helps to better understand how things happen and all the different elements or practices involved and thus helps, for example, when things 'go wrong' (which happens often in the context of healthcare) in that by tracking the multiplicity of orderings involving doctors, pharmacists, nurses, solutions, tubings or bottles, and babies in incubators, these pathways are made visible and can be assessed or queried to see where unravelings may have occurred, or frictions generated, which are never self-evident since they all involve even more complexities such as "the shape of a building, the rhythm of the day, or systems of calculation" (Mol & Mesman, 1996, p. 436).

While this may sound a bit overwhelming or overly complex, it's important to note that in healthcare settings we *already* orient this way under special circumstances – when something goes majorly awry, such as the removal of the 'wrong' kidney during a surgery – through a process called event mapping (Agency for Healthcare Research and Quality [AHRQ], 2022). In this process, the goal is to, literally, map out the event of concern and not assume all elements of the event are already known or established. The goal of event mapping is to "learn about the processes involved in the work around the event… [because] the environment, the technology, the information, and the processes are all critical clues to the context in which the event occurred" (AHRQ, 2022, no pagination). Investigatory tools like "five whys" are used to access a 'deeper' sense of what happened, and thus assumes that the answer to one question will lead to other questions, all of which need to be answered to understand what was going on. This effort is thus based on an assumption that there are multiple processes and practices interacting with each other, even in locations other than where/when the adverse event took place, that could have influenced the making of the adverse event. In this very pragmatic mode of 'figuring out,' there is an assumed fluidity to the event and thus the question becomes not so much 'what thing broke down' but rather how did practices hook up or not in ways that resulted in the adverse event.

Process philosophy

This all suggests that a process orientation to healthcare, including nursing, can and even already does open up new ways of understanding healthcare phenomenon, which is important, especially after unpacking the ways current individual-centered/bounded approaches have been unable do the work of solving the problems we want to solve. The good news is that there is a long and robust philosophical engagement with process thought that can be used to support empirical moves toward process inquiry. Process philosophy is an umbrella term for a loosely connected trajectory of thought going all the way back to the beginnings of Western philosophy in Greece, with Heraclitus saying, "one cannot step twice into the same river" (quoted in Rescher, 1996, p. 9). Gilles Deleuze, a 20th-century French process philosopher, called this thread a "secret society" (Deleuze, 1992, p. 76), a somewhat hidden stream of philosophy asking questions not about "what is… [but about] the where, when and how of happenings as events" (Robinson, 2016, p. 59).

Questions about 'what is' are Aristotelian in presupposing an X and then going about delineating the properties of X (Emerton, 2019), for example, assuming there is such a thing called 'nursing leadership' and then inquiring into its properties/characteristics.

Questions about 'where, when and how' are process ones, and don't assume static things or bounded entities, out there, waiting to be pointed to or characterized. Instead, these questions assume events happen, are 'on the go,' emerge from circumstances and create different circumstances as they happen, and the questions help to focus attention on "how they become entangled, connect, bifurcate, avoid or fail to avoid the foci" (Deleuze in Robinson, 2016, p. 60).

What does it mean to orient to processual events rather than bounded entities (individuals included)? For Alfred North Whitehead, considered by many to be the progenitor of modern process philosophy, what exists is not pre-existing; it is not what is already out there waiting to be discovered, but the process that creates the world. Whitehead puts it this way:

> process is a fundamental fact in our experience. We are in the present; the present is always shifting; it is derived from the past; it is shaping the future; it is passing into the future. This is process, and in the universe it is an inexorable fact.
>
> (Whitehead, 1938, p. 73)

Whitehead defined the process as the becoming of actual occasions. Events are occasions, occurrences by which "the actual world is built up" (Whitehead, 1929/1978, p. 73). Events consist of entangled occasions, or "nexus," that are "inter-related." The modes of relating vary, which can result in more or less "reinforcement," or reproduction, of the entangling. In this way of orienting, 'things' are construed as entangled occasions that are able to "reinforce each other" and hence (re)produce consistency (Whitehead, 1929/1978, pp. 111–112).

Let's take rocks, for example. Rocks are a favorite item that, as Ian Hacking, a philosopher of science puts it, "the curmudgeonly troll of hyperbolic scientific realism" likes to bring out when the "reality of things" are philosophically challenged (1999, p. 195). For 'hyperbolic realists,' rocks are that which represent "the most unquestionable reality" (Hacking, 1999, p. 204) and sometimes they even threaten to hurl them at people in order to construe the resulting forehead gash as unassailable argument for things as unquestionably *there* – bounded, fixed, weighty, thus *real*. Beyond noticing that throwing a rock is an event, it's interesting how Hacking narrates a more nuanced story by demonstrating how a certain kind of rock, dolomite, constitutes a formation and not a thing. Dolomite thus becomes more accurately "dolomitization" (Hacking, 1999, p. 189), a still-contested process by which dolomite is constructed and which is now considered "a centuries-old problem which changes its face to fit each new generation of biologists" (p. 192). Hacking finds that "dolomite is a sorting" (1999, p. 205), which makes the answer to the question, is dolomite a 'natural kind' in terms of having an Aristotelian property that affixes to any and all samples of dolomite throughout the world, no. Dolomite instead appears to be constituted via "messy mixtures formed by mysterious processes… [of which] there is no stability to explain" (1999, pp. 205–206).

The process of dolomitization is one still being worked out by multiple teams of scientists. The story is not yet complete. Deleuze's process philosophy conceptualizes this effort as a practice of "thinking with AND, instead of thinking IS" (Deleuze, in Robinson, 2016, p. 62). Thinking of the world as 'is' conspires to view the world as pre-existing and fixed; complete. Thinking of the world as 'and' conspires to view the world as inter-connected and never complete; there being always more connections to untangle or make.

This all is not to urge that a process philosophy approach comprises the 'best' or 'only' way we should be orienting, but to say that clearly there are other orientations available than an entity approach, and they provide fresh ways to view and mobilize the world. This should be considered a great opportunity in nursing, one that can help move us past the stalemates we are currently involved with regarding how to 'define' ourselves, our practices, and our unique efficacy (explored in more depth in Bender, 2018; Bender & Holmes, 2019).

Nursing conceptualized as a body count has done some good work for nursing; we now know that nurses are vital to hospital functioning if we don't want patients to die in them. Nursing conceptualized as an entity separated from its work environments has made visible work conditions that don't really help nurses nurse. But orienting to nursing as an 'is' seems to only get us so far. What can be achieved if we orient to nursing as a process rather than nurses as particular people with particular competencies?

Nursing leadership as a process

To bring the story back to the focus of this chapter, leadership seems well suited toward being oriented to as a process and not a thing, or a property of an entity such as a nurse. In rethinking phenomenon such as leadership as a process and not a competence, the almost overwhelming number of 'factors' (remember, there were 105 of them) found in the literature review discussed earlier becomes more understandable as contextualities entangled with the multiplicities of nursing practice, all of which can *result* in what we think of as 'leadership.'

Instead of categorizing these factors into discrete buckets such as 'traits and characteristics,' 'roles,' and 'organizational context,' in attempting to find common attributes 'of' leadership, it would be interesting to see if the data could be ordered in different ways, suggesting possible nursing practices conditioned by particular contexts that consistently produce what we want leadership to accomplish. That perhaps, 'staff nurses' with 'over 5 years of experience' but who have no 'managerial work experience' and work in 'Magnet hospitals' without 'union status' tend to become involved in 'shared governance' which increases 'two-way communication' that leads to new practices that address communicated patient issues (quoted words are identified factors in the Cummings et al., 2020 literature review). This is a rich hypothesis designating a process full of potential avenues for inquiry that can help us to better understand what it is about, for example, shared governance at Magnet hospitals that engage staff nurses and how that engagement can lead to beneficial changes. The relationality of the factors becomes what is focused on, not the attributes in isolation from each other.

It might initially be thought that this kind of scholarship would simply take too long, or is categorically unfundable, or cannot lead to generalizable findings easily taken up by nursing schools and health systems clamoring for leadership 'knowledge.' In the next section, I provide an example of an empirical research program inquiring into leadership processes, demonstrating its feasibility and actionable outcomes.

Clinical nurse leader empirical program of research

My empirical program of research can be said to be a direct outcome of the *Future of Nursing* report. I entered my doctoral program in 2010, the same year the report was first announced with much fanfare – it remains the second most downloaded report of the IOM (National Academy of Medicine, 2021). The report called for research to help understand and delineate nursing leadership. Thus, my dissertation focused on a then brand-new nursing education and practice initiative, the clinical nurse leader (CNL). The CNL educational model and curriculum was articulated in a 2007 White Paper published by AACN (2007). It laid out a series of leadership competencies that were considered necessary for "the nurse of the future." These competencies were to be inculcated through a master's level curriculum and degree. A recent analysis of these 'competencies' demonstrated however that they actually constitute an overarching set of *practices* that involve the coordination and improvement of clinical care processes and outcomes, and the assessment and improvement of patient-level care structures (Bender, L'Ecuyer et al., 2019).

Since the CNL educational program was new, there was no body of research to help understand how this model actually functioned in practice, despite the fact that the CNL masters level degree program quickly became a popular mode of entry into the nursing field (Commission on Nurse Certification, 2021). I therefore commenced what is now a 12-year collaborative effort with other researchers, health system leaders, policy leaders, and CNLs to conceptualize CNL practice and determine whether, and if so how, CNL practice functions to improve patient care quality and safety (for details, see Bender, Baker et al., 2019).

The program of research approaches clinical nurse leadership as a process, is focused on CNL practices, and assumes this practice is complex, dynamic, and inherently context-sensitive (Bender, 2017; Kaack et al., 2018). The scholarship has elucidated the ways CNL implementation patterns (the ways health systems integrate CNLs into their nursing models) influence CNL practice patterns and how these entanglements influence what happens in/to the contexts where CNLs practice (Bender, Burtson et al., 2019; Bender & Lefkowitz, 2020).

This (federally funded) effort does not predetermine CNL practice as X and then set out to determine if this black-boxed X is or is not 'efficacious.' Rather the work has been to understand what CNL practice can accomplish, or not, depending on how it is contextualized into clinical settings and what kinds of processes can be made to happen or change for the better related to this contextualization. This has necessitated multiple innovations in participatory-engaged, mixed-methods approaches that don't assume efficacy comes before effectiveness and that can analyze patterns of relations instead of independent variable correlations (Bender et al., 2021; Cruz et al., 2017).

What we are generating is findings with "analytic generalizability" rather than statistical generalizability (Tsang, 2013; Yin, 2013). Statistical generalizability is a calculation about whether the effect size from a study can be expected to 'hold' in situations outside the study. Analytic generalizability is concerned with assessing whether relationships found through inquiry might apply in other circumstances as well. This approach does not involve a statistically significant 'effect' attached to a set of prescriptive actions, but rather involves a conceptualization of what works that's found to be operationalizable under diverse circumstances. The idea here is that empirical research studying care processes does not assume a predicted 'sameness' of result beyond the sample, but is able to 'figure out' whether and if so how processes can connect up with other processes occurring in other locations and with what achievements.

Conclusion and implications

I've told a story in this chapter about different ways of orienting to the world and how what is seen/done is influenced by which orientation is taken up. I've described, with examples, how the nursing discipline has a history of orienting to nursing through an entitative lens rather than process-relational lens. This has resulted in considering elements important to nursing as individualized attributes, such as individualized leadership competencies, nurses as body counts, and nurses as independent from their work environments. While this has achieved important understandings of what nurses are about, the consideration of the nurse as an autonomous individualized entity in control of their knowledge/competence has not led to hoped-for clarity, especially in terms of understanding nursing in/and leadership.

I then explored what a process orientation makes visible, and introduced some ideas constituting process philosophy, which orients to worlding as eventful and always coming into existence, rather than pre-existing and well substantiated. Process philosophy helps to understand how this orientation can be leveraged to support empirical moves toward process inquiry. I described my own empirical program of research which orients to leadership as processual event rather than individualized competency, and which is producing actionable findings about how nursing leadership, in the form of CNL practice, manifests as relational process and how that influences what happens in/to the contexts where CNLs practice and how that makes a difference to patient care quality and safety. The implication is that a process orientation to leadership in/and nursing both can and does produce conceptual clarity about nursing's unique efficacy in terms of its leadership practices in ways that can be taught to nurses and manifested through practice.

Acknowledgments

The author is grateful to Marjory Williams, Martha Feldman, Deborah Lefkowitz, the UC Irvine Practice Theory reading group, and to Keith Robinson for their longstanding ongoing dialogues and generous sharing of insights. Thanks to Martin Lipscomb for inviting this contribution to the handbook.

References

Agency for Healthcare Research and Quality. (AHRQ, 2022). *System-Focused Event Investigation and Analysis Guide.* Rockville, MD: Agency for Healthcare Research and Quality. Retrieved from https://www.ahrq.gov/patient-safety/settings/hospital/candor/modules/guide4.html

Aiken, L. H., Clarke, S. P., Sloane, D. M., Sochalski, J., & Silber, J. H. (2002). Hospital Nurse Staffing and Patient Mortality, Nurse Burnout, and Job Dissatisfaction. *JAMA, 288*(16), 1987–1993. https://doi.org/10.1001/jama.288.16.1987

Aiken, L. H., Sloane, D. M., Cimiotti, J. P., Clarke, S. P., Flynn, L., Seago, J. A., Spetz, J., & Smith, H. L. (2010). Implications of the California Nurse Staffing Mandate for Other States. *Health Services Research, 45*(4), 904–921. https://doi.org/10.1111/j.1475-6773.2010.01114.x

American Association of Colleges of Nursing. (2007). *White Paper on the Education and Role of the Clinical Nurse Leader.* Retrieved from http://aacn.nche.edu/publi catio ns/white paper s/clini calnu rsele ader07.pdf

American Association of Colleges of Nursing. (AACN, 2021a). *AACN Releases Innovative Teaching Tool Designed to Inspire Nurses to Practice with Moral Courage and Compassion.* Retrieved December 20222 from https://www.aacnnursing.org/News-Information/Press-Releases/View/ArticleId/25101/5B-tool-kit-launch)

American Association of Colleges of Nursing. (AACN, 2021b). *The Essentials: Core Competencies For Professional Nursing Education.* Retrieved from https://www.aacnnursing.org/Portals/42/AcademicNursing/pdf/Essentials-2021.pdf

Bender, M. (2017). Clinical Nurse Leader–Integrated Care Delivery: An Approach to Organizing Nursing Knowledge Into Practice Models That Promote Interprofessional, Team-Based .... *Journal of Nursing Care Quality*, 32(3), 189–195. https://doi.org/10.1097/ncq.0000000000000247

Bender, M. (2018a). Models versus Theories as a Primary Carrier of Nursing Knowledge: A Philosophical Argument. *Nursing Philosophy*, 19(1), e12198. https://doi.org/10.1111/nup.12198

Bender, M. (2018b). Re-conceptualizing the Nursing Metaparadigm: Articulating the Philosophical Ontology of the Nursing Discipline that Orients Inquiry and Practice. *Nursing Inquiry*, 21(2), e12243–e12249. https://doi.org/10.1111/nin.12243

Bender, M., Baker, P., Harris, J. L., Hites, L., LaPointe, R. J., Murphy, E. A., Roussel, L., Spiva, L., Stanley, J. M., Thomas, P. L., & Williams, M. (2019). Advancing the Clinical Nurse Leader model Through Academic-Practice-Policy Partnership. *Nursing Outlook*, 67(4), 345–353. https://doi.org/10.1016/j.outlook.2019.02.007

Bender, M., Burtson, P., & Lefkowitz, D. (2019). The Relationality of Intervention, Context, and Implementation: A Prospective Case Study Examining the Adoption of an Evidence-Informed Nursing Care Model. *Proceedings from the 11th Annual Conference on the Science of Dissemination and Implementation*, 14, 27. https://doi.org/10.1186/s13012-019-0878-2

Bender, M., & Feldman, M. S. (2015). A Practice Theory Approach to Understanding the Interdependency of Nursing Practice and the Environment: Implications for Nurse-Led Care Delivery Models. *ANS. Advances in Nursing Science*, 38(2), 96–109. https://doi.org/10.1097/ans.0000000000000068

Bender, M., & Holmes, D. (2019). Reconciling Nursing's Art and Science Dualism: Toward a Processual Logic of Nursing. *Nursing Inquiry*, 40(1), e12293–e12299. https://doi.org/10.1111/nin.12293

Bender, M., L'Ecuyer, K., & Williams, M. (2019). A Clinical Nurse Leader Competency Framework: Concept Mapping Competencies Across Policy Documents. *Journal of Professional Nursing*, 35(6), 431–439. https://doi.org/10.1016/j.profnurs.2019.05.002

Bender, M., & Lefkowitz, D. (2020). Clinical Routines as an Under-Explored Yet Critical Component of Context in Implementation Science. *Proceedings from the 12th Annual Conference on the Science of Dissemination and Implementation*, 15, 25. https://doi.org/10.1186/s13012-020-00985-1

Bender, M., Williams, M., Cruz, M. F., & Rubinson, C. (2021). A Study Protocol to Evaluate the Implementation and Effectiveness of the Clinical Nurse Leader Care Model in Improving Quality and Safety Outcomes. *Nursing Open*, 8(6), 3688–3696.

Bender, M., Williams, M., Cruz, M., Rubinson, C., & Sharifiheris, Z. (2022). Developing Innovative Methodologies with a Participatory Approach to Examine How the Complex Relationality Between Healthcare Interventions, Their Contexts, and Implementation Strategies Produce Positive Outcomes. *Implementation Science*, 17(Suppl 1), S77

Blake, N., Leach, L. S., Robbins, W., Pike, N., & Needleman, J. (2013). Healthy Work Environments and Staff Nurse Retention. *Nursing Administration Quarterly*, 37(4), 356–370. https://doi.org/10.1097/naq.0b013e3182a2fa47

Commission on Nurse Certification. (2021). *Annual Report Fiscal Year 2021*. Retrieved from https://www.aacnnursing.org/Portals/42/CNC/CNC-Annual-Report-FY2021.pdf

Cruz, M., Bender, M., & Ombao, H. (2017). A robust interrupted time series model for analyzing complex health care intervention data. *Statistics in Medicine*, 36(29), 4660–4676. http://doi.org/10.1111/j.1467-9892.1988.tb00459.x

Cummings, G. G., Lee, S., Tate, K., Penconek, T., Micaroni, S. P. M., Paananen, T., & Chatterjee, G. E. (2020). The Essentials of Nursing Leadership: A Systematic Review of Factors and Educational Interventions Influencing Nursing Leadership. *International Journal of Nursing Studies*, 115, 103842. https://doi.org/10.1016/j.ijnurstu.2020.103842

Deleuze, G. (1992). *The Fold: Leibniz and the Baroque*. Minneapolis: U of Minnesota Press.

Donaldson, N., Bolton, L. B., Aydin, C., Brown, D., Elashoff, J. D., & Sandhu, M. (2005). Impact of California's Licensed Nurse-Patient Ratios on Unit-Level Nurse Staffing and Patient Outcomes. *Policy, Politics, & Nursing Practice*, 6(3), 198–210. https://doi.org/10.1177/1527154405280107

Emerton, N. (2019). *The Scientific Reinterpretation of Form.* Ithaca, NY: Cornell University Press.

Hacking, I. (1999). *The Social Construction of What.* Cambridge: Harvard University Press.

Hughes, R., Meadows, M. T., & Begley, R. (2022). American Organization for Nursing Leadership Nurse Leader Core Competencies. *JONA: The Journal of Nursing Administration, 52*(12), 629–631. https://doi.org/10.1097/nna.0000000000001221

Institute of Medicine. (2011). *The Future of Nursing: Leading Change, Advancing Health.* Washington DC: The National Academy Press. doi, 10, 12956.

Kaack, L., Bender, M., Finch, M., Borns, L., Grasham, K., Avolio, A., Clausen, S., Terese, N. A., Johnstone, D., & Williams, M. (2018). A Clinical Nurse Leader (CNL) Practice Development Model to Support Integration of the CNL Role into Microsystem Care Delivery. *Journal of Professional Nursing : Official Journal of the American Association of Colleges of Nursing, 34*(1), 65–71. https://doi.org/10.1016/j.profnurs.2017.06.007

Kantek, F., Yesilbas, H., & Aytur Ozen, T. (2022). Leadership and Care in Nursing Research: A Bibliometric Analysis. *Journal of Advanced Nursing, 79*(3), 1119–1128

Lake, E. T. (2002). Development of the Practice Environment Scale of the Nursing Work Index. *Research in Nursing & Health, 25*(3), 176–188. https://doi.org/10.1002/nur.10032

Lake, E. T. (2007). The Nursing Practice Environment: Measurement and Evidence. *Medical Care Research and Review, 64*(2 suppl), 104S–122S. https://doi.org/10.1177/1077558707299253

Mchugh, M. D., Brooks Carthon, M., Sloane, D. M., Wu, E., Kelly, L., et al. 2012. Impact of nurse staffing mandates on safety-net hospitals: lessons from California. *Milbank Quarterly, 90*(1): 160–186.

Mol, A., & Mesman, J. (1996). Neonatal Food and the Politics of Theory: Some Questions of Method. *Social Studies of Science, 26*(2), 419–444.

Needleman, J. 2015. Nurse Staffing: The Knowns and Unknowns. *Nursing Economics, 33*(1): 5–7.

Needleman, J., Buerhaus, P., Mattke, S., Stewart, M., & Zelevinsky, K. (2002). Nurse-Staffing Levels and the Quality of Care in Hospitals. *New England Journal Medicine, 346*(22), 1715–1722. https://doi.org/10.1056/nejmsa012247

Needleman, J., Buerhaus, P., Pankratz, V. S., Leibson, C. L., Stevens, S. R., & Harris, M. (2011). Nurse Staffing and Inpatient Hospital Mortality. *New England Journal Medicine, 364*(11), 1037–1045. https://doi.org/10.1056/nejmsa1001025

Needleman, J., Buerhaus, P. I., Stewart, M., Zelevinsky, K., & Mattke, S. (2006). Nurse Staffing In Hospitals: Is There A Business Case For Quality? *Health Affairs, 25*(1), 204–211. https://doi.org/10.1377/hlthaff.25.1.204

Northouse, P. G. (2021). *Leadership: Theory and Practice* (9th ed.). Los Angeles, CA: Sage publications.

Petrovskaya, O. (2022). *Nursing Theory, Postmodernism, Post-Structuralism, and Foucault.* London: Taylor & Francis.

Rescher, N. (1996). *Process Metaphysics: An Introduction to Process Philosophy.* New York: SUNY Press.

Spetz, J., Harless, D. W., Herrera, C. N., & Mark, B. A. 2013. Using Minimum Nurse Staffing Regulations to Measure the Relationship Between Nursing and Hospital Quality of Care. *Medical Care Research and Review, 70*(4), 380–399.

Robinson, K. (2016). Gilles Deleuze and Process Philosophy. In Ann Langley, Haridimos Tsoukas (ed), *Handbook of Process Organization Studies* (pp. 56–70), Los Angeles, CA: Sage Publications, Limited.

Tsang, E. W. K. (2013). Generalizing from Research Findings: The Merits of Case Studies. *International Journal of Management Reviews, 16*(4), 369–383. https://doi.org/10.1111/ijmr.12024

Whitehead, A. N. (1929/1978). *Process and Reality. An Essay in Cosmology [1929] Corrected Edition.* New York: The Free Press

Whitehead, A. N. (1938). *Modes of Thought.* New York: Macmillan Press.

sYin, R. K. (2013). *Case Study Research: Design and Methods.* New York: Sage Publications.

46 Technology and nursing

Olga Petrovskaya

Vignette

The setting for the vignette is an outpatient renal dialysis clinic in a mid-sized Canadian city. This clinic serves patients coming two to three times per week for haemodialysis. It also serves patients doing peritoneal dialysis at home overnight, who visit the clinic monthly, for example, Ms T. A clinic nurse knows these patients well, their families, hobbies, dreams, and troubles. She also knows not everyone will live long enough to receive a donor kidney. Let's peek in the room when the nurse starts taking Ms T's blood pressure (BP) and taking time to do this (*very* simple, to some) procedure. "Sit for a few minutes," she tells Ms T whose arm is stretched on a small table and already wrapped in a tonometer cuff. The nurse makes sure Ms T has caught her breath, all BP equipment is heart-level, and the cuff is inflating symmetrically. The first measurement is taken. "Let's carry on with our conversation, and I'll measure the second time in a few minutes." The nurse learns from Ms T that she has been having rough nights lately—the dialysis machine beeps frequently, and her efforts to troubleshoot do not work. The nurse asks a few focused questions to establish a possible reason for the machine's misbehaving and they arrive at a plan that Ms T thinks might work. While talking to Ms T, the nurse inflates the cuff a second time and writes down the numbers in Ms T's paper record. "Please stand now; let's take standing BP." Ms T rises from her chair, and the measurement is repeated. A nurse reads the numbers to Ms T and explains that they look good, as expected; Ms T nods in confirmation that she understands. The remainder of the visit is devoted to a meticulous sterile procedure, flushing of the dialysis tube sewn inside Ms T's abdomen. "This is my lifeline," Ms T says in a tender voice looking at the tube, while the nurse inspects both the tube and the entry portal on the abdomen.

What is technology? Is the "technical" worthy of our attention?

Nursing evolved alongside society and technology. What is technology, and is it worthy of nurses' attention? A useful starting place is to think about technology as an artefact extending the human body.[1] Conceiving of technology as *any* extension of the human body, no matter how simple or mundane an implement is, reflects a political choice highlighted by feminist scholars of technology (Sandelowski, 1997a). These scholars observe that cars, heavy machinery, medical monitors, and computers are readily acknowledged as kinds of technology. These machines, associated in the popular imagination and societal discourses with masculinity, especially at the time of their invention, were perceived as significant and "spectacular." In contrast, baby bottles, catheters, or mechanical hospital

DOI: 10.4324/9781003427407-53

beds, which are often perceived as "low tech, high touch" objects, tend to disappear from societal view and dominant nursing history, partly due to their use by the female-dominated nursing profession (Sandelowski, 1997a). To avoid the misleading dichotomies of masculine versus feminine technology (and "high tech, low touch" versus "low tech, high touch" fields of practice), in this chapter, any implement, instrument, tool, or machine used in nursing practice is a technological object.

Take any entry point into the historical past of the caring vocations—everywhere we find *objects* used for healing purposes. In the monastic Benedictine Catholic religious order established in Italy circa 529, healing practices included purifying baths ("Benedictines," 2023), dried herbs and potions, fruit extracts to ease gastric aches, beds in an infirmary, and special blades for bloodletting (Carter, 2021).

Nursing work, too, has always involved use of the technology of the time. However, according to Nelson and Gordon (2004; Nelson, 2003), some influential nursing scholarship turned its attention away from this aspect of nursing. Nelson (2003) rejects depictions of the history of nursing as "evolving from religious ignorance to [the] sophisticated expertise" (p. 28) of a modern, professional nurse. In the late 19th and well into the 20th centuries, the figure of Florence Nightingale epitomized this evolutionary nursing history from ignorance to light (Nelson, 2003). In the second half of the 20th century, another evolutionary narrative was born. In the 1970s, American academic nursing elites established the field of so-called unique disciplinary nursing knowledge that was envisaged to govern the less sophisticated "technical nursing practice" (Nelson & Gordon, 2004; Petrovskaya, 2022a). These developments left nursing with little attention to mundane nursing work, work that has always involved the use of objects in skilful and inventive ways (Nelson, 2003; Nelson & Gordon, 2004).

This chapter aims to do justice to the materiality of nursing practice. It is my hope that by the end of the chapter, we will have considered perspectives on technology that reveal more complex and interesting nursing–technology relationships than those residing at the extremes of love and hate towards technology. Upholding the non-essentialist view of both technology and nursing, I argue that technology is worth of our attention and can be usefully understood in relational terms (in the sense of *relationality* articulated in material semiotics as opposed to how this term has been used in most nursing sources). The reader of this chapter is invited to put on hold a view positing an ontological rift between the "human body" (or "society") and "technology" and a corresponding rift between "warm touch" and "cold technology."

Nursing's love-hate relationship with technology

Depictions of technology in nursing literature from the 1960s to the mid-1990s fall into two prevalent but contrasting positions, technological optimism and technological romanticism, as dubbed by Sandelowski (1997b; she borrowed these expressions from Mitcham, 1994). Optimists welcomed technology as beneficial and fully compatible with humanistic nursing care. New tools and machines save time, increase efficiency and diagnostic accuracy, enhance traditional practice and make it more scientific, optimists wrote. Romantics rejected technology as antithetical to nursing care and as a bearer of oppressive masculinist tendencies. Let us consider nurses' central objections to an influx of technology.

Sandelowski (1997b) cites a key article by Peplau from the early 1960s, in which Peplau reaffirmed her vision of nursing as an interpersonal counsel between a nurse and a patient whose humanness should be safeguarded and enhanced by nurses. Peplau called on nurses to assess the fit between nursing's central mission and an increasing automation of health care that leads to distancing and depersonalization. If anything positive can be gained from mechanization in nursing—for example, time efficiency—it should be directed by nurses towards minimizing technology's harmful effects by displaying tender concern for the patient (Peplau, as cited in Sandelowski, 1997b). Other influential nurse scholars, Benner and Watson, writing in the 1980s, emphasized the traditional and nontechnological essence of nursing manifesting as humanism, caring presence, human touch, and the holistic conception of a person. Implicitly or explicitly, this "romantic" focus (Sandelowski, 1997b) presented the anti-technology stance.

An oft cited 1980s publication by Gadow contrasted two "paradigms of patient care," touch and technology, and argued nurses should guard human touch (as cited in Forss & Ceci, 2017). While some commentators read Gadow as attributing dehumanization to technology, Forss and Ceci (2017) defend Gadow's position as non-deterministic: "it is rather that the 'technologization of care' and 'patient autonomy and dignity' are two increasingly distinct streams that articulate a pre-existing ethical problem in all health care" (p. 1). At the same time, Gadow's argument was grounded in the "Western modern dualist distinction between (living) subjects and (supposedly inert) objects" (Forss & Ceci, 2017, p. 1), an ontological assumption similarly displayed in nursing scholarship reviewed by Sandelowski in the late 1990s.

For other nurse authors, the traditional essence of nursing was feminine, a unique power related to nature and able to protect the patient's humanity from the encroachment of the technological age (Sandelowski, 1997b). Anxious undertones permeated nurses' questions about whether they would be replaced by machines and whether patients would ever experience human touch. There were also calls by nurse authors to remember the person on the other end of the device (Sandelowski, 1997b). In the 1990s, these questions became more urgent as relentless advances in medical technology and health care's imperative of standardization and objective indicators were felt to "depriv[e] patients of their individuality, subjectivity, and dignity as human beings" (Barnard & Sandelowski, 2001, p. 367).

During the first two decades of the 21st century, as heath organizations were adopting electronic charting, the electronic health record (EHR) garnered critical attention in nursing literature. Gluing nurses' attention to an EHR on a screen, a computer intrudes on the space between the nurse and the patient. This intrusion decreases eye contact, thus distancing—literally and metaphorically—the person of the nurse from the person of the patient and erodes the humanity of health care (Cuchetti & Grace, 2020; de Ruiter et al., 2016; Rentmeester, 2018). Surfacing non-apparent functions of the EHR, de Ruiter et al. (2016) argued that nurses are now spending more time meeting institutional priorities (e.g., collecting information for billing, quality assurance, and accreditation) than engaging in direct patient care at the bedside. A novel and insidious aspect of health care technology largely absent in earlier decades is surveillance of nurses enabled by the EHR. It serves the hospital's business interests by controlling nurses' productivity and their timely completion of procedures (de Ruiter et al., 2016). Moreover, the topic of patient surveillance became prominent in ethical analyses of artificial intelligence (AI) employed, for instance, in smart homes and remote monitoring (Stokes & Palmer, 2020).

While acknowledging the benefits of the EHR and AI, these and other nurse authors criticize digital technologies as incompatible with authentic human caring and presence. These technologies, it is claimed, should be used as the means towards the ethical ends of individual patient care rather than as ends in themselves, be it maintenance of hardware and software or efficiency and productivity of nurses' work as extra-local priorities. Despite the threats of the digital age, nurse scholars remain hopeful that nurses' intentional actions such as presence and touch can uphold the profession's humanistic moral imperative and mitigate technology's negative effects (Cuchetti & Grace, 2020; Stokes & Palmer, 2020). Thus, 25 years after Sandelowski's (1997b) designation of "technological romanticism," this perspective is still traceable in *philosophical* analyses of technology in nursing.

Summarizing her review of the literature, Sandelowski (1997b) stated, "While optimists link technology to the science of nursing, romantics see technology as detracting from the art of nursing" (p. 172). Both positions, she argued, are limited because they essentialize technology and nursing by treating them as unified and stable entities. Instead, "the (ir)reconcilability of nursing and technology may be a function of how devices are used by people in different contexts, or of the (ir)reconcilability of *views* of technology in nursing," Sandelowski (1997b, p. 169; italics added) asserted.

My reading of Sandelowski is that she denies neither the benefits offered by technology, nor the legitimacy of concerns expressed by nurses. After all, who would want to be in an uncaring situation, surrounded by beeping machines, and abandoned by personnel whose attention is fully occupied by maintaining the equipment? Rather, in her multiple publications on the topic, Sandelowski sought to restore complexity to accounts of nursing work that always involves the use of technological objects whose meanings and effects are not predetermined. One way she restores complexity is by viewing technology as both "fact and symbol," or as objects with physical properties *and* texts rich with meanings. Sandelowski (1999a) writes, "For us nurses, to think about and through technology is to think about and through the 'devices' that have shaped and constituted our collective 'desire' for knowledge, autonomy, visibility and power" (p. 145). Thus, approaching technology as a text/symbol (Sandelowski, 1999b, 2000) is one of the ways out of the impasse between nursing technological optimism and technological romanticism.

Technology as a cultural symbol: professionalization and gender relations in nursing

The history of 20th-century Western nursing, inseparable from the emergence of the modern hospital and scientific medicine, clearly illustrates the nursing–technology nexus. In her book *Devices and Desires*, Sandelowski (2000) argues that the relationship between nursing and technology is an important part of the story of the professionalization of nursing in the United States (US) and one marked by issues of gender and class.

As nurses became skilled users of oxygen equipment, thermometers, stethoscopes, and X-ray machines from the 1890s to the 1940s, they were instrumental to the growth of hospitals in the US (Sandelowski, 2000). The introduction of heart monitors and foetal monitors in the 1960s further signalled a departure from the largely craft technology that had prevailed in American nursing since the late 19th century (Sandelowski, 1997c). A highly gendered female profession, nursing struggled to obtain status and visibility. However, nurses themselves were like technology, serving as "doctor's eyes and hands" and utilized for their instrumental value (Sandelowski, 2000). Thus, technology offered one tangible way for nursing to gain recognition. Furthermore, new technology, such as thermometers and, later on, monitors, required advanced knowledge and promised the elevated status usually afforded to scientific activity rather than one sustained by women's caring (Sandelowski, 2000). By enthusiastically embracing new technology, the nursing profession blurred the boundary with medicine and claimed an expanded scope of practice—worthy achievements in the eyes of many.

Paradoxically—and this is the crux of Sandelowski's (2000) argument—this expansion did not lead to the anticipated improvement in nursing's societal standing. Technical skills like venepuncture post-World War II were considered complex as long as physicians performed them. Once this procedure was abandoned by physicians and embraced by nurses, venepuncture's discursive status changed; it was now considered easy (Sandelowski, 1999c). Electronic foetal monitoring presents another example. The manual assessment of contractions was replaced by, or required the validation of, a "high-tech" monitor, which resulted in the loss of a traditional "high-touch" skill. Monitoring was performed by nurses in an unglamourous place, by the bedside; in contrast, the high-status work of interpreting the data and prescribing treatment remained physicians' domain (Fairman, 2002; Sandelowski, 2000). "Technology helped sustain nurses' invisibility, because most of the work nurses took on in management of the technology was [discursively positioned as] of low status, and unstated in the medical record or other patient care documents" (Fairman, 2002, p. 896). Thus, Sandelowski (2000) reveals the deeply ambiguous nature of the relationship between nursing and technology. The enthusiastic embrace of technology and expanded knowledge and scopes of practice led to deskilling nurses in areas of traditional expertise and further devaluing "true nursing," where "true" refers to the unique domain of nursing practice as caregivers by the patient's bedside (Sandelowski, 1997a, 2000). Gendered professional hierarchies remained largely untouched despite nurses' strengthened link with science and technology.

And yet, to observe that professional hierarchies endure is not to deny that technology shapes identities, roles, and relations of human actors. The development of critical care units in the late 1950s and early 1960s shifted, and to some degree levelled, the relationship between nurses and physicians by expanding nurses' knowledge and skills (Fairman, 1992; Melosh, 1982, both as cited in Sandelowski, 1997b). Perhaps perceived more on the hospital floor rather than reflected in the policy documents or recognized by the public, physicians' dependency on nurses had increased with the introduction of machine technology; nurses had to tame these machines for observation and early management of changing patient conditions. Reviewing nursing literature, Sandelowski (1997b) observes that nurses felt that physicians were amazed at their technological expertise.

Socio-materiality: beyond the essentialist view

Theorizing technology in nursing as a cultural symbol offers one way out of the impasse between technological optimism and technological romanticism in nursing philosophical literature. Another way is offered by the theoretical perspectives collectively known as material semiotics, new materialism, or socio-materiality. Actor network theory (ANT) and after-ANT are prominent examples (Latour, 1996, 2005; Mol, 2002, 2010; Pols & Moser, 2009). Surveying these perspectives is beyond the scope of this chapter. A few insightful analyses of health care technologies citing these and related perspectives (Forss & Ceci, 2017; Kiran, 2017; Pols, 2017; Stankovic, 2017) were published in a special issue of the *Nursing Philosophy* journal arising from the 19th International Philosophy of Nursing Society (IPONS) conference. Below, I sketch key understandings of technology as per socio-material perspectives.

Mutual constitution of humans and technologies

In much of nursing philosophical scholarship, technology is conceived of as essentialist (e.g., ontologically unchanging), deterministic (e.g., beneficial because efficient and cost-effective or, in contrast, harmful because dehumanizing and cold), instrumental (e.g., neutral, passive, and as technical means to human ends), and "technical" (e.g., manual versus intellectual or psychological). Socio-material perspectives juxtapose this conception with a non-essentialist, non-deterministic, non-instrumental, and non-technical view of technology.

Sandelowski's (1997a) analysis of gender–technology relationships summarized above is underpinned by such a view:

> Both gender and technology are increasingly conceived as constitutive of each other and reproduced in every social interaction. That is, there is no one Femininity, Masculinity or Technology, but rather there are historically and culturally specific femininities, masculinities, and technologies. Depending on the context, gender is variously conceived as inextricable from, antecedent to, a condition for, and/or a consequence of technological change. Technology is similarly variously conceived as inextricable from, antecedent to, a condition for, and/or a consequence of "doing gender."
>
> (p. 222)

According to this view, technologies and humans operate within a network of heterogeneous elements in which a supposedly passive object acted upon by a supposedly active human subject can switch places, identities, and roles. Technology becomes an agent, an actor among other actors, and produces effects. "Technologies … alter the conditions in which we know and conduct ourselves, [and] the modernist subject–object distinction does not stand" (Forss & Ceci, 2017, p. 2). Networks are often described as relations, mediations, or assemblages.

Haraway (1991, cited in Barnard & Sandelowski, 2001) uses the notion of cyborgs to challenge culture/nature, subject/object, and human/non-human dualisms:

> Pacemakers and artificial joints implanted in living human beings, genetic engineering, and artificial intelligence systems regularly confront us with the reality of and potentiality for living artifacts and vital machines. These cyborgs blur the line between animate and inanimate, and human and machine.
>
> (p. 368)

The human and the technological mutually constitute each other.

The non-neutrality of technology

Discussion in this chapter leads the reader away from the *instrumental* view of technology, that is, technology as neutral and as simply a means to an end (Franssen et al., 2018). The instrumental view has been contested by various philosophical schools on several grounds. For example, investors and engineers designing technology often openly aim to create *better* technology that can generate profit and *improve* the sphere of technology application (Franssen et al., 2018). In other words, technology is viewed by these groups as valuable in itself. This chapter is informed by other philosophical and theoretical perspectives—most notably, cultural and feminist studies of technology (e.g., technology as fact and symbol in Sandelowski's work) and material semiotics and ANT (e.g., the technology-in-practice view exemplified by Pols work and opposing both technological determinism and social essentialism). These perspectives, too, posit the non-neutrality of technology. Let's examine what different authors mean by that. My goal is not to resolve contradictions or treat the topic exhaustively (a separate chapter is required for this) but to point out generative differences in the literature.

De Ruiter et al. (2016) criticized the omnipotence of the EHR that "coerces" (my word) nurses to spend time and effort on collecting and documenting data required for institutional and extra-local purposes but not benefiting a particular patient in bed. In other words, nurses are pulled away from direct patient care while unwittingly serving unclear and morally questionable agendas facilitated by the EHR such as an unauthorized data sharing with commercial firms and governments (cf. Cuchetti & Grace, 2020). De Ruiter et al. (2016), following Winner (1980), asserted that "technology is not a neutral tool that becomes political as a result of the intention of the user, but is political in its very design" (p. 50). This can perhaps mean that technology might be intentionally designed with evil intent, might result in unintended harm (e.g., thalidomide), or, more broadly, is political because it differentially affects lives and represents vested interests. Considering the case of overpass bridges in New York State that barred Black people from accessing scenic beaches (Winner, 1980), in its design, technology certainly reflects political agendas and biases of the time.

Another aspect of a thesis of non-neutrality challenges a purely functional conception of technology. Commonly, technology is perceived as embodying instrumental rationality, that is, existing to help fulfil human needs. This view is criticized in nursing literature by authors drawing on the post-phenomenology of Don Ihde (Barnard & Sandelowski, 2001; de Ruiter et al., 2016; Kiran, 2017; Sandelowski, 1997b). They argue that the functional view masks a profound existential aspect of technology. In a triad, human-tool-the-world, technology "transforms how the world appears to us, and with it, how we behave in it" (Kiran, 2017, p. 7). Traditional boundaries of the body change too, especially in virtual space; the body is bifurcated into the actual and virtual existence (de Ruiter et al., 2016).

Most nurse authors discuss non-neutrality in terms of technology's moral ambivalence, ambiguity, or dual effect, often using these interchangeably. A tool, instrument, or device is neither *tout court* good or bad; its ethical status is ambiguous and depends on the user. Let's look at one example. An electronic patient portal, when used by a patient with proper credentials and an authorized access, is beneficial as it conveniently provides timely information such as latest blood test results. In turn, when accessed by a dishonest stranger who happens to have log-in credentials, the portal assists in the crime of stealing personal information (cf. Antonio et al., 2020). Or a patient can find the portal helpful for viewing test results, but the same portal turns into a nuisance when the medical jargon in it is incomprehensible (Santos et al., 2021). For nurses, the online portal serves well for answering patients' non-urgent questions sent via the portal, yet the phone is the device of choice for time-sensitive communication. Depending on the use and the user, technology can be both good and bad. Thus, in nursing literature, ambivalence refers to a "mixture of … advantage and disadvantage" (Barnard, 2016, p. 10) and, similarly, dual effects encompass challenges and opportunities (Kiran, 2017).

Subtly, the socio-material perspectives go beyond the statement that technology depends on how humans use it. We have encountered the latter sentiment in Sandelowski, and I argued above that her critique is a positive shift in nurses' essentializing view of the nursing–technology relationships. We can now make another step and consider that as "technologically mediated subjects, as subjects made active and coherent through heterogeneous networks of material and human relations, we lose the comfort of the humanist view ... *that it is completely up to humans to decide the use of technologies*" (Forss & Ceci, 2017, p. 2; italics added). On my reading, this links to Latour's (2002) idea about technological objects as *mediators*, which is different from the notion of intermediaries (p. 250). A mediator effects an ontological detour that opens into a different mode of existence. Furthermore, a technological object *enfolds* time, space, and actants (or actors; p. 248). The notions of fold and detour enable Latour (2002) to claim that "technologies belong to the human world in a modality other than that of instrumentality, efficiency or materiality" (p. 248). For him, this mediating (i.e., producing new realities) nature of technology undermines the conception of technology as a simple, neutral thing seen as different from "human" moral choices. In other words, Latour discards the idea that technology and humans are fundamentally different: that the technology is an empty carrier that we control, while the humans own morality and make choices.

Technology in practice

Informed by the work of Latour and after-ANT theorists, sociological literature espousing the socio-material view of technology has shifted away from both technological determinism *and social essentialism* while advocating the so-called technology-in-practice approach (Petrovskaya, 2022b). The key idea here is the analytical and practical shift away from user intentions or actions towards the relations among human and non-human elements in the network. Pols (2017) states that technologies are plural and should be studied "empirically, by analyzing the relations between people and their technologies. These relations are always unpredictable, as it is not given beforehand what values the participants pursue" (p. 1).

In health care practices, the dichotomy "warm touch/cold technology"—circulated in some academic discourses—does not hold (Kiran, 2017; Pols, 2017). Instead of representing ostensibly "warm humanity," nurses can give a cold shoulder to others. Instead of being "cold," technologies can be caring. The studies with therapeutic robots have shown that the robots solicit spontaneous affect; patients feel warmth and sympathy towards the robots (Kiran, 2017; Pols & Moser, 2009). Surprisingly, patients and therapeutic robots have been observed changing the roles—patients enjoyed taking care of their technologies. The robot "alter[ed] the pregiven classifications of who [was] a caregiver and who [was] a care receiver" (Kiran, 2017, p. 5).

The socio-material perspectives do not cultivate an uncritical, sanguine outlook. There certainly is a sense that "the more we embrace technological intervention, choices in practice become less likely" (Barnard, 2016, p 10). Ultrasonography has displaced manual Leopold manoeuvres for determining foetal position in uterus. The implementation of the EHR, accompanied by the administrators' admonitions to stop using paper, makes bedside nurses hide their informal handwritten notes, or "scraps." However, Allen (2015) views nurses' scraps as crucial for the ongoing patient care delivery and for supporting nurses' ability to construct practical knowledge. Often, technological innovation does not become one of the methods, but rather the only way to proceed. Technologies bring about new realities and new subjectivities.

Despite the rhetoric of the time-saving potential, technology in health care creates new demands on nurses' time (Sandelowski, 1997b). Often, nurses must check and triangulate information generated by instruments and machines. Nurses must maintain the equipment and provide psychological and physical comfort for a patient who might be fearful of the equipment (Sandelowski, 1997b). Alarms are a particularly "compelling and sometimes distracting influence upon a nurse's time, physical commitment, and intellectual attention" (Barnard, 2000, cited in Barnard, 2016, p. 13). Socio-material perspectives reveal the complexity of this invisible nurses' work, including the work of material articulation, or the upkeep, gathering, and alignment in time and space of required non-human (and human) actors within the trajectory of patient care (Allen, 2015).

Nurses' practical knowledge

Focusing on the materiality of nursing practice—bodies and technology—adds weight and concreteness to what Carper (1978) named a personal way of knowing and others elaborated on as embodied knowing, knowing how, or practical knowledge. Comparing propositional knowledge, *I know that*, and practical knowledge, *I know how*, Risjord (Martin Lipscomb, 2020) emphasizes the constitutive role of the latter in nursing practice. Risjord explains that practical knowledge, as understood within the ecological model, involves manipulation of the physical environment and objects (Martin Lipscomb, 2020). Not accidentally, the word *ecological* conveys emerging relationships among the elements within a system.

Nursing scholarship has not always paid attention to this important epistemology. How so? Sandelowski (1997a) observes that "Western thought [led to] the subordination of the artistic and manual to the intellectual and verbal, and the resulting subordination of technology to science" (p. 222). Being antagonistic or indifferent to technology in (their accounts of) nursing practice as the above discussion in this chapter demonstrates, nurse authors might have preferred vague notions of "personal knowing" *à la* Carper when referring to non-linguistic, tacit forms of knowing. Furthermore, both bodies and things lost gravity in much of the discourse of American nursing theory (Nelson & Gordon, 2004; Sandelowski, 1997a). This discourse tends to value the cognitive, emotional, and/or spiritual; "critical thinking"; theory-guided practice; and interpersonal relations— all typically theorized as immaterial—over the manual, bodily, mundane, and technical.

Sandelowski (1997a) believes that a robust theorizing of technology that includes embodied ways of knowing (e.g., instrumentation extending the senses and physical capacities) will draw the attention of nurse scholars to the body. The twin belief she expresses is that a robust theorizing of technology will shed light on nursing practical, manual, and other non-verbal knowledges as *not* "simply the robotic completion of procedures following physicians' orders" (p. 221). Consider the first vignette where a nurse measures BP and examines the dialysis tube. The knowledge needed to accurately measure and record physiological indicators by "cajoling" the tool and the patient to "participate" (my words), the tinkering with the objects and the bodies that nursing practice requires (Mol, 2009; Pols & Willems, 2011), is equally important to the knowledge needed to order these procedures (i.e., typically done by physicians and increasingly by advanced practice nurses such as nurse practitioners). Nurses' activities, such as measuring BP, flushing the tube, or navigating inside the EHR to progress the ongoing trajectory of patient care (Allen, 2015), "require practice theories of intervention, approach, deliberation and enactment; they require particularized and 'practically practical' knowledge to direct concrete action, as opposed to general and 'speculative' knowledge of things to be done" (Sandelowski, 1997a, p. 221). For this reason, it is hard to separate "cognitive" from "manual," and "critical thinking" from "technical procedures," in nursing practice vignettes.

Concluding thoughts

The nursing–technology relationship—coloured by the issues of gender and class—is an important part of the story of professionalization of nursing (Sandelowski, 2000). The ambiguous nature of this relationship observed in American nursing around the mid-20th century, still unfolds today particularly in the nurse practitioner role (Sandelowski, 2000). We are witnesses to the processes captured in Sandelowski's old question, whether nursing's search for legitimacy through science and technology and the concomitant move away from the bedside into non-direct care roles will bring about improvements in the profession's status and patient care.

This chapter highlights the difficulty of tearing apart and placing in opposition "technical care and the human side of practice" if technical is *not* considered ontologically and a priori different than human and if humans (or cyborgs) could ever be uncoupled from tools and artefacts.

Critiquing discussions of human caring in nursing literature that contrast it to the technology-enabled or "peripheral work" that takes away from "true caring," this chapter advocates for theories of technology and nursing attentive to the socio-materiality of practices such as ANT and after-ANT perspectives. One nursing-specific example is translational mobilization theory developed by Allen (2015). After all, if the interpersonal component of nursing is valorized, but the skilful manipulation of technological objects (e.g., operating technology or working around it) is taken to be a distraction from "real nursing," how can we ever hope that others (administrators, the public, policymakers) recognize the vital invisible work nurses undertake to keep health care going?

In this chapter, it was not possible to discuss all aspects of health care technology. Developments described as "virtual nursing and vanishing bodies" (Sandelowski, 2002) such as posthumanist and transhumanist enhancements or projects converting the body into a code, is the growing area in scholarly literature and will benefit from a separate analysis.

Nursing philosophical scholarship has been informed by *normative* ethical theories with an aim to instil a critical outlook towards, and the mindful use of, technology. Similarly, nursing literature has helped reduce nurses' naivete about the politics and unarticulated purposes of digital tools. Now we can draw methodological and research implications from this chapter. The best theorizing of nursing–technology relationship avoids essentializing nursing and technology and studies technology in context. Nurse philosophers and researchers are encouraged to observe, describe, and analyse the effects of technology in the future (and of future technologies): what subjectivities are enabled; what assumptions ("scripts"; Akrich, 1992) are embedded in technologies and how they work in intended ways or lead to workarounds; how professional boundaries and "patienthood" are shifting; what conditions, arrangements, and accommodations help enact "ethics with" (Kiran, 2017) technology for patients and nurses. Socio-material perspectives discussed in the chapter call for *empirical* ethics (Pols, 2017), for example, case studies of how technologies and values are understood and enacted in everyday life and health care.

The idea of cyborgs, or the blurring of boundaries between humans and non-humans, will not be accepted by all. Nurses might continue to draw on the humanistic philosophical canon, echoing Whelton's (2016) argument about the essence of humanity resting in "rational capacities of providing meaningful speech and freely chosen actions" that underscores the difference between humans and machines (p. 28). In this view, humans interact with technology, but this does not change the essence of humanity (Whelton, 2016). Others, however, will ask, "What is 'the person' ... when we increasingly, through prostheses and implants, become 'cyborgs,' a fusion between human and machine? What is embodiment in a digitalized health care world and what does this mean for health?" (Forss & Ceci, 2017, p. 2). While it is increasingly challenging to sustain the image preferred by Whelton (2016) of a "common bond between all humans" (p. 28) that excludes other species and assemblages, perhaps we can agree that nursing is formed within, and forms, networks consisting of a range of actors, including humans, technology, and information.

Acknowledgements

I wholeheartedly thank Dr. Madeline Walker for her flexible and sensible editorial assistance, Dr. Martin Lipscomb for his patience and the opportunity to contribute to this important volume, Drs. Deborah Lefkowitz and Mike Rowe for our stimulating ANT reading group.

Note

1 Admittedly, this definition is problematic for Latour (2002), whose work I cite favourably later on. However, I will let this definition stand for now.

References

Akrich, M. (1992). The de-scription of technical objects. In W. Bijker & J. Law (Eds.), *Shaping technology-building society: Studies in sociotechnical change* (pp. 205–244). Cambridge: MIT Press.

Allen, D. (2015). *The invisible work of nurses: Hospitals, organisation and healthcare.* Routledge.

Antonio, M. G., Petrovskaya, O., & Lau, F. (2020). The state of evidence in patient portals: Umbrella review. *JMIR Journal of Medical Internet Research, 22*(11), e23851. https://doi.org/ 10.2196/23851.

Barnard, A. (2016). Radical nursing and the emergence of technique as healthcare technology. *Nursing Philosophy, 17*(1), 8–18. https://doi.org/10.1111/nup.12103

Barnard, A., & Sandelowski, M. (2001). Technology and humane nursing care: (Ir)reconcilable or invented difference? *Journal of Advanced Nursing, 34*(3), 367–375. https://doi.org/10.1046/j.1365-2648.2001.01768.x

Benedictines. (2023, January 4). In *Wikipedia.* https://en.wikipedia.org/wiki/Benedictines

Carper, B. (1978). Fundamental patterns of knowing in nursing. *Advances in Nursing Science, 1*(1), 13–23.

Carter, M. (2021, February 16). *How medieval monasteries laid the foundations of modern medicine.* The Tablet. https://www.thetablet.co.uk/blogs/1/1714/how-medieval-monasteries-laid-the-foundations-of-modern-medicine

Cuchetti, C., & Grace, P. J. (2020). Authentic intention: Tempering the dehumanizing aspects of technology on behalf of good nursing care. *Nursing Philosophy, 21*(1), e12255–n/a. https://doi.org/10.1111/nup.12255

de Ruiter, H.-P., Liaschenko, J., & Angus, J. (2016). Problems with the electronic health record. *Nursing Philosophy, 17*(1), 49–58. https://doi.org/10.1111/nup.12112

Fairman, J. (2002). Devices and desires: Gender, technology, and American nursing [Review of devices and desires: Gender, technology, and American nursing]. *American Historical Review, 107*(3), 896–897. https://doi.org/10.1086/532555

Forss, A., & Ceci, C. (2017). Technology, health care and person centeredness: Beyond Utopia and Dystopia. Thinking the future. *Nursing Philosophy, 18*(1), e12162–n/a. https://doi.org/10.1111/nup.12162

Franssen, M., Lokhorst, G.-J., & van de Poel, I. (2018). *Philosophy of technology, 2.3 The centrality of design in technology.* Stanford Encyclopedia of Philosophy. https://plato.stanford.edu/entries/technology/

Kiran, A. H. (2017). Mediating patienthood—from an ethics of to an ethics with technology. *Nursing Philosophy, 18*(1), e12153–n/a. https://doi.org/10.1111/nup.12153

Latour, B. (1996). *Aramis, or the love of technology.* (Translated by Catherine Porter). Harvard University Press.

Latour, B. (2002). Morality and technology: The end of the means. *Theory, Culture & Society, 19*(5/6), 247–260.

Latour, B. (2005). *Reassembling the social: An introduction to actor-network-theory.* Oxford University Press.

Martin Lipscomb. (5 May, 2020). *Nursing conversations – Mark Risjord.* [Video]. YouTube. https://www.youtube.com/watch?v=HSL1Dn0e01I

Mol, A. (2002). *The body multiple: Ontology in medical practice.* Duke University Press.

Mol, A. (2009). Living with diabetes: Care beyond choice and control. *The Lancet, 373*(9677), 1756–1757. https://doi.org/10.1016/S0140-6736(09)60971-5

Mol, A. (2010). Actor-network theory: Sensitive terms and enduring tensions. *Kolner Zeitschrift fur Soziologie und Sozialpsychologie, 50*(1), 253–269.

Nelson, S. (2003). *Say little, do much: Nursing, nuns, and hospitals in the nineteenth century.* University of Pennsylvania Press.

Nelson, S., & Gordon, S. (2004). The rhetoric of rupture: Nursing as a practice with a history? *Nursing Outlook, 52*(5), 255–261. https://doi.org/10.1016/j.outlook.2004.08.001

Petrovskaya, O. (2022a). *Nursing theory, postmodernism, post-structuralism, and Foucault.* Routledge.

Petrovskaya, O. (2022b). Educational technology: Insights from actor-network theory. Response to B. Garrett. In M. Lipscomb (Ed.), *Complexities and values in nursing education.* Routledge.

Pols, J. (2017). Good relations with technology: Empirical ethics and aesthetics in care. *Nursing Philosophy, 18*(1), e12154–n/a. https://doi.org/10.1111/nup.12154

Pols, J., & Moser, I. (2009). Cold technologies versus warm care? On affective and social relations with and through care technologies. *ALTER –European Journal of Disability Research, 3*(2), 159–178. https://doi.org/10.1016/j.alter.2009.01.003

Pols, J., & Willems, D. (2011). Innovation and evaluation: Taming and unleashing telecare technology. *Sociology of Health & Illness, 33*(3), 484–498. https://doi.org/10.1111/j.1467-9566.2010.01293.x

Rentmeester, C. (2018). Heeding humanity in an age of electronic health records: Heidegger, Levinas, and Healthcare. *Nursing Philosophy, 19*(3), e12214–n/a. https://doi.org/10.1111/nup.12214

Sandelowski, M. (1997a). Exploring the gender-technology relation in nursing. *Nursing Inquiry, 4*(4), 219–228. https://doi.org/10.1111/j.1440-1800.1997.tb00107.x

Sandelowski, M. (1997b). (Ir)reconcilable differences? The debate concerning nursing and technology. *Image: The Journal of Nursing Scholarship, 29*(2), 169–174. https://doi.org/10.1111/j.1547-5069.1997.tb01552.x

Sandelowski, M. (1997c). "Making the best of things": Technology in American nursing, 1870–1940. *Nursing History Review, 5*, 3–22.

Sandelowski, M. (1999a). Nursing, technology and the millennium. *Nursing Inquiry, 6*(3), 145–145. https://doi.org/10.1046/j.1440-1800.1999.00026.x

Sandelowski, M. (1999b). Troubling distinctions: A semiotics of the nursing/technology relationship. *Nursing Inquiry, 6*(3), 198–207. https://doi.org/10.1046/j.1440-1800.1999.00030.x

Sandelowski, M. (1999c). Venous envy: The post-World War II debate over IV nursing. *Advances in Nursing Science, 22*(1), 52–62.

Sandelowski, M. (2002). Visible humans, vanishing bodies, and virtual nursing: Complications of life, presence, place, and identity. *Advances in Nursing Science, 24*(3), 58–70.

Santos, A. D., Caine, V., Robson, P. J., Watson, L., Easaw, J. C., & Petrovskaya, O. (2021). Oncology patients' experiences with novel electronic patient portals to support care and treatment: Qualitative study with early users and non-users of portals in Alberta, Canada. *JMIR Cancer, 7*(4), e32609. https://doi.org/10.2196/32609.

Stankovic, B. (2017). Situated technology in reproductive health care: Do we need a new theory of the subject to promote person-centred care? *Nursing Philosophy, 18*(1), e12159–n/a. https://doi.org/10.1111/nup.12159

Stokes, F., & Palmer, A. (2020). Artificial intelligence and robotics in nursing: Ethics of caring as a guide to dividing tasks between AI and humans. *Nursing Philosophy, 21*(4), e12306–n/a. https://doi.org/10.1111/nup.12306

Whelton, B. J. B. (2016). Being human in a global age of technology. *Nursing Philosophy, 17*(1), 28–35. https://doi.org/10.1111/nup.12109

Winner, L. (1980). Do artifacts have politics? *Daedalus, 109*(1), 121–136.

47 Teaching and learning clinical reasoning

Maximizing human intelligence, expert clinical reasoning, scientific knowledge and decision-making supports

Patricia Benner

The goal of this chapter is to make visible and critique the taken-for-granted Cartesian and Kantian representational views of the mind that hamper understanding and teaching of clinical reasoning in nursing. Research on acquiring clinical reasoning skills in nursing and the research evidence for lack of practice-readiness for most newly graduates to engage in clinical reasoning upon graduation guide this discussion on the problems associated with teaching clinical reasoning in nursing (Benner, 2001; Benner, Tanner, & Chesla, 2009; Benner, Hooper-Kyriakidis, 2011; Chan & Burns, 2021; Brown & Hart, 2022). An outdated representational, taken-for-granted view of the mind guides pedagogies for teaching clinical reasoning, along with a commonly held view by nursing educators that clinical reasoning is a form of scientific reasoning as demonstrated by the Nursing Process which is a linear, scientific problem-solving process (Benner, 2022). Both an outdated Cartesian representational view of the mind and viewing clinical reasoning as a form of scientific reasoning rather than a form of science-using clinical (practical) reasoning create learning problems and a major practice-readiness gap for new graduates ill-prepared to perform clinical reasoning in actual practice (Chan & Burns, 2021; Brown & Hart, 2022).

Clinical reasoning is a form of practical reasoning that uses contextually grounded scientific knowledge. The clinical reasoner encounexers unfolding clinical situations that must be managed across patient changes. Clinical reasoners must be attentive, curious, engaged and responsive to the patient and his or her clinical situation as it changes across time.

Descartes' (1628, 1978) taken-for-granted representational view of the mind includes a separation of mind, body and world, in conjunction with Kant's vision of moral agency, as being constituted by radically free autonomous choice makers, ideally influenced by the will, rather than by emotions, shape folk psychology, social imagination and social practices about teaching and learning and how the mind works in most of academia and in nursing, in particular (Taylor, C., 1984; Sullivan et al., 2008). In contrast to representational Cartesian and Kantian views of the mind, an alternative view of intelligent embodied human agents with socially embedded minds, engaged in the world, with real-world experiential learning, directly experienced, from immersion in the world and not necessarily or even usually mediated by representations such as concepts, ideas and schema, more accurately characterizes human thinking, knowledge development, skill-learning and intelligence (Dreyfus, 1986; Gallagher, 2005; Taylor, 2016; Dreyfus 2017). Concepts and theories usually influence access to explanation and understanding when the person is in an unfamiliar or puzzling situation, rather than being involved actively in familiar situations. This alternative view also accounts for tacit knowledge (Wittgenstein,

DOI: 10.4324/9781003427407-54

1953, 2001; Polanyi, 1958, 2015) and family resemblances or "fuzzy" recognition, based upon past clinical situations associated with the clinical reasoner's experiential learning, skilled know-how and successful or failed clinical reasoning (Wittgenstein 1953, 2001; Dreyfus, 1992; Dreyfus, 2017). In other words, perception is most often guided by attunement and engagement with the situation, rather than detachment and decontextualization of the situation through breaking the situation down into formal concepts or elements. Heidegger (1962) characterizes what is essentially a Cartesian or Kantian view of the mind as a "Present at Hand" mode where there is deep unfamiliarity, such as the completely inexperienced novice, or a situation of extreme breakdown without an understanding of what is going on in the situation, then the person may break the situation down into decontextualized elements, or formal conceptual entities in order to make sense of the "foreign" inaccessible situation void of understanding.

Socially constituted, embedded, embodied, engaged agency, an alternative to Cartesian and Kantian views of the mind

A socially constituted, embodied and socially embedded and engaged view of agency, as developed by Merleau-Ponty (1962) and further described by Dreyfus and Taylor (2016); Dreyfus (2017); Gallagher and Zahavi (2021); Robbins and Ayede (2009); and Lave and Wenger (1991) provide an alternative to Cartesian and Kantian views of agency. This embodied, socially embedded view of the mind provides a less mechanistic, less deterministic and more accurate view of human intelligence.

Both Cartesian and Kantian thoughts about mind, body and world relations, emotions and rationality have become a taken-for-granted basis for many social practices, in academia and nursing education in North America (Taylor, 1984; Taylor, 2004; Dreyfus & Taylor, 2016).

A representational view of the mind is not supported in current learning sciences, nor in philosophy; yet, they are dispersed in almost all areas of Western thought and in social practices, and especially, in a widespread taken-for-granted understanding of emotions, epistemology, ethics, teaching-learning, moral agency and rationality (Merleau-Ponty, 1962; Collins, 1985; Benner & Wrubel, 1989; Lave & Wenger, 1991; Damasio, 1999; Lakoff & Johnson, 1999; Robbins & Ayede, 2009; Gallagher & Zahavi, 2021; Benner, 2022). Critique and rejection of Cartesian representational view of the mind and mind-body dualism (Dreyfus, 1986; Dreyfus & Taylor, 2016; Dreyfus, 2017) and Kant's view of the role of the will guided without emotions, are widespread in learning sciences, philosophy and the human sciences (Zlateve et al., 2008). In nursing, overcoming a representational view of the mind and an outdated understanding of the role of emotions in perception and rationality can clarify and improve teaching-learning of clinical reasoning (Benner, Hooper-Kriakidis, & Stannard, 2011). A socially constituted, embedded, intelligent and embodied view of human thinking and agency characterizes how clinicians, nurses and physicians engage in situational awareness (Endsley, 2018), and situated thinking-in-action when clinical reasoning.

In a socially constituted and embodied intelligence view, human beings are understood as participants who share intersubjective meanings rather than being enclosed, separate subjective minds standing over against a separate, objective world (Zlatev et al., 2008). The mind is embodied in the world and is neither strictly an object, nor a completely a conscious atomistic self (subject) with complete clarity (Heidegger, 1962; Merleau-Ponty, 1962; Taylor, 1971).

Scientific language that attends only to the physical and natural world omits intelligent, human embodied access and involvement in the world that discloses salient clinical and human issues in patient-nurse caring situations. For example, most nursing textbooks give objective, decontextualized statements of "knowing that and about," rather than accounts of "knowing how and when," or actual accounts of "thinking-in action." Naturalistic scientific language leaves out perceptual capacities central to understanding human intelligence (Dreyfus, 1986, 1992). Much can be gained by attending to, teaching and making the most of the characteristics of human intelligence. While human intelligence is fallible and requires disciplined habits of thought and action to address limitations by learning from mistakes, doing careful assessments, avoiding confirmation biases, consultation with other expert clinicians and use of current scientific knowledge and machine intelligence to augment human intelligent capacities that are missing from outside-in objectified approaches.

The mental faculty of "intuition" in Descartes' model of the mind imagines that the person sees mental objects clearly and makes distinctions between idea objects (Lakoff & Johnson, 1999, pp. 94–117). This Cartesian form of intuition can be distinguished from intuition that rests on experientially learned perception, embodied skilled know-how and fuzzy recognition of familiar clinical situations. A point of failure for Old-Fashioned Artificial Intelligence (AI) based on an information-processing model of the mind (Dreyfus, 1992) was this inability to recognize the nature of the whole situation, lack of perceptual grasp of context or frame of the problem, and lack of fuzzy recognition abilities, and the limits of formalism, the inability to make practical situations completely explicit. In contrast to the experienced expert's intuition, the "intuition" to which Descartes refers is not embodied, perceptual, nor does it include a fuzzy quasi-emotional recognition of past similar situations as Descartes explains:

> By intuition I understand, not the fluctuating testimony of the senses, nor the misleading judgement that proceeds from the blundering constructions of imagination... intuition is the undoubting conception of the unclouded mind, and springs from the light of reason alone.
>
> (Descartes, 1628/1970, pp. 19–22)

Emotion-based responses and tacit memory are essential for the development of human-skilled know-how and the ability to make situated judgments and rational thought possible, both of which are required for expert clinical reasoning (Merleau-Ponty, 1962; Cambridge Handbook; Collins, 1985; Benner & Wrubel, 1989; Lave & Wenger, 1991; Damasio, 1999; Lakoff & Johnson, 1999; Noe, 2010; Gallagher & Zahavi, 2021; Benner, 2022).

Human intelligence, rational thought and expertise depend on emotionally imbued, fuzzy recognition and perception (Dreyfus, 1986; Dreyfus, 1992; Benner, 2001). The embodied, socially embedded, person, engaged in the world, is essential for clinical reasoning (Taylor, 2016). Excellent clinical reasoning, a science-using form of practical reasoning, requires embodied, human intelligence that can be augmented, but not replaced by decision supports or machine intelligence. The human ability to "see the big picture" and notice a current clinical situation, in terms of past similar and contrasting cases, exceeds what can be noticed by monitoring of patients' vital signs or studying population statistics, and pathophysiology of diseases alone. These aspects of human intelligence are distrusted and often delegitimized as "acting on instinct" or practicing "anecdotal medicine," fearing that clinicians will act without adequate scientific evidence or succumb to "confirmation bias" that distorts clear and rational explorations of alternative clinical conditions and explanations. These feared "risks" of experience-based embodied intelligence can be mitigated by performing careful, data-based assessments, and consultation with other expert clinicians involved in the patient's care situation. The potential benefits of human intelligence by seeing the big picture, recognizing similarities between similar cases and so on, outweigh the limitations, in terms of early recognition of critical patient changes. Teaching students to develop their situational awareness, tacit understandings, understanding of context and timing in clinical situations allows for astute early warnings to patients' changing clinical condition and astute clinical reasoning that can then be confirmed or disconfirmed.

The advantages and limits of both expert human intelligence and machine-based decision supports need to be considered, and each used to their best advantage to maximize good clinical reasoning. But because we imagine that we can meet all the conditions for scientific reasoning in practical clinical situations, legitimizing tacit knowledge and experience-based ability to recognize subtle and early changes in the patient's clinical condition are not adequately taught or emphasized in nursing education.

Human intelligence, contrary to representational views of the mind, relies on embodied intelligence, engagement in the situation, skilled-know-how, social embeddedness of the thinker along with experience-based learning salient to the situation at hand. Embodied intentionality and intelligence are characterized by Dreyfus and Dreyfus (1986; Dreyfus, 1986) as a "sense of salience" and "understanding without a rationale," and experience-based knowledge, that allows some things to stand out as more or less significant than others, without thinking about it (i.e., analyzing it by breaking the situation down into explicit elements) (Benner, Hooper-Kyriakidis, 2011). With a sense of salience, clinical situations are not encountered as a meaningless collection of clinical data points, but understood as a familiar situation with relevant points of concern. For example, nurses can recognize early or impending shock prior to vital sign changes, during compensatory phases of early shock, or early recognition of pulmonary emboli, based on experience and astute observation. Expert psychiatric nurses are able to recognize signs of extreme escalation in anger that are likely to lead to violence in particular patient situations. Medical-surgical nurses recognize early clinical signs of sepsis; or have perceptual grasp of changes in the patient's color, physical condition, energy or attention levels that signal clinical changes in the patient's conditions (Benner, 2000; Benner, Hooper-Kyriakidis, 2011). Embodied intelligence and skilled perceptual acuity of expert clinicians can be lifesaving. Recognition of experience-based subtle patient changes triggers further assessment and exploration, allowing needed time for rapid interventions (Benner & Wrubel, 1982; Benner, 1984; Benner & Tanner, 1987; Benner, Hooper-Kyriakidis & Stannard, 2011).

The sensing, skillful embodied agents' clinical know-how allows them to negotiate and flourish in the context of the inevitable human condition of ambiguity, despite the inevitability of some misunderstandings and mistakes (Merleau-Ponty, 1962; Dreyfus, 2017). The caveat is that the finite, historical embodied clinician must always be prepared to learn from and prevent mistakes.

Neurocognitive studies (Damasio, 1999: Ennen, 2003) demonstrate that emotion provides an access to the world, opening persons up to emotional and relational contexts that allow for perception, rational thought and judgment:

We propose that emotions provide embodied information about the costs and benefits of anticipated action, information that can be used automatically and immediately, circumventing the need for cogitating on the possible consequences of potential actions. Emotions thus provide a strong motivating influence on how the environment is perceived (Zadra & Clore, 2011).

In Nursing, for example, having experienced and cared for many patients with pulmonary emboli, the clinician has a tacit memory or nuances and aspects of symptoms, distress and contexts associated with pulmonary edema. Coaching nurses in noticing and developing a narrative memory of real unfolding cases, for example, of pulmonary emboli, along with teaching the necessary clinical assessments, and definitive confirmatory tests, can increase the clinician's astute development and use of tacit memory, and narrative understandings of clinical syndromes enhancing their noticing and recognition skills.

A preference for scientific deductive reasoning, and the prevalent representational view of the mind cause a lack of acknowledgment and exploration, along with a failure to teach students to experientially learn and develop and value these human capacities for situational awareness and tacit understandings of whole clinical situations. At the earliest stages of situational awareness and problem recognition in clinical reasoning, indubitable proof is often elusive, but insistence on immediate indubitable proof can hamper exploration and legitimacy of early recognition of changes in patients' clinical condition. Providing more realistic teaching of clinical reasoning, based upon actual situated-thinking-in-action and using human experience-based perceptual capacities for tacit memory, can never substitute for the additional necessary associated steps of verification, but without developing these perceptual capacities, nurses will be unable to detect crucial early clinical changes. Ignoring and dismissing this huge asset of experience-based embodied human intelligence and tacit knowledge can delay and even prevent the nurse's development and focus on experience-based knowledge that guides proficient and expert nursing practice and makes wise clinical reasoning possible (Benner, 2021).

Techne and phronesis

Being an excellent clinical reasoner requires moral imagination, situated thinking-in-action, clinical experience, and skilled know-how. Aristotle called practical reasoning that embodies situated, attuned, skilled know-how, moral responsibility and agency in particular situations *phronesis* (wisdom) (Dunne, 1997). In contrast to *phronesis*, *techne* refers to making things or producing outcomes. *Techne* uses rational calculation or "cause and effect" thinking. *Phronesis is* "characterized as much by a perceptiveness about concrete particulars, as use of universal principles or generalizations" (Dunne, 1997, p. 273). Practice traditions must be self-improving, but can never be without error or misunderstandings, a characteristic of all traditions, including scientific traditions. Practice communities and traditions must engage in innovation and improvement in order to avoid the risk of becoming rote, dead traditions (MacIntyre, 1981). A community of practitioners, collectively, can generate verifiable intersubjective truth open to questioning and disconfirmation. Merleau-Ponty's (1962) notion of intersubjective truth refers to the kind of "objectivity" that can be achieved by considering multiple perspectives from a community (see Zlatev et al., 2008). For example, the use of observation and first-person experience-near narratives can make knowledge embedded in nursing practice visible and public for articulation and evaluation (Benner, 1984, 2000; Benner, Hooper-Kyriakidis & Stannard, 2011). In clinical practice, multiple skilled observers can attest to or raise questions about the nature of the clinical situation, using collective observations and clinical evidence. This kind of team-based assessment is often the only available option for determining validity and accuracy of clinical reasoning in the moment of rapidly changing clinical situations.

The practices of nursing and medicine (and other practice disciplines) require both *phronesis and techne* and as described by Aristotle. *Techne*, or procedural and scientific knowledge, can be formalized in explicit statements and provide a degree of certainty except for timing and individual adjustments required for particular patients. In contrast to *techne*, *phronesis* requires engaged practical reasoning by skillful, excellent practitioners who are member-participants in a community of practitioners, and who practice with a sense of responsibility to patients, with the goal of overcoming mistakes and improving practice (Gadamer, 1960, 1975; MacIntyre, 1981; Dunne, 1997; Benner *et al.*, 1999; Sullivan & Rosin, 2008). The notions of good internal to the practice and concerns for the patient's well-being guide the action of the practitioner, as a member of a community of practice. Wise clinical reasoning (*phronesis*) prohibits separating means and ends, and merely engaging rational calculation (Dunne, 1997). Means and ends are intricately connected in nursing and all health care in many situations, such as assisting with the birthing of infants, caring persons for those approaching death, and any situation where patient/ families must be considered in choosing approaches to nursing and medical care (Benner *et al.*, 1999, pp. 363–403). A local group of practitioners' skillful comportment, habits, practices and dispositions are developed in a dialogue with their larger practice tradition:

> A practice is not just a surface on which one can display instant virtuosity. It grounds one in a tradition that has been formed through an elaborate development and that exists at any juncture only in the dispositions (slowly and perhaps painfully acquired) of its recognized practitioners. The question may of course be asked whether there are any such practices in the contemporary world, whether the wholesale encroachment of technique has not obliterated them – and whether this is not the whole point of MacIntyre's (1981) recipe of withdrawal, as well as of the postmodern story of dispossession.
>
> (Dunne, 1997, p. 378)

Phronesis is interpersonal and relational in ways that *techne* cannot be. In *techne*, means and ends can be separated, with the means often not being given due value leaving room for expediency to rule the day. In *phronesis,* means and ends are inextricably related. "Each bends and responds to the other so that horizons and world are opened and reconstituted so that new possibilities emerge" (Wynn, 1997). Healing and recovery of one's embodied relationship to the world are mysterious, lived rather than mastered and require relationship, openness and trust. Education for *phronesis* provides a way of incorporating the best of human perception, the use of experiential learning from past clinical experiential learning allowing evidence-based science most salient to the particular situation to be used.

Christine Tanner (2006) defines clinical reasoning as follows:

> "Clinical reasoning" is the term I will use to refer to the processes by which nurses and other clinicians make their judgments, and includes both the deliberate process of generating alternatives, weighing them against the evidence, and choosing the most appropriate, and those patterns that might be characterized as engaged, practical reasoning (e.g., recognition of a pattern, an intuitive clinical grasp, a response without evident forethought)... Good clinical judgments in nursing require an understanding of not only the pathophysiological and diagnostic aspects of a patient's clinical presentation and disease, but also the illness experience for both the patient and family and their physical, social, and emotional strengths and coping resources.
>
> (Tanner, 2006, p. 204)

This definition is ground-breaking in that it acknowledges perceptual grasp and notices characteristic of human intelligence in addition to the use of scientific knowledge, and patient assessment and evaluation. For students to learn clinical reasoning, they need realistic rehearsals. Clinical reasoning starts with a perceptual grasp of the nature of the whole clinical situation and situation-awareness about what is most salient in the patient's situation. In acute care situations, the nurse and health care team clinically reason across time, with the goal of getting a better understanding of the clinical situation as it unfolds. Clinical reasoning leads to responsible actions appropriate to the clinical situation. Increased study of front-line knowledge embedded in expert nurse clinicians' actual clinical reasoning is needed in order to better understand situational awareness (Endsley, 2018; Benner, 2022) for rapid clinical reasoning across time on behalf of the patient.

Unfolding changes across time and concern for the particular patient's well-being are excluded in an "outside-in" linear scientific reasoning process such as the Nursing Process. Clinical reasoning does not take the form of "criterial reasoning" nor the application of single algorithms. Such approaches cannot safely guide clinical reasoning because they often conflict with the individual clinical situations such as conflicting clinical interventions, co-morbidities, specific sensitivities to medications or interventions along with practical, contextual considerations of the available health care team, the environment of care and more. Clinical reasoning often uses modus-operandi thinking, i.e., thinking backward much like a crime detective figuring out what and how the chain of events in a crime situation caused the current "M.O." of the clinical situation, i.e., what caused the patient's particular cascade of clinical events.

In our research on skill acquisition, we found that persistent disengaged standing over against situations in an objectified, detached way (a Cartesian social and clinical imagination) limited what nurses noticed in patient care situations (Rubin, 1996, 2009). Disengagement and detachment constrained experiential learning and prevented development of proficient to expert levels of performance. Proficient and expert performance is characterized by the clinician's use of narrative memory of actual whole clinical experiences rather than using lists of signs and symptoms to determine the nature of the clinical situation (Benner, Tanner & Chesla, 2009; Benner, 2021).

William Sullivan and Matthew Rosin (2008) call for a new agenda in higher education, one that focuses on preparing students' minds for a life of practice. This new agenda blends practical reasoning (i.e., clinical reasoning) with critical rationality and addresses the problem of conflating clinical reasoning (practical reasoning) with scientific reasoning or critical thinking. They point out that:

...Practical reason, once central to the educational tradition that stemmed from the rhetorical and humanistic studies of the European Renaissance, has been all but eclipsed by a focus on utility, on the one side, and on analytical reasoning, on the other...For practical reason, the focus is on thinking that is oriented toward decision and action. Because of this, we take exception to the way critical thinking is currently understood and promoted.

...Teaching for practical reasoning is concerned with the formation of a particular kind of person—one who is disposed toward questioning and criticizing for the sake of more informed and responsible engagement. Such persons use critique in order to act responsibly, as it is the common search for ways to realize valuable purposes and ideals that guides their reasoning. Practical reason grounds the academy's great achievement—critical rationality—in human purposes that are wider and deeper than criticism...In the end, practical reason values embodied responsibility as the resourceful blending of critical intelligence and moral commitment.

(Sullivan & Rosin, p. xvi, 2008)

As noted earlier, clinical reasoning, a perfect analogue for practical reasoning, as described and defined by Charles Taylor (1970), a noted philosopher and thinker on practical reasoning:

> Practical reasoning is a reasoning in transitions. It aims to establish, not that some position is correct absolutely, but rather that some position is superior to some other. It is concerned, covertly or openly, implicitly or explicitly, with comparative propositions. We show one of these comparative claims to be well founded when we can show that the move from A to B constitutes a gain epistemically. This is something we do when we show, for instance, that we get from A to B by identifying and resolving a contradiction in A or a confusion which A screened out, or something of the sort. The argument fixes on the nature of the transition from A to B. The nerve of the rational proof consists in showing this transition is an error-reducing one. The argument turns on rival interpretations of possible transitions from A to B, or B to A...The form of the argument has its source in biographical narrative. We are convinced that a certain view is superior because we have lived a transition which we understand as error-reducing and hence as epistemic gain.
>
> (Taylor, C., 1970, p. 72)

The mistaken assumption that clinical judgment mimics scientific reasoning is based upon the taken-for-granted folk psychology that all high-level mental functioning depends upon mental representations (Descartes, 1637, 2016; Ennen, 2003; Dreyfus & Taylor, 2015; Taylor, 2016; Endsley, 2018; Benner, 2022; Dreyfus, S.E.). Research on how proficient to mastery level performers (Benner, Tanner & Chesla, 2009) demonstrates that when proficient to master level clinicians engage in experience-based skillful clinical reasoning in situations where they are deeply familiar and are highly skillful, clinically reason, they use a science-using form of practical reasoning (Benner, Tanner, Chesla, 1996, 2009; Benner, 2022).

Expert clinical reasoners perceptually grasp and attune their perception to the unfolding clinical situation in the concert with what is understood about the particular patient's clinical condition and co-morbidities along with population statistics for patients with similar diagnoses. Expert clinical reasoning is rooted in the notions of good internal to nursing practice, along with the nurse's responsibility for the best outcomes and well-being of the patient. The temptation of cognitivists, holding to a representational view of the mind, is to break the situation down into isolatable elements, and use algorithms and formal criteria for making "yes and no" decisions at particular points in time (what Taylor, 1995 calls "snapshot" reasoning). Clinical reasoning is more like a motion picture than a slide show or "snapshot" reasoning at particular points in time because clinical reasoning requires making sense of changes in the patient's condition across time. Skilled know-how and perception and perspective become invisible to the cognitivist, using an information-processing snapshot reasoning approach to characterize thinking.

Clinical reasoning through transitions by engaged intelligent agents does not follow naturalistic scientific reasoning that bases judgments on formal objective elements or isolatable criteria. The scientific approach oversimplifies and ignores multiple causal sources and knowledge based on an intelligent agent's situated first-hand observations of events, and ongoing feedback about the changes in the patient's condition resulting from their interventions (Taylor, 2016). For example, the need for perceptual grasp by an engaged proficient to expert clinician, the necessity of keeping track of the changes in the patient's clinical condition across time and make the "best call" or best sense of the clinical situation (best account) (Taylor, 1989), in terms of diagnoses and clinical interventions, urgently needed by the patient characterizes expert clinical reasoning in actual rapidly changing clinical situations fraught with ambiguity.

Superior mechanistic reasoning is not sufficient for good clinical reasoning for many reasons, including leaving out the engaged embodied intelligent agent's role in understanding unfolding, often ambiguous clinical events. Mechanistic 17th-century science cannot give an accurate account of how good clinical judgments are made in rapidly changing clinical practice situations. Expert clinical reasoning based upon absorbed coping, in a familiar world of practice, is not the same as "rote" repetitive responses in the thoughtless re-enactment of past situations, nor is it the same as a rote following of guidelines or rules. The actor attends to the context and the situation's demands for sense-making and skillful responses based upon actual sequential changes in the patient across time. Perceptual grasp of the best perspective on the nature of the situation (Taylor, 1989) is essential for appropriate actions attuned to meeting the demands of internal notions of the good and qualitative distinctions of excellent nursing practice relevant to the clinical situation (Benner, Hooper-Kyriakidis, Stannard, 1999, 2010; Sullivan & Rosin, 2008; Dreyfus, H.L. 2017; Benner, 2021).

This perceptual acuity is often accompanied by a coupled experience and science-based knowledge about what to do in the situation along with the rationale for preferred interventions. The expert clinical reasoner attends to changes in the patient's condition across time recognizing the salience of those changes for the patient's treatment, while using the best scientific evidence for clinical reasoning, using expert medical advice, definitive clinical tests for the patient's particular situation. Knowing how, when and why essential aspects of expert are situated thinking-in-action.

Textbook accounts of nurses' knowledge are typically limited to decontextual accounts of "knowing that and about" with no account of "knowing how, when and why, in context," i.e., situational awareness, situated thinking-in-action. Textbook accounts of objectified, decontextualized accounts of "knowing that and about" need to be augmented by narrative accounts and observations of actual situated thinking-in-action and demonstration of "knowing how, when and why, in context" based upon situational awareness paired with a deep-background knowledge of the patient's clinical condition and the relevant scientific knowledge and standards of practice related to the situation. This cannot happen, if we imagine that thinking and learning both begin and end, depending only on formal concepts, theories and ideas lodged in the mind, rather than being augmented and enriched by direct experiential learning from the real world.

References

Benner, P. (2001) *From Novice to Expert: Excellence and Power in Clinical Nursing Practice. Commemorative Edition*. Upper Saddle River: Prentice Hall.

Benner, P. (2021) "Novice to mastery: Situated thinking, action, and wisdom." In Elaine Silva Mangiante, Kathy Peno & Jane Northup (Eds.), *Teaching and Learning for Adult Skill Acquisition: Applying the Dreyfus and Dreyfus Model in Different Fields*. Charlotte, NC: Information Age Publishing.

Benner, P. (2022) *A Rich First-Person Narrative Account of Rapid Clinical Reasoning, Situational Awareness and Situated Thinking in Action.* Posted October 13, 2022, EducatingNurses.com

Benner, P., Hooper-Kyriakidis, P., & Stannard, D. (2011) *Clinical Wisdom and Interventions in Acute and Critical Care, Second Edition: A Thinking-in-Action Approach.* New York: Springer.

Benner, P., Stannard, D., & Hooper, P. (1996) "A thinking-in-action approach to teaching clinical judgment: A classroom innovation for acute care advanced practice nurses." *Advanced Practice Nursing Quarterly,* 1(4), 70–77.

Benner, P., & Tanner, C. (1987) "Clinical judgment: How experts use intuition." *American Journal of Nursing,* January 87(1), 23–31.

Benner, P., & Wrubel, J. (1982) "Clinical knowledge development: The value of perceptual awareness." *Nurse Educator,* 7, 11–17.

Brown, J. D., & Hart, L. (2022) "Improving practice readiness among nurse residents." *The Journal of Continuing Education in Nursing,* 53(9), 411–416.

Chan, G., & Burns, E. M., Jr. (2021) "Quantifying and remediating the new graduate nurse resident academic-practice gap using online patient simulation." *Journal of Continuing Education Nursing,* 52(5), 240–247.

Collins, C. (1985) *The Last Dogma of Empiricism.* PhD thesis, Berkeley, CA: University of California.

Damasio, A. (1994) *Descartes Error: Emotion, Reason and the Human Brain.* New York: Putnam.

Descartes, R. (1628) (1970) "Rules for the direction of the understanding." In E. S. Haldane & G. R. T. Ross (Eds.), *The Philosophical Works of Descartes,* two volumes reprint. Cambridge: Cambridge University Press. Benner, 2022.

Dreyfus, H. L. (1986) "Misrepresenting human intelligence." *Thought,* 61(243) (December 1986), 430–441.

Dreyfus, H. L. (1992) *What Computers Still Can't Do. A Critique of Artificial Intelligence.* Cambridge, MA: MIT Press.

Dreyfus, H. L. (2017) "On expertise and embodiment: Insights from Maurice Merleau-Ponty and Samuel Todes." In J. Sandberg, L. Rouleau, A. Langley & H. Tsoukas (Eds.), *Skillful Performance Enacting Capabilities, Knowledge, Competence, and Expertise in Organizations* (p. 149). Oxford: Oxford University Press.

Dreyfus, H. L., Dreyfus, S. E. with Thom Anthanasiou. (1986) *Mind Over Machine. The POWER of Human Intuition and Expertise in the Era of the Computer.* New York: The Free Press.

Dreyfus, H. L., & Taylor, C. (2015) *Retrieving Realism.* Cambridge, MA: Harvard University Press.

Dreyfus, S. E. (2014) "System 0: The overlooked explanation of expert intuition." Chapter 2. In M. Sinclair (Ed.), *Handbook of Research Methods on Intuition* (pp.15–27). Northampton, MA: Edward Elgar.

Dunne, J. (1997) *Back to the Rough Ground. Practical Judgment and the Lure of Technique.* Notre Dame, IN: University of Notre Dame Press.

Endsley, M. R. (2018) "Expertise in situation awareness." In K. A. Ericsson, R. L. Hoffman, A. Kozbelt & A. M. Williams (Eds.), *Cambridge Handbook of Expertise and Expert Performance* (2nd Ed., pp. 714–741). Cambridge: Cambridge University Press.

Ennen, E. (2003) "Phenomenological coping skills and the striatal memory system." *Phenomenology and the Cognitive Sciences,* 2, 299–325.

Gallagher, S. (2005) *How the Body Shapes the Mind.* Oxford: Oxford University Press.

Gallagher, S., & Zahavi, D. (2021) *The Phenomenological Mind,* 3rd Ed. London & New York: Routledge.

Heidegger, M. (1962) *Being and Time.* Transl. John Macquarrie & Edward Robinson. New York: Harper & Row.

Lakoff, G., & Johnson, M. (1999) *Philosophy in the Flesh, the Embodied Mind and its Challenge to Western Thought.* New York: Basic Books

Lave, J., & Wenger, E. (1991) *Situated Learning. Legitimate Peripheral Involvement.* Cambridge: Cambridge University Press.

MacIntyre, A. (1981) *After Virtue: A Study in Moral Theory.* Notre Dame, IN: University of Notre Dame. Notre Dame Indiana.

Merleau-Ponty, M. (1962) *Phenomenology of Perception.* Transl. C. Smith. London: Routledge.

Noe, A. (2010) *Out of our Heads.* New York: Hill and Wang.

Polanyi, M. (1958, 2015) *Personal Knowledge: Towards a Post-Critical Philosophy,* Enlarged Ed. With Forward by Mary Jo Nye. Chicago, IL: University of Chicago Press.

Robbins, P., & Ayede, M., Eds. (2009) *Cambridge Handbook of Situated Cognition.* Cambridge: Cambridge University Press.

Rubin, J. (1996, 2009) "Chapter 7 "Impediments to the development of clinical knowledge and ethical judgment in critical care nursing." In Benner, Tanner & Chesla (Eds.), *Expertise in Nursing Practice* (pp.171–198). New York: Springer.,

Sullivan, W. M., Rosin, M. S., Shulman, L. S., & Fenstermacher, G. D. (2008) *A New Agenda for Higher Education: Shaping a Life of the Mind for Practice.* San Francisco, CA: Jossey-Bass & Palo Alto, CA: Carnegie Foundation for the Advancement of Teaching.

Tanner, C. (2006) "Thinking like a nurse: A research-based model of clinical reasoning." *Journal of Nursing Education,* 45(6) (June, 2006), p. 2004.

Taylor, C. (1971) "Interpretation and the sciences of man." *The Review of Metaphysics,* 25, 3–34.

Taylor, C. (1984) "Philosophy and its history." In R. Rorty, J. B. Schneewind & Q. Skinner (Eds.), *Philosophy in History. Essays in the Historiography of Philosophy* (pp. 17–30). Cambridge: Cambridge University Press.,

Taylor, C. (1989) *Sources of the Self. The Making of Modern Identity.* New York: Cambridge University Press.

Taylor, C. (1995) Explanation and practical reasoning." In *Philosophical Arguments* (pp. 51–53). New York: Harvard University Press.

Taylor, C. (2004) *Modern Social Imaginaries.* Durham, NC: Duke University Press.

Taylor, C. (2016) *The Language Animal, the Full Shape of Human Linguistic Capacity.* Cambridge, MA: The Belknap Press & New York: Harvard University.

Wittgenstein, Ludwig. (2001) [1953]. *Philosophical Investigations.* West Sussex: Wiley Blackwell Publishing.

Wynn, F. (1997) "The embodied Chiasmic relationship of mother and infant." *Human Studies,* 20(2), 253–270.

Zadra, J. R., & Clore, G. L. (2011) "Emotion and perception: The role of affective information." *Wiley Interdisciplinary Review Cognitive Science,* 2011 November–December; 2(6), 676–685.

Zlatev, J., Racine, T. P., Sinha, C., & Itkonen, E. (Eds.) (2008) *The Shared Mind, Perspectives on Intersubjectivity.* Amsterdam: John Benjamins Publishing Co.

Index

Note: **Bold** page numbers refer to tables and page numbers followed by "n" denote endnotes.

516   *Index*

For Product Safety Concerns and Information please contact our EU
representative GPSR@taylorandfrancis.com
Taylor & Francis Verlag GmbH, Kaufingerstraße 24, 80331 München, Germany

www.ingramcontent.com/pod-product-compliance
Lightning Source LLC
Chambersburg PA
CBHW072006230326
41598CB00082B/6813